both for illustrative material and much technical information. More directly our special thanks are offered to our secretaries, Mrs. L. L. Ewen, Mrs. D. Dinsdale, and Miss J. Forshaw, who have, with great patience and rare skill, transformed our nightmare manuscripts into comprehendible form, and to Mr. R. Schofield and Mr. F. Cutler of the Department of Medical Illustration of the Christie Hospital and Holt Radium Institute for help with so many of the illustrations. Mr. L. G. Owens, B.Sc., of Messrs. John Wright & Sons Ltd. of Bristol, has given us valuable advice, continuous help, and appropriate stimulation as well as showing extraordinary patience in the face of our slowness: we are very grateful to him. Finally, we want to thank our respective wives for having borne, with such good grace, considerable periods of 'book-widowhood': our already inestimable debt to them is thus further increased.

W. J. M.
J. B. M.

Manchester, 1968

PREFACE TO THE FIRST EDITION

'How much physics should a radiographer or a radiologist know?' or 'How much physics should be included in their training?' are questions widely, and often vociferously, discussed amongst those responsible for radiological education. The answer to each question is not necessarily the same and we cannot claim to be able to offer a conclusive answer to either. It is obviously possible to be a good radiologist or a good radiographer and yet have a very small knowledge of physics. Equally such a person would be even better at his or her job if he or she has a working knowledge of the ways in which radiation is produced; of how the rays interact with, and act upon, irradiated material; and of the principles underlying the apparatus being used.

This book attempts to present this type of basic physics of radiology in a logical, if at times unfamiliar, sequence and at a relatively simple level. Although not tied to the syllabus of any particular examination it is hoped that it will be of value to those preparing for the Membership and Higher Examinations of the Society of Radiographers and for the two Diplomas in Medical Radiology. The contents of the courses for these different qualifications differ considerably from one another, but the required level of understanding is not so widely different that the same book cannot be of value to all the students.

The text is divided into four main parts dealing, respectively, with the production and properties of the radiations involved in radiology (primarily X- and gamma rays), their interaction with matter, and their measurement; with diagnostic radiology; with radiotherapy; and with radiation protection. No attempt is made to include details of the physics of electricity and magnetism, which is inevitably the starting point of any course of radiological physics: that subject is excellently covered in *Basic Physics in Radiology* by Kemp and Oliver (published by Blackwell) as well as by numerous school texts designed for the G.C.E. examinations.

It has been our aim to deal with our subject along descriptive lines and we are very much aware that some of our explanations are insufficiently complete to satisfy the purists. For this we make no apology, believing that a simple description understood is far better than a complete truth uncomprehended. In like manner we have largely eschewed the use of much mathematics, not only because of the relatively slight mathematical equipment of many of our potential readers, but, more important, because all too often a veneer of mathematics obscures the underlying physics. Somewhat more originally we stress the importance of radiation energy rather than wavelength, since though the latter has a few uses it is the energy of the photons with which radiology is mainly concerned.

'No man is an island, entire of itself' is a truth of which we have become increasingly aware as our work has proceeded, and we have realized that 'we are a part of all that we have met' and how much we owe to so many people. Our greatest debt is to our past and present physicist colleagues from whom we have learned so much and received such ready help and advice. Generations of M.S.R., F.S.R., and D.M.R. students have been our 'guinea-pigs' and any virtues that this work may possess are partly at least based on their past sufferings! Like all other workers in the radiological field we are very conscious of the help we so often receive from the manufacturers of X-ray and other electro-medical equipment and their representatives

PREFACE TO THE THIRD EDITION

WITH the production of this third edition we have taken the opportunity not only to try, yet again, to remove all the minor errors pointed out to us by our friends, but also, and of greater importance, to endeavour to bring the work substantially up to date by including at least some of the changes and advances that have occurred since the first edition was written.

Conscious of the need to avoid any great increase in the size of the book and of the need to restrict the size of any enforced price increase, we have been somewhat selective and taken notice only of those changes which now form part of accepted clinical practice. To the same end we have reduced, or eliminated, the attention given to items such as the Geiger-Müller counter and 'grid' therapy, the importance of which has waned in the past few years.

The chapter on the clinical use of radioactive isotopes has been revised, recast, and repositioned in the book and a new chapter on the clinical uses of ultrasonic radiations has been introduced. Thermoluminescence and its application to dosemetry receive much more attention than previously whilst new sections have been added on xero-radiography, on computer-assisted tomography and on rare-earth intensifying screens. A short appendix on S.I. units replaces the previous appendix on Symbols, Quantities and Units.

We realize that these new methods, especially those involving radioactive isotopes and ultrasonic radiations, are large in their scope and are rapidly becoming established as separate subjects in their own right. It is not our intention and, in fact, it would be a mistake to deal with them exhaustively in this book. Our aim is to provide a general introduction to them, to set out the basic principles upon which their clinical uses depend, and to indicate their place in the wider context of radiology.

In the revised chapter on gamma-ray sources of plesiotherapy much more attention is given to those radioactive materials which may be used to replace radium or radon, whilst the succeeding chapter on plesiotherapy dosage has been rewritten completely. This latter chapter now gives a more detailed description of and much more tabular information on the Manchester System of mould, interstitial, and intracavitary gamma-ray therapy. We are indebted to Messrs. Churchill Livingstone for permission to use and adapt information previously published in their *Radium Dosage: the Manchester System* (edited by W. J. Meredith) which is now out of print.

As always we are indebted to our many colleagues—medical, scientific and technical—for their guidance and help in matters on which they are far more expert than we. Mrs. M. Greenwood and Miss L. Thompson have given us excellent secretarial help for which we are very grateful, whilst to our respective wives we can only, yet again, express our gratitude for and wonderment at their continued support and tolerance.

W. J. M.
J. B. M.

Lancaster,
Manchester, 1976

FUNDAMENTAL PHYSICS OF RADIOLOGY

By

W. J. MEREDITH
O.B.E., D.Sc., F.Inst.P.

Lately Director of Physics, Christie Hospital and Holt Radium Institute
Withington, Manchester

and

J. B. MASSEY
B.Sc., F.Inst.P.

Regional Physicist, North-western Health Authority,
Christie Hospital and Holt Radium Institute,
Withington, Manchester

THIRD EDITION

A JOHN WRIGHT & SONS LTD. PUBLICATION
Distributed by
YEAR BOOK MEDICAL PUBLISHERS, INC.
35 E. Wacker Drive, Chicago

Distributed in the United States of America, South and Central America, Puerto Rico and the Philippines by

YEAR BOOK MEDICAL PUBLISHERS, INC.

(ISBN 0–8151–5891–2)

by arrangement with
JOHN WRIGHT & SONS LTD,

PRINTED IN GREAT BRITAIN BY JOHN WRIGHT & SONS LTD., AT THE STONEBRIDGE PRESS, BRISTOL BS4 5NU

CONTENTS

Section III.—RADIOTHERAPY

Section IV.—RADIATION PROTECTION

FUNDAMENTAL PHYSICS OF RADIOLOGY

SECTION I. GENERAL PHYSICS

CHAPTER I

MATTER AND ENERGY, RADIATION AND SPECTRA

THE universe in which we live is so vast, and the materials of which it is composed are so apparently infinite in their variety, that it is, at first, astounding to learn that it is all made up of various combinations of about 100 separate and distinct substances called **elements**. In fact, 95 per cent of the earth and its atmosphere is made up of no more than a dozen elements, whilst a mere four (hydrogen, oxygen, carbon, and nitrogen) make up about 95 per cent of the weight of the human body.

An element may be described as a single substance which cannot be made simpler by chemical methods. When one element joins with another, or with several others, the result is a chemical **compound**. For example, the elements sodium and chlorine combine together to form the compound sodium chloride, better known as common salt, whilst the gases hydrogen and oxygen can combine to form that most essential of compounds, water. A slightly more complex compound is limestone, which is made up of the elements calcium, carbon, and oxygen, whilst the tissues of our bodies, though very complex in structure, are compounds mainly composed of the four elements listed above, hydrogen, oxygen, carbon, and nitrogen.

Just as a chemical compound is made up of a number of different elements, so all material is made up of enormous numbers of extremely tiny particles. The smallest particle of an element is called an **atom**, whilst the smallest particle of a compound is a **molecule**. In common salt the molecule consists quite simply of one atom of sodium linked to one atom of chlorine, whilst in water two atoms of hydrogen are attached to one of oxygen. Limestone has a molecule of five atoms—one each of calcium and carbon and three of oxygen—whereas the molecule of a protein, one of the important materials of the body, may be made up of thousands or even millions of atoms.

A molecule may be split into its component atoms, but when this happens the chemical properties of the material will be changed. For example, when an electric current is passed through water the molecules may be split into the constituent hydrogen and oxygen, two gases with properties very different from those of the parent material.

It was, for a long time, believed that atoms were the smallest of particles and that they were indivisible. Now we know that they, too, in their turn are made up of even smaller, simpler particles. Just as a molecule can be separated into its constituent parts, so an atom can be separated into its components (though the process is much more difficult). As with the molecule such separation produces quite different materials and destroys the properties of the original. As will be discussed in greater detail later, an atom is like a miniature solar system having at its centre a **nucleus** wherein is concentrated practically all the weight of the atom, and which carries a

1

positive electrical charge. This central 'sun' is surrounded by a number of very light and negatively charged particles called **electrons**.

Going back from minute particles to the forms which matter usually takes in practice, we find that there are three, namely solids, liquids, and gases. Any material can exist in each of these forms, depending on the temperature. For example, water is normally gaseous at above 100° C., solid below 0° C., and liquid in between. The fundamental difference between the three states is merely the closeness of the constituent atoms or molecules. In a solid these particles are packed very close together, have generally fixed positions, and may, as in a crystal, be arranged in very orderly patterns. In a gas the particles are widely separated and move about quite freely, at random. Liquids have their particles closer together than gases but still have almost the same random movement of particles.

From what has been briefly said it would appear that all matter is made up of **mass** and **electricity**. However, there is a third factor of equal importance, and that is **energy**, a concept with which everyone is familiar and yet which is not easy to define. Though we now know that energy can be converted into mass, and vice versa (and we shall study some examples of this later), for the present it is convenient to keep the two factors apart and to discuss their properties separately.

Life may be regarded as one manifestation of the interaction of matter and energy, whilst radiology is intimately concerned with the relationship of matter with one particular form of energy—radiation. Therefore before embarking upon a detailed study of radiology it is necessary to be familiar with the basic facts about energy and matter.

ENERGY

Energy, in simple terms, can be described as the ability to do work, or as that which is being expended when work is being done. If we carry a case upstairs, work is done; if we compress a spring, work is done; if we pull apart a negatively and a positively charged particle against the electrical attraction that exists between them, work is done. In each of these cases a **force** is involved (the force of gravity, the resistance to compression, or an electrical force respectively), and they have been quoted to illustrate the fact that work usually involves overcoming a force. The amount of work done is proportional to the force and to the distance over which the force has been overcome. It is on this basis that the unit of work, or energy, the **erg**, is defined. Though it is sufficient for our purpose to know that the erg is the unit, the definition of the erg, together with definitions of other fundamental units, is given in an appendix at the end of the book.

Like matter, energy has many forms, the most important of which are probably:

1. *Kinetic Energy.*—This is the energy possessed by virtue of movement. If a piece of material of mass m moves with a velocity v, its kinetic energy is $\frac{1}{2}mv^2$.

2. *Potential Energy.*—This is the energy that a body has because of its position, for example, a weight on a high shelf, or a compressed spring.

3. *Heat Energy.*—Heat is the energy of the movement of atoms and molecules of any material. The level of this heat energy is indicated by the *temperature*. The higher the temperature, the greater is the movement of the particles and hence their energy.

4. *Electrical Energy.*—The energy associated with electricity is measured by multiplying the electrical charge being moved by the electrical force (the potential difference or voltage) against which it has been moved. In practical terms this is the product of the current (amperes), the pressure (volts), and the time (hours, etc.). The so-called 'unit' which is paid for in the electricity bill is a kilowatt-hour (1 kilowatt is 1000 watts, and watts are amperes × volts).

In radiology the electrical charge involved is often that of the electron (e), and a very convenient unit of energy is the **electron-volt** (eV.) or more frequently the kilo-electron-volt (keV.), which is the energy involved when an electron passes through a potential difference of 1000 volts.

5. *Chemical Energy.*—Energy can be 'locked up' in chemical compounds and released under certain circumstances. For example, the detonation of an explosive institutes chemical changes and much energy is released. Or less violently, our ability to walk, climb, or, in fact, undertake any human activity depends upon energy acquired by our bodies through chemical processes.

6. *Nuclear Energy.*—Commonly, and erroneously, called 'atomic energy'. Locked up in the very heart of the atom—in its nucleus—are very large amounts of energy, the controlled release of which could supply all man's energy needs indefinitely. The uncontrolled release could well eliminate him.

7. *Radiation Energy.*—All the electromagnetic radiations—and these include X- and gamma rays, which are our special interest, are travelling electric and magnetic fields, and thus transfer energy from one place to another.

Although apparently quite different, all these forms of energy are closely related and energy in one form can often be readily converted into another. For example, water in a mountain lake has potential energy and as it flows down a river, or through steel pipes to a power station, this potential energy is converted into kinetic energy. This kinetic energy of the water can be transferred to the spinning blades of a turbine which will drive a generator which produces electrical energy. This in turn can supply heat, or light, or recharge an electric 'accumulator' in which the energy is stored chemically. Alternatively, the electricity may operate an X-ray machine and some of the energy be given out as radiation. Some examples of energy conversions are shown pictorially in *Fig. 1*.

Some energy conversions are easier than others and some are just not practicable. For example, the energy undoubtedly contained in 'cold' water, and which has to be removed before the water will freeze, cannot readily be converted into electrical energy, nor can the electricity coming from a battery be converted directly into X-ray energy. But where conversion from one form to another is practicable a most vital condition holds. This is that the total amount of energy in the system remains the same throughout, even though this may not appear to be so. For example, when a car is brought to rest by the application of its brakes, its kinetic energy is lost apparently without trace. In fact, it has been converted into heat energy, as can easily be ascertained by touching the brake drums! Energy is said to be *conserved*.

So also is mass. In chemical changes the form of the different substances may change completely but their total mass does not. These principles of the Conservation of Mass and of Energy were central pillars of nineteenth-century science and are still completely acceptable today, with the one important reservation already hinted at.

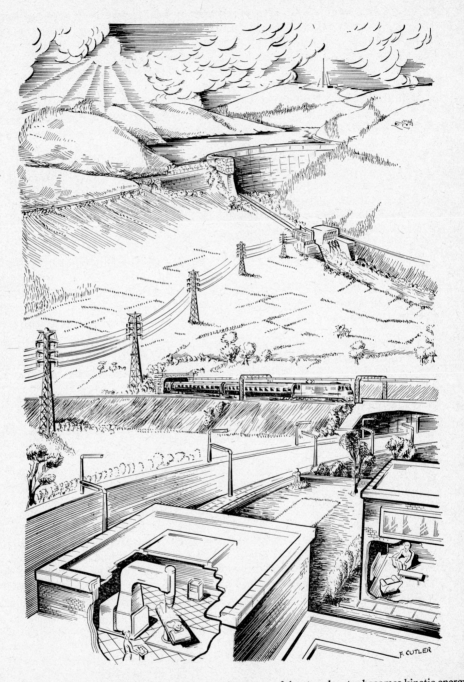

Fig. 1.—Energy transformations. The potential energy of the stored water becomes kinetic energy of the flowing stream, some of which is converted to electrical energy. This drives trains (kinetic energy) or produces X-rays, light, heat, or radio-waves (all are forms of energy). Basically all this energy stems from solar heat which comes from nuclear energy in the sun.

Early in this century Einstein postulated that there was an equivalence of mass and energy, the energy (E) equivalent to a mass (m) being given by the equation:

$$E = mc^2, \quad \text{where } c \text{ is the velocity of light.}$$

This is what might be termed the 'exchange rate' for mass and energy. In international finance exchange rates between all the different currencies are quoted in the daily press but at times they are only of academic interest. During international crises, for example, it may be quite impossible for pounds to be exchanged for roubles, or for dollars, even though the rates are quoted. So too with matter and energy, where conditions for conversion are far more the exception than the rule. In fact for 30 years after it was postulated, the formula remained a theoretical concept only to be dramatically and triumphantly verified experimentally in some of the first 'atom-splitting' experiments carried out under Lord Rutherford at Cambridge. Now it is completely accepted as the unifying link between the two conservation principles.

Intensity.—Before leaving general, for detailed, considerations of energy, a word should be said about the meaning of the term **intensity** as it is applied to energy. This is a term that has been very loosely used in radiology, often with confusing results. Throughout this book every effort will be made to restrict its use to the generally accepted physical meaning, that is, as an indication of the flow of energy. Strictly it is the amount of energy passing per unit time through unit area placed at right-angles to the direction of energy flow. Intensity is therefore measured in *ergs* per square centimetre per second. For example, imagine, as shown in *Fig. 2*, that E ergs of energy pass through the square window whose side measures a cm. The average intensity is then E/a^2 ergs per second.

HEAT

A number of the forms of energy just listed are of particular interest in radiology and deserve more detailed consideration. Heat is one of these, being produced in considerable quantities as a by-product of the X-ray production process. Perhaps the chief radiological interest in heat is, in fact, how to get rid of it!

As already stated, heat is the energy of movement of the atoms and molecules that make up all material and is, in many ways, the simplest form of energy. In most processes involving energy conversion, heat is a partial or complete end-product. The case of the kinetic energy of the braking car being converted into heat has already been quoted. In many chemical reactions the released energy appears as heat, and so we shall find when studying the effect of X-rays on materials that one of the products is heat. The measurement of the heat generated is often a very good method of assessing the amount of energy involved in a process.

The level of heat in a body is indicated by its *temperature*, which can be regarded as a measure of speed of movement of the particles: the hotter the material (that is to say, the higher the temperature) the faster the particles move. Several scales of temperature have been developed but the one most commonly in scientific use is the *centigrade* (or Celsius) scale on which 0° is the temperature of melting ice and 100° that of boiling water. More fundamental, based on the expansion of a gas with increasing temperature, is the Absolute (or Kelvin) scale on which 0° C.—melting ice—is 273° K. The so-called absolute zero, 0° K., is −273° C.

Heat Transfer.—Since, as has been said, energy is always conserved, the cooling of heated material can only be achieved by transferring heat energy to another place, or by converting it into another form. In this transfer, one or more of three different processes will be involved.

Conduction.—The first of the three processes is **conduction**, which is mainly responsible for heat transfer in solids. Atoms in solids are closely packed together, cannot move about freely, and may be regarded as being in frequent collision with their immediate neighbours. Rise of temperature makes the movement faster and these collisions more frequent and violent.

Imagine then that a metal bar has been heated at one end. The local atoms will be moving much more rapidly than their distant cousins in the cooler part of the bar.

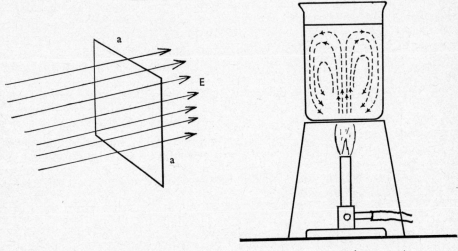

Fig. 2.—The meaning of intensity.   Fig. 3.—Convection currents.

However, these higher energy (hotter) particles will collide with, and hence speed up, some of their slower (cooler) neighbours. At the same time the original particles will lose energy, be slowed down, and hence be made cooler.

In their turn, the newly speeded-up atoms collide with their cooler neighbours, speeding them up, and so on down the bar. Thus gradually energy is transferred along the bar and parts distant from the hot end become warmer. Heat is thus *conducted* along the bar and unless the lost heat is replaced by some outside source, the hot end will be cooled. Conduction distributes throughout the whole bar, but without any actual movement of material, the heat which is initially localized.

Metals are the most efficient conductors of heat, copper being one of the best whilst tungsten, a metal widely used in radiology, is relatively poor, though much better than any non-metal.

Convection.—In a liquid or a gas (that is to say, in a fluid) the constituent particles are much farther apart than they are in a solid, so that they move around much more freely and make far fewer collisions. Conduction, therefore, plays little part in heat transfer in fluids.

The effect of heating part of a fluid is to expand that material so that it becomes less dense and rises through its denser neighbouring material, whilst its place is taken up by the denser, cooler material. If heat is being supplied continuously, as by the Bunsen burner depicted in *Fig.* 3, the process described goes on continuously and the circulation indicated is set up, carrying heated material to all parts of the fluid. This process involving the movement of heated material is called **convection** and can only occur in fluids—liquids and gases—when, in contrast to solids, the material is free to move.

Radiation.—The third mechanism by which heat energy can be transferred from or to any material is by **radiation**, which involves neither particle nor material movement, and in fact does not require material of any kind. In this process the heat energy of particle movement is converted into *infra-red* radiation (of which more will be said later) which travels out through space in all directions. Emission of radiation occurs more readily from black surfaces than from polished ones—a scientific reason to be added to the aesthetic reason why silver teapots should be kept highly polished if hot tea is desired!

Cooling.—Which of the three transfer processes will contribute most to the cooling of a particular object will depend very much on the prevailing circumstances but, as will be seen, each plays an important role in the cooling needed in radiology.

Whatever the circumstances, the rate of cooling depends on the difference in temperature between the hot object and its surroundings. The greater the difference the more rapidly will heat be lost. As far as conduction and convection are concerned the rate at which heat is transferred is directly proportional to the temperature difference. For radiation the amount of energy radiated by a body is proportional to the fourth power of its *absolute* temperature. Therefore if a hot object is at temperature $T°$ C. and its surroundings are at $t°$ C., the rate of cooling by radiation will be $(T + 273)^4 - (t + 273)^4$. One consequence of this difference in the temperature dependence of the various transfer methods is that the importance of radiation loss increases rapidly as the temperature of the hot body increases. This will be seen to be of moment when the cooling of an X-ray target is considered.

ELECTROMAGNETIC RADIATION

Everyone is familiar with the rainbow, that beautiful array (or *spectrum*) of colours into which sunlight is split when passing through water droplets. Just as the separate colours are constituent parts of visible light, so light itself, the infra-red radiation just mentioned, and a number of other radiations are constituent parts of the much wider range, or spectrum, of the so-called **electromagnetic radiations**. Though there are very great differences between the properties of the radio-waves at one end of the spectrum and the X-rays at the other, they all have a number of important properties in common. They are all rapidly fluctuating electric and magnetic fields and, most important, they all travel through free space with the same velocity, the so-called 'speed of light' which is about 3×10^{10} cm. per sec. or 186,000 miles per sec. Before discussing the rest of their common properties and some of their individual features it is desirable to consider some general ideas about this type of radiation.

WAVES AND PHOTONS

Waves.—We usually think of electromagnetic radiations as being waves, such as that shown in *Fig.* 4, travelling through space and carrying energy from one place to another. This type of wave is called a *transverse wave* because, as indicated, the fluctuation is at right-angles to the direction in which the wave travels. A simple example of this type of wave is provided by a rope, one end of which is fastened to a fixed point while the free end is waggled up and down. Waves 'run' along the rope though the material moves up and down.

Transverse waves have four main features, viz.:

1. Wavelength (λ), which, as shown in *Fig.* 4, is the distance between successive corresponding points on the wave.
2. Frequency (v), which is the number of waves produced per second. In the case of the rope this is the number of times a particular point goes up and down per second.
3. Velocity (c), which is the distance travelled per second by the waves.
4. Amplitude (a), which might be described as the 'vigour' of the wave, as indicated in *Fig.* 4.

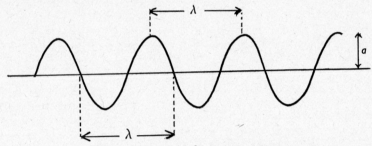

Fig. 4.—Parameters of a transverse wave.

The first three of these features are interrelated since the distance travelled by waves per second (the velocity) equals the number of waves per second (the frequency) multiplied by the length of each wave, i.e.,

$$\lambda v = c.$$

Since all electromagnetic radiations have the same velocity, *the frequency of any such radiation must be inversely proportional to its wavelength.*

Photons.—Though the idea of the radiation being waves is very valuable in that it enables many radiation phenomena to be understood, it is not entirely satisfactory. For example, it implies that energy is flowing continuously and uninterruptedly, whereas we know that this is not so. A beam of electromagnetic radiation delivers its energy as a series of discrete, that is separated, 'packages' of energy, rather like a stream of minute machine-gun bullets. Packages of energy are usually called **quanta** (singular: *quantum*), but to those of electromagnetic radiation the name **photon** is usually applied.

The philosophical reconciliation of these two quite radically different concepts of radiation, neither of which is universally satisfactory, is far beyond the scope of this book. Nor shall we follow the lighthearted suggestion of Sir William Bragg and use the wave theory on Mondays, Wednesdays, and Fridays, the quantum theory on Tuesdays, Thursdays, and Saturdays, and neither on Sundays! We shall simply use whichever seems to be most helpful in a particular instance. Furthermore, there is a link between the two concepts. The energy (E) contained in a photon is linked with the radiation frequency (v) on the wave concept through the formula:—

$$E = hv.$$

'h' is a universal constant, named Planck's constant after the physicist who introduced it into another branch of physics. Using this formula and the already stated relationship between wavelength and frequency (viz., $\lambda v = c$) it follows that

$$E = hc/\lambda,$$

which means that the shorter the radiation wavelength the greater the energy associated with its photons. Short wavelength means high frequency, which means large photon energy—long wavelength means low frequency, which means small photon energy.

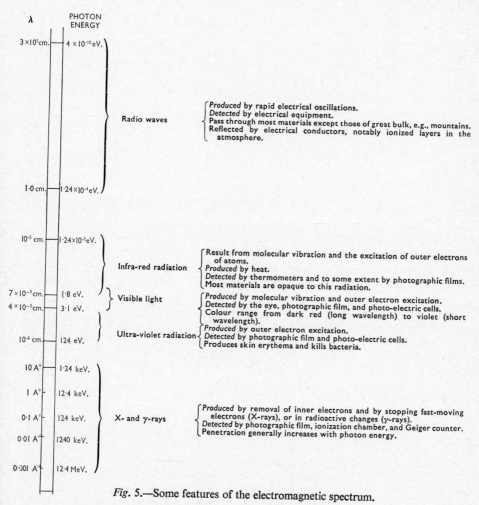

Fig. 5.—Some features of the electromagnetic spectrum.

THE ELECTROMAGNETIC SPECTRUM

The diagrammatic table (*Fig. 5*) sets out the wavelengths, frequencies, and photon energies of the main types of radiation which comprise the electromagnetic spectrum, with some brief indication of the means of their production and of any noteworthy properties. It must be stressed that there are no precise boundaries for any type of radiation, and that except in the case of visible light each radiation type tends to overlap its neighbours. Even in the case of visible light the precise boundaries depend on the eye of the observer and not upon any exact physical effect.

Special attention is drawn to the fact that the lengths of the shorter radiations are given in Å rather than in centimetres. This abbreviation stands for Ångström units.

The Ångström unit (1 Å), which equals 10^{-8} cm., was introduced originally to simplify statements of X-ray wavelengths in the energy range used in X-ray crystallography where wavelengths of 10^{-8} cm. (1 Å) are common. For higher energy, and therefore shorter wavelength radiations, the X unit (1 X unit $= 10^{-11}$ cm.) has been suggested but has never commanded great support.

Fig. 5 has listed some of the individual properties of the different radiations and it should be noted that a number of the properties are common to several of them. In addition, there are a number of other properties—some of which have already been mentioned—which are shared by all electromagnetic radiations, viz.:—

1. They all travel with the same velocity in free space.

$$c = 3 \times 10^{10} \text{ cm. per sec.}$$

2. All transfer energy from place to place, in quanta. The energy (E) associated with a quantum, or photon, is associated with the frequency ν by:

$$E = h\nu.$$

3. In free space they all travel in straight lines.
4. In passing through matter the intensity of the radiation is reduced (**attenuation**), both because some radiation energy is taken up by the material (**absorption**) and because some is deflected from its original path to travel in a new direction (**scattering**). It should be noted that any effect of radiation on matter depends on how much energy that matter receives (absorbs) from the beam.
5. In free space all electromagnetic radiations obey the *inverse square law.* This states that, for a point source, the radiation intensity (I) at any place varies inversely as the square of the distance (d) from the source to the place at which the intensity is being considered:

$$I \propto \frac{1}{d^2} \quad \text{or} \quad I = \frac{k}{d^2},$$

where k is a constant for the circumstances being considered.

The validity of this law can easily be demonstrated by considering a point source giving out radiation equally in all directions (isotropically). If it emits E ergs per sec. then the intensity (that is, the ergs per cm.² per sec.) at a distance d cm. from the source must be E divided by the area of the sphere over which the radiation has spread.

Thus:

$$I = \frac{E}{4\pi d^2} \quad \text{or} \quad I \propto \frac{1}{d^2}.$$

SPECTRA

The separation of light into its component colours—or, more strictly, into its component wavelengths or energies—in the production of the rainbow is the best known example of the production of a *spectrum* (plural: *spectra*). A spectrum may be described, somewhat pedantically it must be admitted, as 'the arrangement of the constituent parts in a progressive series according to their energy or wavelength', and it must be remembered that this can apply equally well to any of the electromagnetic radiations, not simply to light. Or, for that matter, it can be applied to streams of charged or uncharged particles. Nor, as will be shown, is the rainbow type of spectrum the only type that exists.

Continuous Spectra.—In the rainbow there is an unbroken band of colours, gradually changing from dark red at one side to dark violet at the other, literally colour 'as far as the eye can see', though here it is not distance but the wavelength sensitivity

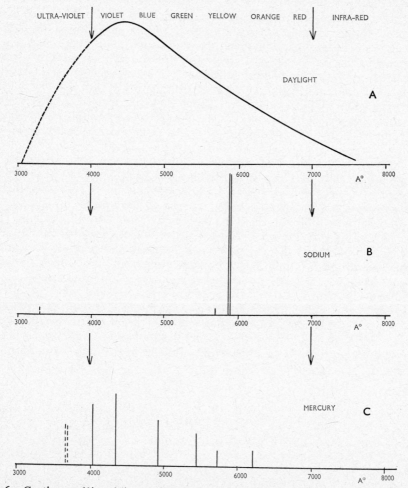

Fig. 6.—Continuous (A) and line spectra (B and C). The height of the curve, or the length of the vertical lines, shows the relative radiation intensities. The arrows show the limits of the visible spectrum, the dotted lines indicating invisible (ultra-violet, in this case) radiation.

of the eye which sets the limits. One colour merges into the next and there are no colour gaps. Since every colour is due to a different wavelength it can be said that all wavelengths, between the extremes, are present.

This is a *continuous* spectrum and, in the case of visible light, is the sort emitted by a heated body. The wavelengths present depend only on the temperature and not upon the heated material. For example, if a steel poker and a brass poker are left in the fire, both become 'red hot' and the spectra of their radiation will be identical. Compared with 'the colours of the rainbow' these spectra will lack the violet and blue radiations, and will be predominantly red. On the other hand, if the pokers are heated to 'white heat', their spectra will be much more close to that of sunlight which, of course, emanates from that extremely hot body, the sun.

Continuous spectra occur for other radiations too, as will be seen later, and have general properties very similar to those outlined here.

Line Spectra.—Mercury- or sodium-'vapour' lights are now a very familiar part of our street lighting. If light from these sources is passed through a prism, spectra are produced which are quite different from the spectra of sunlight or of the light from a heated poker. Instead of a continuous band of colours, one merging into the next, and indicating that all wavelengths are present, the spectra from mercury or sodium lamps, for example, will be made up of isolated colours and many wavelengths will be missing. *Fig.* 6, B and C, shows graphs of the intensity of different wavelengths in light from mercury-vapour and sodium-vapour lamps and a marked difference will be seen between these and the intensity variation in the continuous spectrum of *Fig.* 6 A. The spectrum of sodium vapour consists almost entirely of two nearly equal wavelengths and thus this is a source of almost pure (or monochromatic) yellow light. By contrast, light from the mercury-vapour source is made up of a large number of separate wavelengths, mostly towards the short wavelength end of the visible range. The red end of the spectrum is weakly represented and this accounts for the harsh bluish colour of the light. *Line* spectra, as those of this type are usually called, are emitted by burning substances or, for example, by gases through which an electric discharge is passing. In direct contrast to the continuous spectrum, the wavelengths present in a line spectrum do not depend upon the temperature of the source, provided that this is high enough to cause light to be emitted at all, but entirely upon the chemical substance involved. Because each substance emits its own quite distinctive line spectrum, this type is often called a *characteristic* spectrum, and is the key factor in a very powerful tool for identifying the presence of very small amounts of material.

Emphasis has here been laid upon line spectra of visible radiation: this is because these are more familiar and are most easily demonstrated. However, line spectra, having general properties such as those described here, also occur with other radiations and are very important in radiology.

CHAPTER II

ATOMS AND NUCLEI

IT was in 1897 that J. J. Thomson discovered a negatively charged particle much smaller than any atom and called it the **electron**. This discovery destroyed the view, already referred to in CHAPTER I, that atoms were indivisible and were the smallest possible particles, and it was the first step to the building up of our modern concept of the structure of the atom. Rutherford and Bohr took the next great step when, in 1911, they postulated, and produced irrefutable evidence to support, the existence of an atomic nucleus. As a result of their work we now can say that the atom of any element resembles a minute solar system, in which electrons (negatively charged) circle round a positively charged **nucleus**, where the great majority of the mass of the atom is concentrated. Just as there are vast regions of emptiness in astronomical space, so there are—relatively speaking—in the atom. If the atom were enlarged to the size of a concert hall, an electron would be about as big as a fly and so, interestingly enough for all its greater weight, would the nucleus. Such emptiness (though very surprising when we think how solid matter appears to our limited senses) helps us to understand, to some extent at least, why radiations, for example, can pass unchanged through apparently solid material. Really solid substance is, in fact, extremely rare.

ATOMIC STRUCTURE

The difference between the atoms of different elements is in the number of electrons circling round their respective nuclei and in the weight and positive charge of these nuclei. Hydrogen, the lightest of the elements, has the simplest atom, having only one electron, whereas uranium, the heaviest naturally occurring material, has 92 electrons in its atom. Since complete atoms are electrically neutral, the positive charge on the nucleus of any atom exactly equals the total negative charge on the surrounding electrons. A hydrogen nucleus, thus, has a single positive charge, whilst the uranium has one 92 times as big. The number of electrons circling round the nucleus—and hence its positive charge—is usually called the **atomic number,** to which much greater reference will be made later.

Electron Orbits or Shells.—The electrons can be regarded as moving around the nucleus in a series of *orbits* or '*shells*', at varying distances from the nucleus, in much the same way as the planets of our solar system travel in different orbits at a variety of distances from the sun. Because of very complicated rules, which are beyond the scope of this book, there are limits to the numbers of electrons which can be present in any orbit; these are listed below. However, perhaps more important is the fact that there can never be any electrons in between orbits. The maximum numbers of electrons in the different orbits are as follows: 2 electrons can be accommodated in the orbit closest to the nucleus, the orbit to which the symbol, K, is applied. At a rather greater distance is the L orbit, which can take up to 8 electrons, whilst orbits M, N, and O, each progressively more remote, may contain, respectively, up to 18, 32, and 50 electrons. Just as the planets are held in their courses around the sun by gravitational forces, so electrons are held in their orbits by the electrostatic attraction between their negative charges and the positive charge of the nucleus.

13

In any particular type of atom this attraction, or *binding force*, is naturally greatest for the electrons in the K orbit since they are closest to the nucleus, and it gets progressively weaker for the electrons in the L, M, N, and O orbits which are progressively farther from the nucleus. Furthermore, any particular electron (and we can take a K electron as an example) will be more tightly 'bound' in those atoms with a large positive charge on the nucleus (large atomic number) than those in atoms with a lower atomic number. For example, the K electron in carbon (atomic number 6), sulphur (atomic number 16), and gold (atomic number 79) have binding forces of, respectively, 0·28, 2·5, and 81 units.

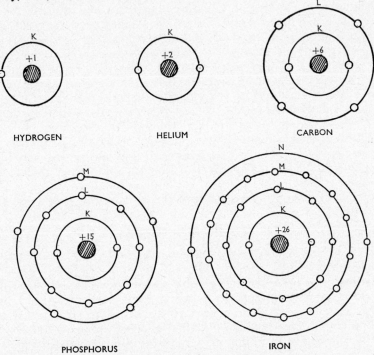

HYDROGEN   HELIUM   CARBON

PHOSPHORUS   IRON

Fig. 7.—The orbital electrons in five different atoms.

Some Examples of Atomic Structure.—As has already been stated, hydrogen, the lightest of the elements, has a single electron circling around its nucleus which, therefore, will carry an electric charge of equal magnitude but of opposite sign to that of the electron. If, for convenience, we regard the electronic charge as the unit of negative charge on the atomic scale, then the charge on the hydrogen nucleus will be a unit of positive charge. It is also customary to regard the mass of the hydrogen nucleus as unity on the atomic scale.

After hydrogen, the next heaviest element is the rare gas helium, whose atom has 2 circling electrons, and hence a doubly charged nucleus. Carbon has 6 electrons in its atom, whilst nitrogen has 7, oxygen 8, phosphorus 15, iron 26, and so on up to uranium with 92. Their nuclei, therefore, have positive charges of these magnitudes. *Fig.* 7 shows diagrammatically the orbital arrangements of some of the simple atoms mentioned.

Energy Levels.—The removal of an electron from an atom is only possible if the attractive force between the electron and the nucleus can be overcome. To overcome a force, as has been stated in CHAPTER I, work must be done, energy must be expended, and so it is in the case of the atom. An electron can only escape if it is given sufficient energy. Most energy is needed for the removal of the electrons in the K shell or orbit, since they are closest to the nucleus and the binding force is greatest. Less and less energy is required respectively for the removal of the L, M, N, and O electrons.

An alternative and very useful representation of the electrons in the atom is the *energy-level diagram* which depicts the electrons as occupying different energy levels, each energy being that required to remove the particular electron from the atom.

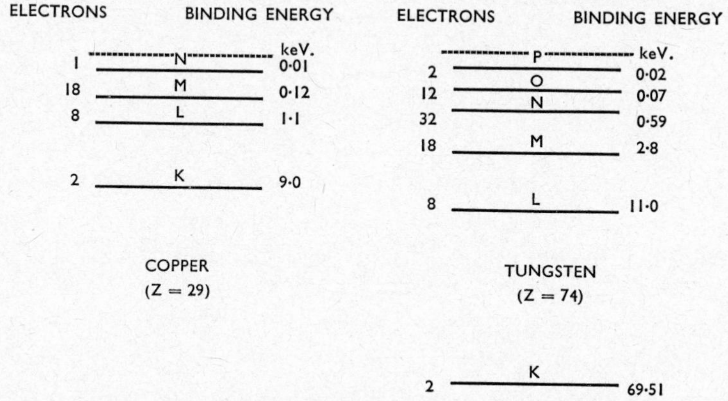

ELECTRONS		BINDING ENERGY
1	N	keV. 0·01
18	M	0·12
8	L	1·1
2	K	9·0

COPPER
(Z = 29)

ELECTRONS		BINDING ENERGY
2	P	keV.
2	O	0·02
12	N	0·07
32		0·59
18	M	2·8
8	L	11·0

TUNGSTEN
(Z = 74)

| 2 | K | 69·51 |

Fig. 8.—The electron energy levels for copper and tungsten.

Fig. 8 shows such diagrams for the copper and tungsten atoms. On the left-hand side of each level is the number of electrons in it, whilst on the right is the energy (in kilo-electron-volts—keV.) needed to free an electron from that level, that is, to remove it from the atom.

This diagram shows that the K electrons are the most difficult to remove, and that the tungsten electrons, at each level, are much more tightly 'bound'—more difficult to remove—than their copper counterparts (because tungsten has 74 positive charges on its nucleus compared with only 29 for copper). It also shows that the outer electrons in each atom are relatively easily removed. This is not only because they are remote from the nucleus, but also because electrons in orbits closer to the nucleus to some extent 'shield' the outer electrons from its attractive effect.

Because they are so easily removed the outer electrons in all atoms play important roles in chemical reactions: the chemical behaviour of any substance is, in fact, controlled by its electrons and their orbital distribution. For example, 2 atoms of hydrogen and 1 atom of oxygen combine together to form water (H_2O). Hydrogen has a single electron, whilst oxygen has 8. Two of these are in the K shell whilst the remainder occupy six of the available eight places in the L shell. When hydrogen and oxygen combine the two remaining places in the L shell are occupied by electrons of 2 hydrogen atoms, and thus the 2 hydrogens and 1 oxygen are bound together.

Or take the case of lithium fluoride, a substance very similar to sodium chloride (or common salt) and of considerable importance in radiation dosemetry. Lithium's 3 electrons are arranged so that 2 are in the K shell and the third is alone in the L shell. On the other hand, fluorine has 2 electrons in the K shell and 7 in the L shell (which can take 8). What more natural then that lithium's lone outer electron should latch into the vacant place in the fluorine outer shell and link the two atoms together.

Though these descriptions are incomplete they serve to illustrate how orbital arrangements control chemical properties.

Ionization and Excitation.—Because its nuclear positive charge balances the total negative charge of the electrons, a normal atom is electrically neutral. Removal of one of these electrons upsets the balance and the resulting particle will have an excess of positive charge. It will, in fact, be a positive **ion**. The removed electron, either alone or when attached to a normal atom, constitutes a negative ion. The process of their production is called **ionization** and, because it is so important in radiology, it will be considered in some detail. By way of example, the removal of a K electron and events subsequent to its removal will therefore be discussed in detail.

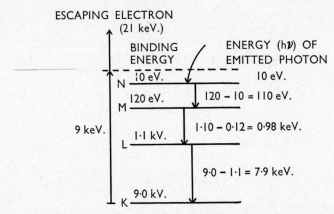

Fig. 9.—The removal of the copper K electron and the consequent electron 'jumps'.

Ionization.—Before an electron can escape from an atom it must acquire enough energy to enable it to overcome the binding force, and, as already shown in *Fig.* 8, the inner electrons need to be supplied with the most energy if they are to be removed. For this example it will be assumed that, by absorbing X-ray energy, for example, a copper K electron has received 30 keV. of energy. This is considerably in excess of its binding energy of 9 keV., so that the extra 21 keV. constitute the kinetic energy with which the liberated electron rushes away from its parent atom. As to its fate we do not here inquire, though it will be of interest later. Now attention will be returned to the positive ion that remains after the electron has been ejected. This positive ion is an unstable particle which can only become a normal atom again by attracting to itself an electron to complete its full complement.

The most obvious place from which the vacancy in the K shell can be filled is from the neighbouring L shell and indeed the most likely immediate consequence of the K electron removal is that one of the electrons in the L shell 'jumps' into the vacated place—and creates a vacancy in the L shell. This, in turn, may well be filled by the M-shell electron, which then is refilled from the N shell, as depicted in *Fig.* 9. These, of course, are but internal electronic rearrangements and the process is only complete when the ion has attracted an electron from outside to restore its charge neutrality.

Just as an electron has to receive energy to escape from its orbit so, when it transfers from one orbit to another closer to the nucleus, it must surrender some energy. It has to give up, in fact, the difference between the binding energies of the two orbits.

For example, since the copper K-electron binding energy is 9 keV. and that for the L electron is 1·1 keV., an electron 'jumping' from the L orbit to fill a vacancy in the K orbit must surrender $9 - 1·1 = 7·9$ keV. of energy, and this it does in the form of a photon of *electromagnetic radiation*.

Electron transitions other than those illustrated in *Fig.* 9 are also possible, following the removal of the K electron. For example, an M-shell electron may move in, with the emission of $9 - 0·12 = 8·88$ keV. of energy, or an electron may come into the K-shell vacancy directly from outside the atom, in which case it surrenders the full binding energy of 9 keV. as a single photon. The transitions shown in *Fig.* 9 are, however, the most likely to occur, and the photon energies indicated are the most intense emitted. For example, if the intensity of radiation arising from the L to K transition is taken as 100, then the radiation intensity arising from M electrons filling the K vacancy is 20, whilst that from electrons coming directly from outside is a

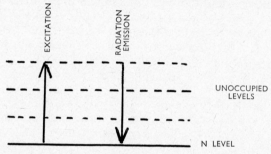

Fig. 10.—Excitation and consequent radiation emission.

mere 0·1. This means that the chance of the K-shell vacancy being filled from the L shell is 1000 times as great as it is of being filled from outside the atom.

More important, however, is it to notice that after an atom has been ionized its return to normal, by the capture of another electron, is accompanied by the emission of a number of photons of different energies.

Now the binding energies of the different orbits depend on the nuclear charge change and therefore will be different for different elements. Furthermore, the differences between these binding energies will vary from element to element and so therefore will the energies of photons emitted following ionization. The energy level values and their differences are characteristic of the element, and the radiations emitted constitute the *line* spectrum, and are usually called the **characteristic radiation** of the element.

Excitation.—Whilst electrons can readily 'jump' inwards towards the nucleus when vacancies occur, movement in the opposite direction—except for the complete removal of the electron from the atom—is only possible for electrons in the outermost shell. By absorbing some extra energy—but insufficient to allow it to escape from the atom—an outer electron can move, where a vacancy exists, into an orbit slightly farther from the nucleus than its normal orbit, and hence one with a slightly smaller binding energy. There are a number of such orbits for each atom and they are said to be 'unstable', since it is unlikely that an electron will remain in one of them for long; rather it will revert, quite quickly, to its normal orbit and in so doing will give out the energy difference in the form of a photon of electromagnetic radiation which, because of the small energy difference involved, will be of low energy or long wavelength, usually visible or ultra-violet light. *Fig.* 10 illustrates this.

The raising of the electron to a rather higher level is the process of **excitation**. No electron is lost by the atom, but one is raised into an unstable orbit and ultimately returns to its normal state with the emission of radiation characteristic of the atoms concerned. Just as ionization is followed by the emission of X-radiation, so excitation ends with the emission of visible or ultra-violet radiation photons.

However, there is another feature which is worthy of attention because it is of some moment as far as the effects of radiation are concerned. Whilst the atom is in the 'excited' state it is often more chemically reactive than normal, so that excitation may enable it to take part in chemical processes into which, in the normal state, it could not enter. 'Excitation' in biological material may, therefore, be an important cause of the biological damage produced by radiation.

NUCLEAR STRUCTURE

Just as the atom, once thought to be indivisible, has an internal structure of its own, so the nucleus is not just a tiny uniform speck of matter but it also has a very complicated structure. Much of the detail of this is far from being understood, and detailed discussion of it is beyond the needs of the readers of this book—and the capabilities of its authors! For what follows, it is sufficient to regard the nucleus as being made up of combinations of two fundamental particles, *protons* and *neutrons*. These particles—they are sometimes called *nucleons*, since they are nuclear particles—are of equal mass (which can be taken as unity on the atomic scale*), but whereas the proton has a single positive charge,* the neutron is electrically neutral. The proton is identical with the nucleus of the hydrogen atom and it may usefully be stressed, in view of oft-observed confusion, that this material particle is very different from the *photon* or 'particle' of electromagnetic radiation.

Compared with these two particles, the other main constituent of atoms, namely the *electron*, is almost weightless, its mass being only 1/1850 of that of the proton or neutron. Surprisingly, however, its diameter is of the same order as that of the proton. Nuclear matter is much more dense than electronic matter.

Table I.—THE CHARGES AND MASSES OF SOME FUNDAMENTAL PARTICLES

PARTICLE	CHARGE (Z)	MASS (A)
Proton	$+1$	1
Neutron	0	1
Electron	-1	1/1850 ⎱ often
Positron	$+1$	1/1850 ⎰ regarded as 0

For completeness, mention can also be made of another particle which, though not a normal constituent of matter, is of considerable importance in radiology. This is the *positron*, or positive electron as it was originally called, which has a mass equal to that of the electron and a charge equal in magnitude, though opposite in sign. By way of summary the charges (usually symbolized by Z) and masses (symbolized by A) of these particles are given in *Table I.*

Atomic and Mass Numbers.—A nucleus is characterized by its charge, which is usually called its *atomic number* (Z) and by its mass on the atomic scale, usually nowadays called its *mass number* (A). The atomic number is thus the number of

---

*In terms of everyday practical units the mass of the proton is 1.67×10^{-24} g., whilst the magnitude of its positive charge, or of the electron's negative charge, is 4.8×10^{-10} e.s.u.

protons in the nucleus (and equally the number of electrons circling round it), whilst the mass number is the sum of the number of protons and neutrons.

Structure and Isotopes.—By way of illustration the nuclear constitutions of some common elements are given in *Table II*, from which it can be seen that, in the elements with the smaller atomic numbers, the number of neutrons exactly or nearly equals the number of protons. On the other hand, those elements with larger atomic numbers seem to need an increasing excess of uncharged particles.

Table II.—THE NUCLEAR CONSTITUTIONS OF SOME ELEMENTS

ELEMENT	CHEMICAL SYMBOL	NUMBER OF NUCLEAR PROTONS	NEUTRONS	ATOMIC NUMBER (Z)	MASS NUMBER (A)
Hydrogen	H	1	0	1	1
Helium	He	2	2	2	4
Carbon	C	6	6	6	12
Oxygen	O	8	8	8	16
Phosphorus	P	15	16	15	31
Iron	Fe	26	30	26	56
Copper	Cu	29	34	29	63
Silver	Ag	47	60	47	107
Iodine	I	53	74	53	127
Gold	Au	79	118	79	197
Lead	Pb	82	126	82	208
Uranium	U	92	146	92	238

One of the great problems of nuclear physics has been to explain what it is that holds the nucleus together. According to the laws of electrostatics the protons should fly apart, thus disrupting the nucleus, because of the electrostatic repulsion between them. Yet they don't! Obviously there is some other force overcoming the repulsion. The most obvious force is that of gravity which is known to pull all bodies towards each other. However, this force is much too small, and there must be another which comes into play when particles are very close together, as are the nucleons in the nucleus. This 'short-range nuclear force' exists between all nucleons, that is to say it tends to pull together proton and proton, neutron and neutron, and proton and neutron. Only in the case of proton-proton interaction is there opposition from the electrostatic force: the other interactions are all 'binding' and it is therefore clear that the neutron plays an important part in the 'glue' that holds the nucleus together. It also becomes clearer why the higher atomic number elements have a greater excess of neutrons—to overcome the greater repulsive forces created by the greater number of protons.

The combinations of protons and neutrons listed in the table above are not, of course, the only ones that can be imagined. Nor are they the only ones that exist in nature. However, for each number of protons Z, the number of proton-neutron combinations that can produce stable nuclei is relatively small. Too few neutrons and—perhaps less understandably—too many neutrons endanger the stability of the structure.

Consider first the number of neutrons that can combine firmly with one proton. In hydrogen a single proton forms the nucleus. An equally stable nucleus can be formed by the combination of a proton and a neutron, and this, to form an atom, would need a single electron circling round it, just as hydrogen has. Now the chemical properties of an atom depend on, and are controlled by, the orbital electrons, so that this new atom (with a proton and neutron for its nucleus) has chemical properties which are identical with those of hydrogen. In fact the substance, for a long time after its discovery in 1932, was called *heavy hydrogen*. It is now called *deuterium*, and its nucleus is called a *deuteron*.

Hydrogen and deuterium are the simplest examples of **isotopes** (literally *isotope* means 'the same place' and indicates that they occupy the same place in the chemical periodic table of the elements). They are substances with the same atomic number but have different mass numbers. Isotopes, therefore, have identical chemical properties, since they have the same number of orbital electrons, but they have different physical properties. For example, they will have different boiling and freezing points, whilst, in the case of the two isotopes specifically mentioned here, the gas deuterium diffuses more slowly than hydrogen because of its greater weight.

As they occur in nature, elements are often mixtures of their various stable isotopes, and not necessarily in equal proportions. Thus when the chemist measures the *atomic weight* (i.e., the weight of an atom of the element compared with that of hydrogen) his answer is not a whole number, since what he measures is the *average* mass number. For example, the atomic weight of chlorine is 35·5: natural chlorine is a mixture of 75 per cent of the isotope of mass number 35 and 25 per cent of the isotope of mass number 37.

Radioactive Isotopes.—A much more striking, and radiologically more important, difference in physical properties is illustrated by the nucleus formed by a combination of a proton and 2 neutrons. This is the nucleus of *tritium*, whose atom will also have a single circling electron and therefore will have chemical properties identical with those of hydrogen with which, like deuterium, it is *isotopic*. However, in contrast with the nuclei of hydrogen and deuterium, the nucleus of this third isotope is unstable. At some time after their formation (on the average after 18 years, but some much sooner whilst others much later) nuclei of this isotope will disintegrate, emitting radiation and changing into a different and stable nucleus—in fact into the nucleus of an isotope of helium.

Tritium thus has a physical property not shared by its two isotopes: it is unstable— it is *radioactive*. It is the simplest example of a radioactive isotope and it is the last of the 'hydrogen' isotopes, for the combination of a proton with 3 neutrons is so unstable that such a nucleus is never formed.

A precisely analogous situation exists with other elements. With any particular number of protons there are usually two or three sets of neutrons which yield stable nuclei. For example, carbon—with 6 protons—has two stable isotopes, the one with 6 neutrons and the second with 7. Nitrogen ($Z = 7$) also has two stable isotopes, whilst oxygen ($Z = 8$) has three. In a few cases only one combination is stable (for example, beryllium's 4 protons and 5 neutrons or phosphorus ($Z = 15$) with 16 neutrons). At the other end of the scale, some substances have many stable isotopes, for example, calcium ($Z = 20$) has six, tin ($Z = 50$) has ten, and mercury ($Z = 80$) has seven.

If, however, a further neutron is added to one of these stable nuclei, or if a neutron is subtracted, an unstable, radioactive nucleus may result. Take the example of carbon: if a neutron is removed from the stable nucleus of the lighter carbon isotope (6 protons and 6 neutrons) the resulting combination of 6 protons and 5 neutrons, which is another carbon isotope but with a mass number of 11, is radioactive. So, too, is the isotope of mass 14 which is produced when 1 extra neutron is added to the 6 protons and 7 neutrons of the heavier stable carbon isotope. A radioactive isotope of every element can be produced and, as a general rule, an excess or a lack of neutrons produces this instability. Nevertheless it must be stressed, in view of the widely held— and persistent—error, that the word 'isotope' is not synonymous with 'radioactive'.

Because of their spectacular properties, and their potential dangers if misused, radio-active isotopes have attracted far more attention than their stable brethren. Nevertheless it must be remembered that these latter, like the poor, have been—and are—always with us and are the stuff from which the vast majority of our world is made.

Some aspects of the use of radioactive isotopes in radiology, and in medicine in general, will be dealt with later. Suffice it here to state that their importance stems from both their being isotopes and their being radioactive. Being isotopes they can take part in exactly the same chemical reactions and processes as their stable counterparts, and so can be introduced into the tissues, and their fate or distribution revealed and studied by means of the radiation they emit. By analogy with the glowing phosphorus that enables the flight of the 'tracer' bullet to be followed, radioactive isotopes have found widespread use in so-called 'tracer' experiments, as well as sources of radiation for therapeutic purposes.

Atomic Symbols.—Chemists have long used single or two-letter symbols to represent the chemical elements. For example, H stands for hydrogen: strictly it stands for an atom of hydrogen, whilst H_2 represents the molecule of hydrogen, the usual form in which the gas occurs, which is made up of two atoms of hydrogen. Similarly, He stands for helium, Al for aluminium, Pb for lead, and so on. The convention has now been extended to enable both the atomic number and the mass number to be indicated if desired. By general, but not complete, international agreement numbers representing these physical factors are entered in front of the chemical symbol, any numbers coming after the symbol being of chemical significance. The atomic number is placed as a subscript and the mass number as a superscript, as in

$$\mathrm{^{12}_{6}C} \quad \text{and} \quad \mathrm{^{14}_{6}C}$$

which are the full symbols for the isotopes of carbon ($Z = 6$) whose mass numbers are respectively 12 and 14. The latter is, of course, a radioactive isotope. In many cases the atomic number subscript is redundant and except in some equations describing nuclear reactions it is normal to omit it. Thus the radioactive isotopes of phosphorus and cobalt, which are widely used in medicine, are usually written ^{32}P and ^{60}Co, without their atomic number subscripts of 15 and 27 respectively. The continued use of the symbols P^{32} and Co^{60}, etc., in textbooks and publications, chiefly of American origin, is, to say the least, unfortunate.

The most frequently used chemical numbering is in the right-hand lower position where the numbers indicate the numbers of atoms of each substance present. Thus H_2SO_4, the chemical formula for sulphuric acid, indicates that two atoms of hydrogen, one atom of sulphur (the figure 1 is usually omitted), and four atoms of oxygen combine together to form this molecule.

Nuclides.—Before leaving the subject of symbols and nomenclature, reference must be made to a term relatively recently introduced and increasingly used. Strictly it is wrong, though quite common, to speak, for example, of ^{32}P as 'an isotope'. It should be described as 'an isotope of phosphorus'. There is a need, however, for a shorter term and to meet this the word *nuclide* was coined, and is defined as follows: 'A nuclide is a species of atom characterized by the constitution of its nucleus, in particular by the number of protons and neutrons in its nucleus.' Thus ^{12}C and ^{14}C are isotopes of carbon and each is a nuclide in its own right.

CHAPTER III

RADIOACTIVITY

SOME of the proton-neutron combinations discussed in CHAPTER II are not stable, and it is found that, sooner or later, in quite a random way, such nuclei will, atom by atom, change so as to achieve a more stable proton-neutron combination. In so doing the atom changes its atomic number (and sometimes its mass number), and hence its chemical identity. The phenomenon is called **radioactivity** and the nucleus is said to be **radioactive**. The change from one nucleus (the parent) to another (the daughter) is called a **disintegration**.

As each nucleus disintegrates, in its effort to find a more stable combination, it emits a charged particle which, because of its kinetic energy, is capable of penetrating solid material. In addition the daughter nucleus may get rid of any excess energy in the form of electromagnetic radiation of considerable penetrating power.

With the passage of time the number of parent nuclei remaining progressively decreases, as does the amount of radiation emitted. The number of atoms (i.e., the amount of radioactive material) remaining, and the intensity of the emitted radiation, are said to **decay**. Hence the term *radioactive decay* refers to the gradual reduction (due to nuclear disintegrations), with the passage of time, of the number of parent nuclei remaining and of the intensity of the emitted radiation.

Radioactive disintegration occurs quite spontaneously—it happens without any known cause, and is completely uncontrollable and unalterable by any known agency, physical, chemical, or anything else. In many instances the daughter nucleus is stable but there are also numerous examples where the daughter is also radioactive. In a few instances a nucleus goes through a whole series of radioactive changes—each giving a radioactive daughter product—before a stable proton-neutron combination is attained. Such series of radioactive changes are often called radioactive '*families*'.

The Radioactive Emissions.—The different emissions that are known to occur from different radioactive substances will first be discussed and then attention will be focused on the other important aspect of radioactivity, namely, the speed with which the material decays, and the laws which apparently govern the decay.

1. *Beta (β) Particles.*—Nuclei which have too many neutrons often move towards stability by emitting high-speed electrons, which are often called beta particles. What apparently happens in the nucleus is that a neutron changes into a proton and a negative electron:

$$\mathrm{^{1}_{0}n} \longrightarrow \mathrm{^{1}_{1}p} + \mathrm{^{0}_{-1}e.}$$

Neutron   Proton   Electron

The electron is then emitted and the proton stays in the nucleus.

An example of this type of radioactivity is provided by the phosphorus isotope of mass number 32 (15 protons and 17 neutrons compared with the 15 protons and 16 neutrons of stable phosphorus). This emits beta particles and the daughter product is sulphur:

$$\ce{^{32}_{15}P} \longrightarrow \ce{^{32}_{16}S} + \ce{^{0}_{-1}e}.$$

It will be noted that the daughter product, which is stable, has an atomic number which is one greater than that of the parent nucleus, and this is what is to be expected since the loss of one unit of negative charge (in the ejected electron) is electrically equivalent to the gain of one unit of positive charge, i.e., a proton. On the other hand, the mass number of parent and daughter is the same since the loss of the electron involves no loss of mass: a neutron was converted to a proton but the total number of these nucleons remains unchanged.

2. *Positrons.*—Whilst nuclei with an excess of neutrons emit negative electrons, those with a lack of neutrons (which is equivalent to an excess of protons) may gain stability by positron (positive electron) emission. In this case one of the excess protons becomes a neutron and a positron, the latter being ejected whilst the neutron remains in the nucleus.

$$\ce{^{1}_{1}p} \longrightarrow \ce{^{1}_{0}n} + \ce{^{0}_{+1}e}.$$

$$\text{Proton} \qquad \text{Neutron} \quad \text{Positron}$$

The carbon isotope of mass 11 undergoes this type of radioactive decay. It has 5 neutrons to its 6 protons, as compared with 6 of each in the common stable carbon isotope. Boron is the daughter product of this radioactive change.

$$\ce{^{11}_{6}C} \longrightarrow \ce{^{11}_{5}B} + \ce{^{0}_{+1}e}.$$

As in beta-particle emission both parent and daughter have the same mass number, but the daughter's atomic number is one less than that of the parent because of the loss of one unit of positive charge on the emitted positron.[*]

3. *Gamma (γ) Rays.*—In very many cases the ejection of the beta particle or the positron from the nucleus completes the radioactive decay process, but in some others the daughter nucleus, when formed, has too much energy for stability (it is said to be in an 'excited' state), and usually it quickly gets rid of that excess in the form of electromagnetic radiation, which is called *gamma radiation*.

An example of gamma-ray emission is the radiologically very important case of cobalt 60 (normal stable cobalt has a mass number of 59). This heavier isotope with its extra neutron emits a beta particle to form a nickel nucleus which has too much energy, which is immediately emitted as high-energy gamma radiation. Pedantically, of course, it is the excited nickel nucleus that is the source of the gamma rays, but their emission is so rapid that they are usually, and certainly more conveniently, regarded as part of the cobalt decay scheme.

$$\ce{^{60}_{27}Co} \longrightarrow \ce{^{60}_{28}Ni} + \ce{^{0}_{-1}e} + \gamma.$$

$$\text{Photon}$$

---

[*] It must be confessed that the picture of beta-particle and positron emission presented here is not complete and this path has been deliberately chosen in the interests of general simplicity. As those who have read rather more deeply into nuclear physics will know, both these types of emission include the emission of another particle, the *neutrino*. Though extremely important to the nuclear physicist, this uncharged particle of practically zero mass has no practical importance in radiology, and therefore will not be referred to again.

It will be noted that the photon emission affects neither mass numbers nor atomic numbers since, of course, photons have neither mass nor charge.

4. *Annihilation Radiation.*—Compared with electrons, positrons are extremely rare particles and they quickly combine with electrons (which are in plentiful supply). When this happens both particles disappear, their masses being converted into two photons of electromagnetic radiation, usually called—for obvious reasons—*annihilation radiation.* This high-energy radiation, which will be described in greater detail in CHAPTER VII, always accompanies positron emission in radioactive decay.

5. *Alpha* (α) *Particles.*—Though they were the first emission from radioactive nuclei to be discovered and studied, alpha particles have very little radiological importance and hence their relegation to a late place in this sequence. They are doubly positively charged, and have a mass of four: in other words they are helium nuclei. Decay through alpha-particle emission only occurs amongst radioactive materials whose atomic numbers are in excess of 80. One very important alpha-ray emitter is radium, which as a result of the ejection of the alpha particle becomes the gas 'radon' (sometimes called 'radium emanation'). Radon is also radioactive and also emits an alpha particle: a good example of a radioactive 'daughter' element.

$$^{226}_{88}\mathrm{Ra} \longrightarrow ^{222}_{86}\mathrm{Rn} + ^{4}_{+2}\mathrm{He.}$$
$$\alpha \text{ particle}$$

6. *K-electron Capture.*—An alternative method of approaching or achieving nuclear stability which is sometimes used by nuclei having too few neutrons (which is equivalent to having too many protons) is for the nucleus to attract into itself one of its own encircling K electrons. One of the excess protons is thereby neutralized (or neutronized!). The vacancy in the K-electron shell will be filled by a process identical with that which follows *photoelectric absorption* (*see* CHAPTER VII). K-electron capture, therefore, is accompanied by the emission of X-rays characteristic of the daughter element.

7. *Isomeric Transitions.*—In certain cases the excited nuclear state following the emission of a beta particle may be a nearly stable state and the nucleus may be able to remain in it for minutes, hours, or even days. The *isomer*, as it is called, thus behaves as a separate radioactive material decaying exponentially by *isomeric transition* with the emission of a gamma ray only. An example of this is provided by technetium 99m which is produced when molybdenum 99 emits a beta particle. Technetium 99m has a half-life of 6 hours, emitting a 140-keV. gamma ray to become technetium 99.

The Properties of the Emissions.—The emissions from radioactive nuclei fall into two distinct groups—charged particles and photons. However, they all share at least one important property, which is that they are all capable of producing *ionization.* That is to say, when they penetrate or pass through any material they are capable of removing electrons from the constituent atoms, thus ionizing the material. Since the removal of electrons requires energy, the production of ionization uses up their energy so that the particles are brought to rest, and the photons disappear.

The Charged Particles.—There are three to consider, the positively charged positron and alpha particle, and the negatively charged beta particle (or electron). Because of their electrical charge they ionize *directly*—that is to say the positively charged particles remove electrons by *attraction*, whilst the beta particles *repel* electrons out of atoms. Thus along the path followed by the particle there will be a trail of ionization, or what is usually called a *track*. These tracks can be revealed under special conditions in a device called the 'Cloud Chamber'. *Fig.* 11 shows some examples of particle tracks revealed in this way.

An important feature of any ionization is its *density*, by which we mean the number of ionizations produced in unit length of the path of the ionizing particle. The greater the charge on the particle, the more ionizations it produces in a unit length. Whilst

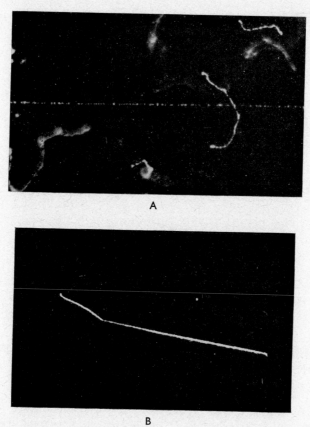

A

B

Fig. 11.—Cloud-chamber photographs of the tracks of ionizing particles: A, The straight track of a beta particle, with the shorter tortuous tracks of electrons set in motion by gamma rays. (*Photo, Science Museum, London.*) B, The particles (a beryllium nucleus and an alpha particle) resulting from the disintegration of a nitrogen nucleus by a neutron. (*By kind permission of Professor Feather.*)

in air millimetres or centimetres are the usual units, in water or tissue the micron (one thousandth of a millimetre) is usually used. The ionization density is also inversely proportional to the velocity of the particle.

There are two important consequences of the dependence of ionization density on particle velocity. Not only do fast particles produce less dense ionization than slow particles, but also the ionization density produced by any given particle varies along its track. At the beginning of its track the particle is travelling at its fastest and therefore produces the smallest ionization density. However, such ionization as it produces reduces its energy, slows it down, and it, therefore, produces a rather greater amount of ionization per unit length. In its turn this slows the particle still more and its ionization density is further increased. And so the pattern rises to a crescendo of increasing ionization density at the end of the track. This ionization *pattern*, which is the same for all charged particles, is represented by the Bragg Curve, so called after the discoverer of the phenomenon.

Fig. 12 shows this initially gradual and finally steep build-up of ionization density along the track of the particle—the Bragg curve—and also indicates that the particle has a definite *range*, in this case about 7 cm. This definite range for charged particles, which depends on their initial energy as well as upon the particle charge, is in distinct contrast with the exponential attenuation of photons, which will be discussed later.

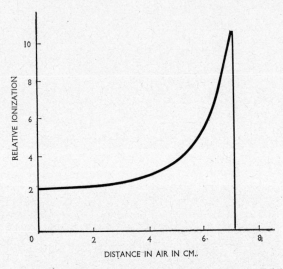

Fig. 12.—The Bragg curve of ionization by a charged particle.

Alpha particles: These are helium nuclei, and therefore have a mass of four and a double positive charge. For any given energy they will, because of their considerable mass, travel relatively slowly which, coupled with their double charge, means that they produce a great deal of ionization per unit length of track, lose their energy quickly and for this reason they have a very short range in solid material. They are completely stopped by very thin layers of solid material and they have no place in clinical radiology except that if an alpha-ray source gets into the body it will irradiate the tissues around it very intensely and constitute a hazard to health.

Beta particles: Being electrons and therefore negatively charged, and of very small mass, beta particles produce far less ionization per unit length of their path than do alpha particles of the same energy. Their range is thus greater, its exact value depending of course on their energy. Beta particles from radioactive strontium or phosphorus, for example, can penetrate through millimetres of tissue and therefore are used, clinically, as external agents for very superficial treatments or for internal therapy when their radioactive parent is introduced into the body.

Positrons: Their properties are exactly the same as those of the electron except that, having a positive charge, they ultimately disappear in annihilation radiation.

The Photons.—Both the gamma rays from the radioactive nuclei, and the annihilation radiations that always accompany positron emission, are electromagnetic radiations of high energy, and apart from their source and means of production, they are identical in properties with X-rays. In most of the discussions that follow in this book the term 'X-rays' will often be used—the stated facts, except where they refer to the method of production, will apply equally well to gamma rays.

Being uncharged, these radiations have much greater penetrating power than charged particles of the same energy, and most of their ionization is produced indirectly. Photons interact with matter to produce high-energy electrons which then behave exactly like beta particles and produce a lot more ionization, as will be seen from the full discussion of the properties of X- and gamma rays which will be given later.

Radioactivity in Practical Radiology.—It is the radiation that comes from radioactive materials that makes them important in radiology, and this radiation is used in two main ways. First, it may be used for treatment purposes in radiotherapy, and secondly, detection of the emission of radiation can be used to reveal the presence of the isotope in any material—this is the basis of 'tracer' uses of radioactivity, which will, like the therapeutic use, be discussed in a later chapter. Obviously for either of these uses, radiation penetration is required to reach either the part to be treated or the detecting instrument. For this reason alpha-particle emitters find no use in medicine, whilst for radiotherapy interest is chiefly but not exclusively centred in gamma-ray emitters. In 'tracer' work, beta rays, positrons, and gamma rays are all of value.

Summary.—*Table III* summarizes the general properties of the radioactive emissions. It must be stressed that the energies and other facts related to them are only examples, and are by no means the only energies possible for the emissions. Each type can be produced at any of a wide range of energy. Note that the ion density and range of the electron and positron of the same energy are the same.

Table III.—RADIOACTIVE RADIATIONS AND SOME OF THEIR CHARACTERISTICS

RADIATION	IONIZATION	IONIZING PARTICLE	SOME EXAMPLES OF TYPICAL		
			Radiation Energy	Mean Ion Density*	Range†
Alpha	Direct	Helium nucleus	5·5 MeV.	3500	40
Beta	Direct	Electron	1·0 MeV.	7·3	4300
	Direct	Electron	100 keV.	12·3	140
Positron	Direct	Positron	1·0 MeV.	7·3	4300
Photon (X- or γ-ray)	Indirect	Electron	1·2 MeV.	8–60	—

* Ion density in ions per micron of water (1 micron = 10^{-3} mm.).
† Range (approximate) in microns of water.

Rate of Decay.—If a radioactive isotope is studied it will be found that the rate at which it is giving out radiation falls progressively with time. Furthermore, it will be found that the amount of the material that remains decreases with time in exactly the same way. Different substances decay at different rates, but all follow the same sort of pattern, and some examples of this are given in *Fig.* 13.

There are a number of important features of this decay and the first is, as already hinted, that it cannot be altered in any way by any known agency. The rate of decay of a particular radioactive material is the same whether the temperature is high or low, whether the material is under high pressure or very low, and is unaltered by any chemical combination in which it may be found. Similarly, the rate of decay is the same for freshly prepared and for very old material. In so far as this means complete predictability of the amount of radiation that will be emitted in any time interval, this property is a considerable advantage. In so far as it means, for example, that the decay can never be halted or the radiation 'switched off', it can be a disadvantage.

Exponential Decay.—A more important feature is, however, revealed when the numerical details of information like that included in *Fig.* 13 are examined closely. It has already been stated that the decrease in the rate of decay and the decrease in the amount of radioactive isotope present follow exactly the same pattern in time.

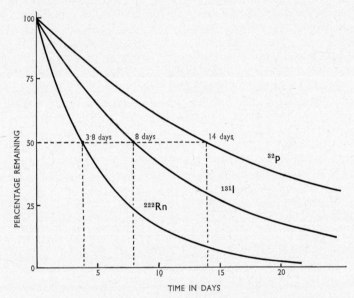

Fig. 13.—Radioactive 'decay' curves for radon 222, iodine 131, and phosphorus 32.

From this it can be concluded that the rate of decay—the amount decaying per second or minute, for example—depends on the amount of the material that is present. Furthermore, it is found that the fraction of the atoms present at any time which decay per second is always constant for any particular material.

For example, imagine that there are 1,000,000 atoms of a particular radioactive isotope present and that 100,000 of these decay in 1 min.; that is to say, $\frac{1}{10}$ of the atoms present decay per min. At the end of the minute 900,000 remain so that during the next minute 90,000 will decay ($\frac{1}{10}$ of 900,000) leaving 810,000 unchanged. During the third minute 81,000 of these will decay, so that at the end of 3 min. 729,000 atoms of the original material still exist. In the fourth minute $\frac{1}{10}$ of these 729,000 atoms will decay, leaving $729,000 - 72,900 = 656,100$ radioactive atoms. And so it would go on: in any given period the same fraction of the material present will decay.

This can be explained by saying that for some reason, which we cannot explain, there is a constant chance that any particular atom of a given material will decay in some stated period of time. For example, in radioactive iodine (^{131}I), each nucleus has roughly one chance in a million of decaying every second. (Though this number sounds small it is, in fact, quite large compared with many met with in radioactivity.) This number can be likened to the death-rate in a human population, though of course that varies with social conditions whereas in radioactivity for one radioactive species the value is absolutely constant.

However, it might be helpful to use the human analogy. The death-rate in England and Wales is about 12 per thousand per year at the moment, so that in a city like Manchester (population 600,000) about 7200 people die every year. In London (population 8,000,000) the number will be about 96,000 annually. In other words, the number of deaths equals the death-rate multiplied by the population. And in radioactivity the decay per unit time equals the number present multiplied by the chance, per unit time, of decay. If, for example, 100,000,000 atoms of iodine were present, the number which would decay in 1 sec. would be:

$$100,000,000 \times \frac{1}{1,000,000} = 100.$$

More generally if N atoms are present and the chance of decay is λ per second, then the number decaying per second will be $N \times \lambda$.

λ, which is the chance, or the likelihood (mathematically it is called *the probability*), that an atom will change in a second is usually called the *transformation constant*, a rather terrifying name for an essentially simple idea.

So far, decay in seconds has been discussed. Mathematically it is usual to consider any length of time, starting from very short ones, in which case the decay formula is written:

$$dN = -\lambda N \, dt,$$

where N and λ are as already described and dN is the number of atoms which decay in the very short time dt. The negative sign indicates that the *change dN* is a reduction. This formula can also be written:

$$\frac{dN}{N} = -\lambda \, dt$$

and is then the mathematical expression of the basic truth already stated, that the *fraction* decaying in any stated time interval is constant.

This very important *physical* fact leads (and the argument is set out in APPENDIX II for those who wish to follow it) to the *exponential law* of radioactive decay, viz.:

$$N = N_0 \, e^{-\lambda t},$$

where N_0 and N are, respectively, the number of radioactive nuclei present initially and after a time t.

This formula applies, of course, to all radioactive materials, each of which will have a different value of the constant λ. The greater the value of λ (that is to say, the greater the chance or 'probability' of decay) the more rapidly will the substance decay and the smaller will be the values of N after any particular time. In *Fig.* 13 are shown the variations with time of amounts of three radioactive materials which are important in radiology, namely, phosphorus 32, iodine 131, and radon 222. For radon, $\lambda = 2 \cdot 1 \times 10^{-6}$ per sec. (or about 2 chances in a million per sec.) and its more rapid decay than phosphorus 32 whose λ is $5 \cdot 6 \times 10^{-7}$ (about four times smaller) can be seen. For iodine 131 the transformation constant is $1 \cdot 0 \times 10^{-6}$ which lies between the other two, as does the rapidity of decay.

Half-life.—*Fig.* 13 hints that, and the exponential formula states that, theoretically at least, a radioactive substance never completely disappears. Its strength gets weaker and weaker but some—admittedly a very small amount—will be left even after a very long time. Rather like old soldiers, radioactive substances never die, they simply fade away. The transformation constant (λ) gives an idea of the speed with which this happens but a more usual indication is the *half-life* or *half-value period*. The latter term is rather outmoded now, but in many ways would seem to be a preferable—being more descriptive—term.

The half-life is simply the time taken for half of any amount of radioactive material to decay (or for the decay, or emission, rate to fall to half its initial value) and the values for the isotopes dealt with in *Fig.* 13 are those indicated. As is to be expected, since both are directly connected with the rate of decay, there is a direct relationship between the half-life ($T_{\frac{1}{2}}$) and the transformation constant and that is:

$$T_{\frac{1}{2}} = \frac{0 \cdot 693}{\lambda}. \; *$$

The half-lives from *Fig.* 13 together with those of some other radioactive isotopes used in radiology are set out in *Table IV*, from which it will be noticed that the value of the half-life does not seem to have any obvious relationship to the atomic or mass numbers of the material. For interest, the emissions from the isotopes are also given.

Table IV.—Some Clinically Useful Radioactive Isotopes

Element	Mass Number (A)	Atomic Number (Z)	Half-life	Radiation
Sodium	24	11	15 hours	β γ
Phosphorus	32	15	14 days	β
Iron	59	26	45 days	β γ
Cobalt	60	27	5·3 years	β γ
Strontium	90	38	28 years	β
Iodine	131	53	8 days	β γ
Iodine	132	53	2·3 hours	β γ
Caesium	137	55	30 years	β γ
Tantalum	182	73	115 days	β γ
Gold	198	79	2·7 days	β γ
Radon†	222	86	3·8 days	α
Radium†	226	88	1620 years	α

† Parents of radioactive series giving also β- and γ-rays.

It should be noted that the 'equal fractions' rule applies just as much to half-lives as to any other fractional decay period, so that one-quarter of the original material will remain after the elapse of twice the half-life, with one-eighth remaining after three half-lives, and so on. For the mathematically minded it can be said that the fraction of the original material remaining after n half-lives will be $(1/2)^n$. For the less mathematically inclined it may be helpful to remember that after ten half-lives (that is to say, after a period ten times as long as the half-life) about one-thousandth of the original material remains. Strictly $(1/2)^{10} = 1/1024$ but $1/1000$ is a very easily remembered approximation which can be very useful when the disposal of radioactive wastes is being considered. Taking this approximation a stage further, after twenty half-lives one-millionth remains.

So much, then, for the general physical properties of radioactive nuclei and their emissions. The next chapter will deal with our sources of these materials.

---

* Mathematically this arises as follows:
Since $N/N_0 = e^{-\lambda t}$, for the half-life $e^{-\lambda T_{\frac{1}{2}}} = 0 \cdot 5$; but $e^{-0 \cdot 693} = 0 \cdot 5$, whence it follows that $\lambda T_{\frac{1}{2}} = 0 \cdot 693$.

CHAPTER IV

RADIOACTIVITY—MATERIALS

ALTHOUGH today every known element can be obtained in radioactive form, radio-activity was first observed in natural uranium. This was by Becquerel in 1896 and a few years later Pierre and Marie Curie isolated a number of other radioactive elements, the most famous being radium, from natural uranium ore. For over thirty years the only known radioactive materials were those occurring naturally and principally the elements with atomic number in excess of 80. However, in 1934 Professor and Mme Joliot-Curie (son-in-law and daughter of the isolators of radium) discovered that normal stable substances could be rendered radioactive by suitable bombardment with nuclear particles. This discovery of what was called 'artificial' radioactivity—to distinguish the substances from those occurring naturally though there is no fundamental difference between them—opened the door to the vast numbers of radioactive materials now available. Numerous bombardment processes have been used to produce 'artificial radioactivity' but only two are of major importance. In all, there are four sources of radioactive material which deserve attention, and these are:—

1. Naturally occurring radioactive materials.
2. Radioactivity 'induced' by neutron bombardment.
3. Radioactivity 'induced' by proton bombardment.
4. 'Fission' products.

NATURALLY OCCURRING RADIOACTIVE MATERIALS

With a few exceptions all the natural radioactive materials have atomic numbers of more than 80 and can be grouped into one or other of three radioactive 'families' starting, respectively, with uranium, thorium, and actinium. Each 'family' is a series of radioactive changes each of which yields a radioactive 'daughter' until a stable substance ends the line. For example, uranium emits an alpha particle and becomes uranium X (an isotope of thorium). This product is radioactive, emitting beta particles and gamma rays to yield uranium X_2, which is a beta-particle emitter having uranium II as its daughter. And so the series goes on through a total of 13 radioactive substances, which include the radiologically very important substances radium and radon, until the final product—a stable isotope of lead—is reached. Radium, radon, and some of their daughter elements will be discussed in more detail later.

The most important of the natural radioactive materials with atomic numbers less than 81 is an isotope of potassium, potassium 40, a beta-particle and gamma-ray emitter, which constitutes about 0·01 per cent of natural potassium. Its gamma rays enable its presence in the body to be detected, and this is the basis for studies of potassium distribution and metabolism, which are of considerable diagnostic value.

RADIOACTIVITY 'INDUCED' BY NEUTRON BOMBARDMENT

At the end of CHAPTER II it was pointed out that an extra neutron might render a nucleus unstable. Being uncharged, neutrons are able to enter nuclei relatively easily and the most prolific method of producing radioactivity 'artificially' is to subject stable materials to neutron bombardment. The most common result of such bombardment is what is called the 'n-γ' reaction, which means that a neutron enters the nucleus (we usually say that the neutron is 'captured') and some energy is liberated therefrom in the form of a gamma ray. It should be emphasized that this is *not* a radioactive gamma ray, because its emission is not spontaneous but the immediate result of neutron capture. The new atom produced in this process has the same atomic number as the irradiated material but a mass number one greater. Though it will often also be radioactive, it must be stressed that n-γ reactions can lead to stable isotopes as well.

A typical example of this type of nuclear reaction is provided by the bombardment of stable phosphorus by neutrons, which results in the production of the phosphorus isotope of mass 32. Similarly, the cobalt isotope of mass number 60 results from the neutron bombardment of normal cobalt (cobalt 59). These reactions are summarized in the following equations:

$$^{31}_{15}P + ^{1}_{0}n \rightarrow ^{32}_{15}P + ^{0}_{0}\gamma;$$

$$^{59}_{27}Co + ^{1}_{0}n \rightarrow ^{60}_{27}Co + ^{0}_{0}\gamma.$$

In each case the daughter product is radioactive and, typical of nuclei having an excess of neutrons, both phosphorus 32 and cobalt 60 are beta-particle emitters, whilst cobalt 60 also emits gamma rays. The details of their radiologically important decay schemes have already been given in CHAPTER III. Because the product has the same atomic number as the parent substance it is impossible to separate them chemically. Hence, using the n-γ reaction, it is impossible to obtain a pure specimen of the radioactive isotope, or, in the jargon of the subject, to obtain a 'carrier-free' sample: there will always be some stable isotope present.

RADIOACTIVITY 'INDUCED' BY PROTON BOMBARDMENT

Just as the capture of a neutron by a nucleus may disturb the stability of that nucleus, so also may the capture of a proton. Because the proton is positively charged its entry into the nucleus is much more difficult than is that of a neutron. There is increasing electrostatic repulsion as it approaches the positively charged nucleus and the proton has to have considerable energy to achieve the desired penetration. For this purpose the protons are usually accelerated to high energies in the machine called a *cyclotron* and isotopes produced in this way are often called 'Cyclotron Produced Isotopes'.

The most common result of proton bombardment of nuclei is the capture of the proton and the ejection of a neutron—the 'p-n' reaction. For example, if sulphur 34 is bombarded with protons the chlorine isotope of mass 34 is produced:

$$^{34}_{16}S + ^{1}_{1}p \rightarrow ^{34}_{17}Cl + ^{1}_{0}n.$$

This chlorine isotope is radioactive and, since it has fewer neutrons than in the stable isotope, it gives out positrons. It should also be noted that the product of this reaction (^{34}Cl) is a different substance than the irradiated material (^{34}S). Because of this, pure samples ('carrier-free') of the radioactive product can be prepared, since sulphur and chlorine can easily be separated chemically.

Uranium Fission and Atomic Energy.—Before the fourth listed source of radio-active materials—'fission' products—can be discussed it is necessary to make a very considerable digression to discuss a most important physical phenomenon. In CHAPTER II the question 'What holds the nucleus together?' was asked but was not answered, though it was indicated that neutrons play an important role in it. So does energy. It has been found that the weight of a nucleus is smaller than the sum of the individual masses of the constituent protons and neutrons, the difference having been given out as energy when the nucleus was formed. The difference is called the *mass defect* and it is generally greater for the medium atomic number elements than for those with low or high atomic numbers. If, therefore, light elements could be fused together to form heavier ones, or heavy elements could be split to produce lighter ones, energy might be given out. And in fact this is just what happens and is the basis of the sources of atomic energy (it would be more accurate to call it nuclear energy) which men are tapping.

Attention will here be concentrated on the second of the two processes, namely the release of energy when a large nucleus splits into two smaller ones. That this happened, and that it could, in fact, be a source of energy on a major scale, was first realized when 'uranium fission' was discovered in 1939. Two German physicists, Hahn and Strassman, observed that, after uranium had been bombarded with neutrons, it was possible to detect the presence of medium atomic number elements in the irradiated material. The reason for this was that uranium nuclei were being split, generally into two roughly equal halves. At the same time considerable amounts of energy were being released and, very important indeed, two or three neutrons were liberated at each fission. A typical fission reaction is:

$$^{235}_{92}U + ^{1}_{0}n \rightarrow ^{137}_{55}Cs + ^{97}_{37}Rb + ^{1}_{0}n + ^{1}_{0}n + energy.$$

Two important principles are illustrated by this equation. Normal caesium has a mass number of 133 while stable rubidium has a mass of either 85 or 87. The two substances produced by the splitting of the uranium have masses considerably in excess of these numbers; they have considerably more neutrons than their stable isotopes and therefore are very likely to be radioactive. The above example is only one of many ways in which the uranium atom may split, but no matter how it splits the fission products are usually radioactive.

The second point to be noted is that whereas 1 neutron was required for the fission, 2 neutrons emerged from it, thus giving the possibility of a 'chain-reaction', provided all the released neutrons can be used to produce further fission. *Fig.* 14 shows diagrammatically what could happen under such circumstances.

Starting with a single neutron and assuming that 2 neutrons are produced at each fission, there will be over 1000 neutrons after ten 'generations' of fissions, and over 1,000,000 after twenty. Therefore, though each fission only produces a minute amount of energy (though a large amount on the atomic scale), soon a very considerable amount would be released in this rapidly expanding process. *Fig.* 14 is, in fact, a diagrammatic representation of an atomic explosion. Since such a process requires the use of practically every neutron produced, the block of material used must be greater than a certain minimum size (otherwise a large number of neutrons escape unused) and, furthermore, natural uranium cannot be used for reasons which are explained below.

For a non-explosive source of power it is not necessary—in fact, it is not desirable—to use every neutron for further fission. So long as one neutron out of each fission can be used to produce another fission, the process can be kept going and a continuing source of power provided. But before this can be affected a major difficulty has to be overcome.

Natural uranium is made up of three isotopes, one of mass number 238 which represents 99·3 per cent of the whole, a second of mass number 235, which makes up about 0·7 per cent of the total, and a third of mass number 233, which is present in such minute amounts that it can be ignored here. When a neutron enters the uranium-235 nucleus, fission always results, but matters are quite different with the heavier isotope. A fast neutron may produce fission, but in many cases instead of fission,

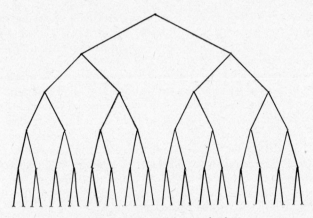

Fig. 14.—A 'chain-reaction'.

straightforward neutron capture will occur, and uranium 239 will be formed. Owing to the relative abundance of uranium 238 this capture process would quickly remove the neutrons produced by any fissions and so bring the chain-reaction to an end. If energy is to be generated by uranium fission a method has to be found of eliminating the uranium 238 or its capturing property.

Since the actual removal of the heavier isotope is not an economic possibility—chemical separation is impossible because the substances are isotopes and physical separation is extremely difficult and very expensive—the solution to the problem depends on the fact that uranium 238 does not react at all with slow neutrons, whereas with uranium 235 they produce fissions. The energy emitted by the fission process is mostly carried away by the neutrons whose consequent high speeds render them likely victims of non-fission capture by uranium 238. Some method must therefore be found of slowing down these neutrons quickly and converting them into 'slow' neutrons which will only react with uranium 235. If this can be done the effect will be the same as if the uranium 238 had been removed.

The only way in which the neutron (which, it must be remembered, is uncharged) can lose energy and thus be slowed down is in collision with other atomic nuclei. In such collisions, the more nearly equal are the masses of the colliding particles, the greater the energy that is transferred, so that ways have to be found to use light atoms for slowing down the high-energy neutrons. Unfortunately, many of the lighter elements are unsuitable for this purpose. For example, hydrogen, lithium, and boron all 'capture' neutrons and would therefore remove them from the reaction just as surely as the uranium 238 would do. Helium, on the other hand, forms no chemical compounds and is only available as a gas, the atoms of which would be too far apart to be effective as a slowing-down agent in an apparatus of reasonable size, whilst beryllium is too rare to be considered. Thus, of the six lightest elements, only deuterium (the hydrogen isotope of mass 2) and carbon are satisfactory. In practice, therefore, either deuterium, in the form of 'heavy water' (i.e., D_2O as compared with ordinary water, H_2O), or carbon, in the form of very pure graphite, is used. Very pure materials are needed because quite small traces of elements which capture neutrons may have an upsetting effect out of all proportion to their quantity.

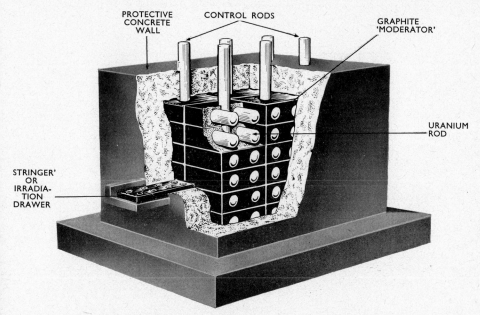

Fig. 15.—Schematic diagram of the nuclear reactor or 'pile'.

The Nuclear Reactor or 'Pile'.—This is the name given to the practical arrangement in which fission neutrons are slowed down so that a continuing nuclear reaction to provide, for example, a source of power is possible using natural uranium. The principles of the construction of the pile are shown in *Fig.* 15. Uranium rods are mounted in—and separated from each other by—a 'moderator' which is, as indicated above, either heavy water or graphite. The whole is surrounded by a thick layer of moderator material which acts as a 'reflector' and this, in turn, is surrounded by a thick wall of concrete to protect workers from radiations generated within the pile.

It is in collisions with deuterium nuclei in the heavy water, or with carbon nuclei in the graphite, that the neutrons are rapidly slowed down and rendered unable to react with the nuclei of uranium 238. The action of the 'pile' and the reasons for some of its features can probably best be understood by studying, as in *Fig.* 16, the fate of a few fission neutrons in a 'pile'.

Imagine that a fission occurs at A in one of the uranium rods. Most probably both fission neutrons (throughout this example we assume two neutrons to be produced per fission) will escape from the rod since, as already pointed out in CHAPTER II, matter is largely space and the uncharged neutron, unaffected by nuclear or electronic charges, can travel considerable distances before making a collision. In the moderator each makes a number of collisions, is slowed down, and deflected from its path many times. Neutron No. 1 actually escapes from the pile whilst No. 2 'wanders' round inside until it enters another uranium rod where it produces a fission and neutrons Nos. 3 and 4. No. 3 follows a path, and has a fate, similar to that of No. 2, producing a fission and hence 2 more neutrons in another rod. Neutron No. 4 behaves similarly but it will be noted that at one stage of its path it was heading out of the pile only to be turned back by a collision in the 'reflector'. Ultimately it, too, makes a fission-producing collision, giving rise to neutrons 5 and 6. One of these, by chance, reaches another rod without undergoing many slowing collisions so that it still has considerable

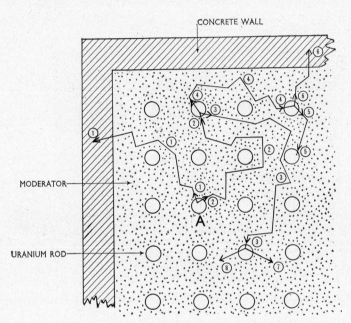

Fig. 16.—The paths of some neutrons in the reactor.

energy when it is captured by a uranium 238 nucleus and is lost. Neutron 6, after a number of collisions in the moderator, escapes from the pile.

Thus, in this short survey which started with a single neutron-producing fission, a total of four fissions have occurred, 2 neutrons have escaped from the pile, 1 has been captured giving uranium 239 (and ultimately, by radioactive decay, the important substance plutonium), and 2 remain to produce further fissions or suffer any of the other fates. The chain-reaction can continue.

From this short sequence the role of the 'moderator' will be clear as well as that of the 'reflector'. It will also be seen why a thick protective wall has to be built round the reactor, for without it the escaping neutrons would be a very serious hazard to those working with or near the 'pile'.

The events described were chosen to illustrate the various possibilities. By chance it could have been that each neutron had gone on to produce another fission, so that the 6 neutrons studied might have produced six fissions and 12 neutrons to carry on the good work. Such a sequence would certainly lead to the pile 'running away' if not exploding, so to guard against such a contingency 'control rods', made of steel which is rich in boron or cadmium, are available to be lowered into the pile. Boron and cadmium readily capture neutrons and so will efficiently remove any neutrons in excess of those needed for the maintenance of the chain-reaction.

It will be noted that the reactor is not only a source of energy but also a source of large numbers of neutrons, many of which can be used for other than the continuation of the reaction. Therefore it is usual to build into the reactor long drawers or 'stringers' into which substances, which it is desired to irradiate with neutrons, can be placed. These may be in the reflector, where they will have very little effect upon the running of the pile, since they will mostly be irradiated by neutrons (like Nos. 1 and 6 above) which would otherwise escape. 'Stringers' going into the heart of the pile will absorb neutrons which might have taken part in the reaction and therefore will play a part in its control. Any substances placed in these 'stringers' will be subjected to much more intense neutron bombardment than if placed in the reflector and more intense radioactive sources will result.

Most of the 'n-γ' reactions discussed earlier are produced in the 'pile', which is therefore a major source of radioactive materials, as well as a most important source of energy.

Before leaving the consideration of the working of the reactor, the very legitimate question concerning where the neutron, that starts off the whole process, comes from must be answered. There are two main sources. Neutrons are present in cosmic radiation, which continuously bombards our world, but probably a more effective source is from the spontaneous fission of uranium. In 1 gramme of uranium about one in 10^{24} atoms spontaneously split every second, but even at this extremely low rate there will be, on the average, about one fission per minute in every gramme of uranium, which is quite enough to 'trigger off' the whole process. And finally it must be added that reactors can also work with other high atomic number materials: plutonium is one of them.

'FISSION' PRODUCTS

We may now return to the fourth of the listed sources of radioactive material.

High atomic number elements have a greater excess of neutrons over protons than do lower atomic number elements (more 'glue' needed to hold the nucleus together). For example, uranium 235 has 143 neutrons with its 92 protons, an excess of 51, whereas, for example, palladium with half the atomic number (46) has 64 neutrons in its heaviest stable isotope, an excess of 18. Thus if the uranium 235 should split into two palladium nuclei, each of these would have considerably more neutrons than are needed for stability. Most fission products are therefore radioactive. When the 'pile' is working radioactive materials are continually being produced in the uranium rods, rather like ash accumulates in a fire. Used rods will therefore become what can only be described as a 'chemical mess' from which many elements can be extracted by chemical means because of their different atomic number, but only with great difficulty because of the intense radiation coming from the radioactivity. Nevertheless the 'pile' is a major source of radioactive isotopes.

The splitting of the uranium nucleus does not follow a fixed pattern but rather there is a matter of chance about the size of the fragments of any particular fission; the whole effect rather resembles the efforts of an inexperienced axeman trying to split logs! Very seldom will a fission yield equal parts, and very seldom will it result in a very small and a very large part. The pattern is that shown in *Fig.* 17, which shows the relative amounts of the different atomic number materials produced.

Notice that the amounts are plotted on a logarithmic scale because of the wide range that has to be presented. Thus only one-hundredth of 1 per cent of all fission results in equal halves whereas mass numbers of 95 and 139 are produced by about 6 per cent of fissions. Among the clinically important radioactive materials produced with

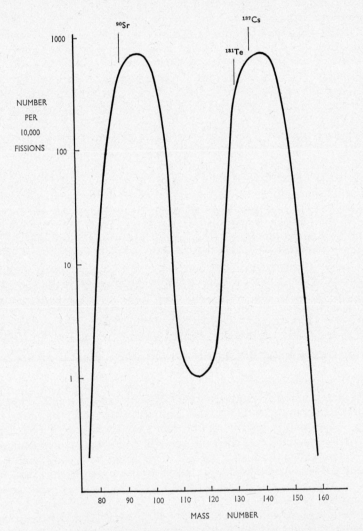

Fig. 17.—Relative amounts of different isotopes among the fission fragments.

relatively high yields are caesium 137, strontium 90, and tellurium 131, the parent of iodine 131. Fission is the main source of these materials.

In all, about 300 different radioactive isotopes accumulate in the uranium rods of a working reactor, some of them coming from radioactive 'families' which stem from direct fission products. An example of one of these 'families' is that coming from the fission product xenon 139. The heaviest stable isotope of this inert gas has a mass number of 136 (54 protons and 82 neutrons), which means that the fission-product isotope has 3 neutrons too many and, as might be expected, it is very unstable, needing three beta-ray emitting radioactive changes before a stable nucleus is achieved.

$$\beta \qquad \beta \qquad \beta$$

$$^{139}_{54}\text{Xe} \longrightarrow \ ^{139}_{55}\text{Cs} \longrightarrow \ ^{139}_{56}\text{Ba} \longrightarrow \ ^{139}_{57}\text{La}$$

0·5 min.   6 min.   86 min.   Stable

The times given below each substance are their radioactive half-lives, and it is not without interest that the value increases from left to right as the radioactive changes carry the nucleus nearer to final stability.

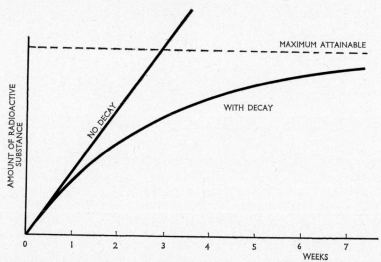

Fig. 18.—The growth of radioactive phosphorus (^{32}P) due to the irradiation of normal phosphorus (^{31}P) by neutrons in the reactor. The straight line indicates the total amount produced, i.e., the amount that would have been present but for radioactive decay.

Radioactive Equilibrium.—Imagine that some material is placed inside the 'pile' which is running at a constant rate. The material will be subjected to neutron bombardment at a constant rate and neutrons will be captured at a constant rate. If this neutron capture leads to radioactive nuclei then radioactive material is being made at a constant rate. However, it must not be assumed that the amount of radioactive material is increasing at this rate, because radioactive decay is also taking place. It will be remembered that the number of radioactive nuclei decaying depends on the number present and therefore initially very few decay because few are present. As the stock increases the number decaying increases, and eventually a state is reached when the number decaying equals the number of new radioactive nuclei being produced. A state of equilibrium is then attained.

Fig. 18 shows the growth of a radioactive isotope (phosphorus 32) and the equilibrium that is attained. It also shows the way in which the amount of phosphorus 32 would have increased had there been no decay.

Those mathematically inclined may be interested to know that the formula for the growth curve is:

$$N = N_{\max} (1 - e^{-\lambda t}),$$

where N is the number of radioactive nuclei which are present after the material has been irradiated for a time t, and N_{max} is the maximum number that can be achieved, i.e., the equilibrium quantity; λ is the transformation constant of the isotope being produced.

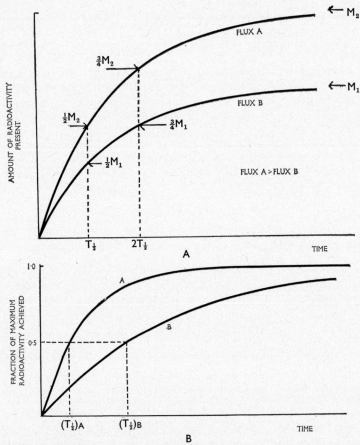

Fig. 19.—How the growth of a radioactive product depends on neutron flux and the material being irradiated: A, The same material irradiated at two different fluxes; B, Different materials in the same flux.

The maximum strength of the isotope (N_{max}) that can be achieved depends upon three factors:

1. The transformation constant λ. N_{max} is inversely proportional to λ.
2. The number of neutrons passing through the material per second.
   This is called the 'neutron flux'.
3. The ability of the irradiated material to capture neutrons.
   This is called its 'capture cross-section'.

By contrast, the rate at which the maximum, or any fraction of it, is attained depends only upon the transformation constant λ. This is illustrated in *Fig.* 19 A which shows the growth of a particular radioactive isotope through bombardment at two different neutron fluxes. The greater flux produces the greater amount of activity but it will be seen that half or three-quarters of maximum activity is achieved at the same rate for each flux.

Fig. 19 B shows a contrasting situation: the irradiation of different materials, and hence the production of different daughter products, in the same neutron flux. In this case the maximum is reached more quickly by the product with the greater transformation constant, that is to say, by the material which breaks down more easily. The slower the product decays (that is to say, the longer its half-life) the longer it takes to reach its maximum, equilibrium value.

These are important observations when the production of radioactive isotope sources is being considered. The ultimate strength of source of any material is controlled by the neutron flux, whilst the rate at which that strength is reached is controlled

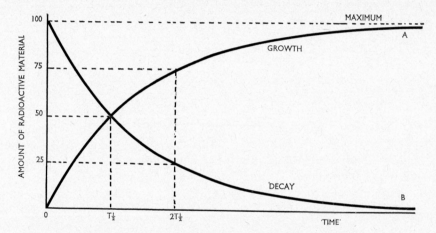

Fig. 20.—The growth and decay of a radioactive isotope.

entirely by the material. Prolongation of irradiation will not produce strengths greater than the equilibrium value. Stronger sources can only be achieved by using greater fluxes.

An interesting feature of the rate of growth is its relationship to the rate of decay of the isotope. They are 'complementary'—the meaning of which term is illustrated by *Fig.* 20. In this diagram are shown the growth of the isotope due to the neutron bombardment (curve A) and the normal decay of this product (curve B). It will be immediately apparent that growth to half the maximum value occurs in the same time as the isotope alone would need to decay to half its starting value—i.e., one half-life. Similarly, whilst in two half-lives decay would be to one-quarter, growth would be to three-quarters. Three half-lives reduce a decaying isotope to one-eighth, whilst in a similar period seven-eighths of the maximum strength is achieved by the neutron irradiation. Finally, as has been pointed out already, in ten half-lives a radioactive material decays to 1/1000 of its starting value: in ten half-lives 999/1000 of the maximum strength is produced by irradiation; or, in practical terms, equilibrium can be regarded as achieved in ten half-lives.

This type of equilibrium—the reaching and maintaining of a constant strength—is called a *permanent* equilibrium, and it can be produced, in theory at least, in a nuclear reactor which can provide a constant neutron flux and hence a constant rate of isotope production.

Radioactive substances can also be produced, as daughter elements, by the decay of a radioactive parent, and in this case, too, the amount of daughter element increases in a way similar to that shown in *Fig.* 18 but with the important difference that the source (the parent substance) in this case is being reduced continuously and so, therefore, is the rate of daughter element production. The precise effect of this source decay upon the growth of the daughter will depend upon the speed with which the parent decays and there are several possible variants on the theme. The only two which are of importance in radiology, however, are illustrated by the growth of radon from radium, and of radium A from radon. *Fig.* 21 shows the two effects.

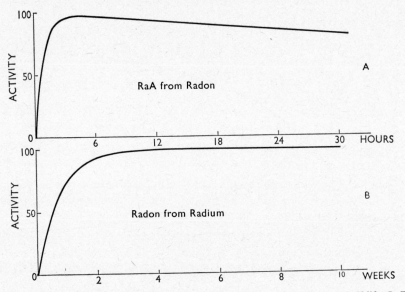

Fig. 21.—Growth of a radioactive daughter element, A, From a parent of short half-life. B, From a parent of long half-life. Note the difference in the time scales.

Radium has a half-life of about 1700 years compared with radon's half-life of 3·82 days. Radon equilibrium is attained in about 40 days (roughly ten half-lives) during which the radium has decayed a mere 0·04 per cent. The equilibrium is effectively permanent, but strictly speaking the source has decayed and therefore the equilibrium is called *secular* to distinguish it from the truly constant situation.

Radium A, on the other hand, has a half-life of about 20 min., and over the 3 or 4 hours required for it to come to equilibrium with its parent radon, that material will have decayed about 3 per cent. The variation of the amount of Ra A with time follows quite a different shape of curve, as is shown, because its parent has a half-life which is not very great. Nevertheless an equilibrium is achieved even here, though it is not lasting and is given the name of *transient* equilibrium.

Quantities of Radioactive Material.—The first radioactive materials to be discovered were solids, so that the obvious unit for their measurement was a unit of weight—the gramme, or more usually some sub-multiple of it like the milli-(1/1000) or the micro-(1/1,000,000) gramme. However, a difficulty quickly arose with the separation of the radioactive gas, radon, for here a unit of weight was obviously unsuitable. A special unit, the *curie*, was therefore introduced, and was originally defined as the amount of radon in equilibrium with 1 gramme of radium. Later the definition was extended to cover any of radium's decay products.

The discovery of artificial radioactivity in 1934 and the subsequent floods of new radioactive isotopes posed a further problem. Many were solid but weight was not a good basis for measurement since many radioactive materials (such as those produced by n-γ reactions) are mixtures of stable and radioactive isotopes. Weight alone would give no indication of the proportion that was radioactive.

After an abortive attempt to introduce a new unit, the Rutherford, it was internationally agreed to redefine the curie so that it would be applied to any radioactive isotope. In its new form the curie is no longer a unit of quantity of radioactive material but is a unit of *activity*. In clinical work the actual amount of radioactive material present is relatively unimportant. Principal interest is in the number of atoms which disintegrate per second, or in the intensity of radiation being emitted (the two are, of course, intimately connected). And this is essentially what *activity* defines—the number of disintegrations per second. An amount of radioactive material in which there are $3 \cdot 7 \times 10^{10}$ disintegrations per second is said to have an activity of 1 curie. This number is the measured disintegration rate for radium, so that the new definition does not upset old quantities but extends the unit's usefulness to all materials.

In June, 1975, the International Committee on Weights and Measures adopted a new S.I. (Système International) unit of *activity* named the *becquerel* after the discoverer of radioactivity. The symbol is Bq. and a source has an activity of 1 becquerel if its disintegration rate is 1 per second. The becquerel is thus a very tiny amount of activity, 1 curie being equal to $3 \cdot 7 \times 10^{10}$ Bq., and even a microcurie is equal to 37 000 Bq.

CHAPTER V

THE PRODUCTION OF X-RAYS

THE X-RAY TUBE

X-RAYS were discovered by Wilhelm Conrad Röntgen in November, 1895, whilst he was experimenting with the passage of electricity through a gas at very low pressure. The vital piece of his apparatus was a long glass vessel from which as much air as possible had been removed and into each end of which a short platinum electrode was sealed. When an electric discharge at high voltage was passed through the almost evacuated tube, Röntgen noticed a glow on a piece of glass, covered with zinc sulphide, which was lying a short distance from the tube. The glow persisted even when the discharge tube was shrouded in black paper, and Röntgen was quickly able to establish that the cause was a hitherto undiscovered radiation. To it he gave the name X-rays, X being the established symbol for the unknown quality.

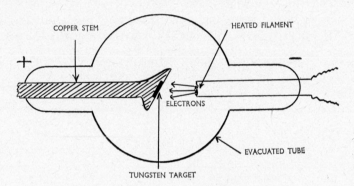

Fig. 22.—An X-ray tube.

Although a modern X-ray tube bears no very obvious resemblance to the discharge tube of Röntgen's apparatus, the basic mechanism of X-ray production remains the same. X-rays are produced whenever high-speed electrons are suddenly brought to rest, some of their kinetic energy, at least, being converted into the electromagnetic radiation. In the original apparatus the source of the electrons was the residual gas in the tube. Accelerated by the applied voltage they were brought to rest by the glass end of the tube, whence the X-rays were emitted. Nowadays the electrons come, by thermionic emission, from an electrically heated filament of tungsten, which means that the supply is much more easily controlled, and they are brought to rest by a block of material of high atomic number, in which X-ray production occurs much more efficiently than in glass.

The basic features of this type of X-ray tube (often called the Coolidge tube, in honour of the American who developed it as a much more efficient alternative to the 'gas-tube' which developed from Röntgen's apparatus) are shown in *Fig.* 22.

The whole tube is evacuated as completely as possible so that the electrons suffer no impediment, and therefore suffer no loss of energy, in their passage from the filament to the 'target'.

If a high voltage is applied between the electrodes of such an 'X-ray tube' so that the filament is the cathode (negative electrode) and the 'target' is the anode (positive electrode), any electrons emitted when the filament is heated will be repelled from it and attracted towards the 'target', where they are abruptly brought to rest. During their passage from filament to 'target' each electron will have acquired energy (E)

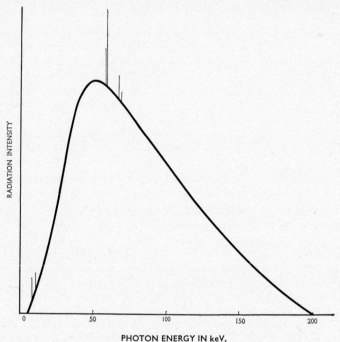

RADIATION INTENSITY

PHOTON ENERGY IN keV.

Fig. 23.—The spectrum of radiation from an X-ray tube.

equal to the product of its charge (e) and the voltage difference between the two electrodes (V):

$$E = eV$$

and this kinetic energy is surrendered to the target and there converted into other energy forms. One form is X-radiation.

Technical details of some practical X-ray tubes will be given later. For present purposes the rudimentary tube depicted in *Fig.* 22, together with an appropriate constant high-voltage supply and a filament-heating current, will be assumed to be available.

THE RADIATION

X-rays are produced by the interaction of the electrons from the filament (the 'cathode stream') with the material of the target, and if the rays coming from any tube are analysed it will be found that they are not all of one energy but constitute a complex spectrum such as that shown in *Fig.* 23.

In fact the spectrum is made up of two distinct parts and is the result of two quite different mechanisms. There is a continuous spectrum containing all energies from a certain maximum downwards, and upon this there is superimposed a 'line' spectrum of a relatively small number of separate energies.

The Continuous Spectrum.—To the continuous spectrum the name *Bremsstrahlung* or 'braking' radiation is often applied, and gives a good clue to the way in which the radiation is produced, i.e., by the slowing down of the cathode-stream electrons by the atoms of the 'target' material.

What happens in the bombarded target is extremely complicated and its explanation beyond the scope of this book. However, it is possible to present a fairly simple mechanistic picture, which though not precise in detail, enables the main features to be understood.

As a generalization it may be said that two types of interaction ('collisions') are involved. In the first the impinging electrons 'interact' with the electrons of the atom (the electron 'cloud'), whilst the second is between the electrons and the nuclei. When electrons approach fairly close to atoms they will be repelled, and therefore deflected, by the 'cloud' and, to some extent, will be slowed down. The small amount of energy so lost will be transferred to the atom involved, so that by this process the target material gains energy; it is heated up. Sometimes, however, an electron will penetrate through the 'cloud' and approach the nucleus itself. In the powerful electrical field of the nucleus the electron behaves rather like a comet entering our solar system; it swings around the sun and departs in a completely new direction. Thus the electron suffers a considerable change in direction and at the same time a large reduction in its speed and, therefore, energy. The energy lost in this type of interaction is emitted as a high-energy photon, that is to say an X-ray. How much energy is emitted depends not only on the details of the 'collision' but also on how much energy the electron retains after any previous 'collisions'. A wide range of photon energies may thus be produced, varying downwards from the 'collision' in which the electron loses its energy in a single 'collision'—a rare but not impossible event. *Fig.* 24 illustrates some of the type of interactions that may occur when electrons strike the target. Electron 1, after slight deflexions by two atoms, penetrates the 'cloud' of a third, suffers a marked change of direction, and emits an X-ray photon. With some residual energy it continues, suffers another minor deflexion before giving up all its residual energy in a final nuclear 'collision'. Electron 2, typical of many, suffers a long series of 'collisions' with the electron 'clouds', which result in small energy losses—and heat production—but no X-ray photons. Electron 3 is quite different. It passes very close to the nucleus and is brought to rest, thus giving up all its energy. Such a 'head-on' type 'collision' produces the maximum energy photon possible. Finally electron 4 makes three nuclear 'collisions', giving up roughly a third of its energy in each.

It must be stressed that *Fig.* 24 only indicates the types of interaction, and does not represent the direction of emission of the photons or how often they occur, both of which features of the X-ray production process depend upon the energy of the electrons—i.e., upon the applied voltage—as will be described later. However, the diagram illustrates the important fact that X-rays are not produced solely at the surface of the target. Electrons penetrate through many atomic layers and the X-rays have therefore to pass through some thickness of target material before emerging into space. This has a marked influence on the spatial distribution of radiation from an X-ray tube, a point to which we will return later.

Applied Voltage, Maximum Photon Energy, and Minimum Wavelength.—In what might be termed the head-on 'collision' between an electron and a target atom the former loses all its energy in one photon. The energy (E) of this photon thus equals the energy of the electron, which is its charge (e) multiplied by the voltage (V) applied to the tube, i.e., $E = eV$. For example, if the tube is working at a constant 200 kV. the maximum photon energy that can be produced will be 200 kilo-electron-volts (200 keV.). Because of this sort of conversion of kinetic energy, acquired from electrical energy, into electromagnetic radiation energy, it is convenient—and increasingly

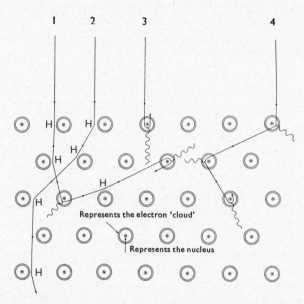

Fig. 24.—Some interactions between electrons and atoms in an X-ray tube target, and their results. H indicates heat-producing 'collision'. ∿∿ indicates photon-producing 'collision'.

common—to speak of photon energies in terms of electron-volts (eV.) or kilo, or mega-electron-volts (keV. or MeV.).

It is also becoming more common to state radiation energies rather than wavelengths, and certainly the newer method is generally more useful, and will mainly be adopted in these pages. However, there are occasions when a knowledge of wavelength can be useful and it is therefore desirable to establish the relationship between the two. In the 'head-on' collision:

$$\text{Electron energy} = \text{Photon energy,}$$
$$\therefore \ E = eV = h\nu = h\frac{c}{\lambda},$$

where e is the electronic charge; V the tube voltage; h is Planck's constant and ν, c, and λ are respectively the frequency, velocity, and wavelength of the emitted radiation. Inserting known values of e, h, and c into this formula, the minimum wavelength that can be produced for a given operating voltage can be found. *N.B.*—Maximum energy gives maximum frequency and therefore minimum wavelength.

$$\lambda_{\min} = \frac{12 \cdot 4}{\text{Applied kilovoltage}} \text{ Å.}$$

For example, the minimum wavelength emitted by a tube working at 80 kV. will be $12 \cdot 4/80 = 0 \cdot 155$ Å.

Because the minimum wavelength is directly linked with the maximum electron energy, and this in turn is linked with the maximum applied voltage, it is always desirable, in X-ray work, to state the maximum applied voltage. In ordinary usage the magnitude of an alternating voltage or current is stated in terms of the so-called Root Mean Square (R.M.S.) value of the voltage or current, because it is this value which is related to the power being delivered. In X-ray work the photon energy is more important than the electrical power being used, so that peak voltages are stated, their designation being in a form such as 200 kV.$_{peak}$. Root mean square and peak values are related by the expression:

$$\text{R.M.S.} = \frac{\text{Peak}}{\sqrt{2}}.$$

For example,   200 kV.$_{peak}$ ≡ 141·4 kV.$_{R.M.S.}$

The Shape of the Continuous Spectrum.—A complete explanation of how the spectral energy distribution of the continuous spectrum arises is beyond the scope of this book and the needs of its readers. The general pattern, however, can be usefully explained in relatively simple terms.

Very few of the electrons bombarding the target of the X-ray tube make the 'head-on' collisions in which they lose all their energy and produce a photon of maximum energy. Most electrons lose their energy in a series of interactions. Some of these result in the production of one or more X-ray photons, the energy of each of which will be less than the maximum: the remainder of the electrons' energy is given up in the production of heat. Apart from the heat production, the overall effect of the bombardment is the production of X-ray photons of all energies from the maximum downwards. The total amount of radiation (the number of photons multiplied by the photon energy) of any particular photon energy that is produced increases steadily as the photon energy decreases. This is shown in *Fig*. 25, by the dotted line, which may be regarded as indicating the continuous spectrum of the *produced* radiation.

There are, however, two other factors which influence the spectrum of the radiation which actually emerges from the tube, that is, the spectrum of the useful beam. These factors are the wall of the X-ray tube (its thickness and its material) and the target itself through which the radiation has to pass. The penetrating power of the X-ray photons falls off quickly as their energy decreases (a fuller discussion of this matter will be found in CHAPTERS VI and VII) which means that the lower the energy of the photons, the fewer will be able to emerge from the target and penetrate through the wall. Hence, in spite of the production of an increasing quantity of the lower energies, the *emergent* radiation quantity falls off markedly at the lower-energy end, as shown by the solid line in *Fig*. 25. The shape of the spectrum is thus due both to the mechanism of X-ray production and its radiation attenuation in the target and in the tube wall: the maximum photon energy, as already described, depends on the maximum applied voltage; the minimum photon energy in the beam wall will depend only on any material through which the photons have to pass. As *Fig*. 26 shows, the minimum energy is the same for all applied voltages.

The Line, or Characteristic, Spectrum.—Whereas the continuous spectrum results, as just described, from the interaction of the cathode-stream electrons with the atom as a whole, or at least its 'electron cloud', the characteristic spectrum arises from interaction with individual electrons in the atom. The immediate result of this type of interaction is the removal of one of the orbital electrons, the energy required being provided from the energy of the cathode-stream electron. Ionization of the target

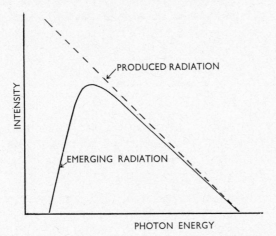

Fig. 25.—The continuous spectrum, produced and emergent.

atom is the first result of this interaction but normality is quickly restored by the sequence of events already described in CHAPTER II. The vacancy in the shell from which the electron has been removed is quickly filled from another shell and the appropriate characteristic photons are emitted.

FACTORS UPON WHICH THE X-RAY EMISSION DEPENDS

A question that may well be asked is: 'How do the applied voltage and the target material affect the X-rays that are emitted?' Briefly, the answer is that the continuous spectrum depends on the voltage and is independent of the target material, whereas the reverse is true of the characteristic spectrum, which does not depend on the voltage but is controlled by the target material. Both these statements, however, require some qualification and deserve some expansion.

Target Material.—

Continuous Spectrum.—Since the continuous spectrum arises from the interaction of the cathode-stream electrons with the 'electron cloud' surrounding the nucleus, it is perhaps not surprising that the precise details of this 'cloud' are unimportant. Just as in the case of the continuous spectrum of visible light emitted by a heated body, where the colour of the light (i.e., the wavelengths or energies of the emitted radiation) does not depend on the material but only on its temperature, so in the case of the continuous spectrum of X-rays the photon energies produced at any particular applied voltage will be the same whatever the target material. For any given generating voltage the peak radiation intensity occurs at the same photon energy, whilst, as already stressed, the maximum energy is controlled entirely by the peak voltage.

It will be shown later that the penetrating power of an X-ray beam (often referred to as its *quality*) depends on the photon energy of its constituent radiation. Therefore the penetrating power of the radiation of the continuous spectrum produced by a given applied voltage is the same whatever the target material. In brief, *quality* depends on kV. On the other hand, the amount of radiation produced (the *quantity*) is not the same for all materials. The higher the atomic number of the target material, the greater will be the amount of radiation produced at a given applied voltage (assuming the same tube current). *Fig.* 26 A illustrates this for targets of tungsten and tin, the areas under the curves representing the total quantities of radiation produced in each case.

Though, at first sight, there seems to be a marked difference between the two curves, closer inspection shows that they are essentially the same. For each the

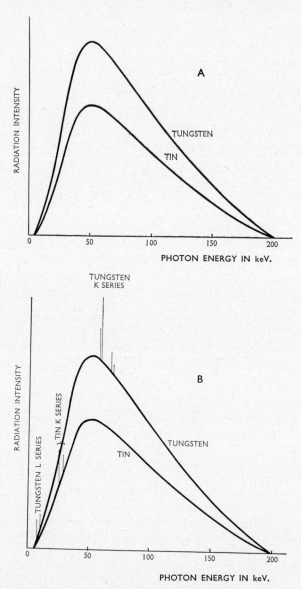

Fig. 26.—A, The continuous spectrum with tin and tungsten targets. The same kilovoltage in each case. B, As in A but with the characteristic radiation added.

maximum and minimum energies are the same, and the maximum intensity occurs at the same energy in each case. In fact, if the curve for tin were 'scaled up' by multiplying its intensity values at any energy by a factor of 74/50, it would fit exactly on to the tungsten curve. There is, of course, nothing magical about this factor, 74 and 50 are, respectively, the atomic numbers of tungsten and tin.

As far as the continuous spectrum is concerned the quality of the beam is independent of the target material, whilst the quantity of radiation (I) produced is proportional to its atomic number, i.e.,

$$I \propto Z.$$

Line Spectrum.—Turning to the 'line' or 'characteristic' spectrum, quite a different state of affairs is found. The energies of the characteristic lines change with the target material, as is to be expected since they are 'characteristic'. For any particular group of lines (say, for example, the K series) their energy is progressively greater the higher the atomic number of the target. For example, in tin the K lines have energies between 25 and 29 keV., whilst in tungsten the corresponding values are from 57 to 69 keV. Lead, whose atomic number is higher still, has K lines at energies between 72 and 88 keV.

The intensity of each line spectrum follows the continuous spectrum pattern, that is to say it is proportional to the atomic number. This, together with the different energies, is shown on *Fig.* 26 B, in which the appropriate characteristic lines are superimposed upon their continuous spectra. The L series for tin have energies round about 4 keV. and do not appear in the spectrum because radiations of very low energy such as this are removed as they try to pass through the tube wall.

The importance of the contribution of the characteristic spectrum to the total radiation output of an X-ray tube depends upon a number of factors, but mainly upon the kilovoltage applied and the tube wall and any 'filters' through which the beam has to pass. Only K radiation need be considered since the L lines are, even for the highest atomic number elements, of too small an energy to get out of the normal tube and hence, since tungsten is the almost universal target material, there is no characteristic radiation contribution to the useful beam for generating voltages below 70 kV. For higher voltages, broadly speaking it can be said that characteristic radiation contributes up to about 10 per cent of the dose in the range 80–150 kV., after which it becomes steadily smaller in importance and is quite negligible at 300 kV. and above.

Applied Voltage.—It has already been stated, many times, that the maximum photon energy emitted from an X-ray tube equals the maximum energy of the cathode-stream electrons which, in turn, depends on the peak applied voltage. Changes, therefore, in the voltage applied to an X-ray tube will alter the maximum photon energy and, in fact, will alter the whole spectrum pattern, as is illustrated in *Fig.* 27, which shows the effect on the total spectrum of increasing the applied voltage from 60 to 90 and finally to 120 kV.

Fixing attention, first, upon the continuous spectrum, the movement to higher values of the maximum energy will be noted, together with a general move of the whole spectrum. The peak intensity, for example, also moves over to higher energies: the only part of the continuous spectrum which does not change markedly is the low-energy end, and this because the low energies emitted are controlled more by the thickness and material of the tube wall than anything else. The *quality* of the beam, therefore, changes with applied voltage, but not only quality but *quantity* also. The area under the curve indicates the total amount of radiation emitted, which is obviously greater at the higher voltages. In fact, the amount of radiation emitted increases as the square of the kilovoltage, i.e.,

$$I \propto kV^2.$$

In contrast, the energies of the lines of the characteristic spectrum cannot be changed by changes in the applied voltage because of the method of this production, provided, of course, that the energy of the cathode-stream electrons (i.e., the applied voltage) is enough to excite them. For example, it will be seen that the lines of the

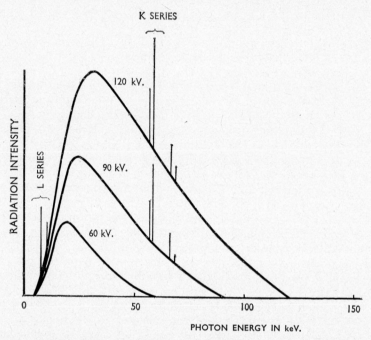

Fig. 27.—X-ray spectra from a tungsten target at different operating kilovoltages.

K series do not appear in the radiation generated at 60 kV. because the removal of the tungsten K electron calls for an energy of nearly 70 kV. The L-series lines appear in all three spectra because the removal of an L electron only needs 11·7 keV.

'Wave form' of the Applied Voltage.—Up to this point it has been tacitly assumed that a constant voltage has been applied to the X-ray tube; however, this is far from universally true in practice, many X-ray tubes being operated on so-called 'pulsating' voltage supplies. These are mainly of two forms, produced respectively by 'full-wave' and 'half-wave' rectification of the alternating voltage produced by the high-tension transformer, and their variations with time are shown in *Fig. 28.*

The mechanism of X-ray production will be the same for all wave forms of the voltage supply, and the maximum energy—as already stated—depends on the peak voltage. However, the intensities of the various photon energies will all tend to be less with pulsating than with constant potential and especially at the higher energy end of the spectrum. In general, therefore, the *quality* of a beam produced by a pulsating voltage supply will be less (the beam will be less penetrating) than that of a beam produced by a constant potential equal to the peak of the pulsations. But there will be no quality difference between 'full-wave' and 'half-wave' supplies, since the voltages present are the same in each case.

Similar differences occur in the *quantity* of radiation produced. Not only is the beam produced by a constant potential supply harder than that produced by 'full-wave' and 'half-wave' rectified voltages, but it has a higher output for the same tube current. This is shown in *Fig.* 29 and arises, of course, from the fact that for much of the operating time voltages less than that supplied by constant potential are being applied to the tube.

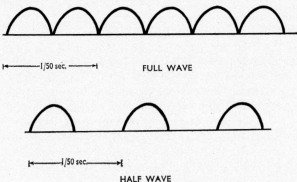

FULL WAVE

HALF WAVE

Fig. 28.—X-ray tube voltage wave forms.

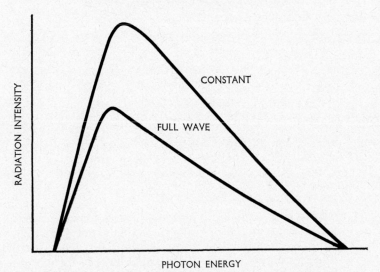

Fig. 29.—The effect of voltage wave form on the spectrum.

The Tube Current.—Besides depending on the factors already mentioned above, the total X-ray emission will obviously depend upon the number of electrons hitting the target, that is to say, it will depend on the tube current (or milliamperage). The greater the current, the greater the number of electrons and, therefore, the more radiation produced.

$$I \propto mA.$$

Radiation quality, on the other hand, is unaffected by the magnitude of the current.

Summary of Influencing Factors

The *quantity* of X-rays generated is proportional to $Z \times kV.^2 \times mA. \times sec.$, and depends upon the wave form of the applied voltage.

The *quality* of the X-ray generated depends almost entirely on kV. and the applied voltage wave form.

THE EFFICIENCY OF X-RAY PRODUCTION

It has already been mentioned that heat is produced, as well as X-rays, when electrons bombard the target. At relatively low applied voltages many of the interactions of the cathode-stream electrons will be with the outer electrons of the target atoms, and will generally result in the generation of heat rather than X-rays. The efficiency of X-ray production, by which we mean the fraction of the energy of the cathode-stream electrons which is converted into X-rays, is thus rather low. At 200 kV., for example, only about 1 per cent of the cathode-stream energy reappears as X-rays, the other 99 per cent being converted into heat. When it is realized that the energy associated with an X-ray set working at 200 kV. and 10 mA. is equivalent to the energy associated with a large electric fire, and that the heat is concentrated on an area of much less than 1 sq. cm., the magnitude of the cooling and target design problems that have to be overcome can be imagined.

Table V.—HEAT PRODUCTION AND X-RAYS

OPERATING VOLTAGE	PER CENT ENERGY IN: HEAT	X-RAYS	HEAT UNITS PER 100 UNITS X-RAY ENERGY
60 kV.	99·5	0·5	19.900
200 kV.	99	1·0	9900
4 MV.	60	40	150
20 MV.	30	70	43

However, the efficiency of X-ray production increases as the generating kilovoltage is increased. For example, about 40 per cent of the electron energy goes into X-rays at 4 MV. whilst at 20 MV. the value is nearly 70 per cent, with only 30 per cent being converted into heat.

This increase in production efficiency has, as it were, a doubly beneficial effect on the cooling problem, for not only is less heat generated but there are proportionately more X-rays as well. Thus, as *Table V* shows, the amount of heat produced for the same amount of X-ray energy emitted (taken here as 100 units) falls rapidly as the kV. increases. The need for efficient cooling in diagnostic (60 kV.) and 'conventional' therapy (200 kV.) apparatus is obvious. It will also be clear why quite simple target cooling suffices for the linear accelerator (4 MV.).

The variation of X-ray production efficiency with target atomic numbers has been implied, at least in an earlier section, when it was pointed out that the higher atomic number elements produce more X-rays than do lower atomic number elements, for the same applied voltage and tube current. Production efficiency is proportional to atomic number.

THE DISTRIBUTION OF X-RAYS IN SPACE

So far nothing has been said about the directions in which X-rays are emitted from the target and how much radiation goes in each direction, yet this is obviously very important to the designer and to the user of X-ray equipment. It is, in fact, a very complicated business, which depends upon the target thickness and material, as well as upon the applied voltage. A complete analysis is beyond our scope and capabilities, but the relatively simple case of the very thin target gives a useful guide to what might be expected in practice. *Fig.* 30 shows how the radiation intensity varies with direction around a thin target for several applied voltages. The length of any radius is a measure of the radiation intensity in that direction. This, of course, only shows what happens in one plane: rotation of this diagram about the line of the electron stream would give the three-dimensional distribution.

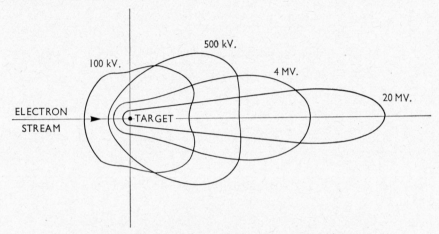

Fig. 30.—The spatial distribution of X-rays around a thin target.

It will be seen that, for applied voltages in the 50–150-kV. range, X-rays are emitted more or less equally in all directions, whereas in the megavoltage range the main emission is concentrated more and more in a 'forward' direction, that is to say, in the direction of the cathode stream. A further point, which cannot so readily be shown diagrammatically, is that whereas the 'quality' of the radiation is also more or less the same in every direction at the lower energies, the most penetrating radiation in the megavoltage emission, like the maximum intensity, is in the 'forward' direction. It is, therefore, reasonable at the lower voltages to use the 'reflection' type of target like that shown in *Fig.* 22, since this has many technical advantages, and to use the rays emitted at or about right-angles to the cathode stream. To do this for very high applied voltages, on the other hand, would be extremely inefficient and, as will be seen later, megavoltage tubes use the 'transmission' type of target in which the electrons bombard one side of the target and the useful beam is that passing through the target and emerging from the other side.

The Thick Target.—In practice the target will not be 'thin' (by which is meant that the cathode-stream electrons make only a few collisions in passing through it) but will be thick enough to bring all the electrons to rest, and the X-ray distribution from such a target will be somewhat different from the picture just given. This is partly because the electrons do not only produce their rays on the surface of the target but many penetrate into the metal and produce radiation below the surface. One such event is shown in *Fig.* 31.

Now even at the lower energies there is rather more radiation produced in forward than in other directions, as a closer consideration of *Fig.* 30 shows, and therefore there will be more radiation in direction OC than in direction OB, which in turn has a higher intensity than OA. On the other hand, the radiation travelling in the former direction has to traverse a greater thickness (OY) of target material than does radiation travelling along OB and OA. Since passage through any material reduces the intensity —by attenuation processes to be described in CHAPTER VI—of the radiation and the reduction is greater the greater the distance traversed, radiation along OC will suffer

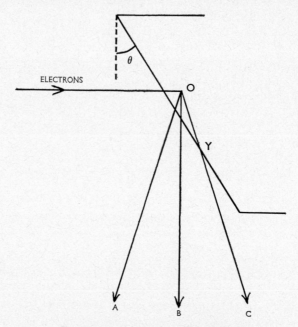

ELECTRONS

Fig. 31.—X-rays from a thick target.

the greatest reduction, and that along OA the least. The two effects therefore tend to cancel each other out—the natural tendency to send more radiation along OC being counteracted by the greater target thickness it has to travel through—and by appropriate choice of the angle of the target face (angle θ of the diagram) nearer equality can be achieved for radiation travelling in the different directions. Some of the practical consequences of the general principles, which have been presented here in simplified form, will be dealt with later, and especially the alterations of radiation distribution that may come about as the target face becomes roughened with use.

CHAPTER VI

THE INTERACTION OF X- AND GAMMA RAYS WITH MATTER—I

ATTENUATION AND SCATTERING

As was originally shown in *Fig.* 5, p. 9, the gamma rays emitted by radioactive nuclei or the X-rays produced electrically as described in CHAPTER V are really the same. Their different names are only useful in indicating their different sources. A photon of X-rays and a photon of gamma rays of the same energy are indistinguishable as far as their properties are concerned. Therefore, in this and subsequent chapters, properties attributed to X-rays are equally attributable to gamma rays of the same energy: only one name is used for reasons of brevity.

When a beam of X-rays passes through matter its intensity is reduced. The beam is *attenuated* and some of the energy that it originally contained is taken up, or *absorbed*, by the irradiated material. Other energy is simply deflected out of the beam, to travel on in some new direction. This is *scattered* radiation. Each of these processes plays an important part in radiology. Different attenuation in different tissues produces the radiographic pattern: absorption produces the radiograph and the biological effects needed in radiotherapy, whilst scattered radiation brings problems to both diagnosis and radiotherapy. It is therefore vital that the processes should be understood by those using radiation.

Because the processes are quite complex, attention will primarily be fixed upon what happens when narrow beams of mono-energetic (or monochromatic) radiation pass through material. The effects of different materials and of different photon energies will be considered. An experimental arrangement such as that shown in *Fig.* 32 might be used. An instrument for measuring X-rays is exposed to the narrow beam and a reading taken. When a sheet of material is placed across the beam at A the reading of the instrument is reduced, whilst the greater the thickness of the material the greater the reduction. Repetition of this sort of observation with another material will produce similar results though the actual change produced by a given thickness will not be the same for the two materials. Similarly, if the original material is used with radiation of a different energy, the general pattern of results will be repeated but will again be different in magnitude. Some typical results are shown in *Fig.* 33 A and B and their significance may be summarized as follows:

1. The *greater* the thickness of material, the *greater* the attenuation.

2. The *greater* the atomic number and/or the density of the material, the *greater* the attenuation produced by any given thickness.

But in contrast:

3. The greater the photon energy, the *smaller* the attenuation produced by a given thickness of a particular material.

Exponential Attenuation.—A closer inspection of the curves shown in *Fig.* 33 reveals the rather striking fact that equal increases in thickness of the inserted material produce equal fractional reductions in the amount of radiation transmitted through

57

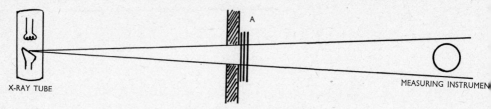

Fig. 32.—The measurement of X-ray attenuation.

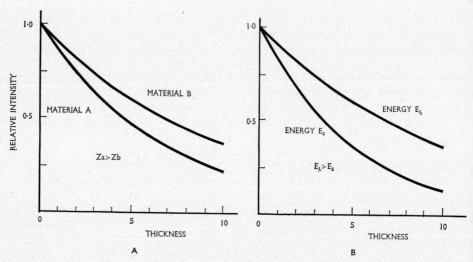

Fig. 33.—The effect, on X-ray attenuation, of A, Atomic number; B, Radiation energy.

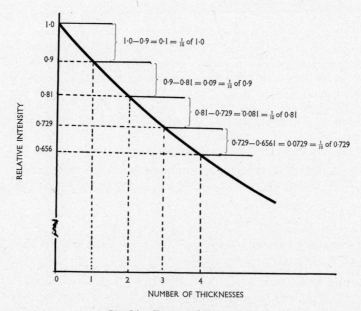

Fig. 34.—Exponential attenuation.

the material. For example, if 1 mm. of substance A reduces the beam by one-tenth (and hence the instrument reading from, say, 100 to 90) then the addition of a further millimetre will remove one-tenth of the remaining beam, and hence reduce the reading to $(90 - \frac{1}{10} \times 90) = 81$; 3 mm. of substance A will reduce the reading to 72·9 (i.e., $81 - \frac{1}{10} \times 81$) and so on, as shown in *Fig.* 34.

An effect of this sort may, at first, strike the reader as being rather strange, for in most of our experience the amount abstracted usually does not depend on the amount present. For example, the price of a particular type of cinema seat does not depend on the size of one's purse; on the other hand, the amount 'absorbed' by income tax usually does! However, it must be remembered that a beam of radiation is made up of large numbers of photons, and that the removal of some of these by attenuation is essentially the 'death' of these photons as far as the beam is concerned. The similarity between photon attenuation and radioactive decay then becomes apparent: in each case there is a constant fractional change in number for equal change in another factor—thickness or time—and it is not surprising that the same type of law covers both phenomena.

Attenuation Coefficients.—The essential physical fact in photon attenuation is that, for a given material, constant fractional reductions are produced, in any one beam, by equal added thicknesses. Therefore it follows that:

$$\frac{\text{Fractional reduction}}{\text{Added thickness}} = \text{Constant},$$

or, in words, the fractional reduction per unit thickness (usually per centimetre) is constant for any given material.

This formula should apply to any X-ray attenuation, and it is of interest to use it in connexion with the values used in *Fig.* 34. There the addition of 1 mm. of material reduced the beam by 1/10 (from 100 to 90), the fractional reduction being

$$\frac{100 - 90}{100} = 0·1,$$

so that the fractional reduction, *per centimetre*, would be

$$\frac{0·1}{0·1} = 1·0.$$

If, however, the attentuation produced by 2 mm. is considered, the reduction is from 100 to 81 and the fractional reduction per centimetre is:

$$\frac{100 - 81}{100} \times \frac{1}{0·2} = 0·95.$$

Finally, for the purpose of this example, the effect of 3 mm. of material is to produce a fractional reduction of:

$$\frac{100 - 72·9}{100} \times \frac{1}{0·3} = 0·90_3$$

per centimetre.

The value therefore is far from constant but decreases with increasing material thickness: does this mean that the formula is not a true representation of the observed facts, or is there some aspect of its use that has been overlooked? The answer can be seen by considering *Fig.* 35, which shows the effect of a 2-mm. thick piece of material which, for purposes of illustration, is divided into two pieces each 1 mm. thick.

One hundred units of radiation reach the material and of these only 90 reach the second millimetre since 10 were removed in the first. Hence the second millimetre has only 90 units to 'work on' and removes 9 of these ($\frac{1}{10}$). The first part of any material always upsets the beam for subsequent layers and therefore the formula only holds as stated when thin layers are considered. In this case the fraction is indeed constant and is called the *linear attenuation coefficient* (μ):

$$\frac{\text{Fractional reduction in a thin layer}}{\text{Thickness in cm. of thin layer}} = \text{Constant} = \mu.$$

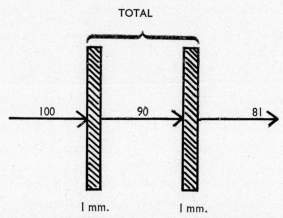

Fig. 35.—'Equal thicknesses remove equal fractions.'

The linear attenuation coefficient, μ, is, then, the fractional reduction per unit thickness of material *as determined by considering a thin layer of material.* Since it is purely a matter of chance whether or not a particular photon gets through a given piece of material, the linear attenuation coefficient can also be regarded as expressing the probability (that is to say, the chance or the odds) of it being removed—or the odds against getting through. For example, if μ were 0·03 per cm. (or 0·03 cm.$^{-1}$), it would mean that, in a thin layer, there would be a 3 per cent chance, per centimetre, of the photon being removed, or roughly a 32 to 1 chance, per centimetre, of its getting through.

The importance of considering thin layers has been stressed because it is only thus that statements, such as, for some materials or radiation energy, μ is, say, 15 per cm., can be comprehended. At its face value it would seem that this means that there is a 1500 per cent chance of removal in a centimetre—15 times certain! This is obviously nonsense, and it arises because a centimetre, in this case, is a very thick layer—even $\frac{1}{10}$ mm. would remove about 15 per cent of the beam—and the formula already quoted only applies to very much thinner layers.

The Exponential Formula.—Strictly speaking the effects of any thickness of material can only be found via the formula that mathematically expresses the physically observed fact that equal fractions are removed by equal added thickness. That formula, which is similar in form to that for radioactive decay, is:

$$I = I_0 e^{-\mu x},$$

where I_0 and I are, respectively, the reading when there is no material between source and measuring instrument, and when a thickness x cm. is interposed; μ is the linear attenuation coefficient for the material and the radiation energy concerned.

Other Coefficients.—Since X-ray attenuation, as will be discussed in more detail later, is a random process of interaction between photons and atoms, the amount of attenuation will obviously depend upon the number of atoms in any thickness of material. For example, the compression of a layer of material to one-half its thickness would not affect its power of attenuation. For this reason the *linear attenuation coefficient* depends on the density of the material, as well as on other features, and is less fundamental than another coefficient which takes the density factor into account.

This is the *mass attenuation coefficient* and numerically it is the linear attenuation coefficient divided by the density (ρ) of the material. Still more fundamental are the *atomic* and *electronic attenuation coefficients* which indicate the chance of removal per atom or electron (respectively) present per square centimetre of material. *Table VI* shows the relationship between all these coefficients and, by way of example, their numerical values for 200-keV. photons in aluminium.

Table VI.—The Relationship between the Attenuation Coefficients

Coefficient	Relationship	Unit of Measurement	Value for 200-keV. Photons in Aluminium
Linear (μ)	—	Per cm.	0·33 cm.$^{-1}$
Mass	μ/ρ	Per g. per cm.^{2}	0·122 cm.^{2} g.$^{-1}$
Atomic ($_a\mu$)	$\mu/\rho \cdot Z/N_0$	Per atom per cm.^{2}	5·45 × 10^{-24} cm.^{2} atom^{-1}
Electronic ($_e\mu$)	$\mu/\rho \cdot 1/N_0$	Per electron per cm.^{2}	4·2 × 10^{-25} cm.^{2} electron^{-1}

N_0 = Number of electrons per g. Z = Atomic number.

Half-value Layer.—One consequence of the exponential attenuation is that it is impossible to reduce an X-ray beam to nothing. No matter how thick the material inserted into the beam, there will always be a chance, albeit very small, of some photons getting through; that is to say, of some radiation being transmitted. Therefore, as also may be seen from the shape of the attenuation curve in *Fig.* 34, it is impossible to state a thickness for the 'range' of the radiation as can be done for particle radiation such as alpha or beta radiation. Nevertheless, the penetrating power, or **quality**, can be defined, quite conveniently, in terms of a thickness. This thickness is the so-called **half-value layer** (H.V.L.), sometimes called the half-value thickness, and is the thickness of a given material which will reduce a narrow beam of X-rays to one-half of its original value.

The materials usually chosen for H.V.L. measurement vary with the energy of the radiation being measured. There are no sharp boundaries or firm rules, but the following may be taken as a general guide:

Radiation generated at up to 30 kV.	Cellophane
Radiation generated at 30–150 kV.	Aluminium
Radiation generated at 120–600 kV.	Copper
Radiation generated at 500 kV.–2 MV.	Lead

Above 2 MV. the concept has relatively little meaning, for reasons which may be clearer later, but if a H.V.L. is being measured, lead is usually used.

The general technique of H.V.L. measurement is to use apparatus similar to that indicated in *Fig.* 32. Various thicknesses of the test material are inserted into the narrow beam and an attenuation curve like those shown in *Figs.* 33 and 34 obtained. From this curve the H.V.L. can be read off in the same way as the thicknesses for other fractional reductions in *Fig.* 34. Measuring the H.V.L. is, in fact, equivalent to measuring the penetrating power of the beam, and therefore the linear attenuation coefficient, since obviously penetration and attenuation are interrelated. It is, therefore, necessary to prevent—as far as possible—any scattered radiation from reaching the measuring instrument, because if this happens the beam will appear to be more penetrating than it actually is, as *Fig.* 36 indicates. To reduce this unwanted scatter to a minimum the beam (as in *Fig.* 32) is just large enough to cover the measuring instrument, and the inserted materials are placed half-way between the instrument and the source.

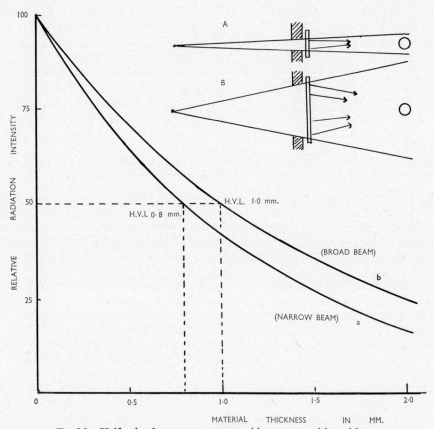

Fig. 36.—Half-value layer measurement with narrow and broad beams.

H.V.L. and μ.—It will be apparent, from what has been stated already, that there must be a close relationship between the H.V.L. and the attenuation coefficients. This may be found through the exponential formula. If the symbol $D_{\frac{1}{2}}$ is used for the H.V.L. then we have:

$$\frac{I}{I_0} = 0.5 = e^{-\mu D_{\frac{1}{2}}}.$$

Since, as can be read off from tables of the exponential function, $e^{-0.693} = 0.5$, it follows that $\mu D_{\frac{1}{2}} = 0.693$, i.e., the product of the linear attenuation coefficient and the H.V.L. equals 0.693.

To illustrate this an example may be given. The H.V.L. for the radiation from an X-ray tube working at 200 kV. is found to be 1·5 mm. of copper. Hence the linear attenuation coefficient of copper for this radiation is given by:

$$\mu = \frac{0\cdot693}{D_{\frac{1}{2}}} = \frac{0\cdot693}{0\cdot15} = 4\cdot62 \text{ cm.}^{-1}.$$

It will be noted that the coefficient, as is customary, is quoted 'per centimetre' and that is why the H.V.L. quoted in millimetres was converted to centimetres when used in the formula.

Quarter, and other, Value Layers.—Because, for a monochromatic beam, equal added thicknesses produce equal fractional reductions it follows that if a thickness $D_{\frac{1}{2}}$ reduces the beam to a half, then the addition of an equal thickness, making $2D_{\frac{1}{2}}$ in all, will reduce this half by a further half, and the whole beam to a quarter of its original value. The quarter-value layer is therefore twice the thickness of the H.V.L.— at least for a beam of photons of one energy. By the same token, a thickness of $3D_{\frac{1}{2}}$ reduces the beam to one-eighth, and $4D_{\frac{1}{2}}$ brings it down to one-sixteenth. The mathematically minded will see that a thickness of $n \times D_{\frac{1}{2}}$ will reduce the beam to $(\frac{1}{2})^n$ of its original value. If $n = 10$ (i.e., we use ten times the H.V.L.) the beam is reduced to $(\frac{1}{2})^{10}$ or roughly to $1/1000$ of its original value—a useful simple rule in connexion with protection problems.

ATTENUATION AND ABSORPTION

So far attention has been focused on the radiation passing through matter. Nothing has been said about the radiation removed from the beam, or how it was removed, or what effects such removals have upon the material, or the fate of the energy removed from the beam.

Four possible types of fate await the photon on its attempted passage through matter. It may:

1. Be deflected from its original path and henceforth proceed in a new direction but with unchanged energy.

2. Be deflected, as before, but also lose some of its energy.

3. Disappear altogether.

4. Be transmitted unchanged—nothing happens to it.

To the first two of these possible fates the name *scattering* is usually applied, whilst in possibilities (2) and (3) there will be a change of energy. In these, energy is transferred to the attenuating material, or it may be said that the material *absorbs* energy from the beam. The first three possibilities, of course, contribute to the *attenuation* of the beam, since in each of them photons are removed from the beam.

'Bound' and 'Free' Electrons.—Before going on to consider the detail of the interaction processes listed above, it is necessary to say what is to be understood by the terms 'bound' and 'free' electrons, which will be used from time to time. Strictly speaking there are normally no 'free' electrons in matter. Each electron is 'bound' in the atom by the electrostatic attraction between itself and the positive charge on the nucleus, and it can only become 'free' if it receives enough energy to overcome this binding force. As described in CHAPTER II, an electron is freed from the atom if it receives energy in excess of its 'binding energy'. For the outer electrons of any atom this 'binding energy' is only a few electron-volts, which is not only small compared with the binding energies of the inner electrons, but also very small compared with the energy of X-ray photons.

This leads to the concept that an electron may be considered to be 'free' *when its binding energy is small compared with the energy of a photon with which it interacts.* For practical purposes all electrons in the elements which make up the greater part of the soft tissues of the body may be regarded as 'free' for all X-ray energies met in radiology. In the higher atomic number elements, however, the situation is somewhat different. For example, whilst the M and N electrons in lead, with binding energies of about 3·0 and 0·25 keV. respectively, may be regarded as 'free' when interacting with a 100-keV. photon, the K electrons (binding energy 88 keV.) are certainly 'bound'. On the other hand, even the K electrons are 'free' for radiation in the megavoltage range.

ATTENUATION PROCESSES

Twelve different methods of interaction between X-ray photons and matter have been postulated, some of which have not yet been observed (!) whilst others occur so infrequently as to be of little importance. For example, the interaction of radiation with the so-called 'meson field' around the nucleus only occurs for radiation energies in excess of 150 MeV., and then only infrequently. It will not be mentioned here again! Only five of the twelve methods are sufficiently important to attract attention here and only three of these are of any practical importance in present-day radiography or radiotherapy. The five can be divided into two sets, the Photon-scattering and the Photon-disappearance phenomena (CHAPTER VII).

PHOTON SCATTERING

By this term is understood the deflexion of the photon from its original path and hence its being lost from the beam. In this deflexion the photon may, or may not, lose energy.

Elastic Scattering.—This is the name given to the process by which radiation is deflected without losing any energy. Because it was the subject of many studies in the early days of X-ray work it is also known by a number of other names—coherent, unmodified, classical, Thomson and Rayleigh scattering are names that have been applied to it. It is one of the processes that can be more easily described by considering the radiation as waves rather than as photons, and is also one of the processes where the interaction is with 'bound' electrons.

X-rays passing close to an atom cause 'bound' electrons momentarily to vibrate at a frequency equal to that of the radiation. These vibrating electrons in turn emit X-rays of this same frequency but in all directions. Thus energy is taken from the beam and is scattered in all directions. No energy is permanently taken up by the irradiated material: it all remains electromagnetic energy. The process is thus one of *attenuation* without *absorption*.

Since the process involves 'bound' electrons it occurs more in higher atomic number materials and also more with low-energy radiations, since these are the conditions for which the number of 'bound' electrons is greatest. The mass attenuation coefficient (which is a measure of the probability of the process occurring) for elastic scattering is directly proportional to the square of the atomic number ($\propto Z^2$) and inversely to the radiation energy $\left(\propto \dfrac{1}{h\nu}\right)$.

Because it never contributes more than a few per cent to the total attenuation of X-ray beams used in radiography or radiotherapy, and nothing to energy absorption from them, elastic scattering is unimportant to the medical or industrial radiologist, but it is vital to the X-ray crystallographer. 'X-ray diffraction' or 'X-ray crystallography' which has produced such important information about the structure of materials (including, recently, some most important information about the basic structures of living materials) is possible because of the 'interference' between the X-rays elastically scattered from the orderly arrays of atoms in crystals. This 'interference' produces patterns from which the positions of the scattering atoms can be deduced.

Inelastic Scattering.—Though also known as modified or as incoherent scattering, this process is best known as **Compton** scattering, in honour of the United States physicist who first elucidated the mechanism by which it occurs. Henceforth, in this book, this—Compton scattering—is the name that will be applied to it. Unlike elastic scattering, Compton scattering is an interaction of photons with 'free' electrons, and

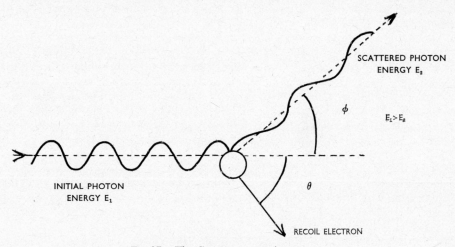

Fig. 37.—The Compton scattering process.

what happens can best be visualized as billiard-ball-like collisions. In each of these the photon hands on some of its energy to the electron and itself continues in a new direction (i.e., it is *scattered*) but with reduced energy and hence with increased wavelength. As shown in *Fig.* 37, the electron 'recoils' with the energy lost by the photon.

The angle through which the photon is scattered, the energy handed on to the electron, and the energy lost by the photon (and hence its wavelength change) are all interconnected. For example, if the angle ϕ, through which the photon is scattered, is small (the electron having, as it were, been struck a 'glancing blow') a very small share of the energy is given to the electron, and therefore the photon loses very little. The scattered photon has, therefore, almost the same energy, and wavelength, as the original. On the other hand, in a 'head-on' collision, in which the photon is turned back along its original track (it is scattered through 180°), the maximum energy is transferred to the recoil electron. In this situation the wavelength change is also a maximum. Most collisions will, of course, lie somewhere between these two extremes and in each case the change of wavelength (often denoted by the symbol $\delta\lambda$) is given by the formula:

$$\lambda_2 - \lambda_1 = \delta\lambda = 0\cdot024(1 - \cos\phi) \text{ Å}.$$

3

It will be noted that the wavelength *change* depends neither on the material being irradiated nor on the radiation energy (or wavelength). It depends only upon the angle through which the radiation is scattered.

The Scattering Coefficient (σ).—In contrast with elastic scattering, the Compton process results in both *attenuation* of the beam, and also in the transfer of some radiation energy to the irradiated material (that is, *absorption*). For clarity it is desirable to consider these two aspects of the problem separately, though they are obviously connected.

Variation with Photon Energy and Material: The linear scattering attenuation coefficient is usually symbolized by σ, and therefore the mass coefficient is σ/ρ, and their magnitudes decrease steadily with increasing radiation energy. In other words, *and this is most important*, high-energy radiation is less scattered than is lower-energy radiation. As will be seen in the next chapter, when the other interaction processes have been considered, the *relative importance* of scattering, as an attenuation process, increases steadily, at least up to energies of several million electron-volts, but the *absolute amount* of scattering steadily decreases.

Compton scattering involves interaction between photons and electrons and therefore the amount that occurs depends on the number of electrons present. With the exception of hydrogen (which has about twice the normal number) all elements contain approximately the same number of electrons per gramme, that is to say, they all have practically the same electron density. For example, the electron densities of oxygen ($Z = 8$), calcium ($Z = 20$), and lead ($Z = 82$) are respectively 3·01, 3·006, and 2·38 × 10²³ electrons per gramme: a small range for such a wide range of atomic numbers. Hydrogen, in contrast, has 5·997 × 10²³ electrons per gramme.

This means that, except for hydrogen and materials containing hydrogen, the mass scattering coefficient (σ/ρ) is practically the same for all substances. In hydrogen and in hydrogenous materials (of which water and soft tissue are radiologically important examples) the Compton effect will be greater in proportion to the amount of hydrogen present.

The Recoil Electrons and Scattered Photons: As already stated, the result of the Compton process is that the energy of the initial photon is shared between the scattered photon and the recoil electron, and this division may be represented by the equation:

$$\sigma = \sigma_{\mathrm{s}} + \sigma_{\mathrm{a}},$$

where σ_{s} and σ_{a} are respectively the fractions of the total energy removed by the process which are taken respectively by the scattered photon and the recoil electron. A question to be answered, then, is how much goes to each? For this answer we must look more closely at the scattering process.

The simple, yet rather surprising fact that the *wavelength* change produced by Compton scattering depends only on the angle, and neither upon the material nor upon the radiation energy, must not be allowed to obscure the much more important fact that the change in energy suffered by the photon steadily increases as the photon's initial energy is increased. The higher the photon energy the more the recoil electron receives for any particular scatter angle. This is illustrated in *Table VII*, which refers to radiation scattered through 90°. The same pattern applies to all angles. In this table the conversion from photon energy to wavelength or vice versa is made via the formula already given, viz.:

$$\lambda = \frac{12\cdot4}{\mathrm{keV.}} \text{ Å.}$$

Table VII.—WAVELENGTH CHANGE AND ENERGY TRANSFER TO THE
RECOIL ELECTRON FOR 90° SCATTERING

PRIMARY PHOTON		SCATTERED PHOTON		RECOIL ELECTRON	
Energy (E_1)	Wavelength (λ_1)	Wavelength $(\lambda_1 + 0.024)$	Energy (E_2)	Energy $(E_1 - E_2)$	Percentage of Initial Energy
12·4 keV.	1 Å	1·024 Å	12·1 keV.	0·3 keV.	2·4
124 keV.	0·1 Å	0·124 Å	100 keV.	24 keV.	19
1,240 keV.	0·01 Å	0·034 Å	365 keV.	875 keV.	71
12,400 keV.	0·001 Å	0·025 Å	496 keV.	11,904 keV.	96

That the amount of energy transferred to the recoil electron should increase with increasing initial photon energy is to be expected. What is not so predictable is the very important fact that an increasing *share* of the total energy removed from the beam is absorbed by the recoil electron. Consequently the energy of the scattered photon is a smaller fraction of the total. In other words, not only is high-energy radiation

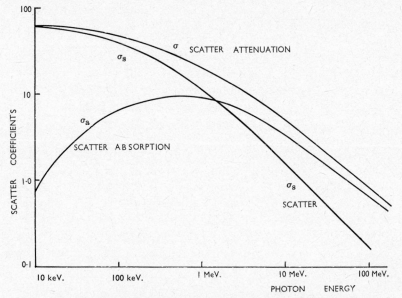

Fig. 38.—Scattering attenuation and absorption coefficients.

less likely to be scattered but also it yields a smaller scattered radiation intensity. *Fig.* 38 shows how σ (the probability of scatter) varies with photon energy and also shows how this energy is divided between the scattered photon (represented by σ_s) and the recoil electron (σ_a). It will be seen, for example, that at 100 keV., 86 per cent of the energy is retained by the scattered photon, whereas at 10 MeV. the recoil electron takes the lion's share (68 per cent) leaving only 32 per cent to the photon.

Thus in Compton scattering most of the energy goes into the recoil electron (i.e., is *absorbed*) with high-energy radiation, whereas at low energies most of the photon energy is scattered. The importance of these facts in radiology will be discussed later.

Direction of Scattering and of the Recoil Electrons: Although any photon can be scattered in any direction, the general pattern of scattered radiation in space changes with photon energy, as shown in *Fig*. 39. In general it may be said that, for low-energy photons, there is roughly an equal chance of their being scattered in any direction, whereas as the photon energy increases, the scattered photon is more and more likely to be travelling in a 'forward' direction. For high energies scattering through large angles is more and more unlikely. At low energies 'back' scatter—scattering through more than 90°—is almost as common as forward scatter.

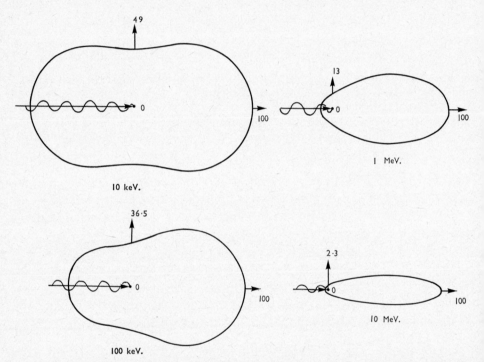

Fig. 39.—The spatial distribution of scattered radiation for various photon energies. The length of any radius from the point of scattering, 0, indicates the relative amount of radiation scattered in that direction. Thus the amounts scattered through 90° are: 49, 36·5, 13, and 2·3 per cent of the forward amount, respectively, for 10 keV., 100 keV., 1 MeV., and 10 MeV. photons. Note the reduced total scattering as energy increases.

From their mode of production the recoil electrons always travel in a forward direction, their energy—as already stated—being linked with the angle through which the photon is scattered. The fastest electrons are associated with large angle scattering: for high photon energies, however, even recoil electrons associated with small scattering angles acquire considerable velocities.

Summary of the Compton Effect.—In this process energy is lost when a photon is scattered by interaction with a 'free' electron. The energy with which the electron 'recoils' depends (as does the change in wavelength of the photon) upon the angle through which the photon is scattered. At high energies the fraction of the energy which goes to the recoil electron (i.e., is absorbed) is much greater than at low energies.

The mass scattering attenuation coefficient (σ/ρ) decreases with increasing photon energy and, except for those containing hydrogen, is practically the same for all substances.

CHAPTER VII

THE INTERACTION OF X- AND GAMMA RAYS WITH MATTER—II

THE DISAPPEARANCE PHENOMENA

The Photo-electric Effect.—In this effect a photon disappears altogether when interacting with a 'bound' electron, some of the energy being used to remove the electron from its 'shell' (that is, to overcome the 'binding' energy) whilst the rest is the kinetic energy with which the electron (usually called a photo-electron) leaves the atom:

$$h\nu \quad \longrightarrow \quad W \quad + \tfrac{1}{2}mv^2.$$

| Photon energy | Binding energy | Kinetic energy |

An example may help to make this clear. Assume that 100 keV. photons are passing through lead, and that one of them interacts with and ejects a K electron (binding energy 88 keV.). This photo-electron will, therefore, leave the atom with $100 - 88 = 12$ keV. of kinetic energy. If another of these photons ejects one of the L electrons, 15 keV. will be used up in overcoming its binding energy. The photo-electron, in this instance, would have kinetic energy of $100 - 15 = 85$ keV.

This is not, however, the end of the matter. By the ejection of the electron the atom has become *ionized* and in a highly unstable state. Very quickly the orbital vacancy caused by the electron's ejection will be filled by the sort of reshuffling process that was described in CHAPTER II, and the original neutrality and electron balance are finally restored by an electron from outside being attracted into the ionized atom. During this rearrangement process, of course, radiations characteristic of the atom will be emitted, in exactly the same way as they were following the ejection of an electron in the production of X-rays, as described in CHAPTERS II and V.

Thus the photo-electric process takes place in two distinct parts. First, the photon completely disappears, its energy being completely absorbed by the atom. Then the energy W (which was initially used up to overcome the binding energy of the ejected electron) is reradiated in the form of characteristic radiation. The process is therefore attenuation and partial absorption (the kinetic energy of escape of the photo-electron).

Just how important the characteristic radiation is, and how much energy is involved, depends upon the circumstances. *Fig.* 40, for example, which is very similar to *Fig.* 9, summarizes the events which follow the ejection of a K electron from a lead atom and a tin atom. Other sequences are possible, of course, but those shown are, in fact, those most likely to occur.

From this diagram it will be seen that, even for a high atomic number element, such as lead, much of the characteristic radiation is of low energy. For low atomic number elements, such as those which comprise most of biological material, all the characteristic radiation is of low energy. In such cases the characteristic radiations have so little energy that they are immediately absorbed by atoms neighbouring on those from which they are emitted. For example, the binding energy of the K electron in carbon (a very common constituent of all tissues) is about 0·3 keV. When one electron is removed by, let it be assumed, a 50-keV. photon, 49·7 keV. goes into kinetic energy whilst the ionized atom temporarily retains the remaining 0·3 keV. This is then reradiated as characteristic radiation of such low energy that it is immediately re-absorbed, quite probably in the same cell as that in which the initial event occurred. In biological materials, therefore, the photo-electric process results in all the energy removed from the beam being *completely absorbed* by the materials.

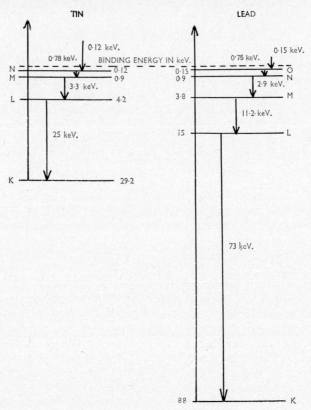

Fig. 40.—Electron energy levels in tin and lead, and typical electron transition following the ejection of a K electron. The number alongside each arrow indicates the photon energy associated with that transition.

In materials of higher atomic number such as are used in X-ray filters and in photographic emulsions the energy reradiated as characteristic radiation is of considerable importance, as will be seen in later chapters.

The Photo-electric Coefficient (τ).—Since the process involves 'bound' electrons, the chance that a photon will interact in this way with matter can be expected to increase with atomic number and to decrease with photon energy. As a general rule the mass photo-electric attenuation coefficient (τ/ρ) is directly proportional to the cube of the atomic number of the attenuator and inversely proportional to the cube of the radiation energy.

The variation, with photon energy, of (τ/ρ) for both lead ($Z = 82$) and for aluminium ($Z = 13$) is shown in *Fig.* 41. It should be noted that both co-ordinates have logarithmic scales, a mathematical device which enables a wide range of values to be shown in a limited space, but which may give a false impression unless its significance is realized. From this diagram a number of important features can be seen. The first is that, over a wide range of energy, the value of (τ/ρ) for lead is some 250 times as great as the value for aluminium—the ratio of the cubes of their atomic numbers is 251 : 1. The second feature to be noted for both materials is the rapid general decrease

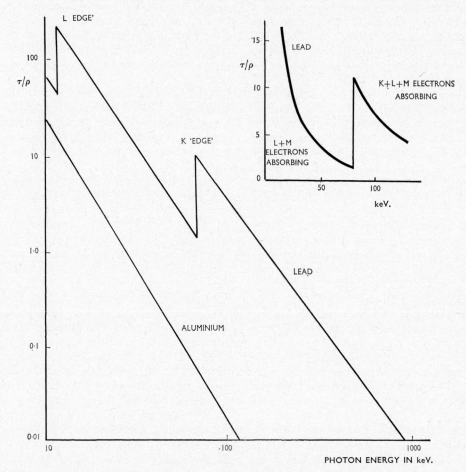

Fig. 41.—Variation, with photon energy, of the photo-electric effect in aluminium and lead. Insert shows the absorption 'edge' in greater detail.

of the attenuation coefficient as the radiation energy is increased, the rate of fall being in accordance with the stated dependence on the inverse of the cube of the radiation energy. A third important and unexpected feature is also revealed. This is the sudden breaks that occur and produce sudden departures of the smooth variation so far implied.

Absorption 'Edges'.—These sudden changes in the attenuation of the radiation occur at photon energies equal to the binding energies of the different electronic shells. For example, there is a break in the lead curve at 88 keV., which is the binding energy of the lead K electron, and another at 15 keV., which corresponds to the binding energy of the L shell. There is no break in the aluminium curve in the range covered by *Fig.* 41 since the aluminium K shell binding energy is only 1·5 keV.

The reason for the breaks is as follows. In the case of lead, for example, photons with energy in excess of 88 keV. have sufficient energy to remove any electron from the atom, so that all the 82 electrons can play a part in beam attenuation. On the other hand, a photon whose energy is, say, 87·5 keV. would be unable to remove a K electron so that for this, and lower energies, the K electrons take no part in beam attenuation and energy absorption. At 88 keV. there is, therefore, a sudden break in the photo-electric attenuation curve; at, and above, that energy all 82 electrons can take part in the photo-electric effect; below it the 2 K electrons have no effect and only 80 electrons take part in attenuation.

Simple arithmetic does not, however, explain the magnitude of the 'break'. The numbers above would suggest a drop in attenuation of about 2 per cent whereas *Fig.* 41 (and more especially the insert which shows the 'edge' in greater detail) shows an approximately sevenfold change in attenuation. This greater effect is because the likelihood, or probability, of an electron interacting with a photon increases the nearer the energy of the photon is to the binding energy of that particular electron. Thus at, say, 90 keV. any photo-electric effect will be almost entirely with K electrons—in fact near the 'edge' the 2 K electrons will be removing about seven times as much radiation as all the other electrons put together, and thus when they cease to function, there is a big reduction in the total effect.

Absorption 'edges' have two important consequences. The first is that in their neighbourhood lower-energy photons are less attenuated, and are therefore more penetrating, than higher-energy photons, in direct contrast to the general situation. Secondly, any substance is relatively transparent to its own characteristic radiation, the energies of which are always at least a little less than the corresponding binding energies. These effects are especially important when filter materials are considered, but they are unimportant when the energy of the 'edge' is small compared with the maximum energy of the beam. For example, since even in the highest atomic number elements the absorption edge energy does not exceed 116 keV., the phenomenon is of no consequence for beams generated at more than 400 kV., no matter what filter is used.

Summary of the Photo-electric Effect.—Here a photon disappears when it interacts with, and ejects from the atom, a previously 'bound' electron. Part of the energy is used up in overcoming the binding energy and the rest becomes kinetic energy of the ejected photo-electron. The former portion is ultimately reradiated as characteristic radiation when the ionized atom returns to normal.

The mass attenuation coefficient of the photo-electric effect is directly proportional to the cube of the atomic number of the atoms concerned, and is generally inversely proportional to the cube of the radiation energy. τ/ρ, however, changes considerably at absorption 'edges' which occur at photon energies equal to the binding energies of the various electrons.

$$\tau/\rho \propto Z^3$$

$$\text{and} \quad \tau/\rho \propto \left(\frac{1}{h\nu}\right)^3.$$

Pair Production.—When a photon whose energy is in excess of 1·02 MeV. passes close to the nucleus of an atom, the photon may disappear, and in its place a positive and a negative electron appear. Mass has thus been produced from energy whilst the total amount of charge remains unchanged by the simultaneous production of equal positive and negative charges.

In the nineteenth century Joule demonstrated the equivalence of heat energy and mechanical work (the so-called 'mechanical equivalent of heat') whilst in the early years of this century Einstein postulated that should it ever be possible to convert matter into energy or vice versa the 'energy equivalent of mass'—if we may use a term similar to that used by Joule—would be according to the equation:

$$E = mc^2,$$

where E is the energy associated with a mass m, and c is the velocity of light.

Pair production is a striking confirmation of the accuracy of this theory for, on the basis of this equation, the mass of either a positive or a negative electron is equivalent to 0·51 MeV. of energy. The process should, therefore, have a 'threshold' of 1·02 MeV. and this indeed is the minimum energy at which it occurs. Photons with less than this energy cannot produce the effect: for those with energy in excess of 1·02 MeV. the extra energy will be shared, as kinetic energy, between the two created particles. Once again all the energy removed from the beam (attenuation) has been absorbed.

However, this is not the whole story—the process thus far described is not complete. As has already been mentioned in CHAPTER III, whilst electrons are very common in nature, positrons are very rare and have no permanent place in its scheme of things. The created positron, therefore, soon links up with another negative electron and they 'annihilate' one another, changing back into the energy equivalent of their masses, that is into *two* photons each of 0·51 MeV. energy. This is the so-called *annihilation radiation* which is always an accompaniment of positrons, and which can be regarded as the 'characteristic radiation' of the pair-production process. Of the energy (E) originally removed from the beam, the amount *absorbed* is thus ($E - 1·02$) MeV.

The Pair-production Coefficient (π).—Since pair production is caused by the nuclear field, the likelihood of its occurrence increases with the magnitude of that field, and hence with the nuclear charge, or the atomic number of the irradiated material.

In marked contrast with the other attenuation processes described, pair production *increases* with radiation energy. For reasons already given it can only start at 1·02 MeV. but its effect steadily increases above that figure. However, for the materials of most interest in radiology—the tissues of the body—the relative importance of pair production is small for beams generated below about 30 to 40 million volts.

Summary of Pair Production.—Here photons with energy greater than 1·02 MeV. disappear on passing close to a nucleus; 1·02 MeV. is needed to create the electron-positron pair and is ultimately reradiated as two 0·51-MeV. photons of annihilation radiation, when the positron combines with an electron. Energy in excess of 1·02 MeV. is permanently absorbed by the material, initially as kinetic energy of the electrons.

$$\pi/\rho \propto Z,$$

and π/ρ increases as (photon energy in MeV. $- 1·02$) increases.

Photo-nuclear Reactions.—If a photon has an energy greater than the binding energy that holds the neutrons and protons together in the nucleus, it can enter that nucleus and eject a particle from it. This could be either a neutron or a proton but is more likely to be the former. In such an interaction the photon would disappear altogether, and any energy that it possessed, in excess of that needed to remove the particle, would be the kinetic energy of escape of that particle.

For the majority of atoms the 'threshold' energy for this effect is about 10 MeV. and the chance of it occurring increases rapidly with increasing energy, until a maximum is reached at about 5 MeV. above the threshold. After this the chance falls off with equal rapidity. In other words, photo-nuclear reactions affect a relatively small range of radiation energies and furthermore, even within this range, they are very rare events, at most contributing a few per cent to the total attenuation by a given material.

Because a nuclear particle has been ejected, the resulting nucleus may be radio-active, and in the early days of the use of megavoltage radiation there was some fear that this induced radioactivity of the irradiated material might make the patient something of a radiation hazard to others or, at any rate, add considerably to the radiation dose delivered by more familiar processes. These fears have proved ground-less and the process may be dismissed as being of no importance in radiology.

TRANSMISSION

All the above processes lie in wait, as it were, to trap the unwary photon as it passes through material. In any beam there will be some photons which avoid them all and these will be *transmitted*. Nothing will have happened to these photons—they are entirely unaffected by their passage. They are not, as sometimes seems to be imagined, a battered remnant of the fine healthy beam that set out to cross the attenuating barrier. Their energy, and hence their penetrating power, are unaltered: passage through the barrier has reduced their numbers but not affected the 'survivors'.

A Summary of Attenuation.—The different relationships that have already been given can be summarized as follows:

Scattering: $\dfrac{\sigma}{\rho}$ decreases as $h\nu$ or keV. increases and is mainly independent of Z.

Photo-electric effect: $\dfrac{\tau}{\rho} \propto \left(\dfrac{1}{h\nu}\right)^3 Z^3$ or $\left(\dfrac{1}{keV.}\right)^3 Z^3$.

Pair production: $\dfrac{\pi}{\rho} \propto Z$ and increases as (photon energy in MeV.$-1\cdot02$) increases.

The total attenuation will be the sum of the attenuations due to each process:

$$\frac{\mu}{\rho} = \frac{\sigma}{\rho} + \frac{\tau}{\rho} + \frac{\pi}{\rho},$$

The question now to be answered is: 'How does the importance of these contributions vary at various energies?' and an indication is provided by *Fig.* 42, which shows how the *percentage* contribution of each process to the total attenuation changes with photon energy for two materials, one of fairly high, and the other of low, atomic number. From this diagram three main features emerge:

1. That the photo-electric effect dominates the attenuation scene at low photon energies, especially in the higher atomic number materials.

2. That pair production takes command for very high energies and, again, especially for high atomic number elements.

3. That for medium photon energies, and especially in elements of low atomic number (such as those of greatest importance in biological materials), the Compton scattering process is the main method of attenuation. It will be noted that the region of Compton process importance covers much of the energy range of interest in radiology.

Fig. 42 shows the *relative* importance of the processes but gives no indication as to how the total mass attenuation coefficient varies with photon energy or with the atomic number of the attenuator. As far as the latter is concerned, the answer is straightforward. The greater the atomic number, the greater is the mass attenuation coefficient.

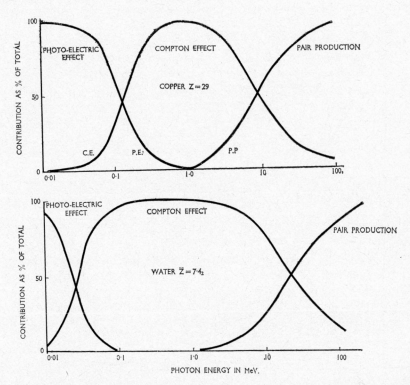

Fig. 42.—The *relative* importance of the different attenuation processes at various photon energies.

As to variation with energy, some typical values are shown in *Fig.* 43 in which the variations of the various mass coefficients with photon energy are given for copper. It will be noted that, in order to show a wide range in a relatively small space, the scales for this graph are logarithmic and therefore have the disadvantage that they may mislead the casual, though not the careful, observer. For example, at 10 keV. the scatter contribution is about 1/500 of that of the photo-electric effect, whereas a casual glance at the diagram might suggest that it was about 1/5!

Nevertheless, the main general features of the attenuation picture emerge quite clearly:

1. That the photo-electric effect falls off rapidly, with increasing energy.

2. That scattering *decreases* as photon energy increases.

3. That scattering is the predominant process over the medium-energy range (as already stressed in *Fig.* 42).

4. That the penetrating power of an X-ray beam increases with increasing energy until energies well in excess of 1 MeV. are reached. (*Note*: The smaller the attenuation coefficient the more penetrating the beam.) Later *increasing* pair production reverses

the trend and, somewhat astonishingly to most of our ideas, very high-energy radiations are *less* penetrating than some of lower energy.

Note: All that has been said, and will be said, in this chapter concerns beams of photons of one energy. The principles enumerated apply to all energies but their

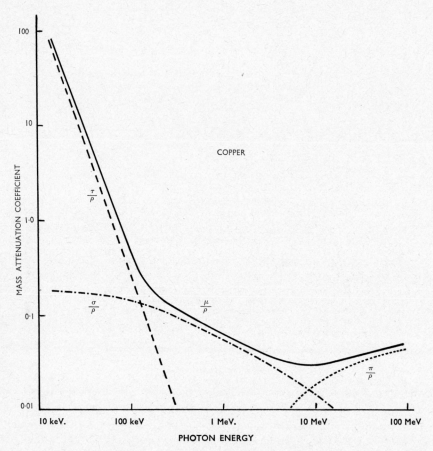

Fig. 43.—Variation with photon energies of the individual and total attenuation coefficients for copper.

application to the range of energies such as are present in the spectrum of radiation emitted by an X-ray tube introduces complexities which are best avoided at this stage. The attenuation of practical beams will be dealt with later.

ABSORPTION

So far attention has been focused mainly upon the removal of radiation from the beam—*attenuation*—by matter. Important as this subject is, the taking up of energy from the beam by the irradiated material—*absorption*—is at least as important, since it is upon this absorbed energy that all the effects of X-rays depend. Absorption must, therefore, now be considered.

First to recapitulate what has already been stated.

We know: (1) that unmodified scattering involves no absorption; (2) that in Compton scattering part of the energy removed from the beam is absorbed, and that as the photon energy increases more and more of the removed energy is absorbed, and less and less scattered; (3) that the photo-electric process is not one of complete absorption, since part of the energy of the photon originally removed is reradiated as characteristic radiation. However, in elements of low atomic number this radiation is of such low energy that it is immediately reabsorbed, and therefore the photo-electric effect can be regarded as providing complete absorption; (4) that for pair production all but 1·02 MeV. of the abstracted energy is absorbed.

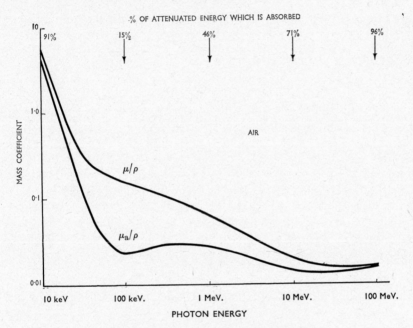

Fig. 44.—Attenuation and absorption in air.

These facts are summarized in *Fig.* 44, which shows how the mass attenuation (μ/ρ), i.e., the fraction *removed* per gramme, and mass absorption coefficients (μ_a/ρ), i.e., the fraction *absorbed* per gramme of air, vary for radiations from 10 keV. up to 100 MeV. At low energies where the photo-electric effect predominates the two coefficients are almost identical, as they are in the very high-energy range where most of the attenuation is by pair production. On the other hand, there is a marked difference between the coefficients in the range 40 keV. to 4 MeV., where the Compton process is the main cause of attenuation. Especially in the lower part of this range, the scattered photons retain much of the original energy, so that a relatively small part of the energy removed from the beam is absorbed by the air. For example, only 15 per cent for 100-keV. photons.

A noteworthy, if somewhat minor point concerning the absorption curve for air is its relative independence of photon energy over a wide range. For a hundredfold range of energy (100 keV. to 10 MeV.) the coefficient varies by little more than a factor of two.

Variation with Material.—*Fig.* 45 gives the same sort of facts about absorption as *Fig.* 44 but for a range of materials, and it shows a number of points of considerable importance. First, there is the shape of the curve for hydrogen. In the photon energy range covered by this diagram attenuation in hydrogen is practically entirely due to the Compton process. The low absorption value for low photon energies shows the effect of the scattered photon retaining most of the available energy, whilst the falling value at high energies is due to the steady reduction of σ/ρ with energy.

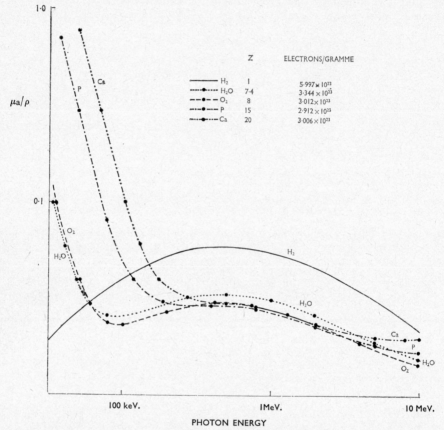

Fig. 45.—Absorption variation with photon energy for some materials. The absorption per gramme is practically the same for all materials not containing hydrogen over a wide energy range.

Next, attention should be transferred to the curves for oxygen ($Z = 8$), phosphorus ($Z = 15$), and calcium ($Z = 20$) and to the most vital fact that over a wide range of intermediate energies the mass absorption coefficients are practically identical. This is the energy range of Compton process predominance and that process, as already stressed, does not depend on atomic number but only on electron density. Since the electron density of all elements except hydrogen is practically the same, all substances which do not contain hydrogen will have nearly the same mass absorption, and attenuation, coefficients in the energy range in which the Compton effect predominates. *Fig.* 45 shows a representative sample: other substances would show the same effect.

Hydrogen having roughly twice as many electrons per gramme, as *Fig.* 45 indicates, also has roughly twice the mass absorption coefficient in the range under discussion.

At either end of the energy range the absorption coefficients for the three materials are quite different, for there either photo-electric absorption or pair production is important and the effect of atomic number makes itself felt.

The final topic for comment is the curve for water. At low energies its mass absorption coefficient is less than that of oxygen because its average atomic number (about 7·4) is rather less than that of oxygen and so it has a slightly smaller photo-electric effect. This disadvantage is offset, however, at higher energies by the fact that, because water contains hydrogen, its electron density exceeds that of non-hydrogenous materials. Therefore, over the majority of the range shown, water absorbs more than the other materials. That its mass coefficient exceeds that of oxygen even at the high-energy part of this range simply means that pair production plays a very minor role in both oxygen and water up to 10 MeV. At, say, 100 MeV. this would not be so and oxygen would again be the more absorbent.

The Spatial Distribution of the Secondary Radiations.—As a result of the inter-action of radiation with matter some electrons are freed from their parent atoms and set in motion, and X-rays will be found travelling in every direction. Some of this radiation will be scattered radiation, some characteristic radiation, and some, possibly, annihilation radiation. It can all conveniently be described as *secondary* radiation. To call it all *scatter* is plainly inaccurate and undesirable.

The relative amounts of each of these results of radiation interaction with matter have already been discussed; their consequences will be discussed later. At this stage all that remains is to say a few words about the directions in which the various secondary radiations travel.

First to deal with the electrons. As already pointed out, recoil electrons—by the very nature of the method of their production—travel forward, never making an angle of more than 90° with the direction of the initial photon, and generally at a much smaller angle. Photo-electrons and electron pairs, though more randomly emitted, also tend to travel forward, especially for higher energy radiations.

Of the secondary X-rays, characteristic and annihilation radiations are generally given out equally in all directions, that is to say their distribution is *isotropic*, and so, roughly—as has been shown—are the scattered photons for low-energy beams. In the megavoltage range principally used in radiotherapy (1–10 MeV.), however, the vast majority of the secondary radiation will be Compton-scattered photons and, at these energies, they will travel in a generally forward direction, having suffered comparatively small angle scattering. Very little of this radiation suffers 180° scatter, i.e., there is very little 'backscatter'. The importance of these facts in radiography and radio-therapy will be described later.

CHAPTER VIII

THE EFFECTS OF X-RAYS

THE last two chapters have shown that the primary effect of the interaction of X-rays with matter includes the production of high-energy, and hence high-speed, electrons. These electrons are the main agents through which all the effects of X-rays arise and it is, therefore, necessary to study, in some detail, what happens to them and to the energy they have received, as they pass through matter.

Heat, Excitation, and Ionization.—Our purpose is probably best served by considering a concrete example. What happens to a photo-electron as it passes through the material surrounding the atom from which it was ejected? This particle, it must be remembered, has a negative charge, and the atoms close to, or 'through', which it will be moving have 'clouds' of negative charges surrounding their nuclei. Therefore the photo-electron will continuously be subjected to repulsions which deflect it from its original path and also slow it down. Its path is therefore tortuous and quite quickly it loses all its energy. Thus brought to rest it is quickly captured by one of the many atoms which have been ionized by the radiation.

At the same time, of course, there will have been effects upon the atoms of the material. One of these is that the photo-electron may have repelled a whole atom: it will have given it, as it were, a 'push', thus transferring some of its energy to the atom. Since the kinetic energy of the atom is the manifestation of its temperature, the slowing down of the photo-electron in this way is associated with the generation of some *heat*.

Under other circumstances there will be interaction between the photo-electron and one of the individual electrons of the atom. This may involve the transfer of enough energy to an orbital electron to 'raise it' from its normal orbit to one of slightly higher energy. As a result an *excited* atom is produced, in which state that atom may be very reactive chemically, or it may break away from other atoms with which it is in chemical combination. The alternative fate of the excited atom is that it reradiates the excess energy, usually as ultra-violet radiation or visible light.

A more dramatic alternative is that the photo-electron may repel an individual electron sufficiently violently to eject it completely from its parent atom. *Ionization* is, therefore, a consequence of the passage of electrons through matter. Again chemical changes may be a consequence, since the electron ejected may have been responsible for a chemical bond in a compound, which would therefore be destroyed by the removal of this bond. Or the positive ion formed when the electron was ejected may be chemically very active and enter into chemical reactions, not previously possible to it, with neighbouring atoms or molecules.

Should no such chemical reactions occur, and they are by no means inevitable consequences of ionization, the positive ion quite quickly (in no more than a millionth of a second) will regain an electron and return to its normal state. Much ionization ends in *recombination*, and the emission of characteristic radiation.

Finally, there is a possibility that the photo-electron will suffer the sort of 'collision' that was described in CHAPTER V with the result that an X-ray photon is produced. In materials of high atomic number this *Bremsstrahlung* production would be the most important of all the processes, but for materials of interest in clinical radiology it occurs but seldom and need not be further considered. (It will be recalled from CHAPTER V that the efficiency of X-ray production depends on the atomic number of the 'target' material.)

In one or other, or all of these ways, the photo-electron loses energy until it is finally brought to rest and recaptured by a positive ion. The consequences of its brief life are summarized in *Fig.* 46 and it is fair to say that all the effects of X-rays stem from one or other of the processes there displayed, which of course are also produced by Compton and pair production electrons.

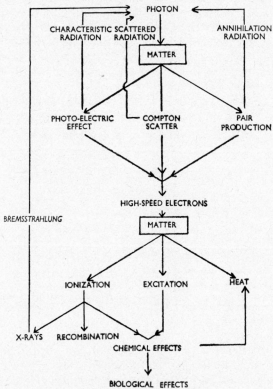

Fig. 46.—The effects of X-rays.

Ionization.—From many points of view this is the most important of the three processes and the most easily observed and measured. Ionization, excitation, and heat are produced in the same proportions over a wide energy range, so that measurement of ionization gives a good measure of the total energy being absorbed. On the average, for every ionization that it produces in the low atomic number elements which are of interest in radiology, the electron loses 34 eV. of its energy. (To ionize an atom of, say, oxygen requires less energy than this, but the figure includes the energy used up for the accompanying excitation and heat production.) Therefore an electron, on average, produces about 30 ionizations for every 1 keV. of its energy. A 100-keV. photo-electron can, therefore, produce about 3000 ionizations before it is brought to rest: or the recoil electron set in motion when a 124-keV. photon is scattered through 90° by the Compton process, and which thus acquires 24 keV. of energy (*see Table VII*, p. 67), will produce about 700 ionizations. In other words, each primary electron (photo-electron, Compton electron, or pair-production electron) produced by the interaction of an X-ray photon with matter produces hundreds more ionizations, as well as excitation and heat. The effects of X-rays are largely due to these *secondary* processes.

Electron Range and Ionization Pattern.—How far can an electron penetrate into, or through, any material? Are the effects that have been described produced close to or at some distance from the place at which the initial electron-liberating event took place? These are questions the answers to which are of importance when the biological consequences of irradiation are being considered and one part of the answer to both is that they depend on the initial energy of the electrons. *Table VIII* shows the range in water—that is to say, the distance travelled—of electrons of different energies, and it clearly shows that, for many electrons liberated by X-rays in general clinical use, all the processes enumerated and all their consequences occur very close to the point of initial interaction between photon and atom. It is only with electrons associated with X-rays of 1 MeV. or more that effects can be produced more than 1 mm. from the

Table VIII.—ELECTRON RANGES IN WATER

ELECTRON ENERGY	RANGE IN WATER	PHOTON ENERGY*
10 keV.	0·0002 cm.	80 keV.
50 keV.	0·004 cm.	220 keV.
100 keV.	0·014 cm.	350 keV.
500 keV.	0·17 cm.	1·1 MeV.
1 MeV.	0·43 cm.	2 MeV.
5 MeV.	2·5 cm.	8·5 MeV.
10 MeV.	4·9 cm.	18 MeV.

* A photon of any energy may give rise to a wide range of electron energies—for example, its Compton recoil electrons may have energies from zero up to some maximum controlled by the photon energy. The energies stated in the first column are the *average* energies of electrons produced by photons listed in this column.

original event. For higher energies still more and more of the final effect will be 'remote'.

In passing, note must be made of the fact that the range of a particle is not necessarily synonymous with the thickness of material through which it can penetrate. By the *range* we mean the total distance that the particle can travel in the material, and not the straight-line distance between the beginning and end of its track. Electrons, as has been said, follow a very tortuous track and in general will only penetrate a layer whose thickness is about half their range.

For the high-energy electrons the distribution of events along their tracks also becomes important in practice. Ionizations do not occur regularly along the tracks of ionizing particles, their spacing being different at different parts. This is because the chance of an ionization occurring in any length of track depends not only on the charge on the particle but also, inversely, on its speed. (Note that it is speed that matters and not energy, as such.) Thus a high-speed electron is less likely to produce ionization than a slower one, and at the beginning of its track—where it is travelling fastest—any electron will produce fewer ionizations per unit length (will have a lower 'specific ionization') than towards the end (where it is considerably slower).

The Bragg curve, already described in CHAPTER III, shows this as illustrated in *Fig.* 47, which demonstrates the way that the pattern changes along the track.

With electrons whose range is very short this general pattern, which applies to all particles, is of no practical importance, since their whole effect is so close to their point of origin. However, it means that for higher-energy electrons not only is their effect spread over some distance—about 5 mm. in the case of 1-MeV. electrons—but that most of the effect is at the track end and at a distance from the origin. This is of considerable significance in megavoltage X-ray therapy, as will be discussed later.

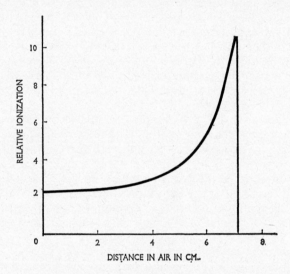

Fig. 47.—The Bragg ionization curve.

Chemical Effects.—The outer electrons in atoms play important roles in chemical combinations and therefore any disturbance of them may produce chemical changes. As has already been indicated, these changes could be disruptive, as when an electron which holds the molecule together (a chemical bond) is removed, or an atom may become much more chemically active and so produce changes which would not have occurred without the aid of the radiation. For example, changes can be brought about in solutions which are otherwise perfectly stable, because the action of radiation on water is to produce highly active 'radicals' which react with the solute in a way in which normal water cannot.

From the many examples which are available only two, each of which is of considerable radiological interest, will be quoted. These are the changing (oxidation) of ferrous sulphate into ferric sulphate when a solution of the former is irradiated, and the destruction, by radiation, of the fermenting powers of some enzymes.

Ferric sulphate absorbs ultra-violet radiation quite differently from ferrous sulphate, so that if a solution of the latter is studied, after irradiation, by ultra-violet spectroscopy, the amount of ferric sulphate produced can be measured. This amount is proportional to the dose of radiation received by the solution and therefore, although large radiation doses are needed to produce measurable amounts of ferric sulphate, the reaction has been quite widely and successfully used as a method of measuring X-ray dosage.

Enzymes are substances which are vital to the working of our bodies as a whole and to the metabolism of cells of all living materials. The fact that their peculiar chemical activity can be prevented by X-rays is not only a good example of a disruptive chemical effect of radiation but also a possible clue as to why, if not as to how, X-rays are able to affect living tissues. If irradiation destroys vital substances, then tissues and processes dependent upon them must suffer.

One other aspect of the chemical effects of X-rays is worthy of comment. As was first discovered during studies of the effects of radiation on enzyme solutions, it is possible to provide some degree of protection for irradiated materials. The addition of another substance, for example, glucose, to the solution to be irradiated cuts down the effect on the solute because the 'protector'—in this case glucose—competes for, and takes, some of the radicals which would otherwise damage the solute. Considerable research has been carried out to try to find a material that could be taken by people likely to be irradiated, so that any effects could be reduced. So far the only materials found to offer much protection have undesirable side-effects. Nevertheless the matter is by no means ended.

Biological Effects.—That X-rays can produce biological effects was realized soon after their discovery, but the dangers from their indiscriminate use, and the benefits from their carefully controlled use, were only recognized more slowly. The earliest observed effect was probably the reddening of the skin (erythema production) after prolonged exposure. A continuation of exposure produces ulceration or even complete destruction (necrosis) of the tissues. Another sequel of excessive irradiation—and especially long-continued (chronic) irradiation with relatively small doses—is the induction of cancers of the skin or of the blood (leukaemia), both of which caused the deaths of many pioneers in the radiological field.

X-rays always damage living tissues, and though this can be put to good effect (for example, cancer cells are more readily damaged and killed than are normal cells, so that X-rays can be used to cure cancer), in general, exposure to X-rays should be avoided unless special advantage accrues from such exposure. A particularly good illustration of this is the taking of a radiograph: the very small amount of biological damage produced by the radiation is trivial compared with the potential benefit that may come from the information from the radiograph.

Physico-chemical Effects.—

1. *Photographic Action*: Perhaps the most widely used of all X-ray effects is that on photographic material. Photographic film, or paper, exposed to X-rays and then developed, will be found to be 'blackened'—the irradiation has so affected the photographic emulsion of silver salts that, after the chemical process called 'development', metallic silver is released and the film or paper appears blackened.

The amount of silver released, and therefore the density of the blackening, or the opaqueness of the film to light, depends upon a number of factors which may conveniently be listed. They are:

a. The amount of radiation to which the film is subjected—the 'exposure'.

b. The quality of the radiation. This will be discussed more fully in a later chapter, but it can be said now that because of the relatively high atomic number elements present in the film, the sensitivity to X-rays varies quite markedly with radiation quality.

c. The characteristics of the film. In general the larger the size of the crystals which, embedded in gelatin, make up the photographic emulsion, the more sensitive (i.e., 'faster') is the film. This feature can be, and is, deliberately used by the film manufacturers to produce different types of film for different jobs. However, there is also a variation, though much smaller, in sensitivity between different batches of the same film type, and this is not so controllable. For radiographic purposes this variation is unimportant, but it must be borne in mind if film is used for precise *measurement* purposes.

d. The type, strength, age, and temperature of the developer; and

e. The length of the development time.

Careful control of the conditions of use and processing of films, together with experience, however, will enable consistent and reproducible results to be obtained, and certainly the rather forbidding-looking list has not prevented the photographic effect of X-radiation from becoming its most widely used property.

More detailed descriptions of the photographic action of X-rays, of the properties of the X-ray film, and of its processing are given in CHAPTERS XV and XVI.

2. *Induced Colour Changes*: Several substances, or their solutions in water, undergo colour changes when irradiated by X-rays. For example, a solution of the dye methylene blue is bleached, or barium platinocyanide changes, as irradiation proceeds, from apple green through darker shades to light brown and eventually dark brown if enough radiation is used.

Such changes have no practical application today, though in the early days of radiology they were used as the basis of dose measurement. The *pastille dose* served radiology well until more satisfactory methods, such as are to be described in the next chapter, were developed.

Physical Effects.—

1. *Heating Effect*: Although the production of heat is one of the initial results of the slowing down of the primary electrons, it also arises as an end-product of the chemical reactions induced by the radiation. Even so the total amount of heat produced, by the X-irradiation of any material, is very small, and it can only be detected by the most sensitive instruments, whilst its accurate measurement calls for extremely refined experimental methods. Some idea of the smallness of the amount of heat produced may be obtained from the fact that a dose of radiation which would undoubtedly prove fatal to anyone exposed to it would raise his or her temperature by little more than two-thousandths of 1° C.

2. *Fluorescence*: When X-rays fall upon certain material visible light is emitted: such material is said to *fluoresce*. It will be recalled that it was this phenomenon which led to the discovery of X-rays, when Röntgen noticed that some potassium platinocyanide, near his gas-discharge tube, glowed whenever the electric current was being passed through that tube. Since this happened even when the tube was shrouded in black paper, Röntgen realized he must be producing a hitherto undiscovered radiation. Fluorescence is one aspect of the larger topic of luminescence which is of sufficient importance in radiology to deserve special attention.

LUMINESCENCE

There are many different ways in which materials may be made to emit light. The general name of **luminescence** is given to a wide range of different phenomena, all of which result in the emission of light as a result of varying kinds of stimuli.

The luminescent materials which emit light as a result of X-irradiation are conveniently divided into three groups which are:

1. **Phosphorescent Materials.—**With phosphorescent materials the light emission continues for a period of time (which can be considerable) after the X-ray absorption has taken place. Clearly such materials are not suitable for fluoroscopy when it is desired that any change in X-ray beam

pattern (such, for instance, as can be seen when the passage of barium compounds through the stomach is being observed) shall be seen immediately. Delay in light emission would also tend to blur the pattern because of the inevitable movement of the patient. Even in radiography phosphorescence, or *afterglow*, as it is usually called, which lasts for more than a very short time, is to be avoided since carry-over of the pattern of one exposure to that of the next would spoil the second film. Although materials which exhibit phosphorescence are of no use for X-ray screens, they have other uses and can be seen every day on advertisement hoardings, where they lend a very striking brilliance to the colours.

2. **Fluorescent Materials.**—In fluorescent materials, on the other hand, the emission of light is so quickly completed following the X-irradiation that it can be regarded as instantaneous. It does, of course, take a little time and there is no sharp dividing line between phosphorescence and fluorescence, though it will be clear that the latter phenomenon, with its short 'afterglow', is that which is needed for X-ray purposes, rather than phosphorescence with its long 'afterglow'. For the materials in common use the 'afterglow' lasts only for a fraction of a second or so, which is short enough even when rapid serial exposures are being made.

3. **Thermoluminescent Materials.**—The luminescence of phosphorescent and fluorescent materials occurs during irradiation under normal room temperature conditions. The emission of light starts immediately the X-irradiation commences and stops instantaneously with the termination of exposure in the case of fluorescence but fades off slowly in the case of phosphorescence. There are other materials, however, which will also emit visible radiation during or after irradiation by X-rays but only if heated to a few hundred degrees centigrade. Because this light emission is associated with heating they are called thermoluminescent materials. Many substances exhibit the phenomenon but perhaps the most widely used, in radiology, is lithium fluoride.

THE MECHANISM OF FLUORESCENCE

The explanation of the phenomenon of fluorescence is to be found in the fact that fluorescent materials are crystalline. In such a material there are electron levels just as there are in simple, isolated atoms. In the description of photo-electric absorption and the emission of characteristic radiation, given in CHAPTER V, it was pointed out that if an electron is removed from a normally occupied level and the vacant space (a *hole* as it is called) so created is subsequently filled by an electron moving into it from an outer level, a photon of electromagnetic radiation is emitted. The quantum energy of the emitted photon is equal to the difference in energy of the two levels. If the lower-energy level concerned is an inner level of a comparatively high atomic numbered material then the emitted photon is an X-ray, whereas if the lower level is an outer one, the photon is likely to be one of visible light.

In the previous discussion of characteristic X-rays, main attention was focused on the inner (K or L) levels which, it will be recalled, had definite, single values of energy, each being characteristic of the particular type of atom concerned. In fluorescence the emphasis is on the outer electron level, since it is the emission of visible light which constitutes this process. In order to discuss some of the details of

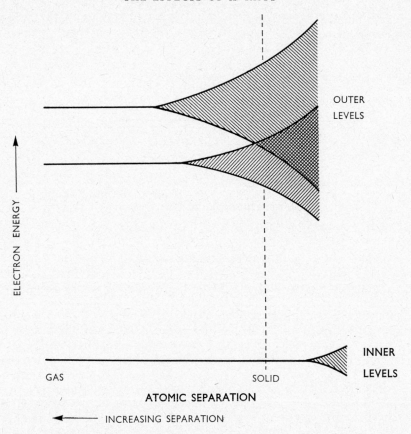

Fig. 48.—The spreading of energy levels into energy bands as atoms get closer together.

fluorescence it is necessary first to describe in a little more detail the pattern of energy levels which exist in a solid material.

Strictly speaking the pattern of discrete energy levels (K, L, M, etc.) given in CHAPTER II is true only for an isolated single atom (e.g., in a gas). In a solid the inner levels (K, L, etc.) of each of the atoms comprising the solid are exactly the same as for the single atom and the nearby presence of all the other atoms of the solid has no effect on these levels. These inner levels are, of course, completely filled with electrons. For the outer levels (O, P, etc.), many of which are empty, the situation is different. Instead of each electron being restricted to a definite energy value, the presence of the other atoms makes it possible for each electron to have any energy within a small but definite range. This range is sufficiently wide, however, that the previously separate single levels now overlap to form a quite wide band of possible electron energies.

This is shown diagrammatically in *Fig*. 48, where the shaded region represents the range of energy values which it is possible for an electron to have. At the left of the picture the situation in a single atom is depicted, and at the right that in a solid is shown. Thus in a solid the large number of single, separated, outer electron energy levels are replaced by a few *bands* of energy, within the lower and upper energy of which it is possible for an electron to have any value of energy.

For the kind of crystal being discussed the energy-level pattern has the form shown in *Fig*. 49.

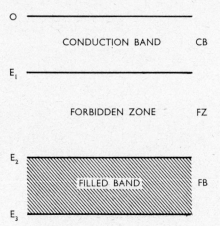

Fig. 49.—The electron band structure of a perfect, and pure, crystal of an insulating material.

This energy diagram is interpreted as showing:

   a. The Conduction Band (OE₁).—Between the level O (which represents the energy level at which an electron can leave the material) and the lower level E_1, there is a band of energy formed from some of the broadened outer energy levels of the atoms constituting the crystal. This band is called the *conduction band*, since any electron which may happen to be in this band can move freely about the material and in so doing can exhibit the phenomenon of electrical conduction. In fluorescent materials this band is, as shown in the diagram *Fig*. 49, empty of electrons and the material is therefore an electrical non-conductor (insulator).

   b. The Forbidden Zone.—Over the energy range E_1–E_2 there are no energy levels and electrons cannot exist in this region of energies. This region, which is called the *forbidden zone*, corresponds to the region between the energy levels of a single atom.

   c. The Filled Band.—Between E_2 and E_3 there is a continuous band of energy levels and electrons can have any energy between these two limits (E_2 and E_3). All these levels are full and there is normally no room for any more electrons in this band. It is therefore called the *filled band*. Electrons can, however, be removed from this band and so leave behind vacant positions or *holes*, into which other electrons can subsequently move.*

---

   * *Electrical Conduction.*—As has already been indicated, electrical conduction occurs when there is a steady drift of any electrons in the conduction band. In a good conductor—a metal—there are many electrons in the conduction band and in fact there is usually no forbidden zone between the conduction band and the upper filled band.

   In an insulator there are no electrons in the conduction band and the forbidden zone is wide so that movement of electrons—conduction—is not possible. There are some materials called **semiconductors** which, although they normally have no electrons in the conduction band and are therefore insulators, can acquire some and thus become (rather poor) conductors. The forbidden zone is not too wide and for this and other reasons it is possible in many ways (heat, light, X-rays, etc.) to lift some electrons into the conduction band. Semiconductors also have traps similar to those described below, which contribute to their properties. These properties are varied and complex and the well-known *transistors*, of which there are several kinds, are made of semiconductors.

d. *The Inner Levels.*—Below E_3 there are other bands, forbidden zones, and eventually the unmodified discrete, single inner energy levels. None of these has any importance in the discussion of fluorescence and so can be ignored.

Electron Traps.—The situation described by *Fig.* 49 is that which would exist in a pure and perfect crystal. The presence in an actual crystal of impurities and faults results in there being some extra electron energy levels in the forbidden zone, E_1–E_2. These levels are localized at definite places within the crystal and should an electron occupy such a level then it will be held at this place in the crystal. The electron is said to be trapped and these localized energy levels are called electron *traps*. Two such traps are shown at *T* on *Fig.* 50. In fluorescent materials the trap is normally occupied by an electron.

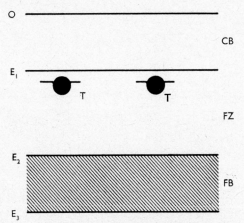

Fig. 50.—Energy bands in a fluorescent material, showing electron traps (T) with energies near the top of the forbidden zone.

These traps are very similar to the electron trap which is responsible for the sensitivity speck in the photographic silver bromide crystal. The manufacture of fluorescent materials involves the production of very pure materials to which very definite amounts of deliberate 'impurities' are added. The exact way in which this is done determines the exact nature and extent of the fluorescence.

The process of light emission can be described by reference to *Fig.* 51. If there is an electron in a trap (*T*) and also a hole (*H*) in the filled band, then these two may combine, the electron trap so becoming empty and the hole being filled. When this happens a single photon of visible light is emitted. The energy ($h\nu$) of this photon is equal to the energy difference between the level of the trap and the hole ($E_T - E_H$). Within the crystal there will be many such traps, not all of which will be at exactly the same energy level (E_T). Furthermore, the energy level of the hole (E_H) may have any value within the band (E_2–E_3). Hence, although each photon (like characteristic radiation) has a definite energy wavelength, the value may be any one of quite a wide range. Hence the spectrum of visible light emitted as the result of very many of such events will be a continuous one extending over a certain, not too large, range of wavelengths.

Fluorescence.—In fluorescence some or all of the energy of a photon of X-rays is absorbed by the crystal and a fast-moving Compton or photo-electron is produced. This electron moves through the crystal and gradually dissipates its kinetic energy by liberating more electrons from the filled band and lifting them to the conduction band, at the same time creating a corresponding number of holes in the filled band. In this way the hole in *Fig.* 51 A was formed. These holes will very quickly be filled

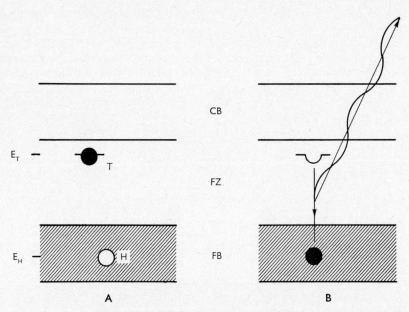

Fig. 51.—The emission of light from a fluorescent material. A, Removal of an electron from the filled band creates a hole (H). B, The hole is filled by an electron from a trap, and a visible photon is emitted.

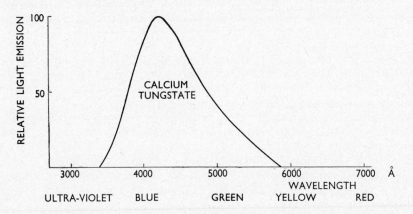

Fig. 52.—The spectrum of the light emitted from a typical intensifying-screen fluorescent material.

by electrons moving from the traps (*T*) and, in so doing, emitting the visible fluorescent light photons. The electrons raised to the conduction band will eventually fall into the emptied traps and so refill them ready for the next time. It can be seen, therefore, that the fluorescent material does not wear out and cease to work after being once used, since the traps are automatically 're-set'.

Since many holes are created by each absorbed photon there are many visible light photons emitted for each X-ray photon absorbed. The final and almost instantaneous result of the absorption by the fluorescent material of X-ray photons is therefore the emission of a large number of visible light photons extending over a small continuous range of wavelengths. The spectrum of the fluorescent light from an intensifying screen is shown in *Fig.* 52. It should be noted that the colour of light is not dependent on the energy of the X-ray photon but depends only on the crystal's properties (in an exactly similar way to the characteristic radiation which is emitted subsequent to photo-electric absorption where wavelength and energy do not depend upon the original photon energy).

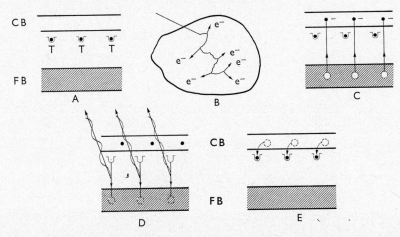

Fig. 53.—Fluorescence—immediate emission. A, The original state of the material. B, Each X-ray photon produces many electrons. C, Electrons lifted to the conduction band and holes produced in the filled band. D, The holes filled from the traps and visible photons emitted. E, Electrons from CB refill the traps and restore the original situation.

There is an alternative mechanism for fluorescence which does not depend upon the existence of such traps, and which can occur instead of, or together with, the process already described. In the type of materials used in radiology it is, however, not as important as the process involving traps. What happens is that an electron raised to the conduction band goes directly to fill a hole in the filled band and in so doing emits the visible fluorescent light.

Summary of Fluorescence (*Fig.* 53).—

1. Some X-ray energy is absorbed and a secondary (photo- or Compton) electron is produced.
2. The secondary electron, in moving through other atoms, creates many holes in the filled band, and so lifts many electrons to the conduction band.
3. Electrons already in traps (T) combine very quickly with the newly created holes and so emit visible fluorescent light photons.
4. Alternatively (but uncommonly) electrons fall directly from the conduction band to fill the holes and so emit visible fluorescent light photons.
5. The vacated traps are refilled by electrons from the conduction band.
6. Many X-ray photons are absorbed and as a result of each many visible light photons are emitted and their spectrum is a continuous one.

Phosphorescence.—In some materials there can be traps of a different type. Such a trap is shown at *R* in *Fig.* 54. Unlike the type of trap (*T*) involved in fluorescence, this type of trap (*R*) is normally empty, although such a trap can be filled by an electron falling into it from the conduction band. Furthermore, once in the trap the electron cannot (for reasons too complex to be dealt with here) move to the filled band to fill any hole which may exist there. The trapped electron can, however, move back to the conduction band, provided it can acquire the small amount of energy necessary to do this. From the conduction band the electron can fall into a hole in the filled band and so generate a visible light photon.

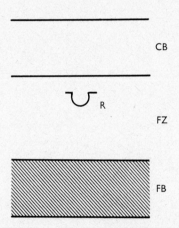

Fig. 54.—A phosphorescent material has empty traps (R) at energy positions near the top of the forbidden zone.

The acquisition of this small extra amount of energy necessary to return the electron to the conduction band is not too difficult and is obtained from the heat (kinetic) energy of the atoms making up the crystal. If the temperature is low then, on the average, the electrons will stay for a long time in the trap (*R*), whereas if the temperature is higher they will move up to the conduction band more quickly. The length of time involved depends, of course, on the depth of the trap below the conduction band (i.e., in the material) as well as on the temperature. The electrons do not all leave the trap after the same length of time; some come out quite quickly and some stay in the trap for a very long time. The process is what is known as a statistical one rather like radioactive decay, which was discussed in CHAPTER III. The average length of time which the electrons spend in the trap will determine for how long, after the initial X-ray irradiation has ceased, the visible light will continue to be emitted. If the traps are very close to the conduction band the time will be small but if they are well below, the emission may well continue for a considerable time (minutes or hours).

Summary of the Phosphorescence Process (*Fig.* 55).—
1. X-ray energy is absorbed and a secondary (photo- or Compton) electron is produced.
2. The secondary electron creates many holes in the filled band of atoms through which it passes, and so lifts many other electrons to the conduction band.
3. These electrons fall into traps (*R*), where they stay for a period of time.

4. When and if an electron in a trap acquires sufficient energy (from the atoms of the crystal) it will move back into the conduction band.

5. From the conduction band the electron falls to fill a hole in the filled band and so emits a visible light photon.

6. The time interval between (3) and (4) determines how long the light continues to be emitted after the X-ray irradiation has finished.

7. Many X-ray photons are absorbed and as a result of each, many visible light photons are emitted, and their spectrum is a continuous one.

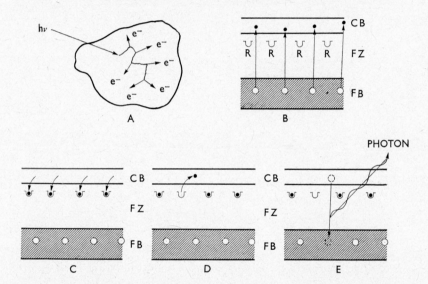

Fig. 55.—Phosphorescence—delayed emission. A and B, Photon-liberated electron raises more electrons to CB and makes holes in FB. C, Electrons from CB fall into traps. D, Electron returns to CB having acquired some energy. E, This electron returns to fill hole in FB and emits photon of visible light.

Luminescent Materials.—These descriptions of the processes involved in the phenomena of fluorescence and phosphorescence are very much simplified accounts of what is a very complex situation. Several other types of mechanism can also, and do, exist, but the account given does indicate how the detailed properties of a luminescent material depend very critically on exactly of what, and how, it is made. Of particular importance are the added impurities which control to a large extent the character of the traps.

In all luminescent material there will be a tendency for traps of both kinds (T and R) to exist and therefore for the material to exhibit both fluorescence (quick light emission) and phosphorescence (delayed light emission). In radiology minimum phosphorescence (afterglow) is required and this can be achieved by careful control of manufacture and by the addition of minute amounts of other impurities, which tend to prevent ('kill') the formation of phosphorescent traps (R), or at least to ensure that they are only a little way below the conduction band, so that any phosphorescence is sufficiently quick to be acceptable.

Thermoluminescent Materials.—In these materials there are traps which, like those in phosphorescent materials, are normally empty. However, unlike those in phosphorescent materials, the traps are well 'below' the conduction band so that there is practically no chance, at ordinary temperatures, of any electron which may enter them ever being lifted back into the conduction band. Only if the material is heated to a temperature of 200–300° C. can the trapped electrons acquire sufficient energy to reach the conduction band whence, as in phosphorescence, they can fall back to refill the holes in the filled band, emitting light in the process.

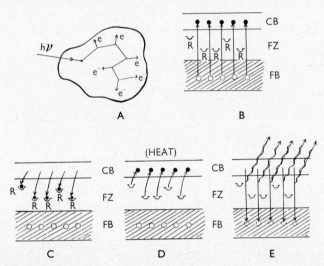

Fig. 56.—Thermoluminescence—light released by heat. A and B, Photon-liberated electron raises more electrons to *CB* and makes holes in *FB*. C, Electrons fall from *CB* into traps (*R*) in *FZ*. D, By heating, the trapped electrons are raised back to *CB* whence (E) they return to *FB* emitting visible light.

Summary of the Thermoluminescence Process (*Fig.* 56).—

1. X-ray energy is absorbed and a secondary (photo-electric, Compton or pair-production) electron is produced.

2. The secondary electron causes many holes in the filled bands of atoms through which it passes and so lifts many electrons into the conduction band.

3. These electrons may fall back into traps (*R*) where they are held.

4. When the material is heated to a temperature of 200–300° C. the trapped electrons can acquire sufficient energy to escape back into the conduction band.

5. From the conduction band the electrons can fall back to fill holes (not necessarily the holes from which they individually came) in the filled band, visible photons being emitted in the process.

6. It will be noted that the traps occur at different 'levels' in the forbidden zone. Escape from some is easier (i.e., is possible at a lower temperature) than from others. Light is emitted over a range of temperatures, as is illustrated by the 'glow curve' shown in *Fig.* 57. Some light is emitted at quite low temperatures, most at 70–100° C., whilst to empty all the traps heating up to 300° C. is necessary. The total amount of light emitted (indicated by the area under the curve) is proportional to the amount of radiation energy absorbed, so that the phenomenon is potentially the basis

of a method of radiation dosemetry. In practice, as will be described later
(p. 127), the area under the upper parts of the curve is used since the lower
parts can be subject to fading to an extent depending on the length and
condition of storage between irradiation and 'read-out'. For some applications when less accuracy is required the peak emission is sometimes used
as the measurement.

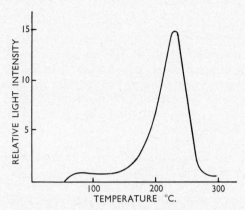

Fig. 57.—A thermoluminescent glow 'curve'.

Luminescence in Clinical Practice.—The principal uses of fluorescence in clinical
radiology (as will be described in a later chapter) are to enhance the photographic
action of X-rays (using 'intensifying screens') and to provide a means of converting
invisible X-rays into visible light so that, in fluoroscopy, the radiologist can 'see' the
X-ray image. Another application of great and increasing importance is based on the
fact that a number of transparent materials, notably sodium iodide and some plastics,
fluoresce (or 'scintillate') when irradiated with ionizing radiations. Though the
amount of light emitted may be quite small, the photomultiplier tube enables it to be
measured and form the basis of a very sensitive detector ('the scintillation counter')
which will be described in CHAPTER XI. Thermoluminescence is the basis of a very
convenient method of comparative radiation dosemetry.

CHAPTER IX

THE MEASUREMENT OF X-RAY QUANTITY

FOR many years after their discovery, X- and gamma rays were used quite empirically in medicine, but it was gradually realized that this approach was both dangerous and was hampering progress, especially in radiotherapy but to some extent also in diagnostic radiology. If the full potentialities of any agency are to be harnessed, a quantitative relationship between the agency and its effects must be established. Or, in other words, some means of measuring X-rays had to be found, and a unit of X-ray quantity defined and accepted.

The Measuring System.—Radiotherapy, using either external sources of radiation or internally administered radioactive materials, is concerned with the deliberate use of the radiation to cause biological effects in the tissues of the human body. X-ray diagnosis and *in vivo* radioactive isotope diagnostic investigations inevitably also involve—as a side-effect—irradiation of the tissues. The magnitude of the biological effects—desirable in the case of therapy and undesirable in the case of diagnosis—depends upon how much radiation energy is absorbed by the irradiated material. Therefore the object of X-ray dosemetry is *the measurement of energy absorbed in any material*, and, in particular, *in the different tissues of the body*. Although the magnitude of the biological effect depends, as stated above, on the quantity of the absorbed energy, many other factors are also of relevance. The volume of tissue irradiated, the pattern of the absorbed energy distribution, the length of time over which radiation is given, the type of tissue, the quality of the radiation, etc., all have their effect and need to be borne in mind when considering the relationship between a biological effect and the energy absorbed by the tissues. These considerations are, however, in the realm of radiobiology and radiotherapy and do not concern us further here.

Direct measurement in the irradiated person is impracticable and, therefore, a system has to be selected which will, as nearly as possible, simulate the material of interest. Any of the effects of X-rays described in CHAPTER VIII might, in principle at least, be used to measure what is loosely called X-ray 'dose'. However, any measuring system (no matter what is being measured) must satisfy certain criteria, and, therefore, each effect that might be used must be scrutinized to see whether or not it has the desired features.

First there are some general criteria. The system should be:

1. Reproducible. The measuring system, particularly the materials involved, should be obtainable in constant form everywhere and at any time.
2. Repeatable. Repeated measurements of the same amount of radiation should give the same reading wherever and whenever they are performed.
3. Sensitive. Small amounts should be sufficient to obtain an acceptable reading.
4. Objective. As far as possible personal subjective judgement should not be involved in obtaining an answer.
5. Linear. The response should be simply proportional to the quantity being measured.

Then, turning to the more specific requirements of X-ray dosemeter, the method used should be independent of the intensity (Exposure rate) of the radiation to be measured and should be capable of measuring very small and very large amounts of radiation and of operating over a wide range of radiation quality. CHAPTERS VI and VII have shown that the amount of radiation absorbed from a beam depends upon the energy of the radiation and on the atomic number of the material. Since, as already stated, the measuring method has to be indirect, and since we usually cannot know the radiation quality very precisely, it is important that the variation of absorption with radiation energy in the test material should be as nearly as possible the same as for the material of interest. This is achieved if the two substances have the same atomic number, for then, at any radiation energy, they will absorb equal amounts of energy per gramme regardless of their physical state, be it solid, liquid or gas.

Many of the effects of X-rays have been tried as a basis of dosemetry. None has all the desirable features listed but that which most nearly satisfies them is the *ionization of air*, which is now the internationally accepted basis of standard X-ray dosemetry.

Ionization of Air.—CHAPTERS VI and VII have already shown that ionization is a major product of the energy-absorption process and in CHAPTER VIII it was pointed out that a constant fraction of the energy absorbed from the beam goes into ionization. Therefore to measure ionization is essentially to measure energy absorption.

Air is chosen as the material in which measurements are made, for several reasons. Not only is it readily available everywhere, and inexpensive, but also because its composition is universally almost constant, a fact that those dwelling in allegedly more salubrious places find hard, but have to accept! The material is, therefore, reproducible. Measurement of the ionization is carried out electrically, and methods of adequate accuracy and sensitivity can be devised. Furthermore, the answer can be read off a meter dial or a number counter so that the amount of personal judgement needed is reduced to an absolute minimum. Air ionization, therefore, satisfies the primary criteria set out above.

Very high dose rates may present technical difficulties of collecting all the ionization produced, whilst very high or very low doses present measurement problems, but all these can be solved and the method can therefore be said to be independent of intensity and total dose. Furthermore, as *Fig.* 44, p. 77, shows, the absorption coefficient for air, and hence the ionization do not change much over a wide range of photon energies.

However, the main advantage of air as the medium for measurement lies in none of these features but in the fact that its atomic number is almost identical with that of muscle tissue. The atomic number of air—the average of its several components—is 7·64 whilst that for muscle is 7·42. Thus, for radiation of any energy, the energy absorbed per gramme of air will be practically the same as the energy absorbed per gramme of muscle tissue. Measurements of ionization of air, therefore, give direct information about ionization, and hence energy absorption, in the most important type of body tissue.

Ionization of air does not, however, run parallel at all radiation qualities with the ionization and absorption per gramme in materials of different atomic number. Thus, as will be discussed later, the evaluation of radiation energy absorption in bone ($Z \approx 13$) on the basis of air ionization measurements is a more complex matter.

THE ROENTGEN

Ionization in air has been internationally accepted as the basis for X-ray measurement, and for the definition of a unit of X-ray quantity since the second International Congress of Radiology in 1928, when it was also agreed to call the unit the *roentgen*. Subsequent congresses modified the definition, though that accepted in 1937 remained unchanged for many years, and, though it has now been superseded by wording which is strictly more correct, the 1937 version is more descriptive of what happens and is more readily understood by those more interested in utility than in pedantic correctness.

It states that the roentgen is 'That amount of X, or gamma, radiation such that the associated corpuscular emission, per 0·001293 gramme of air, produces in air ions carrying 1 electrostatic unit of charge of either sign'.

0·001293 gramme is the weight of 1 c.c. of air at 0° C. and 760 mm. of mercury pressure (i.e., at N.T.P.), whilst the 'associated corpuscular emission' refers to the photo-electrons, Compton recoil electrons, and/or the pair-production electrons set in motion by the primary interactions between the radiation photons and the air. These electrons, as described in CHAPTER VIII, produce large numbers of further ionizations before being brought to rest, and if the total charge liberated by electrons originating in 1 c.c. of air amounts to 1 e.s.u., then the air has been exposed to 1 roentgen.

It will be noted that the wording of this definition is such that, strictly, it defines the radiation. The roentgen is an amount of radiation, according to this definition, and not a measure of the energy taken from that radiation, which is what we really want. Plainly, however, the unit is based on the energy extracted from the beam and, in fact, the amount of energy absorbed per roentgen can easily be calculated.

For many years the roentgen was used in this dual role—both as a unit of radiation quantity and as a unit of absorbed energy (dose). However, the two roles are not always compatible, especially for very high-energy radiations and, of course, the roentgen does not indicate directly the absorbed dose in materials like bone, whose atomic number is quite different from that of air. Pedantically, too, the roentgen is only a unit of X- or gamma rays and cannot be used for other ionizing radiations like beta rays or neutrons. For these, and other reasons, therefore, an additional unit, the *rad*, was introduced in 1956, and in 1962 it was decided that henceforth the roentgen shall be the unit of *exposure*, whilst the rad should be the unit of *absorbed dose*.

At the same time (1962) a considerable revision of dosemetric terminology was undertaken by the I.C.R.U., in an effort to produce a more logical and more strictly accurate series of definitions. In this they have succeeded, though the new definitions are possibly less comprehensible than the old to many in radiology who are not expert in dosemetric matters. At the same time it is unfortunate that a word like 'exposure', which has a widely understood and useful, if ill-defined, meaning in radiology, should have been taken and given a very special meaning in a closely allied context. Confusion is almost certain to be caused. In an attempt to avoid such confusion here, the radiation quantity will be written with a capital E (i.e., Exposure) whilst the radiological procedure will be given as 'exposure'.

The special meaning of *Exposure* (X) has to be defined, of course, and it is 'the quotient ΔQ by Δm, where ΔQ is the sum of all the electrical charges on all the ions of one sign produced in air, when all the electrons (negative electrons and positrons) liberated by photons in a volume element of air whose mass is Δm are completely stopped in air:

$$X = \frac{\Delta Q}{\Delta m}.$$

'The special unit of Exposure is the roentgen (R):

$$1 \text{ R} = 2 \cdot 58 \times 10^{-4} \text{ coulomb per kilogram of air.'}$$

Though the words used are so different from those in the 1937 definition, their meaning is the same, though more precise. Also, the numerical value of the new roentgen is identical with the old one.

THE RAD

'Exposure' is fundamentally a property of the beam, and therefore does not fulfil our stated purpose of measuring absorbed energy. *Absorbed dose* is what we want to measure, and it has been defined by the I.C.R.U. as 'the quotient of ΔE_D by Δm, where ΔE_D is the energy imparted by ionizing radiation to the matter in a volume element, and Δm is the mass of matter in that volume element:

$$D = \frac{\Delta E_D}{\Delta m}.$$

'The special unit of absorbed dose is the *rad*:

$$1 \text{ rad} = 100 \text{ ergs per gramme.'}$$

It will be noted that no particular material is specified in this definition: it applies to any material, whereas, of course, the roentgen measures ionization in air. The roentgen can be regarded as the amount of radiation incident upon the material and the rad as the amount of energy absorbed as the result of this exposure. Direct measurement of rads is, however, very difficult and the usual procedure for their estimation is to measure the Exposure in roentgens and then calculate the rads through known factors which depend on the material irradiated and on the radiation energy. This conversion is very straightforward for soft tissue (it will be recalled that the atomic numbers of air and soft tissue are almost identical) but is complex for materials like bone. A full discussion of the conversion will be given later after methods of measuring Exposure have been described and discussed.

THE GRAY

In June, 1975, the International Committee on Weights and Measures adopted the *gray* (symbol Gy) as the S.I. unit of absorbed dose:

$$1 \text{ gray} = 1 \text{ joule per kilogramme} = 100 \text{ rad.}$$

Dr. L. H. Gray, after whom the new unit is named, made fundamental contributions to radiation dosemetry.

Other Measuring Methods.—Although the ionization of air is the preferred basis for standard measurements of X-rays, many of the other effects described can be, or have been, used successfully as detectors of radiation and to some extent as measuring methods. It is useful to survey some of these and to consider their strong, and weak, points.

Biological Methods.—Some of the earliest attempts to measure X-rays were based on their biological effects, and one of the most used of these was erythema production. The Threshold Erythema Dose (T.E.D.) was the amount of radiation which would produce a just perceptible reddening of the skin in 80 per cent of those exposed. Unfortunately, not only is there considerable variation from person to person (cf. the variation in individual sun-tanning) so that the reproducibility is not high, but the effect depends very much upon the dose rate, and also upon radiation quality in a complicated way. The erythemata and other reactions produced by radiation are, of course, of great importance to the radiologist and may provide useful dosage guides, but they are not suitable for exact and standard measurements.

Chemical Methods.—Over the last decade or so considerable attention has been paid to the use of the oxidation of ferrous sulphate to ferric sulphate, in dilute solution, as a dosemeter. (Often called the Fricke dosemeter after the man who first studied its possibilities.) The method, which depends on the measurement of the change in ultra-violet absorption caused by the oxidation, is especially useful where very large doses have to be measured. However, the relative insensitivity and the fact that the purity of the chemicals is extremely important to the precise effect that will be produced have meant that an otherwise very attractive method cannot be regarded as sufficiently sensitive or robust to displace the established method.

Physico-chemical Methods.—The photographic effect of X-rays is a very obvious basis for a measuring method since it is very sensitive, and over a limited range, at least, the blackening produced is proportional to the radiation energy absorbed. However, as outlined in CHAPTER VIII, the blackening also depends on a number of extraneous factors such as the development conditions, film type, and also to a marked extent upon radiation quality. The latter variation, because the film contains elements of high atomic number, is quite different from the variation in the low atomic number tissue and it is this, coupled with general lack of reproducibility, that disqualifies the method from acceptance as a standard. In a later chapter it will be shown that, provided great care is taken, the photographic film can be used as a very satisfactory dosemeter for the amounts of radiation encountered in protection work. Here the variation of sensitivity with radiation energy can actually be turned into an advantage.

Another physico-chemical effect which was widely used in the early days of radiology was the colour change induced in barium platinocyanide, which, as already mentioned, was the basis of the pastille method of Sabouraud and Noiré. Small pastilles (about the size of aspirin tablets) were placed half-way between tube and patient and irradiation was continued until a desired colour change (in the range apple-green to dark brown) was produced. Apart from the fact that the measurement depended upon the subjective, and very variable, process of colour matching, the colour change was influenced by prevailing atmospheric humidity, the past history of the pastille (colour changes disappeared after a short time so that pastilles could be used over and over again), and, even more important, with radiation quality, once again because of the high atomic number materials present. The pastille method and the pastille dose served developing radiology well, but were dependent upon too many factors beside the dose being measured to retain acceptance as the standard dosemetric method.

Physical Methods

a. Fluorescence: The intensity of visible light emitted by a fluorescent material depends primarily on the amount of X-ray energy absorbed by it and, therefore, also on the intensity of the X-rays falling upon it. Fluorescence would, therefore, seem to offer a method of measuring radiation dosage since the measurement of visible light is quite straightforward. Unfortunately many fluorescent materials used in radiology (e.g., zinc sulphide or calcium tungstate) contain elements of high atomic number so that the variation, with radiation energy, of their absorption will be very different from that of soft tissue. This difficulty might, however, be overcome by using some organic materials, such as anthracene or one of a number of transparent plastics all of which fluoresce when irradiated with X-rays and also have atomic numbers close to those of air and soft tissue. Using a photomultiplier tube to amplify the effects of the tiny amounts of light ('scintillation') produced by the individual X-ray photons, a method has been developed—and is described in CHAPTER XI—which has high sensitivity but, unfortunately, unless careful precautions are taken, does not necessarily have a high reproducibility. Fortunately, for any given piece of equipment the repeatability of measurements is very good.

The amount of light emitted by any fluorescent material depends, to a considerable extent, on the presence or absence of minute amounts of impurities—perhaps more correctly called *additives* since they are deliberately introduced—in the basic material. Only a few parts in a million are needed yet they enhance the light emission out of all proportion to their relative amounts. Clearly, however, it is extremely difficult to ensure absolute constancy of additive content and of substance response. The phenomenon is, therefore, unacceptable as the basis of standard dosemetry though it can provide an excellent method of radiation detection and, under carefully calibrated conditions, of measurement.

b. Thermoluminescence: A very wide range of dosages can be measured by using the thermoluminescent phenomenon. Lithium fluoride, which shows this effect well, has an atomic number close to that of soft tissue, and therefore the variation, with radiation energy, of energy absorption in both materials will be very similar. Since only 10 or so milligrams of lithium fluoride powder are needed for measurements the method is very suitable for dosage investigations during treatments, since the tiny capsules can readily be inserted into body cavities and sites not normally accessible to more conventional measuring methods. The *relative* values of doses at a number of sites can be readily obtained, for example, but not, without much more difficulty, their absolute values. Like fluorescence, thermoluminescence depends on tiny amounts of impurities in the crystalline material and it is not possible to produce a universally constant material. Therefore, the method, again like fluorescence, cannot be the basis of standard dosemetry. Nevertheless, it is most valuable for comparisons and has, of recent years, been quite widely used for comparing dosage standards between centres and countries, especially those without their own standardizing laboratory. Details of a dosemeter using thermoluminescence will be given in CHAPTER XI.

c. Calorimetry: The most direct, and to the physicist the most satisfactory, method of measuring the energy deposited in any material is to measure the heat generated. It will be recalled that heat is one of the initial products of the slowing down of the primary electrons and it is also the end-product of many of the radiation-induced chemical reactions. Therefore to measure heat would be the most direct method of achieving our stated object. Unfortunately, the amounts of heat generated are extremely small and can only be measured accurately by the most careful and highly sensitive techniques. These have been developed and have proved very valuable in fundamental research but are insufficiently robust and far too complicated for general adoption.

Conclusion.—Therefore our methods of dosemetry are generally indirect—we measure *Exposure* by ionization in air, and from this calculate *absorbed dose* in any other material. How these are done will be the subject of the next two chapters.

CHAPTER X

THE ROENTGEN AND ITS MEASUREMENT

THE defining of a unit may not, in itself, be of great practical value; it must be possible to realize the unit and to calibrate practical instruments in terms of it. Thermometers are calibrated by using steam in contact with boiling water under specified conditions, and by means of melting ice; distance-measuring devices are compared with the separation of two marks on a standard piece of metal (or, for more exact work, with the wavelength of a particular type of radiation), whilst weights are compared with standard blocks of metal. The comparable device for the roentgen is the *standard* or *'free-air'* ionization chamber.

THE STANDARD OR 'FREE-AIR' CHAMBER

To fulfil the definition of the roentgen (1962 or 1937 variety, though the requirements of the latter are probably clearer), the ionization produced in air by the irradiation of a known amount of air must be measured. *Fig.* 58 shows, diagrammatically, the apparatus used for such measurements. A narrow beam of X-rays is produced by

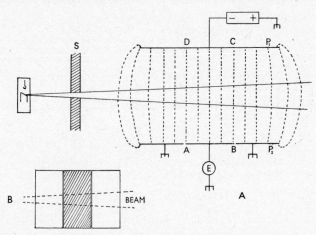

Fig. 58.—A, The general principles of the 'free-air' chamber. B, Plate P_2, showing central collector plate.

a collimating system (S), and passes between two parallel metal plates, P_1 and P_2, which form the electrodes of the ionization 'chamber'. P_1 is kept at a high negative potential with respect to P_2 which is 'earthed' through the electrical measuring device E (which will measure the charge liberated by the ionization). Plate P_2 is not, however, a simple metal plate but, as shown in *Fig.* 58 B, it consists of a central collector plate (AB in *Fig.* 58 A and 'hatched' in *Fig.* 58 B) which is separated from the outer portions by narrow, and insulating, air gaps. The outer portions are directly earthed and act like a 'guard ring' for the collector plate.

This particular design is necessary because of the need to measure the ionization produced in a precisely defined volume of air. As *Fig.* 58 A shows, the electric field

—indicated by the dotted lines—spreads out beyond the confines of the charged plates, but to a rather indefinite extent. Furthermore, though there is some electric field outside the plates, its strength falls off quite rapidly. It should be remembered that an electric field is any region where electric forces may be felt by charged particles and the 'lines of force' are the paths followed by these particles. Thus, if the whole of plate P_2 were used as the collector for negative ions produced by the ionization, some from the region beyond the plates would be collected, but it would be impossible to define precisely the volume from which this collection was taking place. Also, the efficiency of collection would be doubtful, because of the falling off of field strength at the edges of the plates. On the other hand, the collector plate AB is in a region of uniform field and there is no doubt about the volume from which charge will be collected. Any ions formed in the section ABCD, *and no others*, will be attracted to the collector plate AB and measured by E.

It has already been pointed out that the electrons, produced by the primary inter-actions between X-rays and matter, have considerable energy and may produce hundreds of ionizations before being brought to rest. For example, a 100-keV. photo-electron travels some 12 cm. in air and produces about 3000 ionizations,

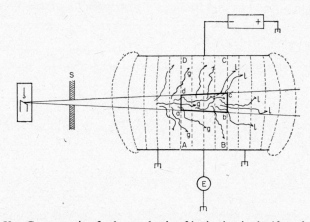

Fig. 59.—Compensation for loss and gain of ionization in the 'free-air' chamber.

whilst the Compton electrons set in motion when a 100-keV. photon is scattered through 90° can travel about 1 cm. and produce nearly 500 ionizations. Therefore ions collected from zone ABCD may well have been produced by primary electrons originating outside ABCD. The tracks of such electrons are labelled 'g' (for 'gain') in *Fig.* 59, which shows a representative selection of the ionizing particles crossing the zone of interest. In contrast with the electrons entering ABCD, there will be others that will start in the irradiated section abcd but will produce most of their effect out-side the collection zone, so that some of their effect will be lost. Such tracks are labelled 'l' (for 'loss') in the diagram.

In practice, provided that before arriving at the collecting volume the beam has traversed a thickness of air which is, at least, equal to the range of the most energetic electron the beam can produce, the gain and loss described will be equal. Therefore we can regard the ions collected by the collector plate AB, and measured by the electrometer, as being the ionization produced by the electrons arising from the irradiation of the volume represented by abcd.

The volume is known—it is the cross-sectional area of the beam multiplied by the length AB of the collector plate—all the ionization has been collected, and it was all produced in air. Hence the exposure, in *roentgens*, has been measured, provided the conditions discussed below have been fulfilled.

Plate Spacing and Other Distances.—The distance needed between the beam-defining diaphragm and the measuring volume, to ensure that there is compensation for loss and gain of ionization, has already been stated. A further design requirement is that the distance of each plate from the beam should also be greater than the range of the fastest electron generated. Fulfilment of this condition ensures that every electron expends all its energy in air and produces all the ionization of which it is capable, rather than colliding with the plate whilst still having some energy. In practice, plate separations are not usually as great as strict compliance with the rule would demand, simply because the maximum range is that of the photo-electrons, and in air, for 100 keV. and upwards, these are responsible for such a small part of the total ionization that the error introduced by failure to use the full-plate separation that they would demand is negligible. Some relevant information on this subject is given in *Table IX*.

Table IX.—THE IONIZATION CAUSED BY AND THE RANGES OF THE PHOTO- AND COMPTON ELECTRONS LIBERATED BY X-RAYS

The plate separation used in the appropriate 'free-air' chamber is shown in the last column

X-RAY GENERATING VOLTAGE	PHOTO-ELECTRONS		COMPTON ELECTRONS		PLATE SEPARATION USED
	Range in Air	% of Total Ionization	Range in Air	% of Total Ionization	
100 kV.	12 cm.	10	0·5 cm.	90	} ~12 cm.
200 kV.	37 cm.	0·4	4·6 cm.	99·6	
1000 kV.	290 cm.	0	220 cm.	100	4 metres

Care must also be taken to see that the X-ray beam does not fall upon any material other than air at a distance, from abcd, of less than the electronic range. Should, for example, some high atomic number material at a closer distance be irradiated, extra electrons would reach the measuring volume.

The Voltage applied between the Plates.—Unless the negative and positive ions produced in the ionization processes are quickly separated they will recombine and the conditions laid down for the measurement of roentgens will not be fulfilled. Recombination will tend, however, to be prevented by the applied electric field between the plates, since this pulls each kind of ion in opposite directions—the negative ions to the anode and the positive ions to the cathode. For any given irradiation the amount of charge collected by the collector plate and measured in E (*Fig.* 59) depends upon the strength of the electric field, which in the case of the standard chamber is simply the voltage between the plates divided by their separation. *Fig.* 60 shows how the collected charge varies with the voltage. With no voltage—no electric field—there is no collection of charge, since all the ions produced quickly recombine. Increasing the voltage (and hence the electric field) steadily increases the amount of the liberated charge collected, since the increasing field more and more prevents recombination, until ultimately the state is reached when further increase of voltage produces no further increase in collection. *Saturation* has been achieved, in which every ion formed is being collected: none recombine and no further increase in collection is possible. It is obviously essential to the proper working of the Standard Chamber—and, in fact, for any ionization chamber—that the applied (or polarizing, as it is often called) voltage should be sufficient to produce saturation conditions. Then the charge (Q) collected is independent of the applied voltage (V) and depends only on the exposure (R). For beam intensities usually met in radiology electric fields

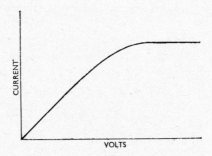

Fig. 60.—The variation of ionization current with applied voltage.

of 100–200 volts per centimetre between the plates of the standard ionization, or the collecting electrodes of another chamber, are adequate.

Temperature and Pressure.—The definition of the roentgen requires the measurement of the charge liberated by the irradiation of a given *mass*, not volume, of air. This means that in an open chamber, such as that described, and in most practical ionization chambers, except those deliberately sealed, the prevailing temperature and pressure must be taken into account, and their differences from normal temperature and pressure (N.T.P.) (760 mm. mercury pressure and 0° C.) allowed for. For example, if a reading M were obtained when the temperature was $T°$ C. and the pressure P mm. Hg, the true reading R is given by:—

$$R = M \times \frac{T+273}{273} \times \frac{760}{P}.$$

It will be recalled that 0° Centigrade is 273° on the gas, or absolute, temperature scale.

DEPARTMENTAL CHAMBERS

The 'Thimble' Chamber.—The 'free-air' chamber, of which only a small number exist in the world, is a standard, and a standardizing instrument, and, measuring nearly a cubic yard in volume, is obviously quite unsuitable for use in the X-ray department, the measurement of dose within a patient, or the assessment of the dose of radiation received by a radiographer during his, or her, work. For these purposes the so-called 'thimble' ionization chamber has been developed. To understand how it works, a few points of theory must be considered.

Imagine that a large volume of air is being uniformly irradiated by a wide beam of X-rays, and consider, specifically, the ionization in a small circumscribed part of this air—say a sphere 1 c.c. in volume. This small volume will, as shown in *Fig.* 61 A, be criss-crossed by electron tracks. The large majority of these tracks will originate outside this volume of interest, whilst tracks starting inside it will produce much of their ionization beyond its confines. On balance, as in the 'free-air' chamber, these lost ionizations will be exactly compensated for by those gained from tracks starting outside—provided that the air volume being considered is surrounded by air to a thickness to the maximum range (R) of electrons set in motion by the X-rays. If all the ionization in the little volume could be collected and measured, the answer would give the Exposure in roentgens since the process takes place entirely in air. In passing it must be noted that the great bulk of the ionization produced in the volume arises from electrons which were liberated in its surrounding air.

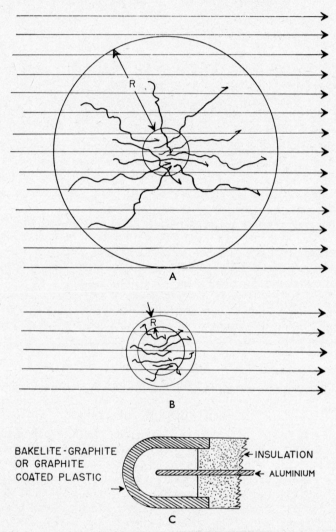

Fig. 61.—The development of the 'thimble' ionization chamber. A, Ionization in air; B, the solid air wall; C, the 'thimble' chamber.

Now the situation within the little volume would not be altered if the surrounding air, out to range R, were 'solidified' to give a 'wall' to the air volume (*Fig.* 61 B). The measurement of the ionization in an air cavity of known volume, surrounded by an appropriately thick 'wall', still satisfies the requirements for the measurement of roentgens.

Neither of the arrangements described is, to say the least, particularly practicable! But they do indicate the essential requirements for an ionization chamber to measure roentgens, viz., a known volume of air, enclosed within a wall of material identical, as far as radiation is concerned, with air, and of thickness at least equal to the range of the most energetic primary electrons liberated by the X-rays. They also stress that the 'wall' of the ionization chamber is of paramount importance, since it contributes the bulk of the ionization that is to be measured. Solid air is obviously unsuitable (!) and therefore a substitute has to be found. This must not only have an atomic number as nearly as possible equal to that of air, but at the same time it must be an electrical conductor, since the 'wall' has to serve as one electrode in the charge-collecting system. *Fig.* 61 C shows the most common—though not the only—form of ionization chamber. The 'wall'—or cap—is shaped rather like a sewing thimble—hence the name. Into it, but insulated from it, protrudes a rod of some material whose atomic number is also close to that of air. This is the other electrode of the charge-measuring system (usually called the 'central electrode') and this simple arrangement constitutes one of the most important items in radiation dosemetry. All that remains is to provide some method of measuring the liberated charge—not, in fact, an easy but by no means an insuperable problem, which will be discussed later.

Wall or Cap Material.—The average atomic number of air is 7·62 and in practice ionization chamber walls have been made either of conducting mixtures of bakelite and graphite, sometimes with other slightly higher atomic number materials added to get the right atomic number 'balance', or of bakelite or some other plastic (mainly made of hydrogen, oxygen, and carbon) coated on the inside with a conducting layer of carbon, in the form of graphite. These latter walls generally have an average, or effective, atomic number which is closer to that of carbon ($Z = 6$) than air. Therefore, because the ionization depends on the interaction of radiation with the material and generally depends on atomic number, these wall materials tend to contribute less ionization to the cavity than would an air wall. Such a chamber is less sensitive than it should be. However, there is a second electrode which also plays a part, and it can be used to provide compensation for the lower-than-air atomic number of the wall. This is done by choosing, for this central electrode, a material whose atomic number is greater, though not too much greater, than that of air. Aluminium ($Z = 13$) is usually used, being the conducting material whose atomic number is closest to that of air and yet greater than it. The relatively small amount of this high atomic number material, used in conjunction with the much larger surface of graphite with its rather too low atomic number, can produce an ionization chamber which behaves almost as if it were entirely made of air.

Chamber Size.—The amount of charge liberated in an ionization chamber depends on the product of two quantities, the chamber volume and the amount of radiation; 1 roentgen gives 1 e.s.u. of charge in 1 c.c. of air; 1 roentgen in 1 litre of air (1000 c.c.) gives 1000 e.s.u.; 20 roentgens in 5 c.c. give 100 e.s.u., and so on. The electrostatic unit of charge is a very small amount of charge and difficult to measure, so that it would seem reasonable to ease the measurement problem by using large ionization chambers. Unfortunately this is seldom possible. For example, the ionization chamber that is used to measure the distribution of radiation in a patient, or in a block of material ('phantom') simulating a patient, has to be small in order to detect the rapid changes of dose that may occur from one point to another. In such cases chamber volumes of from half to one cubic centimetre are usual. For measuring the small amounts of radiation that radiographers may receive during their work, chambers of a few cubic centimetres' volume may be used, whilst for surveying departments for stray radiation, volumes up to a litre are employed. Even in the latter case, however, the amounts of charge that have to be measured are very small, so that sensitive instruments have to be used. Many examples of these could be given, starting with the simple, and sensitive, gold-leaf electroscope which was so valuable in the early days of radiology. Nowadays electronic circuits of considerable sensitivity and reliability are almost always used.

The Measuring System.—Just as a motor-car has two indicators connected with its movement, namely, an odometer which indicates the total distance travelled, and a speedometer which indicates the speed at any instant—in miles or kilometres per hour —so, in radiology, there is a need for two distinct types of measuring instrument. The first, corresponding to the odometer, is the Exposure meter (still usually called the dosemeter) which adds up the total Exposure, in roentgens usually, to which the place has been subjected, whilst the second is the Exposure-rate meter (doserate meter) which measures the Exposure per unit time, in roentgens, or fractions of roentgens, per hour, minute, or second.

The Exposure Meter.—The general principles of the circuit used in this type of instrument are shown in *Fig.* 62 A. A highly insulated lead connects the central electrode of the 'thimble' chamber to one plate of a condenser F, whilst the chamber wall is connected through the polarizing battery to the other plate of the condenser. The voltage supplied by the battery must be high enough to 'saturate' the ionization chamber, and about 200 volts per centimetre of gap between central electrode and wall are usually provided.

Irradiation of the chamber produces ionization in its air, and the negative ions are attracted to the central electrode, whilst positive ions are pulled towards the chamber wall. As soon as the irradiation starts, therefore, the liberated electrical charge (Q) starts to flow through the circuit into the condenser (F), which is thereby charged up to a voltage (V). The three quantities are related by the simple formula:

$$V = Q/F, \text{ where } F \text{ is the condenser capacity.}$$

Measurement of the voltage is thus essentially measurement of the charge liberated, and hence of the Exposure. The increase of the voltage continues until the end of the irradiation, and then the voltage reading indicates the total Exposure used. Having made such a reading the switch S is closed to discharge the condenser, and then reopened for the next irradiation.

The measurement is not easy. In the first place the magnitude of the liberated charge is small, so that the condenser capacity has to be small if reasonable voltages are to be produced. This in its turn means that the measuring instrument must have an even smaller capacity and, furthermore, it must have a very high resistance, if it is not to discharge the condenser continuously. Such conditions can only be achieved with very special electrometers or with electronic circuits using thermionic valves or transistors. These are often complex in their details but fortunately this need not concern us: the principle of their use is the simple one shown in the diagram.

The Exposure-rate Meter.—If the condenser F, in the circuit just described, is replaced by a resistance R (*Fig.* 62 B) the device is converted from an Exposure to an Exposure-rate meter. The collection of the ions produced by the irradiation of the chamber causes a current I to flow in the circuit, and this current generates a voltage $E (= IR)$ across the resistance R through which it flows. Electric current is the rate of passage of charge, and hence the current in this case depends on the rate of liberation of charge in the chamber, and this in turn depends on the radiation Exposure rate therein. Since E is proportional to I, which in turn is proportional to the Exposure rate, then the measurement of E is essentially the measurement of Exposure rate.

Such measurement, as in the Exposure meter, is not easy. The smallness of the ionization current has already been mentioned several times, and a measurable voltage can only be obtained by using, at R, very high resistances—of the order of 10^{10} or 10^{11} ohms. This in itself is not specially difficult but the measurement of the generated voltage is. It must be recalled that a voltmeter must have a resistance which is high compared with the resistance across which the voltage is being measured, and usually

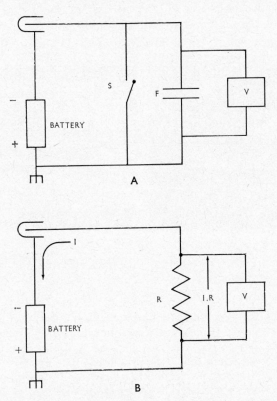

Fig. 62.—The basic circuits of A, the Exposure meter and B, the Exposure-rate meter.

there is a factor of about 1000 between the two. In this case, therefore, the voltmeter would have to have a resistance of 10^{13} or 10^{14} ohms, which is quite out of the question with a moving-coil, or any other, meter of the dial and pointer type. As for the Exposure meter, such a high-resistance voltmeter is now usually achieved by the use of electronic circuits, or so-called 'valve voltmeters'.

One final minor point might be mentioned. In the Exposure meter the instrument reading increases continuously as long as the irradiation continues, because that instrument is adding up (integrating) the charge liberated. With the Exposure-rate meter, the reading instantaneously comes up to the appropriate value and—assuming that the irradiation is constant—stays at that value, no matter how long the Exposure, because it is measuring the rate of flow. When the irradiation ceases the reading immediately falls to zero because the current has ceased to flow: there is therefore no need to have a switch in the Exposure-rate meter to perform this function performed by *F* in the Exposure meter.

Practical Instruments.—In practice the circuits of Exposure and Exposure-rate meters can be quite complicated in order to achieve the sensitivity and reliability demanded for clinical use. Nevertheless, the principles of their operation are simple as already shown, and they are also simple to use. *Fig.* 63 A shows an example of a widely used commercial instrument, with its ionization chamber at the end of a long lead, which enables the operator to be outside the treatment room whilst taking the readings. The relative simplicity of the controls, and the voltmeter on which the answer (in this case, Exposure) is revealed, should be noted.

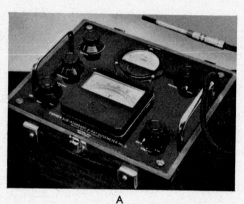 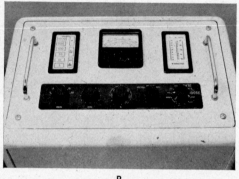

A   B

Fig. 63.—A, A simple and accurate practical Exposure meter; B, The control panel of a multi-range instrument.

It is often convenient to be able to measure different ranges of Exposure, or Exposure rate, or both on the same instrument. This simply means a complication of the details but not of the principle of the instrument. For a number of condensers of different capacity may be available, and selected by appropriate switching so that 0–1, 0–10, or 0–100 roentgens could be measured. Or, by having a selection of resistances, a similar range of Exposure rates could be dealt with. *Fig.* 63 B shows the control table of an instrument that offers the possibility of a range of both Exposure and Exposure-rate measurements merely by the manipulation of a few switches.

The Condenser Exposure Meter.—For the instruments so far described the ionization chamber is permanently connected to the measuring system by a highly insulated lead. For some purposes this is advantageous but, for others, it is convenient to be able to detach the chamber. This is done in what is often called the *condenser* meter, in which the ionization chamber is permanently attached to—and is often an integral part of—an electrical condenser.

Two simple examples of 'condenser' chambers are illustrated in *Fig.* 64, which shows, diagrammatically, cross section details of the construction of the BD.11 and BD.2 chambers originally designed by physicists working under the aegis of the British Medical Research Council. They are made of a bakelite and graphite mixture to which a small amount of vanadium pentoxide has been added, to give a material which is closely 'air-equivalent'. The larger chamber is about 5 cm. long and 1·5 cm.

in external diameter, and is mainly used for personal radiation protection measurements, whilst the smaller chamber is suitable for measurements on patients or even in body cavities. It is 1·3 cm. long and has a diameter of 9 mm.

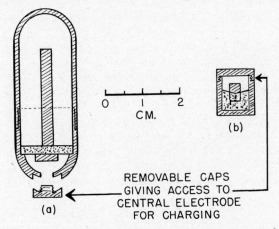

REMOVABLE CAPS
GIVING ACCESS TO
CENTRAL ELECTRODE
FOR CHARGING

(a)

Fig. 64.—Two types of 'condenser' chamber.

Both these ionization chambers are concentric cylinder condensers, the capacity of the BD.2 being considerably increased by the dielectric which fills half of the interior. In use the central electrode is charged up to a certain voltage, detached from the charging device, and irradiated. When the irradiation is complete the residual voltage is measured. The *loss* of voltage is a measure of the Exposure to which the chamber has been subjected.

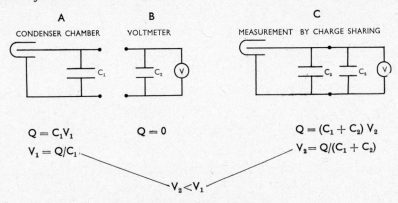

Fig. 65.—The 'charge-sharing' process.

The charging process can be regarded as the storing of a certain amount of charge (assume it to be positive charge) on the central electrode. Irradiation of the chamber liberates positive and negative ions and the latter are attracted to the positively charged central electrode, where they neutralize some of the stored charge. This loss of charge lowers the electrical potential, the change in potential being proportional to the loss of charge which equals the charge liberated by the irradiation. Thus if the change of voltage can be measured, the Exposure is measured.

Charge Sharing.—Whilst the voltage to which the condenser is charged initially can be known indirectly from the voltage of the source, the voltage residual after irradiation has to be measured directly from the chamber. This is usually done by the 'charge-sharing' method.

The condenser chamber, as has already been said, is both ion chamber and electrical capacity (C_1) and it may be represented diagrammatically by separating the two features, as is done in *Fig. 65 A*. Similarly a voltmeter will have some, albeit small, electrical capacity (C_2) and may also be represented by a separation, as in *Fig. 65 B*, into an indicator and a condenser. Imagine now that the chamber is at some unknown voltage and has to be connected to the voltmeter so that the voltage may be measured (*Fig. 56 C*). Assume the chamber voltage to be V_1, so that it stores a charge $Q\,(=C_1V_1)$. The voltmeter is initially uncharged, and when the chamber is connected to it the charge Q is shared between the meter and the chamber. Since the connexion puts the two 'condensers' in parallel the total capacity is now ($C_1 + C_2$) and therefore the voltage (V_2) resulting from the charge Q is $\{Q/(C_1 + C_2)\}$. Since $V_1 = Q/C_1$ it will be clear that the voltmeter indicates a voltage *lower* than the true

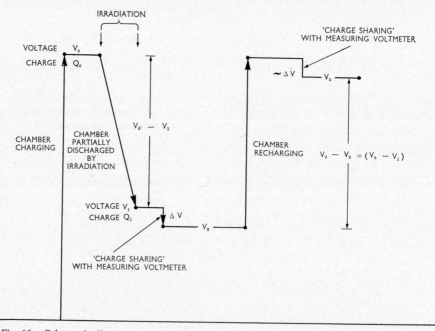

Fig. 66.—Schematic diagram of the results of charging, irradiation, charge sharing, etc., of a 'condenser' chamber for the measurement of the voltage change due to irradiation.

value which was to be measured. The difference can be minimized by keeping the voltmeter capacity as low as possible relative to the chamber capacity, but it cannot be eliminated entirely. Fortunately, it can be allowed for fairly easily, as may be seen by considering, with the aid of *Fig. 66*, the steps actually taken in the use of one of these 'condenser' chambers to measure radiation.

It will be recalled that in order to measure the Exposure it is necessary to determine the charge liberated by the radiation in the chamber, or the charge lost by the central electrode, and that this can be done by measuring the voltage change.

Initially the chamber is charged to a voltage V_0, and stores a charge of Q_0. If it is then irradiated its stored charge falls, say, to Q_1, and its voltage to V_1. The value of $(V_0 - V_1)$ is a measure of the Exposure. The residual chamber voltage is measured by charge sharing with a suitable voltmeter which, for reasons given, gives a reading of V_2 which is less than V_1 by an amount, which is unknown in magnitude, of ΔV. However, if the chamber is recharged to V_0 and immediately, without irradiation, has its voltage measured by the charge-sharing method, a value of V_3 will be recorded. Since the voltage change in this case will be practically the same as that, ΔV, in the measurement of the residual voltage, it can be assumed that the observed difference $(V_3 - V_2)$ equals the required difference $(V_0 - V_1)$.

Now the Exposure is measured by the charge liberated per unit volume at N.T.P.

$$\therefore \text{Exposure} = \frac{Q_0 - Q_1}{\text{Chamber volume}} = \frac{C_1(V_0 - V_1)}{\text{Chamber volume}} = \frac{C_1(V_3 - V_2)}{\text{Chamber volume}}.$$

Since in general neither the chamber volume nor its electrical capacity is known, most chambers are first calibrated by recording the voltage changes following irradiation to known Exposures, and from a calibration curve any other Exposure can be determined.

Chamber Voltage.—In this sort of device it is essential that the voltage between the central electrode and the outer case should always be sufficient to 'saturate' the chamber. This means that the charge initially stored on the central electrode must be large compared with the charge that will be liberated by the Exposure to be measured. It is for this reason that the chamber has to have a large electrical capacity—that it must be a condenser as well as an ionization chamber.

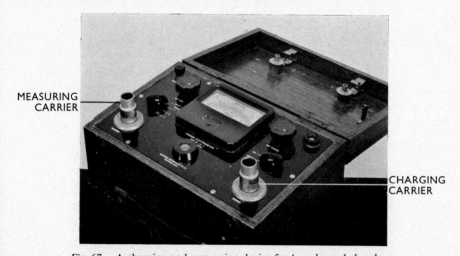

MEASURING CARRIER

CHARGING CARRIER

Fig. 67.—A charging and measuring device for 'condenser' chambers.

Practical Instruments.—Fig. 67 shows the charging and measuring device used with the BD.11 and BD.2 chambers already mentioned. For charging the chamber is placed, as shown, in the right-hand carrier, whilst for charge sharing it is placed in the left-hand carrier and the shared voltage read on the meter—a compact, sturdy, reliable, and sensitive instrument.

The Victoreen Exposure Meter, long the mainstay of radiological dosemetry, is another example of a condenser meter.

THE INSTRUMENTS IN PRACTICE

Wall Thickness.—One of the stated conditions that has to be fulfilled before an ionization chamber measures roentgens is that its wall thickness must be at least equal to the range of the electrons produced by the radiation that is being measured. Now, that thickness will be different for different radiation energies. For example, assuming for simplicity that the wall is of graphite, a fraction of a millimetre will suffice at 50 kV., whereas 5 cm. would be needed for 20-million-volt radiation. In practice, it is customary to use a wall which is about 1 mm. thick, since this is not only reasonably strong to withstand ordinary handling, but it is also suitable for radiations up to about 300 kV. Where higher-energy radiations have to be measured, it is usual to supplement the original wall thickness with close-fitting caps of perspex or other plastic, which bring the total wall thickness up to that needed for the radiation in question.

There is, however, another wall effect that must not be forgotten. Not only does the wall contribute the bulk of the ionizing particles to the air volume, but it does so by attenuating the beam being measured. In other words, the measurement process disturbs the very thing that is being measured. Such disturbance must, obviously, be kept to a minimum, and the ideal ionization chamber has a wall thickness which is no more than an electron range thick. Even the effect of that thickness, however, may have to be taken into account.

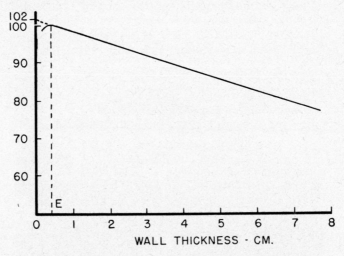

Fig. 68.—The effect of wall thickness on ionization chamber response.

The influence of wall thickness on measured ionization is shown in *Fig.* 68. A wall thinner than *E* contributes too few electrons, whilst if the thickness is greater than *E* the measured effect is reduced because of attenuation of the beam in the wall. Even the required thickness *E* reduces the beam to a small extent, the true Exposure being a per cent or so greater than that indicated. An idea of the magnitude can be found, for any particular radiation quality, by making measurements with caps of various thickness slipped over the normal cap, and then extrapolating back to zero thickness as shown in *Fig.* 68.

As will be seen below, this wall effect is usually allowed for in the calibration of any instrument, but it must be remembered that because a practical Exposure meter must have a compromise wall thickness (it would be impracticable to have a different cap for every radiation energy to be measured) the wall attenuation effect will be most marked at low energies. Normally an ionization chamber has a wall thickness suitable for 200–300-kV. radiation—unless it is designed specifically for some softer radiation—and caps are slipped over it when great wall thickness is called for in the measurement of higher-energy radiations.

Calibration.—The response of a radiation meter to a given Exposure or Exposure rate is influenced by a number of material factors like the air volume, the wall thickness, the air equivalence of the material of the wall and of the central electrode, and the sensitivity of the electrical measuring system. Clearly it is impossible to forecast precisely the exact magnitude of so many different factors, especially for a variety of radiation qualities. The makers—whether commercial or private—of this sort of equipment do the best they can, often making provision for some adjustments to be made, and generally producing instruments whose readings can be accepted, without further investigation, as being correct to a few per cent. For higher accuracy (and it is desirable in many cases to be accurate to 1 per cent) it is usual for an instrument to be compared with the 'free-air' standard chamber, and to be given factors by which readings should be multiplied to give roentgens or roentgen rates. These calibrations should be carried out for each radiation quality at which the instrument is likely to be used, and they should also be repeated at regular (say two-yearly) intervals to check the constancy of the equipment. In between these major calibrations, meters should receive local constancy checks at monthly or two-monthly intervals. Such checks are best carried out by placing the ionization chamber in an easily, and accurately, reproducible position relative to some radioactive source providing a known radiation Exposure rate.

Table X.—CALIBRATION FACTORS FOR AN EXPOSURE METER

The instrument reading is multiplied by the appropriate factor from the second row, to give the Exposure in roentgens

Generating voltage	300 kV.	200 kV.	175 kV.	150 kV.	100 kV.	75 kV.	50 kV.	40 kV.	30 kV.
Multiplying factor	1·02	1·02	1·01	1·00	1·02	1·06	1·13	1·18	1·27

The Calibration Factors.—*Table X* shows a set of factors such as might be given by a standardizing laboratory for a departmental meter. They are the factors by which the instrument reading has to be multiplied for radiations of various energies, and their variation over the energy range is of considerable interest.

At the high-energy end of the quality range covered by this table, the ionization produced is almost entirely due to Compton scattering, and is largely independent of the materials used in the chamber wall and the central electrode. The effect of wall attenuation will also be very small, so that the factor indicates any effect of chamber volume, and/or measuring section sensitivity. In this case the chamber volume is slightly too small, or the instrument sensitivity is a shade too low or, of course, there is a combination of these effects, and any reading has to be slightly increased to give the true value. These errors will, of course, be the same at all radiation energies.

With decrease of radiation energy the photo-electric effect plays an increasingly important part in the interaction of the component parts of the chamber, and in the production of ionization. Since the photo-electric effect varies with the third power of the atomic number, the precise composition of this wall and central electrode becomes increasingly important at the lower energies. The reduction in the correction factor, indicating that the instrument becomes more sensitive for lower-energy radiations, also indicates that the effective atomic number of the chamber is somewhat greater than that of air.

There is, of course, a further important factor which comes increasingly into play at the low-energy end of the range under review. This is the wall attenuation of the X-ray beam. If this effect had no influence the atomic number effect would increase the sensitivity of this chamber more and more, and correspondingly reduce the factor —as the radiation energy was reduced. However, this factor reduction is reversed because the compromise wall thickness (*see above*) is greater than is needed at low energies, and its effect is to cut down the beam as described by *Fig.* 68. The lower the radiation energy the greater is this effect, and hence the greater the value of the correction that has to be used. For very low-energy radiation—such as the 10-kV. 'Grenz' rays—special ionization chambers, with very thin walls, have to be used. 'Thimble' chambers of the conventional type are far too thick walled for this range.

CHAPTER XI

THE GEIGER-MÜLLER AND SCINTILLATION COUNTERS AND THE THERMOLUMINESCENCE DOSEMETER

COUNTERS

As was pointed out in the last chapter, the charge liberated in an ionization chamber depends upon the radiation Exposure and upon the volume of the ionization chamber. Therefore, if very small Exposures have to be measured, it is usual to use chambers of considerable volume. For example, the ionization chamber that might be used to survey an X-ray department for 'stray' radiation, and thus measure Exposures of a few milliroentgens per second (1 milliroentgen (m.R) is one-thousandth of a roentgen), might have a volume of about 1 litre. By way of comparison it will be recalled that the ionization chamber used to measure patient doses in radiotherapy may have a volume of about 0·2 ml.

Even with the large volume, however, the charge liberated is quite small; 1 m.R per second would liberate 1/1000 e.s.u. of charge per ml. per second, or 1 e.s.u. per litre per second, and this latter would constitute a current of about 3×10^{-11} amp. This tiny current calls for very sensitive apparatus for its measurement and yet it arises from a huge number of actual events. The charge on the electron, and therefore on the singly charged ion, is $4·8 \times 10^{-10}$ e.s.u., which means that the charge liberated, and collected, per second in our example must have come from about 2×10^9 ions. An early chapter has already described how the large bulk of the ionization produced by X- or gamma rays is secondary ionization produced by the primary electrons liberated when the photons interact with matter. Assuming that each primary electron produces about 1000 ionizations before it loses all its energy, the observed current must come from about 2×10^6, that is about 2 million photon interactions.

Now it is seldom necessary to measure Exposure rates much below a few milliroentgens per second, and therefore the ionization chamber can be said to do all that is required of it at this low-rate end of the range. However, it may be necessary to detect and record much smaller amounts of ionization than those mentioned. For example, it is often necessary to know the rate at which radioactive atoms are decaying (in order, for instance, to assess the number present in some material). Each time a radioactive nucleus decays radiation is emitted: for example, a beta particle possibly accompanied by a gamma ray may be given off. The latter ionizes like an X-ray photon, by producing a primary electron which produces much secondary ionization. The beta particle is, of course, a fast electron and ionizes just like the primary electron produced by the photon. Each agent is therefore responsible for a considerable amount of ionization. From radioactive phosphorus (^{32}P), for example, come beta particles of average energy about 0·65 MeV. and since, on the average, 34 eV. are required for each ionization, such a particle will produce about 20,000 ionizations before it is brought to rest. This, by most standards, is a very large number, but it is small compared with the two thousand million (2×10^9) ionizations produced by the small Exposure rate discussed above, in the 1 litre-chamber, and it would certainly not be able to produce a measurable effect in an ionization chamber of practical size. In order to detect and record the ionization due to a nuclear disintegration—that is to say to be able to *count* nuclear events—some device other than an ion chamber is needed. There are two main alternatives.

THE GEIGER-MÜLLER COUNTER

This once almost universally used device depends on the enormous amplification of charge that can be obtained in a gas under appropriate conditions. An electron liberated in a gas between two charged electrodes will be attracted towards the anode gaining speed as it goes until checked by collision with a gas atom. Then either it is attached to the atom to form a much heavier negative ion which then continues to drift, but much more slowly, towards the anode, or, having lost practically all its speed, it starts all over again and gradually regains speed. No high-speed particles are, therefore, produced. At reduced gas pressure the chances of collision are very much less and if one of the inert gases is used the chance of the electron attaching itself to a gas atom is also considerably less. Therefore, the electron can attain greater velocity and energy between collisions and if the electric field is strong enough it may acquire enough energy to ionize any atom with which it collides. The electron continues on its way with temporarily reduced but increasing speed accompanied by the extra liberated electrons. The corresponding positive ions drift slowly towards the cathode. This is 'ionization by collision' and is the basis of the *gas-amplification* in the Geiger-Müller counter.

Though there are many shapes and sizes of Geiger-Müller counter, depending on the purpose for which the device is being used, the basic design is that shown in *Fig.* 69.

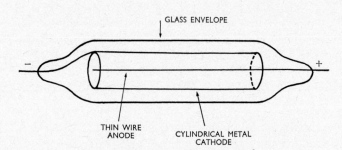

GLASS ENVELOPE

THIN WIRE
ANODE

CYLINDRICAL METAL
CATHODE

Fig. 69.—The basic design of a Geiger-Müller counter.

Essentially it consists of a cylindrical cathode with a very thin wire anode stretched along its axis. These electrodes are mounted inside a usually thin envelope—often made of glass—containing gas at low pressure. Common dimensions are a cathode 2 cm. in diameter and 5 cm. long and a central wire of 0·2 mm. diameter. The gas is usually a mixture of 9 parts of an inert gas, such as argon, with 1 part alcohol vapour at a pressure of about 10 cm. Hg., the exact value depending on the counter design and dimensions. Alternatively, a halogen gas is used to replace the alcohol. This type of counter has the advantage that it operates at a lower voltage (*see below*) and has a rather longer life. The potential difference across the counter is usually between 900 and 1500 volts for an alcohol-filled tube and between 200 and 400 volts for a halogen-filled tube. However, within these ranges, the value is not critical since there is a 'plateau' in which region the counting rate is almost independent of the value of the voltage.

The high voltage produces a very intense electric field in the vicinity of the thin-wire anode whilst the low gas pressure gives the electrons the freedom from collisions needed for their attaining ionizing speed and energy. Not only the initial electrons liberated by the radiation being detected, but also their secondary electrons, surge inwards towards the anode liberating yet more electrons and, by complex processes which need not be detailed, yield an amplification over 10^8, i.e., for every electron produced initially somewhere between 100 million and 1000 million reach the anode. A single electron releases a veritable avalanche of charge; the immeasurably small charge liberated by the initial photon or ionizing particle, therefore, results in a 'pulse' of charge which is readily measurable. Thus the Geiger-Müller counter can be used to detect and count the passage through it of single photons or ionizing particles.

The Geiger-Müller counter has now been largely superseded by the scintillation counter, and the reason for this can be understood by a rather close look at some features of the operation of the Geiger-Müller counter. Firstly, it is not very efficient in the detection of high-energy beta particles and of gamma rays. This is due to the fact that the envelope wall and cathode are usually thin and with the low-pressure gas offer relatively little absorption possibilities to high-energy radiation. For gamma rays an ordinary Geiger-Müller counter is about 1 per cent efficient, whilst if it is fitted with a lead cylinder as its cathode, the efficiency rises to 5 per cent.

The second feature to be noted is that the magnitude of the charge 'pulse' produced by ionization in the counter is independent of the event initiating it, be it a photon interaction, the passage of a beta or an alpha particle or any other cause. The Geiger-Müller counter cannot, in other words, discriminate between different types of radiation. Finally when the 'avalanche' is started it persists for about 300 millionths of a second (300 microseconds or 300 μsec.). This may seem negligibly short in our common experience but it can be of importance at high counting rates because during that period (the 'dead time' as it is called) the counter will not record any other particles which may arrive and, therefore, may give too low a reading.

SCINTILLATION COUNTING

Though very sensitive and though invaluable in the past for radioactivity measurements, the disadvantages of the Geiger-Müller counter, which are outlined above, led to a search for an alternative. Attention, in particular, returned to one of the earliest methods used in the detection of ionizing radiations, namely using their fluorescent effect.

Very early studies of radioactivity revealed that zinc sulphide, for example, 'scintillated' when irradiated with ionizing radiations, and the phenomenon was used for some of the earliest counting methods. It was used, for example, in experiments which led Rutherford to the concept of the nuclear atom. Since the tiny amounts of light were extremely difficult to see and the method extremely tedious it was abandoned in favour of the Geiger-Müller counter. However, the development of the photo-multiplier tube as well as the discovery of new scintillators or 'phosphors', as they are often called (though they fluoresce rather than phosphoresce), has enabled a very powerful new method to be developed on the basis of the old one.

Suitable Scintillators.—As has been described in CHAPTER VIII, many materials fluoresce when irradiated with ionizing radiations but very few are suitable for the radiation counting method to be described, the desirable features for which are that the materials should readily absorb ionizing radiations and should be transparent to the fluorescence photons produced. High atomic number materials are, of course, the best absorbers but they are seldom transparent. They can only be used in thin layers, since only surface scintillations can be seen, and as such they are not particularly suitable for detecting hard gamma rays. For such radiation a fairly thick detector is necessary to ensure there is a good chance of photon interaction. It is essential that the thick phosphor is transparent to the light produced. Materials which satisfy these criteria include crystals of anthracene, naphthalene, and of sodium and potassium iodides. Nowadays many plastic phosphors, often in very large pieces, are also used and for some important applications scintillating liquids are used.

The Photomultiplier Tube.—The detection and measurement of the emitted light depend on the photomultiplier tube, an electronic device originally developed for the 'talking-picture' industry. Electrons can be ejected from some materials by light photons (the photo-electric effect with visible light). Furthermore, if an electron strikes certain materials with sufficient energy it may cause several electrons to be emitted. These two phenomena are the basis of the photomultiplier tube which is shown diagrammatically in *Fig.* 70. At one end of the highly evacuated tube is the photocathode, an electrode coated with some light-sensitive material which emits electrons when photons of light fall on it. Along the tube at intervals is a series of electrodes, usually called *dynodes*, made of a material which readily emits electrons under electron bombardment (an alloy of caesium and antimony is such a material). Each of these electrodes is at a progressively higher positive electrical potential compared with its neighbour, from which it is shielded.

Mode of Action.—Assume that a visible photon produces a single electron at the photocathode. This electron is accelerated by the electric field to the first dynode where, on striking, it liberates, say, two electrons. In their turn they are pulled to dynode number 2 where they produce four electrons, which liberate eight at dynode 3, and these go on to give sixteen at dynode 4, and so on. With 10 dynodes over

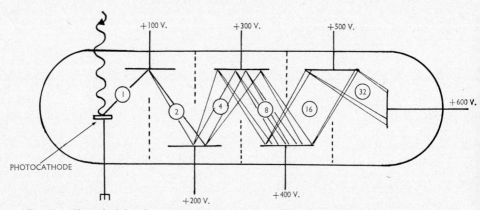

Fig. 70.—The principle of operation of a photomultiplier tube. The numbers in the circles indicate the amplification being produced at each stage of this example.

1000 electrons would reach the tube anode. For a practical photomultiplier tube the secondary emission coefficient is about 5, so that starting from a single electron liberated by a photon, a current of 5^{10} electrons would reach the anode, an amplification of nearly 10 millionfold.

The Counter and its Mode of Action.—To use the scintillation effect for counting radiation the phosphor is placed in close proximity to the photocathode end of the photomultiplier tube (e.g., see *Fig.* 292, p. 402) so that as much as possible of the light produced reaches the photocathode. To aid this the side of the phosphor is polished or whitened to reflect back any light that might otherwise have escaped unused. Of course, all external light must be excluded from the system since any light reaching the photomultiplier tube is inappropriately measured: as if it had been radiation induced. The photomultiplier tube and phosphor are usually housed inside a thick metal shield for both mechanical and radiation protection, but naturally the outer face of the phosphor cannot be so shielded without excluding the very radiation to be measured. This face is made lightproof by a layer of some very thin opaque material which excludes light but allows all but the lowest energy beta particles to pass through. It must be remembered, of course, that this film is very fragile and great care must be taken to ensure that it is not punctured.

When very low-energy radiations have to be measured or in some cases when extreme sensitivity is called for, use is made of a liquid scintillator. In this case the sample to be counted is mixed with the scintillating fluid in a glass tube which is then placed close to the photomultiplier tube, all contained in a lightproof enclosure.

Being a solid (or liquid), the detector of a scintillation counter has nearly 10,000 times as many atoms per unit volume as the low-pressure gas in the Geiger-Müller counter, so that the likelihood of interaction with incident radiation is very much greater. As a result, much smaller amounts of radiation can be detected per unit volume of detector.

The size of each pulse of light produced in the scintillator depends on the amount of energy absorbed from the incident photon or particle and hence on the photon energy. Since the output of the photomultiplier tube depends on the amount of light reaching its photocathode, the size of the electrical pulse from the anode will be proportional to the energy of the photon or particle. The higher the energy the larger the pulse, the lower the energy the smaller the pulse, which is in marked contrast to the behaviour of the Geiger-Müller tube the pulses from which are all of the same size regardless of the radiation energy. With both the Geiger-Müller counter and the scintillation counter the *number* of pulses is a measure of the number of photons or particles interacting.

It is because the pulse size is dependent upon the radiation energy that the scintillation counter can be used to 'discriminate' between different radiations. This is achieved electronically. The circuit detecting the output pulses from the photomultiplier tube can be set to reject all pulses of below or of above a pre-set size or to accept only pulses falling between selected upper and lower size limits. A 'window' is produced, the size and place of which (in the energy range) can be varied. Such a window can reduce the amount of stray or 'background' radiation (*see below*) being counted and is particularly valuable for counting one radioactive isotope in the presence of another. For example, chromium 51, which emits 322 kV. gamma rays, and serum albumin 'labelled' with iodine 125 (which emits 28 and 35 kV. gamma rays) can be used in blood studies to measure, respectively, the red-cell and plasma 'volumes'. By setting the 'window' to accept pulses produced by radiation of between say 250 and 350 kV., the chromium 51 alone will be counted. A 'window' set for 20–40 kV. will measure the iodine 125, though it will also count some scattered radiation from the 322-kV. photons and allowance must be made for this.

Finally, there is the question of 'dead time', a phenomenon which exists for the photomultiplier tube but is very much shorter than in the Geiger-Müller counter. It has two components—the duration of the light flash and the passage of the electrons down the photomultiplier tube. The latter is of the order of one-hundredth of a microsecond (10^{-8} μsec.); the former is considerably longer, being of the order of 1 μsec. in naphthalene and ten times that in zinc sulphide. Even so, the total time during which the system is unable to detect a second scintillation is small compared with the Geiger-Müller counter 'dead time'.

Because of its greater counting efficiency, its shorter 'dead time', and, perhaps above all, its ability to discriminate between different types and energies of radiation, the scintillation counter has largely replaced the Geiger-Müller counter for the detection and measurement of radioactive radiation.

Counting Problems

'*Dead time*' *Correction.*—If a counter, with a 'dead time' of τ records a count rate of N counts per second allowance can be made, using the formula given below, for any counts lost by particles or photons arriving during those periods when the counter was 'dead', having just received another particle or photon. The true count rate (N_T) is given by:

$$N_T = N/(1 - N\tau).$$

The formula is based on the assumption that—on the average—the rate is constant.

For most clinical situations (recorded count rates up to 10 per sec.) no correction is really necessary even with the Geiger-Müller counter ($\tau = 3 \times 10^{-4}$ sec.). If $N = 10$, then

$$N_T = 10/(1 - 10 \times 3 \times 10^{-4}) = 10 \cdot 03.$$

However, with an intense source, an observed Geiger counter count rate of 1000 counts per sec. would mean a true rate of:

$$N_T = 1000/(1 - 10^3 \times 3 \times 10^{-4}) = 1429.$$

A nearly 50 per cent correction indicates that the Geiger-Müller counter is not satisfactory for such high rates. With the scintillation counter ('dead time' of, say, 5×10^{-5} sec.)

$$N_T = 1000/(1 - 10^3 \times 5 \times 10^{-5}) = 1050,$$

a much more acceptable situation.

Background Counting Rate.—A counter set up to detect radiation records some counts even when no source is apparently near it. The counts are partly due to cosmic rays and partly due to radiation from traces of radioactivity in the earth, the atmosphere, the materials of our buildings, or even the materials from which the counter itself is made. There may also be radiation from radioactive materials contaminating the equipment from previous measurements, though scrupulous care should be taken to avoid this. 'Background' is the term usually used to describe this effect. Nearby sources of radiation, being stored or used for other purposes, may also contribute to 'background'. In such cases it is essential that such sources should be kept stationary during any measurements and their contribution, therefore, kept constant. Allowance must always be made for 'background' when making measurements, especially of weak sources. For example, if N counts per minute are recorded when a source is being measured and n counts per minute are observed when the source is removed (i.e., this is the 'background' counting rate) the source alone must be producing ($N - n$) counts per minute. 'Background' varies from place to place and it can usually be reduced considerably, though not entirely eliminated, by screening the counter with lead and, in the case of the scintillation counter, by a suitable discrimination procedure. Many measurements can be carried out in protected enclosures or 'castles' made of slabs of lead two or so inches thick. *Fig.* 71 shows one such enclosure with a Geiger-Müller counter.

Statistical Fluctuations.—When a series of, say, 1-minute observations are made with a counter exposed to a given source, the readings obtained show fluctuations, a typical sequence of 10 being:

102, 99, 97, 112, 100, 101, 88, 101, 95, 104.

This does not, necessarily at least, reflect upon the stability of the instrument because such fluctuations are inherent in the nature of the emission of radiation from radioactive sources which, it will be recalled from CHAPTER III, is a random process.

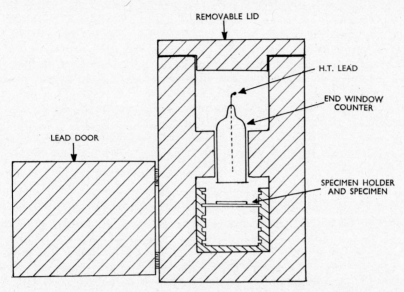

Fig. 71.—A protective 'castle' to reduce the background radiation reaching a counter.

Although 'on the average' radioactive decay (and hence radiation emission) proceeds at a constant rate, the number of nuclei disintegrating in any short interval of time will fluctuate according to statistical laws. A discussion of these can involve a knowledge of mathematics beyond that expected of the readers of this book, but certain fairly simple rules can be given.

If a total of N counts is recorded in, say, 1 minute, then it is very likely though not actually certain that the average counts per minute from the source lie in the range:

$$N \pm \sqrt{N}.$$

$\sqrt{N}$ is called the *standard deviation* of the observation. Thus, if in 1 minute 100 counts are observed, it can be said that the average count rate very probably lies in the range $100 \pm \sqrt{100} = 100 \pm 10$, i.e., between 90 and 110. The accuracy of the observation is therefore ± 10 per cent. On the other hand, if the record had been 10,000 counts the average could be said to be likely to lie in the range $10,000 \pm \sqrt{10,000}$ or $10,000 \pm 100$, the accuracy now being ± 1 per cent. The greater the number of events counted, the smaller is the uncertainty or error due to statistical fluctuations.

It is for this reason that ionization chamber readings—in contrast with counter results—are not subject to noticeable statistical fluctuations. At the beginning of this chapter a particular observation was said to be due to 2×10^6 interactions. Following the line of argument outlined above the average for the source is likely to lie in the range $2 \times 10^6 \pm \sqrt{(2 \times 10^6)}$ or roughly $2 \times 10^6 \pm 1400$, an error range of about seven parts in ten thousand or ± 0.07 per cent.

Statistical fluctuations of the sort described must be especially remembered when measurements are being made to decide whether two sources are of equal, or unequal, strength. If source *A* gave 144 counts per minute, whilst source *B* gave 132 counts per minute (after due allowance has been made for any 'background' counts) it would be tempting to conclude that source *A* was the stronger. In fact they could very well be equal, for all that we can conclude from these readings is that the average value for *A* lies between 144 ± 12, that is to say between 156 and 132, whilst the value for *B* is likely to lie somewhere between 132 ± 11·5 or roughly 143 and 121. Since the two ranges overlap there is a good chance that the sources are equal—or, to be more precise, there is no evidence of any difference between them. Before two readings can be taken as being 'statistically significantly different' it is usual to require that the difference between them shall be twice the standard error of their average. In this example, for the case of the readings given above, the average is (144 + 132)/2 = 138 and the standard error is, therefore, $\sqrt{138}$ or approximately 11·7. Thus, if the two readings were separated by about 23 they could be considered as providing evidence that the two sources were of different strength. Since the difference is only 12, no such difference can be assumed.

THE THERMOLUMINESCENCE DOSEMETER (TLD)

Whilst ionization chambers continue to be used for the majority of X-ray dose measurements an increasing number are now being done with thermoluminescent materials. This is particularly so for measurements of the actual dose received by patients as a result of radiography or radiotherapy exposures. Since the amount of material, and therefore the size, is small and since it also causes very nearly the same attenuation of the X-ray beam as does soft tissue, the TLD can very easily and without detriment be placed on the skin or in a body cavity during exposure.

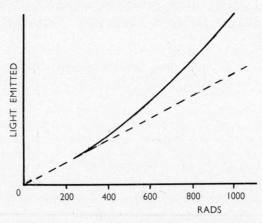

Fig. 72.—The relationship between light emitted and absorbed dose, showing the increase in sensitivity for higher doses. The dotted line shows a strictly linear relationship.

The effect which is used to measure the absorbed dose is, as described on p. 94, that when certain specially prepared crystalline materials, having been previously exposed to ionizing radiation, are subsequently heated, the amount of light emitted is proportional to the absorbed dose in the material resulting from the exposure. In practice it is found that:

1. The total amount of light emitted (called the response) is not perfectly proportional to the absorbed dose. Rather surprisingly the response per rad is greater at higher dose levels. This arises because the exposure creates additional traps and hence makes the material more sensitive at the higher dose levels. The effect is known as supralinearity and results in the variation of response versus dose shown in *Fig.* 72.
2. The response per rad for most TLD systems is dependent on radiation type and quality. For X-rays the variation over the quality range of interest (50 kV.–20 MV., say) is smooth and small, which is to be expected since the TLD material (e.g., activated lithium fluoride) has almost the same average atomic number and electron density as soft tissue, i.e., it is tissue-equivalent.
3. The indicated response (i.e., the value of the read-out instrument reading), as would be expected, depends upon the detailed construction of the equipment used to measure the emitted light.

For these various reasons the TLD system used has to be calibrated appropriately, and the method of doing this is described below (p. 127).

The TLD Reader.—The equipment used to heat the exposed material and measure the emitted light is called a 'TLD Reader'. The reading given by the equipment is used as a measure of the absorbed dose to which the material was subjected. The reader comprises three main parts.

a. *The Heater.*—The irradiated TLD sample is placed on a stainless-steel tray (planchet) and a heater element brought into close contact with the underside of the tray. The temperature of the sample is raised, in a reproducible way, to approximately 300° C by passing an electric current through the element.

b. *The Photomultiplier Tube.*—The amount of light emitted from the heated sample is measured by a photomultiplier tube which is held with its sensitive surface vertically

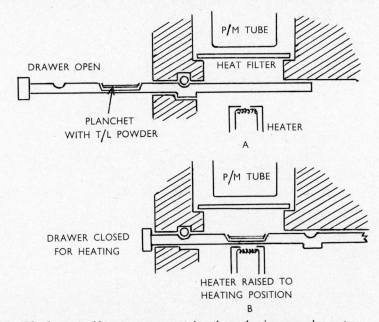

Fig. 73.—The drawer and heater arrangements in a thermoluminescence dosemeter.

above and parallel to the sample (*Fig.* 73). Since it is important to keep the photo-multiplier tube cool so that there will not be an unacceptably large 'dark current', it is usual to fit a 'heat' filter between the photomultiplier tube and the heated sample. This filter allows transmission of the visible light but stops the infra-red radiation coming from the heated tray. If very low doses are being measured it is sometimes necessary to cool the photomultiplier tube using liquid nitrogen, but this is rather inconvenient and is therefore not often done.

During the heating of the sample and the measurement of the emitted light, the photomultiplier tube, heated tray, sample, and heater must be in a lightproof enclosure since, otherwise, the ambient light would contribute to the instrument reading and so invalidate it. A sliding drawer system similar to that shown in *Fig.* 73 is often used. In the open position (A) the planchet containing the TLD sample is placed in the hole in the slide which is then pushed in to bring the sample directly underneath the photo-multiplier tube (*Fig.* 73B). As soon as the slide is closed the heating element is raised and the heating started.

c. The Electronic System.—The amplification effected by the photomultiplier tube is critically dependent on the value of the high voltage applied to its electrodes. There must, therefore, be a very stable high-voltage power supply.

It is the total charge (current × time) produced at the output of the photo-multiplier tube which is proportional to the amount of light incident on its input surface. There must, therefore, be a circuit which integrates (i.e., adds up) the current during the heating period and which displays this value as the output reading or response. It is usual nowadays for it to be displayed digitally.

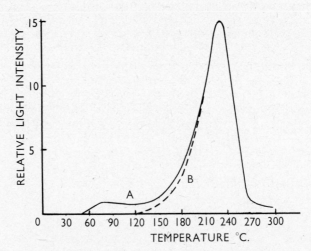

Fig. 74.—A thermoluminescence 'glow curve'. A, Produced shortly after the material was irradiated. B, Produced after storage for about a day.

The Glow Curve.—An example of the variation of the intensity of light emitted as the TLD material is heated up from room temperature to 300° C. is shown in *Fig.* 74 A. Such a curve is known as a 'glow curve'. It will be seen that quite a lot of light is emitted at temperatures below 150–200° C. However, if the irradiated material is stored at room temperature before 'read-out', it is found that the glow curve is changed to that shown in *Fig.* 74 B. The reason for this difference is that electrons stored in the more shallow traps have leaked away during storage. The response is therefore dependent on the period of time between irradiation and read-out and this is unacceptable. The response is said to 'fade'. Fortunately the large majority of this fading takes place in the initial 24 hours and after this time the response is fairly constant. In fact the TLD material can 'store' the dose for many years. This ability to store the signal and permit read-out at a later date is a very useful property of TLD material.

In practice, therefore, it is usual to delay the read-out for at least 24 hours so that the response is independent of the actual time between exposure and read-out. Alternatively, the material, after exposure but before read-out, may be pre-heated to 100° C for about 5 minutes, and this has the same effect as storage for 24 hours.

Calibration.—There are many different kinds of TLD material and each has its own characteristic properties: indeed each batch of material which is nominally the same as another differs (slightly). As has already been stated, it is, therefore, necessary to calibrate each batch of material so that its sensitivities, i.e., response per rad for the range of radiation qualities and dose levels over which it is to be used, are known. Fortunately, for a given type of material the change in pattern of sensitivities from batch to batch is not large so that, although it may be necessary to perform a very full calibration on the initial batch, for subsequent batches a simple check at a single radiation quality (often cobalt-60 gamma rays) and a few dose levels will suffice. This latter check calibration is, with benefit, incorporated into the practical routine of dose measurement described below.

Practical Measurement.—In practice, TLD material is used to measure radiation dose by comparing the response associated with the unknown dose with the response of samples of identical TLD material which have been given known doses of approximately the same magnitude. Although the details of the measuring scheme adopted by different workers may differ slightly, a satisfactory system of working is as follows:

1. A batch of about 20 grammes of the chosen type of TLD material is placed in an oven and kept at a temperature of 400 °C for 1 hour followed by 80 °C for a further 24 hours. This process is called annealing and ensures that all the usable electron traps have been emptied.

2. Since the sensitivity depends on the size of the crystals it is necessary to sieve the material so that only those of sizes between approximately 0·05 and 0·2 mm. are used. As will be stated below, after use it is possible and economic to re-use the TLD material. Unfortunately, during use the crystals disintegrate somewhat and the purpose of the sieving is chiefly to discard those which have become too small for satisfactory use.

3. For each dose measurement about 50–100 mg. of material are normally used. Although the material can be weighed this is a rather time-consuming process, so that it is more usual to dispense it by volume, which is satisfactory. For exposure the material is contained in some kind of plastic sachet. Sufficient sachets for the dose measurements to be made are prepared plus about three or four more which are to be exposed to known doses and so act as calibration standards. These calibration exposures are arranged so that the doses given to the standards cover the expected values of the unknown doses to be measured.

4. After irradiation the sachets are kept for 24 hours to allow the low temperature traps to empty. Alternatively they are held at 100 °C for about 5 minutes.

5. For read-out the contents of each sachet are divided into four or five equal read-out samples. To ensure that all samples have the same mass (and it is very important that they should since the response is proportional also to the mass of TLD material heated) an automatic dispenser is often used. Each sample weighs about 15 mg.

6. In turn each sample is placed on the stainless-steel tray of the read-out apparatus. The lightproof drawer is closed and the heating element raised to be in contact with the tray. The heating now takes place. Nowadays it is usual for the equipment to ensure that the sample is subjected to a constant heating pattern for a definite time during which the sample is raised to 300° C. At the end of the heating cycle the heater is switched off automatically and note is taken of the read-out value which is usually displayed digitally. The average of the four or five samples from each sachet is taken as the response value for that particular sachet.

7. Some TLD read-out machines are fitted with a standard, constant light source which can be placed in the same position as the TLD sample. Its purpose is to enable the overall sensitivity of the photomultiplier tube electronic system to be adjusted to a constant value; i.e., with the light source in place the sensitivity is adjusted until a specified read-out is obtained in a specified time. In spite of having this facility, it is still worth while to calibrate the whole system in the manner described by the use of sachets irradiated to known doses.

8. A calibration curve of average response versus known dose is drawn using the values obtained for the calibration samples. This curve is then used to deduce the unknown doses being measured.

9. After read-out of each sample has been completed the TLD material is tipped into a container in which is stored all the used material. When the original batch of powder has all been used it is washed in methyl alcohol to remove any accumulated dirt, dried and then re-annealed as described above. It is now ready as a fresh batch for re-use.

Solid TLD Materials.—The description given above has been of TLD material in the form of a powder. An alternative is for the TLD crystalline material to be in the form of either discs or rods. These are manufactured either of compressed TLD material or of TLD crystals incorporated into a plastic (e.g., Teflon). Such discs or rods are a few millimetres in cross-section and are very convenient in size. They are annealed, calibrated, exposed, read out, and re-used in exactly the same way as for the powder. They have, however, the advantage that there is no problem of either sieving or weighing irradiated samples. However, one does have to rely on the manufacturer providing discs or rods of equal sensitivities, of the sensitivities remaining constant, or changing in the same way after use.

Application

Radiotherapy.—As previously stated, TLD material is very useful and convenient for measuring doses received by patients whilst actually undergoing the treatment exposures. The presence of the sachets has an insignificant effect on the patient dose. Furthermore, the dose level usually being measured, i.e., a few hundred rads per exposure, is a very convenient level at which to do the measurement.

Radiodiagnosis.—With the increasing importance being placed on minimizing the dose received during radiography, TLD is assuming an important role. As in radiotherapy the thin, virtually tissue-equivalent sachet is almost invisible on the radiograph and therefore does not disturb the investigation. Of particular importance is its use in the measurement of dose to critical organs such as the lens of the eye. The dose levels encountered are usually only (or should be only!) a few hundred millirads up to a maximum of about one or two rads. The accuracy of measurement is, therefore, rather less than is the case with radiotherapy measurements unless very great care indeed is taken with the measurement. Fortunately, in this field of work high accuracy is not usually required. One of the problems associated with the measurement of very low doses is that of light being emitted for reasons not associated with radiation dose. This results in a random background emission of light which reduces the accuracy of measurement. In circumstances where the maximum accuracy is required, some help can be obtained by passing a steady stream of nitrogen over the sample during read-out. This has the effect of suppressing the emission of the unwanted light.

Personnel Monitoring.—The ability of TLD material to store dose over long periods of time makes it very suitable for use as an alternative to photographic film for personnel dose measurement. Furthermore, since the read-out is directly electrical in nature it is eminently suitable for use in an automated system capable of dealing quickly with a very large number of personnel monitors. For these purposes the solid Teflon disc is normally used. As with the film badge-holder used for the same purpose, filters can be incorporated and the pattern of dose observed by the TLD discs behind the various filters used to estimate radiation quality and type. An important advantage of TLD compared with film is that even a system designed to measure low values of dose (say 10 mR) is capable, in the unhappy case of an accidental over-exposure, of measuring up to very large values of dose.

Attractive Features of TLD as a Dosemeter.—It is useful to summarize the attractive features of the TLD dosemeter system.

1. Small in size and chemically inert.
2. Almost tissue-equivalent.
3. Small change in sensitivity with radiation quality.
4. Usable over a wide range of radiation qualities.
5. Usable over a wide range of dose values (1 mR–1000 R).
6. Sensitivity independent of dose rate.
7. Read-out system consistent and suitable for automation.
8. Read-out simple and quick (less than 1 minute per sample).
9. Apart from initial fading can store dose over long periods of time.
10. Exposures can be made 'in the field' away from the measuring laboratory.

CHAPTER XII

ABSORBED DOSE AND THE RAD

EXPOSURE, as the name suggests, is intended to refer to the X-ray beam itself—to be a measure of the amount of radiation at any particular point. This was more clearly laid down in the old definition of the roentgen (the unit of Exposure) than in the new, for the former states that the roentgen is 'That amount of X-, or gamma radiation . . . etc.'. Exposure measures (via absorption in air) the radiation coming to a place, but it tells nothing about what would happen if that place were in any material other than air.

Now in radiology and, as a further example, in radiobiology, interest is not centred in the beam of radiation, as such, but in the amount of energy that it deposits in its passage through the material of interest. Prime interest is in *absorbed dose*, and the problem to be solved is how to measure it.

Fig. 46 (p. 81) shows that much of the absorbed energy ultimately becomes *heat* and, therefore, to measure this heat—by measuring the temperature rise produced by the irradiation—would provide the most direct, and absolute, since the answer would be directly in energy units (ergs), method of absorbed dose determination. Unfortunately, as has already been pointed out, the heat generated is extremely small and its accurate measurement fraught with difficulty, as will be appreciated from the fact that the rise in temperature associated with a full radiotherapy treatment—say an Exposure of 5000 roentgens—would only be about one-hundredth of 1 degree Centigrade. For this reason calorimetry has never, and probably will never, become established as a routine method of dosemetry, though recent technical developments have placed it in a position from which it may challenge ionization methods as a standard method of X-ray measurement, especially in the megavoltage range, where the 'free-air' chamber cannot be used. However, it must be stressed that calorimetry requires very special apparatus and facilities and is unsuitable for ordinary clinical use.

The method adopted for absorbed dose determination, therefore, is the direct method of deducing the absorbed dose in *rads* from the Exposure in *roentgens*. This is possible in the first place because the roentgen represents the same amount of energy absorbed from the beam, by air, no matter what the radiation energy, or quality. To produce an ion pair, in air, needs a few electron volts of energy (somewhere between 10 and 15 eV.) but, of course, ionization is not the only consequence of irradiation; there is also excitation and direct heat production. However, it has been found that, *on the average*, a total of 33·7 eV. are always extracted from the beam for every ion pair produced, no matter what the radiation energy. This energy absorbed per ion pair produced (i.e., 33·7 eV.) is usually symbolized by W. If, for example, the ionization requires 15 eV., the remaining energy of 18·7 eV. goes into energy of excitation and into heat. But the important fact is that ionization is directly, and quantitatively, linked with total energy absorption. Measure the former and the latter can be deduced. On this basis it can be calculated that the energy absorption associated with 1 roentgen is:

86·9 ergs per g. of air.*

---

* See footnote on p. 131.

In air, therefore, 1 roentgen corresponds to an absorbed dose of 0·869 rad since 1 rad is 100 ergs per g.

There is thus a direct link between the roentgen and the rad for air. But what is their relationship, i.e., the relationship between Exposure in roentgens and absorbed dose, in any other material? How, for example, can the absorbed dose in soft tissue or bone, or any other tissue, be determined when the Exposure to which they are subjected is known?

Conversion Factors for Roentgens into Rads.—If the Exposure in roentgens is known then so is the amount of energy absorbed, by a gramme of air, from the beam. The question to be answered is: 'How much energy will be absorbed per gramme of any other material subjected to the same Exposure?' In each case the energy absorbed depends on the mass absorption (*not* attenuation) coefficient of the substance concerned, so that:

Absorbed energy per gramme = energy in the beam × mass absorption
coefficient

$$= E\left(\frac{\mu_a}{\rho}\right).$$

Thus

$$\frac{\text{Absorbed energy per gramme of substance}}{\text{Absorbed energy per gramme of air}} = \frac{E(\mu_a/\rho)_{\text{substance}}}{E(\mu_a/\rho)_{\text{air}}}.$$

But, as shown above, the absorbed energy per gramme of air = 0·869 × R rads, where R = Exposure in roentgens.

Hence

$$\text{Absorbed energy per gramme of substance} = \frac{0·869 \, R(\mu_a/\rho)_{\text{substance}}}{(\mu_a/\rho)_{\text{air}}} \text{ rads}$$

$$= fR \text{ rads},$$

where the factor f, the factor for converting roentgens into rads, can be seen to be 0·869 (the energy associated with a roentgen) multiplied by the ratio of the mass absorption coefficients of the substance under review and air. These coefficients are known for most substances, so that f can readily be calculated. *Table XI* shows some values for three substances of interest in radiology, namely water, muscle tissue, and bone, and from this table it will be seen that the factor varies not only with the material but also with the radiation energy.

The Variation of f with Radiation Quality and with Material.—

Muscle: The values of f given in *Table XI* are shown graphically in *Fig.* 75, which reveals a number of important points more clearly than does the table. First, perhaps, is the close relationship between the factor for air (which is constant for reasons

---

For those who are interested, the figure of 86·9 ergs per g. of air (*see* p. 130) is arrived at as follows:

1 R produces 1 e.s.u. of charge per 0·001293 g. of air or 1/0·001293 e.s.u. per g.

The charge on the electron is $4·8 \times 10^{-10}$ e.s.u. so that 1 e.s.u. is the charge on $2·08 \times 10^9$ electrons.

$W = 33·7$ electron-volts per ion pair and $1 \, \text{eV.} = 1·602 \times 10^{-12}$ ergs.

Therefore energy associated with 1 roentgen is:

$$\underbrace{33·7 \times 1·602 \times 10^{-12}}_{\text{Energy, in ergs per ionization}} \times \underbrace{2·08 \times 10^9/0·001293}_{\text{Ion pairs per g. per roentgen}} = 86·9 \text{ ergs per g.}$$

Table XI.—THE ROENTGEN TO RAD CONVERSION FACTOR (f) FOR WATER,
MUSCLE, AND BONE, FOR A RANGE OF RADIATION ENERGIES

PHOTON ENERGY	f VALUES		
	Water	Muscle	Bone
20 keV.	0·879	0·917	4·23
40 keV.	0·879	0·920	4·14
60 keV.	0·905	0·929	2·91
80 keV.	0·932	0·940	1·91
100 keV.	0·949	0·949	1·46
150 keV.	0·962	0·956	1·05
200 keV.	0·973	0·963	0·979
500 keV.	0·965	0·957	0·925
1 MeV.	0·965	0·957	0·919
1·5 MeV.	0·964	0·957	0·921
2·0 MeV.	0·963	0·955	0·929

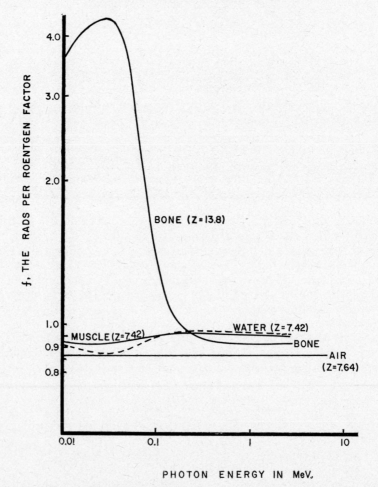

Fig. 75.—The variation, with photon energy, of the factor used to convert roentgens into rads
for some materials of radiological importance.

explained above) and that for muscle tissue. This, of course, is the physical reason why ionization in air forms such a good basis for radiological measurements: it runs so close to ionization in the soft tissues over the whole energy range of radiological interest. Thus 1 R at any quality means almost the same energy absorbed per gramme by muscle, which is usually the tissue being treated.

A second important feature is the closeness in the values of f for water and muscle tissue. This, along with the fact that their mass attenuation coefficients, as well as their mass absorption coefficients, are so closely similar over the whole radiation quality range, justifies the use, as will be described later, of water as a substitute for exposure measurements for clinical purposes. It is seldom practicable to make measurements directly on the patient and they are therefore made in some substitute material (a 'phantom'). Water, for the reason given, is usually chosen as the standard material, and values obtained in it are directly applicable to soft tissue.

Bone: Bone behaves quite differently. Except at high energies, its factor bears very little relation to those of air, water, or soft tissue. This is, of course, because bone has an atomic number (about 13) which is markedly different from that of air, which is 7·6, or of muscle tissue and water, for both of which $Z = 7·4$. The f factor is the ratio of absorption coefficients and whilst, as shown in CHAPTER VII, the coefficient for air remains fairly constant over a wide range of radiation energy, the absorption coefficient for bone (as well as its attenuation coefficient) will increase rapidly towards the lower energy end of the range, because of the increasing predominance of the photo-electric effect. At high energies, where the Compton effect is all-important, the factors for all the substances are roughly the same, since the Compton effect does not depend on atomic number.

In passing it is worth noting that this variation in f factor for bone and its marked difference from that of air is a major reason why the roentgen has been superseded by the rad as the preferred dose unit in radiology. A mere statement of the Exposure in roentgens, whilst giving a good idea of the muscle tissue dose in rads, gives no real indication of the absorbed dose in bone, as the values in *Table XII* clearly show.

Table XII.—ABSORBED DOSES, PER 100 R, IN MUSCLE AND BONE
FOR SOME TYPICAL RADIATION BEAMS

GENERATING VOLTAGE OR RADIOACTIVE SOURCE	RADS (PER 100 ROENTGENS) IN	
	Muscle	Bone
100 kV.	92	414
200 kV.	94	191
250 kV.	94·9	146
^{137}Cs	95·7	92·5
^{60}Co	95·7	92
4 MV.	95·6	92·1

The fourth point arising from *Fig. 75* is, at first sight, quite puzzling. Of the materials dealt with, muscle tissue and water have the lowest atomic number, each being slightly lower than that of air, whilst the atomic number of bone is almost twice as great as those of the others. Therefore the greater absorption (and f factor) for bone at the lower energies is what would be expected, but what is somewhat unexpected is that water and muscle should both absorb more than does air in spite of its slightly higher atomic number. Even more unexpected is the fact that at high energies the factor for bone, although greater than that of air, is *less* than the factors for muscle tissue and water.

How do these apparent anomalies arise? The cause is hydrogen. As has been pointed out in CHAPTER VI, though the Compton effect does not depend on atomic number, it will vary from element to element because it depends on the number of electrons per gramme (the electron density) in the substance. Now this is almost the same in all elements except hydrogen, which has twice as many electrons per gramme as anything else. Hence hydrogen has a Compton effect per gramme which is twice as great as any other element. By the same token the Compton effect in substances containing hydrogen will be greater than in those with no hydrogen, the excess being dependent upon the amount of hydrogen present.

Air contains no hydrogen, whilst water, muscle, and bone contain, respectively, 11, 10, and 6 per cent by weight, so that their electron densities are as follows: air, 3·007; bone, 3·193; muscle, 3·307, and water, 3·344, each multiplied by 10^{23}. In the energy range where the Compton process predominates, therefore, it is to be expected that water and muscle should absorb more energy per gramme than bone and that all three should absorb more than air—which is precisely what is found. At the lower energies the greater photo-electric effect in bone more than compensates for its inferior electron density, whereas the slightly higher atomic number of air cannot overcome the handicap of a 10 per cent electron density, since there is not a great deal of photo-electric absorption in air, water, or muscle even at the lower energies. Therefore the factor for water and muscle remains above that of air.

If very high energies were considered then the absorption in bone would again become greater than that for muscle and water, because there is increasingly more pair production in bone than in the other materials. It will be recalled that the amount of pair production is proportional to the atomic number of the attenuator.

Roentgen to Rad Conversion—A Summary.—Given the Exposure in roentgens at a point in any uniform material the absorbed dose in rads (i.e., the energy absorbed per gramme of material) can be found by multiplying the roentgens by a factor f, the values of which are available in published tables for a variety of substances and a wide range of photon energies. However, it must be noticed that the word 'uniform' is very important in the previous sentence. The fact that bone (that is, solid bone) absorbs less, per gramme, at certain energies than muscle tissue is physically true, and clinically unimportant!

Bone Dosage—A Complex Problem.—The bone, whose absorption has been discussed above, is solid inorganic bone, which is made entirely of the material which is familiar to us in the dry bones of the skeleton. It is made up principally of mineral salts like calcium phosphate. In the living body the bones are not as simple as that, the mineral substance serving as a three-dimensional framework within which are many cavities of varying size filled with the soft-tissue components of the Haversian system, osteocytes, and blood-vessels. These are the living elements of the bone and are extremely important to the functioning of the body as a whole, as well as to the bone itself. Because of their close proximity to the inorganic bone, these soft-tissue elements, and any soft-tissue elements attached to the outside of the bone, will receive a higher absorbed dose than soft tissues remote from bone. They are thus more liable to radiation damage, and it is important to have some idea just how great this higher dose is. The effect of radiation on the inorganic bone is not likely to be important.

Therefore, from absorbed dose in uniform material, attention must be turned to consider what happens in isolated islands of soft tissue embedded in a mineral bone matrix. What is learned in this case will also help to show what dose is absorbed by muscle tissue growing in contact with bone surfaces.

Dosage in Cavities.—Consider then a tiny volume of soft tissue (a 'soft-tissue element') embedded in bone—one of the inclusions listed above—and consider what happens to it compared with an equal soft-tissue element which is entirely surrounded by soft tissue, when they are both subjected to the same exposure. In other words, what is the absorbed dose in soft tissue growing inside bone, compared with the absorbed dose in an ordinary piece of muscle?

The situation is very comparable with that discussed in CHAPTER X when the principle of the 'thimble' ionization chamber was being considered. In that case a volume of air was surrounded by a wall of another material: here the soft-tissue element is surrounded by a 'wall' of either bone or of other soft tissue. As in the ionization chamber the ionization in the enclosed material is partly due to electrons (photo-electrons, recoil electrons, or pair-production electrons) produced by the interaction of photons in the 'wall', and partly due to electrons similarly produced in the material itself. The precise contributions from these two sources depend on the size of the enclosed volume—in the case being considered, on the size of the soft-tissue element.

Small Cavities.—These present the simplest problem, for when a cavity is small (by which is meant that its dimensions are small compared with the range of the electrons liberated by the X-rays being considered) the ionization arising from photon interactions in the cavity can be ignored. Any effects on the soft-tissue element are due to electrons (photo-, recoil, or pair-production) coming from the surrounding 'wall' material. Under these conditions the soft-tissue element is crossed by *the same number of electrons as would cross an equal volume of the surrounding material*. The presence of the small cavity does not alter the electron pattern any more than a small 'pot-hole' on a road alters the flow of traffic.

Since the energy delivered to any material comes from the photo-, recoil, or pair-production electrons crossing it, the absorbed dose must be proportional to the number of these electrons crossing it, which in the case of the soft-tissue element under review is the same, per unit volume, as in the surrounding material. The absorbed dose in the soft-tissue element is therefore proportional to the ionization per unit volume in the surrounding material.

Now the ionization per gramme of any material depends on the mass absorption coefficient (μ_a/ρ), and the ionization per unit volume will be proportional to the mass absorption coefficient multiplied by the density, i.e., $\mu_a/\rho \times \rho = \mu_a$, that is the linear absorption coefficient. Thus, in the small cavity being considered *the absorbed dose is proportional to the linear absorption coefficient of the surrounding material*. For the example being considered:

$$\frac{\text{Absorbed dose in soft-tissue element surrounded by bone}}{\text{Absorbed dose in soft-tissue element surrounded by soft tissue}}$$
$$= \frac{(\mu_a)_{\text{bone}}}{(\mu_a)_{\text{soft tissue}}} . S_{\text{B}}^{\text{ST}},$$

where S_{B}^{ST} is a constant called the linear electron stopping power ratio (ST = soft tissue; B = bone). For soft tissue and bone it is about 0·64.

Table XIII gives both the mass and linear absorption coefficients for bone and soft tissue over a range of energies. It shows that, because of greater density, the linear coefficient for bone always exceeds that of soft tissue, so that, as the last line shows, soft-tissue inclusions in bone always receive a larger dose than is received by soft tissue remote from bone. The excess decreases with increasing radiation energy because of waning photo-electric effect in bone.

Table XIII.—MASS AND LINEAR ABSORPTION COEFFICIENTS FOR BONE AND MUSCLE FOR A RANGE OF RADIATION ENERGIES

The ratio, given on the last line, gives the ratio of the dose in a soft-tissue cavity surrounded by bone to the dose in ordinary soft tissue

PHOTON ENERGY		10 keV.	50 keV.	100 keV.	200 keV.	500 keV.	1 MeV.	2 MeV.
$\dfrac{\mu_a}{\rho}$	Bone	19·0	0·16	0·039	0·030	0·032	0·030	0·025
	Muscle	4·96	0·041	0·025	0·030	0·033	0·031	0·026
μ_a	Bone	32·3	0·27	0·066	0·051	0·054	0·051	0·042
	Muscle	4·96	0·041	0·025	0·030	0·033	0·031	0·026
$\dfrac{(\mu_a)_B}{(\mu_a)_{ST}} \cdot S_B^{ST}$		4·16	4·22	1·66	1·19	1·05	1·04	1·02

Large Cavities.—By no means can all soft-tissue-containing cavities in bone be regarded as small according to the definition given above, for many have dimensions greater than the fraction of a millimetre, which is the range of the electrons liberated by the lower-energy X-rays. To see what happens in such cavities, the case of a soft-tissue element whose diameter is greater than the electron range will now be considered.

Such a cavity is depicted in *Fig.* 76, and, for simplicity, it will be assumed that all the electrons produced by photon interaction have a single range R. Therefore there will be soft tissue in the centre of the cavity which is beyond the range of any electrons generated in the surrounding bone; for this soft tissue the 'wall' will be other soft tissue, and its absorbed dose will be the same as if it were part of a continuous piece of muscle. In contrast, the soft tissue close up to the bone will be very like that in the small cavity already discussed, and will get an absorbed dose closely related to that in the small cavity. The absorbed dose pattern across the cavity will, therefore, as shown in the lower part of *Fig.* 76 A, be high close to the wall, and will fall to what might be termed the normal soft-tissue level at the centre. For comparison purposes *Fig.* 76 B shows the electron tracks across a small cavity and the dose pattern across it, which, as described already, is everywhere raised.

Muscle growing on Bone.—The question of the absorbed dose at the muscle–bone interface, i.e., where muscle is attached to bone and growing in contact with its surface, is also of importance. Here the ionization pattern is rather similar to that in a large cavity, as can be seen from *Fig.* 77. The tissue immediately in contact with bone will receive a considerably higher absorbed dose than tissue further away because of the higher ionization per unit volume in the bone. However, any dose increase can only extend to a depth away from the bone equal to the range of the primary electrons. At distances beyond this, normal soft-tissue doses are received.

The Magnitude and Extent of the 'Bone' Effect.—Although the mineral bone may receive absorbed doses which, at some radiation energies, are less than those received by soft tissue, any soft tissue growing close to or within the bone will *always* receive a greater absorbed dose than would soft tissue distant from bone. Since the soft-tissue elements are the essential living features of bone, this extra dosage—and hence the greater possibility of radiation damage—must always be remembered.

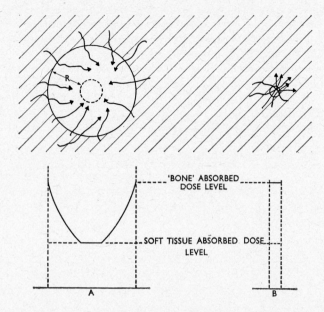

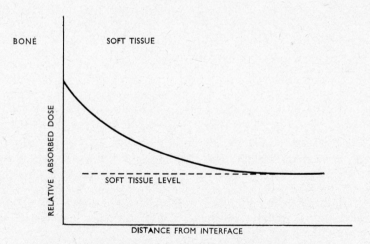

Fig. 76.—Cavity dosage. The shaded area represents a piece of bone in which there are a large and a small cavity, each filled with soft tissue. Electrons generated in the bone by radiation pass right across the smaller cavity (B) but only affect the outer parts of the larger cavity (A). The absorbed dose pattern across each cavity is shown in the lower part of the diagram.

Fig. 77.—The extra absorbed dose to soft tissue close to bone.

In the foregoing, however, no real indication has been given of how much tissue is likely to be involved and only passing reference to the magnitude of the excess dose. Both the amount of tissue receiving increased absorbed dose and the size of the excess depend on the energy of the radiation being used, since this controls both μ_a and the electron range.

And therein lies a conflict, since low-energy radiation means high values of the linear absorption coefficient (μ_a) but, at the same time, low values of the electron range. Reference to *Fig.* 78 will show how these two facts affect the dose in soft tissue in or near bone. In this diagram are shown two soft-tissue-filled cavities in a piece of bone, and a bone–tissue interface CD. The cavities have diameters of 10 and 100 microns respectively. (The micron is a unit of measurement widely used in microbiology and is 1/1000 mm.) Below are shown examples of how the absorbed dose produced across

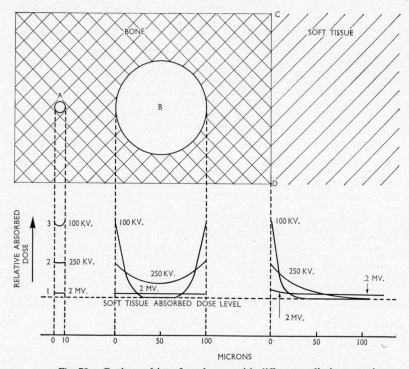

Fig. 78.—Cavity and interface dosage with different radiation energies.

the cavities and near the interface varies when the system is irradiated with radiations generated at, respectively, 100 kV., 250 kV., and 2 MV. For simplicity it is assumed that all the electrons set in motion by one type of radiation have the same range.

Cavity 'A' has a diameter that is smaller than the electron range of any of the radiations and, therefore, it is effectively uniformly dosed even by the 100-kV. radiation, for which the dosage level is highest because, as already indicated, the values of μ_a increase with decreasing energy.

The diameter of cavity 'B' is smaller than the range of the electrons associated with the 2-MV. radiation and therefore is uniformly dosed at a level higher than that received by soft tissue remote from bone. However, the excess is small since μ_a for bone is not greatly different from that for soft tissue at this high energy. In contrast the diameter is considerably greater than the range of the 100-kV. electrons so that while the soft tissue lining the cavity surface receives high dosage, that in the centre gets the dose level received by soft tissue remote from bone. Finally, the electrons associated with 250-kV. radiations have a range about equal to the cavity diameter so that they raise its dose to a higher level than does the 2-MV. radiation but not as uniformly.

The dosage in soft tissue in contact with bone shows a similar pattern. The tissues in intimate contact with the bone receive higher doses than those remote from it, the highest doses being received from the low-energy radiation, but the effect of this falls off tapidly because of the small range of the primary electrons. With the high-energy radiations the electron range is much greater, so that the higher doses due to bone extend deeper into the soft tissues, but of course the magnitude of the excess is quite small.

Fig. 78 has illustrated what happens in three considerably used therapeutic energy ranges, i.e., about 100 kV. (the so-called 'superficial' therapy), about 250 kV. (once called 'deep' but now often called 'conventional' therapy), and about 2 million volts (which is representative of commonly used radiotherapy with 'megavoltage' radiations, including those from radioactive cobalt 60). Higher energies still have not been dealt with because they are seldom used therapeutically. However, it is worthy of mention that the trend here noted, i.e., lower doses with higher energy but the effect being spread over greater distances, is not continued at very high energies. Because of the phenomenon of pair production the value of μ_a, which steadily decreases with increasing energy up to about 10 MeV., above that value starts to increase again. Therefore, for the very high energies, the interface and cavity doses start to increase again, and because of the great range of the electrons, more uniformly irradiate the bigger cavities and give high doses at much greater distance from a bone interface.

Bone-absorbed Dose—A Summary.—Whilst the calculation of absorbed dose in uniform materials is simply a matter of multiplying the Exposure in roentgens by an appropriate tabulated factor, the computation and statement of dosage in the soft-tissue elements growing in or on bone are very complex. The reader will probably have been more impressed by the complications of the problem than by any other feature, yet the foregoing descriptions have dealt with deliberately simplified situations. The effects in practice are considerably more complicated!

Table XIV.—RATIO OF AVERAGE ABSORBED DOSE IN BONE SOFT-TISSUE ELEMENTS TO DOSE IN SOFT TISSUE DISTANT FROM BONE

GENERATING VOLTAGE OR RADIOACTIVE SOURCE	H.V.L.	RATIO
140 kV.	3 mm.Al	2·5
200 kV.	1·5 mm.Cu	1·9
300 kV.	2·5 mm.Cu	1·4
^{137}Cs	—	1·05
^{60}Co and 4 MV.	—	1·03
20 MV.	—	1·15

However, certain relatively simple generalizations emerge. And the first is that soft tissues growing within, or on, bone receive greater absorbed doses, for a given Exposure, than do soft tissues remote from bone. Secondly, this increment of dose is greater at the lower voltages than for radiation in the 1- to 10-million-volt range, for which the effect is at its minimum, though it extends over smaller distances. This fact is one of the great advantages of megavoltage therapy since the greater liability of bone to damage by radiation is thus least in this range. Both the lower voltages and the very high megavoltages produce greater bone effects. Finally, *Table XIV* gives average factors by which the absorbed dose in the bone soft-tissue system—which is the effective bone-absorbed dose—exceed those in ordinary muscle.

CHAPTER XIII

FILTERS AND FILTRATION

IT has already been shown, in CHAPTER V, that the radiation emitted by an X-ray tube is made up of photons of many different energies. The maximum photon energy, it will be recalled, depends only upon the kilovoltage used to generate the radiation, whilst the minimum energy present depends upon the nature and thickness of the material of the wall of the X-ray tube. A typical spectrum is shown in *Fig.* 79. It is for X-rays generated, at 200 kV., in a tube with a very thin wall. Because they do not affect the principles being discussed in this chapter, the characteristic radiations indicated in *Fig.* 79 will be omitted from subsequent diagrams.

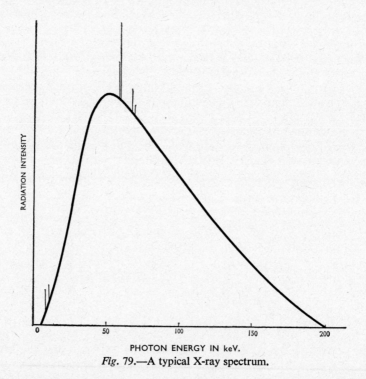

PHOTON ENERGY IN keV.

Fig. 79.—A typical X-ray spectrum.

Because of their different energies the component radiations of a beam of this sort will have very different penetrating powers. Take, for example, radiations of energy 20 and 150 keV. respectively, which are present in roughly equal amounts in the spectrum shown. Their linear attenuation coefficients (μ) in soft tissue are, respectively, 0·79 cm.$^{-1}$ and 0·15 cm.$^{-1}$, which means that only about 0·03 per cent of the 20-keV. photons will penetrate through 10 cm. of the material, compared with 22 per cent of the higher-energy photons. Alternatively, it may be noted, as many of the 20-keV.

photons are removed by about 2 cm. of tissue as would be lost from the 150-keV. photons in 10 cm.

From facts such as these it follows that when a beam of radiation such as that depicted by *Fig.* 79 is incident upon a patient, the bulk of the low-energy photons is absorbed in the superficial layers and very few of them reach the deeper parts of the body (which are often those to be treated by radiotherapy), or emerge from the far side of the patient (and thus play any part in the production of a radiograph). Such radiations therefore serve no useful purpose in these applications of the beam, and in fact they are worse than useless, because they produce unwanted effects where they are absorbed. Their removal from the beam, before they reach the patient, is desirable, and this is the purpose of **filtration.**

Ideally, 'filtration' should remove the unwanted radiation completely and leave the wanted radiation undiminished. As in *Fig.* 80 A, it would be most desirable, say, to remove all the radiation to the left (low-energy end) of the vertical line, and to retain all the high-energy end of the spectrum (to the right of the line). This sort of filtration is possible, for example, with visible light where coloured glasses may give beams of any desired hue from a beam of white light. Unfortunately, a similar effect

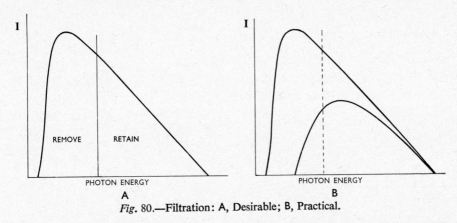

Fig. 80.—Filtration: A, Desirable; B, Practical.

is not possible with X-rays, where any material introduced in the beam will affect photons of all energies to some extent. The best that can be hoped for is that a method can be found that will affect the low-energy photons much more than it affects those of high energy and thus achieve the selective filtration effect shown in *Fig.* 80 B.

The Effects of Filtration.—From *Fig.* 80 B it can be seen that the introduction of a filter into an X-ray beam has two effects. In the first place it removes unwanted radiation, and so 'hardens' the beam or increases its penetrating power, whilst at the same time it reduces the beam intensity. If progressively thicker layers are introduced and their effects studied, it will be found that initially there is a substantial increase in quality (or half-value layer) accompanied by a substantial reduction in beam intensity or, in what is more usually measured, Exposure rate. With thicker layers both effects are less marked but the reduction of Exposure rate continues with increasing filter thickness even when no further increase in quality is being produced. As will be shown later, there is a certain thickness of any given filter material beyond which no further 'hardening' of the beam occurs. This would be the maximum useful filtration. In many cases in practice a filter rather thinner than this is used, in order to have available a rather higher Exposure rate.

Filter Materials.—The role of a filter, then, is to remove the unwanted low-energy radiation as efficiently as possible whilst having the smallest possible effect in the wanted higher-energy photons. It must, in other words, discriminate against the low-energy photons. This, it will be recalled from CHAPTER VII, is exactly what the photo-electric process does: the attenuation due to this effect is inversely proportional to the cube of the photon energy $(1/h\nu^3)$. Scattering, on the other hand, varies inversely only as the first power of the energy $(1/h\nu)$. Therefore a filter material in which the photo-electric effect predominates is clearly needed, and this means a material of high atomic number (Z) since the photo-electric effect varies with Z^3.

Of the materials that are readily available lead $(Z = 82)$ has the highest atomic number and would therefore seem to be the material of choice for our filter.

Lead Filtration.—*Fig.* 81 shows the effect of introducing 0·2 mm. of lead into the beam depicted in *Fig.* 79—a 200-kV. beam—and it will immediately be seen that the

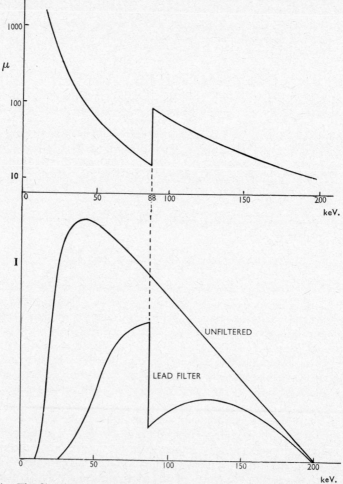

Fig. 81.—The filtration of a 200-kV. X-ray beam by lead. In this, and several following diagrams, the upper part shows the variation with photon energy of the linear attenuation coefficient for the filter metal concerned, whilst the lower part shows the spectra of the filtered and unfiltered beams.

result is very different from that desired. The lead, although discriminating to a certain extent against the low-energy photons, also has a marked effect on some of the higher-energy photons and, in fact, in the middle of this energy region can be seen to be transmitting low-energy photons more readily than those of higher energies.

Why this should be so can be seen from the curve of attenuation coefficient against photon energy shown in the upper part of *Fig*. 81. The K-absorption 'edge' for lead occurs at 88 keV. so that photons whose energies lie between about 60 and 88 keV. are much less attenuated that those between 88 and 110 keV., with the net result that more soft radiation than is desirable is transmitted and the higher-energy photons are excessively reduced.

Filter Material Requirements.—With this experience in mind it is possible, and useful, to list the requirements of a filter material, before going on to consider filters found to be satisfactory in practice. Three principles can be listed:

1. The material chosen must attenuate principally by means of the photo-electric effect in the photon energy range being dealt with—in order to discriminate against the lower-energy photons.
2. The material must not have an absorption 'edge' at an energy close to the energies of the photons that it is desired to use.
3. A requirement not previously mentioned and often overlooked—the thickness of material required must not be too small. If only a tiny fraction of a millimetre of any material is all that is needed, the uniformity of thickness of the foil becomes a matter of great importance. Irregularities in thickness, which might be very difficult to avoid, would produce excessive non-uniformities in the beam, whilst tiny 'pin-holes' which could easily occur would produce tiny completely unfiltered, and unacceptable, beams. One-quarter of a millimetre can be regarded as a minimum acceptable thickness.

Tin Filtration.—For filtration of beams generated between about 200 and 300 kV. tin is accepted as the most efficient material to use. The lower part of *Fig*. 82 shows what happens when 0·4 mm. of tin is introduced into the beam depicted in *Fig*. 79, p. 140, and shows that the type of filtration effect envisaged in *Fig*. 73 B is, with one exception, achieved. The discriminating attenuation of the tin can be readily seen—there is, for example, about a 15 per cent reduction of the 150-keV. component, compared with a reduction of over 90 per cent in the 50-keV. photons. However, there is the exception—a considerable amount of radiation is transmitted in the region of 29 keV. and just below—and this is most undesirable.

Why does the 'leak' occur? Why is tin suddenly less efficient as a filter, in this photon energy range?

The answer is partly provided by the attenuation against energy curve which occupies the upper part of *Fig*. 82, and which shows that tin has its K-absorption 'edge' at about 29 keV. Photons with rather less than this energy will therefore be transmitted much more readily than those whose energy is somewhat in excess of 29 keV. For example, the attenuation coefficient for 25-keV. photons is only about one-fifth of that for 34-keV. photons. Hence the anomalous transmission in this region. However, it must be noted that this does not occur at an energy that is wanted in the beam, and it does not necessarily invalidate tin as a filter material.

However, anomalous transmission *through* the filter is not solely responsible for the extra radiation in this region. The filter itself *adds* radiation to the beam by the very nature of its main attenuation method, the photo-electric effect. It will be recalled that the final act of this attenuation process is the emission of characteristic radiation, and this inevitably occurs here, and these extra photons will be added to those anomalously transmitted, as shown by the two 'spikes' in *Fig.* 82.

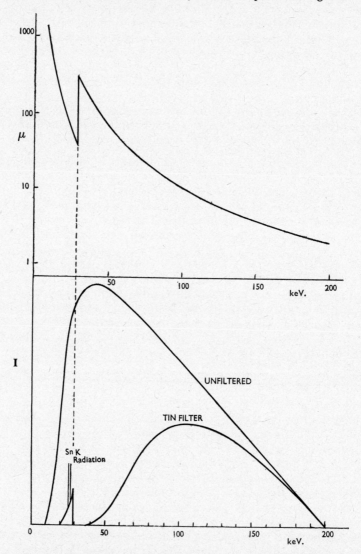

Fig. 82.—Filtration by tin of the same spectrum as shown in *Fig.* 81.

This unwanted low-energy radiation can, however, be removed by 'backing' the main tin filter with a thin layer (usually about a quarter of a millimetre) of copper and this, in turn, with half to one millimetre of aluminium. Copper very readily removes photons with energies in the region of 29 keV. (for the photo-electric effect in copper at round this energy is considerable), but it has an absorption 'edge' at 9 keV. and will add its own characteristic radiation (8–9 keV.) to the beam. This, however, is efficiently removed by aluminium, and any characteristic radiation from that material is of such low energy that it is removed by the air through which the beam has to pass between the tube and the patient. Of course, the 'backing' layers of copper and aluminium reduce the high-energy radiations of the rest of the spectrum, but only to a small extent, and this is a small price to pay for the complete removal of the unwanted 'soft' radiation. The final spectrum produced by this example of a **compound filter** is shown in *Fig.* 83 on which, for comparison, the spectrum produced by the tin filter alone is shown as a dashed line.

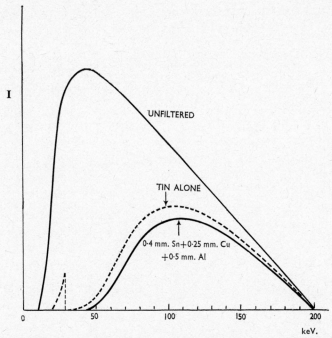

Fig. 83.—The effect of a compound filter. The dashed curve shows the spectrum produced by tin alone as shown in *Fig.* 82.

Copper Filtration.—Another material widely used for the filtration of 200–300-kV. beams is copper $(Z = 29)$ which is also backed by aluminium for the removal of the anomalously transmitted and characteristic radiation of round about 9 keV. Because of its lower atomic number copper shows less photo-electric effect at any energy than tin and therefore discriminates less effectively against the lower-energy photons. Copper is therefore a less efficient filter than tin, by which is meant that if tin and copper compound filters are used to produce a beam of the same half-value layer from the same initial beam, then the tin filter gives the more intense or higher Exposure-rate beam.

The most famous tin filter is that due to the Swedish physicist Thoraeus and consists of 0·4 mm. tin, 0·25 mm. copper, and 1·0 mm. aluminium. It produces the same half-value layer, with a 200-kV. beam, as a 2-mm. copper plus 1·0-mm. aluminium filter but yields a 20 per cent higher Exposure-rate beam. In passing it may be noted that whilst nowadays all tin-copper-aluminium filters are called Thoraeus filters, the name strictly applies only to the combination cited above.

Aluminium Filtration.—Copper is less efficient than tin as the main filtering agent in the 200–300-kV. range because of its lower atomic number and it is therefore to be expected that aluminium ($Z = 13$) would be even less effective, and this is borne out in practice, as *Fig.* 84 shows. In this diagram the result of inserting 15 mm. of aluminium into the beam shown in *Fig.* 79, p. 140, is given, together with the result of using the compound tin filter already discussed; 15 mm. was chosen because it gives a beam of the same Exposure rate as that given by the tin filter, and the diagram

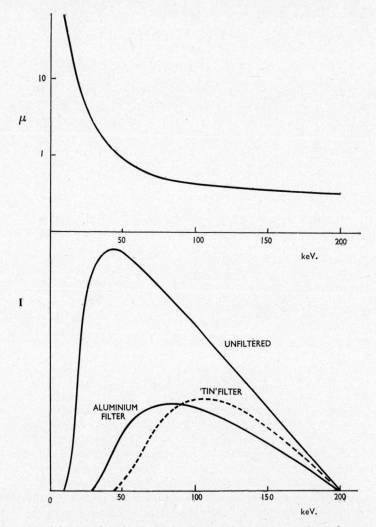

Fig. 84.—Aluminium as a filter for the 200-kV. beam. The dotted curve shows, for comparison, the result of using the compound filter illustrated in *Fig.* 83.

clearly shows that there are relatively far more low-energy photons, and less high-energy photons, in the aluminium-filtered beam.

This is really to be expected since much of the attenuation in aluminium is by the Compton effect ($\alpha\,1/kV.$) rather than the photo-electric effect ($\alpha\,1/kV.^3$) in this energy range. The variation of attenuation with energy curve shown in the upper part of *Fig.* 84 is naturally less steep than those for other materials shown in other diagrams. The aluminium filter therefore produces a much less penetrating beam in this energy range.

Low-energy Beams.—So far attention has been concentrated on 200–300-kV. beams. For lower-energy beams the choice of filter material will be rather different. The spectrum of a typical diagnostic radiology beam is shown in *Fig.* 85. It is generated at 80 kV. and two important points can immediately be made about it. The first is that quite a lot of the radiation has an energy of 20 keV. or less and therefore, as shown at the beginning of this chapter, has very little chance of penetrating through the patient to play a part in the production of a radiograph. These low-energy photons should therefore be removed by suitable filtration. Secondly, many photons have

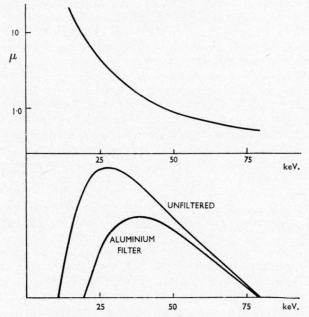

Fig. 85.—Aluminium as the filter for an 80-kV. beam.

energies between 25 and 50 keV., in which region tin will show anomalous attenuation properties owing to its 29-keV. K 'edge'. Since these photons are wanted for radiography, tin is not suitable as a filter material in the diagnostic range.

Aluminium, on the other hand, has no such drawback. Its K level, at 1·6 keV., is well below the lowest photon energy in this spectrum, whilst in spite of its low atomic number (13) aluminium has a considerable photo-electric effect, especially below 50 keV. For example, nearly half the attenuation at 50 keV. is by this effect and nearly two-thirds at 40 keV. For these reasons aluminium is very suitable for, and is widely used as, a filter material for the diagnostic X-ray-generating voltage range.

In *Fig.* 85 the effect of 2-mm. aluminium on the beam is shown, together with the variation of its attenuation coefficient with photon energy. No 'backing' filter is required because of the very low energy of the aluminium K 'edge' and because, as stated earlier, any characteristic radiation is readily absorbed by air. A general 'hardening' of the beam is produced by this filter, but the effect is less marked than that produced, say, by the tin filter on the 200-kV. beam. This is because the photo-electric effect in aluminium, even at these lower energies, is not so great as that in tin in the higher-energy range. For example, at 40 keV. (half the maximum energy of the spectrum shown in *Fig.* 85) the photo-electric effect in aluminium accounts for about 65 per cent of the total attenuation, whereas at 100 keV. (half the maximum energy of the spectrum in *Fig.* 79) the photo-electric effect in tin represents nearly 88 per cent of the total. Aluminium has, in fact, rather too low an atomic number for full filtering efficiency, especially at the higher end of the generating voltage range now used in diagnostic radiology, though it is the best material available for the bulk of the range.

Copper, with its K 'edge' at about 9 keV., would actually be quite acceptable as a material from at least 60 kV. upwards, though at 60 or even 80 kV. the thicknesses needed for adequate filtration would be impracticably small. Some workers, however, use copper filters for voltages of the order of 90–100 kV. upwards.

Very Low-energy X-rays. Grenz Rays.—Although X-rays with energies below 30 keV. have too little penetrating power to be of much clinical use, such low energies are a positive advantage when it is desired to treat superficial layers of the body whilst, at the same time, inflicting the minimum dose—and damage—upon anything below, say, a centimetre deep. Such is the aim of Grenz ray therapy using radiations generated at voltages going down to 10 kV. With such voltages a major problem is the getting of adequate amounts of radiation out of the tube, since, for example, glass of any thickness adequate to maintain the vacuum inside the tube would attenuate the beam far more than can be accepted. The problem here is really the reverse of what has been discussed previously: it is not a matter of finding some high atomic number material which will remove unwanted radiation, but rather a material which can serve as a 'window' for the X-ray tube and yet give maximum transmission. A low atomic number material is obviously called for, and that used is the metal beryllium ($Z = 4$).

A tube fitted with a beryllium 'window' and used at kilovoltages of 30 kV. or upwards has really enormous outputs (20,000 R per min, as opposed to 20 R per min. for a similar tube with a conventional glass 'window') because the beryllium hardly attenuates the beam at all. Great care must therefore be taken to ensure that the correct kilovoltage is used, or that appropriate additional filtration is inserted into the beam when the tube is run at higher voltages, otherwise considerable harm to a patient may ensue.

High-energy Beams (500 kV. to 10 MV.).—The photo-electric effect, upon which good filtration depends, varies inversely as the cube of the radiation energy, and this must be expected to be much smaller for high-energy radiation than for low. Since it also depends upon the cube of the atomic number of the material concerned, it is amongst the high atomic number elements that possible filtering materials for high-energy beams (say up to 1 million volts) must be sought. Of the few possible materials, lead ($Z = 82$) has been most used. In this material the photo-electric effect makes up 50 per cent of the attenuation of 500-keV. photons and 25 per cent even for 1-MeV. photons.

Fig. 86 shows the spectrum of radiation emerging from a 1-million-volt X-ray machine, and the modified spectrum resulting when this beam is passed through 5 mm. of lead backed by tin, copper, and aluminium. In this case the X-ray tube had a fairly thick steel wall so that much of the low-energy radiation produced at the target never escaped from the tube but was completely stopped by the wall. Thus there is no 78-keV. radiation to be anomalously transmitted by the lead: nevertheless, the 'backing' materials are needed to remove the characteristic radiations inevitably added to the beam through photo-electric absorption in each filtering metal.

For X-rays generated at megavoltages in excess of two or three, the situation is again different. Over the energy range of 2 to about 6 MeV. the attenuation coefficients for most materials change remarkably little. For example, the linear coefficient for

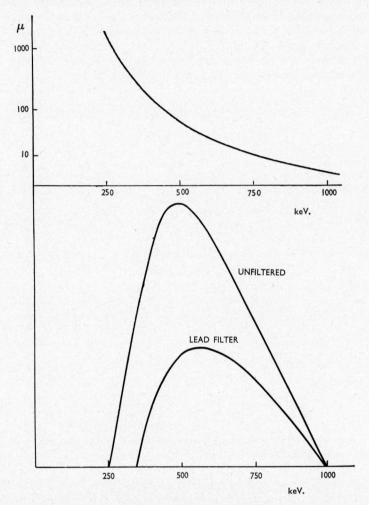

Fig. 86.—Lead as a filter for a 1-million-volt beam. The upper and lower parts correspond to those in previous similar figures.

lead decreases by a mere 9 per cent, whereas it changes by over 80 per cent between 200 and 600 keV. There is, therefore, unlikely to be any great filtration effect (that is to say, discrimination against the lower-energy radiation) when any material is put into the beam. All that would happen is that the beam intensity would be reduced without any useful alteration in the spectral distribution. For radiations generated at above 2 or 3 million volts, therefore, no useful purpose is served by the use of added filtration. The word 'added' should be noted. Megavoltage radiations are produced at a transmission target (as indicated in CHAPTER V) and the passage of the rays through this removes softer radiations which might otherwise be present. There is inevitably a considerable amount of 'inherent' filtration in this type of equipment.

Very High-energy Beams (Above 10 MV.).—Turning finally to even higher-energy radiations it is found that to try to filter them is a positive disadvantage. To understand why this is so it is necessary to look again at the reason behind the use of filtration. Clinical radiology (whether diagnostic or therapeutic) calls for radiations which will penetrate to the desired place (the film or the tumour) and for the removal of those radiations which do not do this efficiently. For radiations below a few MeV. in energy this means the removal of the lower-energy photons because in that energy range the higher the energy the greater the ability to penetrate *all* materials.

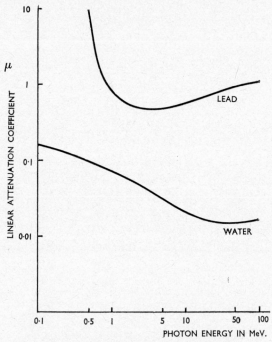

Fig. 87.—The variation of the linear attenuation coefficients of lead and water with photon energy. *N.B.*—Both scales are logarithmic.

However, this is not so for very high-energy beams where, as will be recalled from CHAPTER VII, the pair-production effect plays an important role. Therefore in striking contrast to what happens below 1 MeV., above 1 MeV. attenuation coefficients for all materials eventually increase with increasing photon energy. Because pair production is greater in materials of high atomic number than in those of low Z, the reversal takes place at lower energy in materials of high Z, such as lead, than in those of low Z, such as water, as is shown in *Fig.* 87. In that diagram it will be seen that the minimum attenuation coefficient (maximum penetration) occurs at about 50 MeV., whereas for lead it occurs at about 4 MeV., above which energy it rises steadily, though admittedly slowly.

Now consider what happens to beams incident upon lead and upon body tissues (here assumed to be water). Clearly, from *Fig.* 87, 30-MeV. photons penetrate through water more readily than 20-MeV. photons do, whereas the reverse is true for lead. Using a lead filter for, say, a 40-million-volt beam, in which 20- and 30-MeV. photons will be present and prominent, would therefore tend to *decrease* the beam's penetrating power in tissue by removing more of the higher-energy radiation than of the lower. Filtration is thus to be avoided for very high-energy beams, and any material that has to cross such beams should, wherever possible, be of low atomic number.

Suitable Filter Materials—A Summary.—Whilst there are no hard-and-fast boundaries which divide up the X-ray range and the materials suitable for filters, the following is fairly generally accepted:

Generating Voltage	Filter	
30 to 120 kV.	Aluminium	
100 to 250 kV.	Copper	
200 to 600 kV.	Tin	with appropriate 'backing'
600 to 2 MV.	Lead	
Above 2 MV.	None	

Suitable Filter Thicknesses.—It has already been mentioned that in addition to 'hardening' the beam, a filter also reduces its intensity, and that a compromise may have to be made to achieve an acceptable tube output as well as an acceptable beam penetration. How a decision can be made about what thickness should be used will probably be more easily understood after consideration has been given to the measurement of penetrating power or 'quality'.

RADIATION QUALITY

Physically the two fundamental properties of an X-ray beam are its intensity and the energies of its constituent photons. However, in radiology, interest is centred more in the energy abstracted from the beam (absorbed dose) rather than in intensity, and more upon the penetrating power (quality) than on precise photon energies, and it is the measurement and statement of this 'quality' which will be considered.

Half-value Layer (H.V.L.).—The most commonly used method of measuring radiation quality is to find the half-value layer, which has already been mentioned briefly in CHAPTER VI. Because of the importance of this measurement, not only in connexion with determination of attenuation coefficients, but also in practical

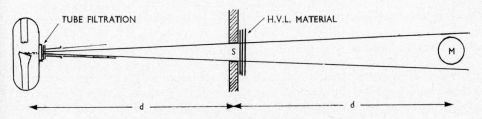

Fig. 88.—The measurement of the half-value layer.

radiology, no apology is offered for reiterating some things that have already been said. The H.V.L. is the thickness of a specified material which reduces the exposure rate at a particular point to half of its initial value. A diagrammatic representation of the method of measuring the H.V.L. is shown in *Fig.* 88.

Various thicknesses of the chosen material are introduced into the beam in front of the beam-defining 'stop' S and measurements of the Exposure rate are taken in each case by the measuring instrument M. A graph such as the lower of the two shown in

Fig. 89 is obtained by plotting Exposure rate against material thickness, and from it the thickness to reduce the Exposure rate to half of its original value (the H.V.L.) can be read off as indicated.

   Narrow and Broad Beams.—It will be noted in *Fig.* 88 that the beam used is narrow, being restricted by the 'stop' S to be just large enough to cover the measuring instrument adequately. This precaution is necessary in order to keep to a minimum the amount of scattered radiation reaching the measuring instrument M. What happens when a

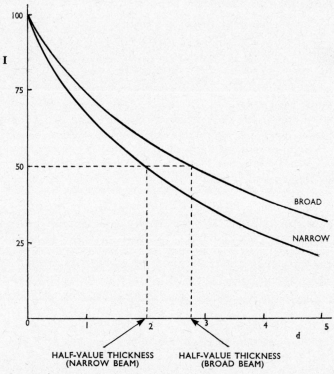

Fig. 89.—Attenuation curves and half-value layers for narrow and broad X-ray beams.

broad beam is used is illustrated in *Fig.* 90. Attenuation reduces the amount of radiation reaching M directly but this loss is compensated to some extent, in the case of the broad beam, by radiation scattered from other parts of the inserted material A. Thus for a broad beam the meter reading is greater than it would be for a narrow beam (when there is practically no compensatory scatter reaching M) and thus the radiation appears to be more penetrating than it actually is. To get a realistic measurement of penetrating power (which is what the H.V.L. gives) the modifying effect of scatter must be eliminated and hence a narrow beam is used. The difference in apparent attenuation for broad and narrow beams is illustrated in *Fig.* 89, the upper curve of which refers to the broad beam and shows the apparently greater penetrating power of the broad beam. Reference will be made again later to 'broad-beam' attenuation or transmission, which is very important in protection work.

   Reverting again to *Fig.* 88, it should be pointed out that the half-value layer material is placed half-way between the source and the measuring instrument because it has been established that in such an arrangement the minimum amount of scatter reaches M.

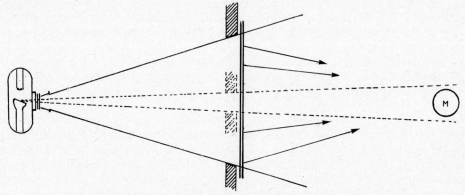

Fig. 90.—Why broad beams appear more penetrating than narrow beams.

Half-value Layer Materials.—The materials usually used for H.V.L. measurements have already been listed in CHAPTER VI, and using the appropriate materials the half-value layers given in *Table XV* were obtained for the beams represented by the spectra illustrated in *Figs*. 79 to 86, pp. 140–149.

Table XV.—HALF-VALUE LAYER AND FILTRATION

Note the superiority of the 'hardening' by the tin–copper–aluminium filter for 200-kV. radiation—each of the four filters passes the same amount of radiation

GENERATING VOLTAGE	ADDED FILTER	H.V.L.
80 kV.	0 2·0 mm. Al	3·2 mm. Al 5·4 mm. Al
200 kV.	0 15 mm. Al 1·5 mm. Cu Sn–Cu–Al compound 0·2 mm. Pb	0·7 mm. Cu 1·4 mm. Cu 1·6 mm. Cu 2·0 mm. Cu 1·2 mm. Cu
1000 kV.	0 5 mm. Pb	4·4 mm. Pb 5·0 mm. Pb

The 'hardening' effect of the filters can readily be seen for each beam as can the the superiority of the compound filter over the others for the 200-kV. beam.

It will be noticed that the same kind of material is often used for half-value layer measurements as is used as a filter material in that range, and this sometimes leads to confusion. The material introduced into the beam for the purpose of H.V.L. determination has nothing to do with the tube filter, even though they are of the same material. The filter is a permanent feature of the tube—the half-value layer material is part of the measuring apparatus, just as is the measuring instrument M. When the measurements are completed M, the 'stop' S, and the half-value layer material are all removed: the filter remains, since it is part of the working tube.

Other Methods of Quality Statement.—A valid objection to the half-value layer as a measure of beam quality is that, because different materials are used in different energy ranges, comparisons of the penetrating powers of two beams are not always easy. Whilst it is clear that a beam whose H.V.L. is 3 mm. of copper is more penetrating than one whose H.V.L. is 1·5 mm. copper, it is by no means clear whether a beam whose H.V.L. is 4·0 mm. of aluminium is more or less penetrating than one with an H.V.L. of 0·15 mm. copper. Or, alternatively, does a half-value layer of 5·0 mm. of copper indicate a harder beam than one of 1·5 mm. of lead? (In fact, the quality of the first pair of beams is the same, whilst the beam whose H.V.L. is 1·5 mm. of lead is considerably harder than that with 5·0 mm. of copper.) Several other methods which do not change their criteria from one energy to another have therefore been suggested.

1. *kV. or kVp., etc.*—The maximum photon energy in any beam, as has frequently been stated, depends upon the maximum voltage applied to the X-ray tube. This would be the kV. or the MV. for a constant-voltage supply and the peak kilo or megavoltage (kVp. or MVp.) when the supply is pulsating. However, in the range of generating voltages from about 100 to 1000 kV. a simple statement of the voltage—kV. or kVp.—is not a very good indication of radiation quality since it ignores the considerable alterations that can be produced by filtration. Below about 100 kV., i.e., in the diagnostic radiology range, provided that there is adequate filtration (1 or 2 mm. aluminium) to remove really low-energy radiations, and in the megavoltage range, where filtration is either ineffective or positively harmful, simple statements of generating voltage are adequate.

2. *Equivalent Energy.*—As already indicated in CHAPTER VI, the half-value layer and the linear attenuation coefficient are closely related, i.e.,

$$\mu = \frac{0 \cdot 693}{\text{H.V.L.}}.$$

Thus if μ is known it is possible, from standard tables of attenuation coefficients, to find a single energy for which photons would have the same value of μ. This, then, is the *equivalent energy* (in keV. or MeV.) of the beam—that is to say, the single energy whose photons would be attenuated to the same extent as are those of mixed energy of the actual spectrum.

By way of example, *Table XVI* shows the half-value layers, linear attenuation coefficients, and equivalent energies of the beams discussed above. The relative penetrating powers are much more obvious from the values of the equivalent energies than from the H.V.L.

Table XVI.—HALF-VALUE LAYER, LINEAR ATTENUATION COEFFICIENT, AND EQUIVALENT PHOTON ENERGY

H.V.L.	LINEAR ATTENUATION COEFFICIENT	EQUIVALENT PHOTON ENERGY
4·0 mm. Al	1·73 cm.$^{-1}$ Al	38 keV.
0·15 mm. Cu	46·2 cm.$^{-1}$ Cu	38 keV.
1·5 mm. Cu	4·62 cm.$^{-1}$ Cu	96 keV.
3·0 mm. Cu	2·31 cm.$^{-1}$ Cu	140 keV.
5·0 mm. Cu	1·39 cm.$^{-1}$ Cu	200 keV.
1·5 mm. Pb	4·62 cm.$^{-1}$ Pb	290 keV.

A useful generalization arising from calculations of this sort is that, for a reasonably filtered beam, the equivalent kilovoltage is about 40 per cent of the applied kilovoltage.

For example, a stream of 80-keV. photons would have the same penetrating power as a beam generated at 200 kV. and filtered with about 1 mm. of copper.

Equivalent Wavelength.—An alternative, but nowadays not so widely used, approach is to find that wavelength for which μ is the same as that calculated from the H.V.L. This can be done either from tables relating attenuation coefficient and wavelength, or by finding the equivalent kilovoltage and then using the relationship between wavelength and energy, viz.:

$$\lambda = \frac{12\cdot4}{kV.}\ \text{Å}.$$

Beam Homogeneity.—A beam of photons of one energy is obviously homogeneous: to use a single energy or wavelength value to describe an X-ray spectrum implies that that radiation is behaving as a homogeneous beam. Such an assumption hardly seems justified when it is remembered what a range of energies there are even in a well-filtered beam. It is useful, therefore, to have some indication of the extent to which the assumption is justified.

Mono-energetic photons are attenuated according to the exponential attenuation law. A homogeneous beam obeys the law: a beam that obeys the law can be said to be behaving as if homogeneous. One feature of exponential attenuation is that if a

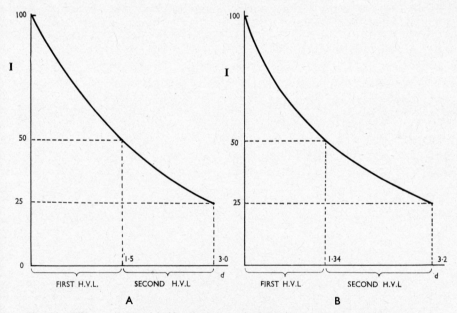

Fig. 91.—First and second half-value layers, A, With a homogeneous, and B, With an inhomogeneous, beam.

certain thickness (the H.V.L.) of a material reduces the beam to half, the addition of an equal thickness will bring it down to a quarter. The *added* thickness, over the half-value layer, to reduce the beam to a quarter is called *the second half-value layer*, and for a homogeneous beam the first and second half-value layers are equal, as illustrated in *Fig.* 91 A.

When the beam is not homogeneous the first material introduced in the half-value layer measurement will harden the beam so that the second half-value layer will be greater than the first (*Fig.* 91 B). The greater the inhomogeneity the greater will be the second H.V.L. compared with the first. The ratio of these two half-value layers, i.e.,

$$\frac{\text{First H.V.L.}}{\text{Second H.V.L.}}$$

is sometimes called the *homogeneity coefficient*. For a homogeneous beam its value is unity: for an inhomogeneous beam it will be less than one—the smaller the fraction, the greater the inhomogeneity.

The 'Semi-log Plot'.—(This section may be omitted, without serious handicap, by those with a limited knowledge of mathematics.)

A more elegant method of revealing the homogeneity—or otherwise—of a beam is to present the data obtained in the H.V.L. determination rather differently from the method used up to now. As has been stated many times, a homogeneous beam obeys the exponential attenuation law, i.e.,

$$I = I_0 e^{-\mu d} \quad \text{or} \quad I/I_0 = e^{-\mu d}.$$

If, instead of plotting I/I_0 against d (as, for example, in *Fig.* 91), the logarithm of (I/I_0) is plotted against d, the graph becomes a straight line if *the exponential law is being obeyed*. (This method of presentation is often called the 'semi-log plot' since one of the axes is scaled logarithmically). A homogeneous beam, therefore, gives a straight-line graph. If the exponential law is not being obeyed—which means that the beam is not homogeneous—the line is not straight. Examples of both these types of

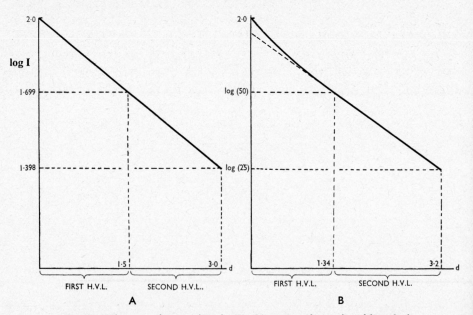

Fig. 92.—The same data as given in *Fig.* 91 presented on a 'semi-log plot'.

graph are shown in *Fig.* 85 which presents, on a 'semi-log plot', the same data as that used in *Fig.* 91. *Fig.* 92 A shows the straight line of the homogeneous beam, whilst the inhomogeneity of the beam represented in *Fig.* 92 B is quickly revealed by the curvature of that line. The semi-logarithmic presentation immediately shows up inhomogeneity, and also its degree, from the curvature of the graph. Furthermore, it also shows whether the beam can be made effectively homogeneous by filtration, for if this state can be reached the curve becomes a straight line.

Such a state of affairs is revealed by *Fig.* 92 B, where the line is straight for thicknesses greater than 1 mm. of copper. This indicates that the beam is made effectively homogeneous by passing through 1 mm. of copper, and therefore that the copper filtration needed to give a homogeneous beam is 1 mm. thick.

Desirable Filtration.—Attention may now be turned to the question of what degree of filtration should be used in practice. Is it necessary to achieve an effectively homogeneous beam such as has been described? As so often happens in radiology, the answer is that a compromise has to be made. On the one hand, filtration increases quality and therefore penetrating power, but, on the other, it reduces the beam intensity.

The maximum filtration that should be used is that needed to produce an effectively homogeneous beam. For example, in the beam illustrated in *Fig.* 92 B the only effect of using a copper filter of thickness more than 1 mm. would be to reduce the beam intensity. No extra 'hardening' occurs because after passing through 1 mm. of copper the beam is effectively homogeneous.

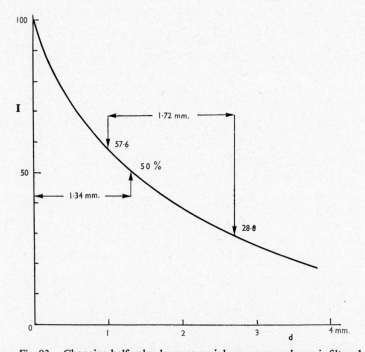

Fig. 93.—Changing half-value layer as an inhomogeneous beam is filtered.

But is the maximum filtration necessary? Would not rather less filtration be acceptable? These questions can only be answered by considering how the penetration of the beam in water or soft tissue varies with half-value layer.

From *Fig.* 92 B, or more easily *Fig.* 91 B, the half-value layer of the beam for various filtration conditions can be evaluated as is shown in *Fig.* 93, the curve of which is identical, as far as data are concerned, with *Fig.* 91 **B.** The half-value layer for the initial beam is clearly 1·34 mm. of copper. However, the beam which has passed through 1 mm. of copper has a different quality which can be determined by finding that thickness (2·72 mm.) for which the beam reading (28·8) is half the beam reading for 1 mm. copper (57·6). From these values it will be seen that the half-value layer for the beam that has passed through 1 mm. copper is 1·72 mm. copper. In a like manner the half-value layers of the beam after it has passed through various copper thicknesses have been found and their values are given in *Table XVII*, which shows

Table XVII.—THE CHANGE OF HALF-VALUE LAYER, OUTPUT, AND LINEAR
ATTENUATION COEFFICIENT FOR WATER, WITH INCREASING FILTRATION

ADDED FILTER (mm.Cu)	H.V.L. (mm.Cu)	EXPOSURE RATE (unfiltered rate 100)	μ WATER
0	1·34	100	0·178
0·2	1·52	88	0·173
0·5	1·66	73	0·170
1·0	1·72	57	0·169
1·5	1·72	47	0·169
2·0	1·72	41·5	0·169

a considerable change in half-value layer before effective homogeneity is attained. Nothing like so great a change occurs in the values of the attenuation coefficients of the beams in water over this quality range owing, of course, to the fact that water attenuates mainly by scattering in this energy range, whereas the photo-electric effect

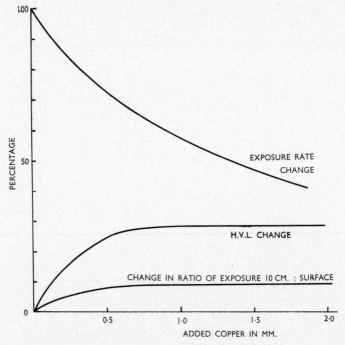

Fig. 94.—Some of the effects of increased filtration.

is still important in copper. The practical effect of this is that the penetration of radiation into water or a patient does not change as much as the half-value layer, and this is of considerable importance in filtration selection.

The effect of these attenuation coefficient changes on the relative depth doses* at 10 cm. in a patient is shown in *Fig.* 94, together with the percentage changes in half-value layer and the fall in beam intensity which would be produced by filters of various thicknesses. Thus a 1-mm. copper filter (which gives the homogeneous beam) gives a depth dose 9 per cent greater than that given by the initial beam, but, on the other hand, it reduces the beam by 43 per cent. An almost equal increase in depth dose (8·0 per cent) can be achieved by using only 0·5 mm. copper as filter, and this cuts down the beam by 27 per cent. From considerations of this sort, the most suitable filter for the beam being discussed would seem to be 0·5 mm. of copper (with appropriate backing), for though the beam is not quite homogeneous according to the standards discussed, it has almost the same penetrating power in water as the homogeneous beam, and its intensity is over 25 per cent greater.

Such are the considerations usually taken into account when deciding upon the filtration to be used, which may be less than that needed to give an effectively homogeneous beam.

Quality Specification.—In a recently published report (Report 10d entitled *Clinical Dosimetry* and published as Handbook 87 of the United States National Bureau of Standards) the International Commission on Radiological Units and Measurements recommended the following methods of quality specification for X-ray beams:

1. For radiotherapy up to 2 MV., state the kilovoltage or megavoltage at which the tube is operating and the H.V.L. of the beam.

2. For radiations generated at above 2 MV., and in the diagnostic range, state the kilovoltage or megavoltage only.

---

* Depth doses will be discussed in greater detail later. Here the term is used to describe the ratio of the Exposure rates at the depth (10 cm.) and the surface.

SECTION II. DIAGNOSTIC RADIOLOGY

CHAPTER XIV

THE PHYSICAL BASIS OF DIAGNOSTIC RADIOLOGY

THE aim of Diagnostic Radiology is to produce a picture in the form of shadows of various sizes, shapes, and degrees of blackness (greyness). From this picture the radiologist attempts to deduce the anatomical structure of the patient responsible for the shadow pattern, and in particular to infer any departure from normality.

In the production of the radiographic picture, complicated apparatus and a sequence of complex processes are involved. This chapter will present a general survey of the whole procedure, which is also shown schematically in *Figs*. 95 and 96. The immediately following chapters will consider individual items separately and in some detail, whilst later chapters will show how the different practical requirements dictate the design of the apparatus and the way in which it is used. Whilst this book is principally concerned with the physical aspects of the subject, of necessity some practical, clinical aspects will, and should, intrude. For complete detailed descriptions of actual techniques, however, the reader must refer to more specialized books.

In surveying the stages which lead up to the making of a diagnosis from the completed picture it is convenient to recall, briefly, the physical facts and principles described in detail in earlier chapters. Theory and practice can, thus, be firmly related and the influence of practical demands on apparatus design more clearly shown.

It will be recalled that X-rays are produced when a beam of fast-moving electrons is stopped by a tungsten target in an X-ray tube (5*). In this process the kinetic energy of the electrons is converted into a small amount of X-rays together with a very large amount of heat. The region of the target where X-rays, and the heat, are produced is called the **focal spot** and since sharp shadows are needed in the picture, this focal spot must be small—often 1 mm. square or less. This, in its turn, makes essential the provision of some efficient cooling system for the removal of the unwanted heat which could otherwise lead to a damaged or useless target. The rate at which X-rays may be produced and the time for which X-ray production may continue without interruption (usually called the **rating** of the tube) depend upon the efficiency of the cooling, and also upon the design of the tube, and especially of the target and its associated parts.

The electron current ('the milliamperes' or 'mA.' in common parlance) is provided by an electrically heated filament, whilst the required kinetic energy results from the high potential difference (kilovoltage) applied between the target and filament. A special power unit or generator (3) must therefore be provided to convert the mains voltage available in the X-ray department to the required kilovoltage, and also to give the heating current. The electrical supply to the department (4) must be adequate to meet demands for large amounts of power, usually over short times,

---

* The numbers refer to the correspondingly numbered items in *Figs*. 95 and 96.

160

especially where modern equipment is used. From earlier chapters it will be remembered that the applied kilovoltage is the main factor in controlling the penetrating power of the beam, whilst the quantity of radiation depends on both the kilovoltage and the total number of electrons hitting the target. This number of electrons is usually measured as the product of the tube current (milliamperes) and the exposure time (seconds), i.e., in milliampere-seconds (mA.s.). The calibrated controls on the control desk (1) enable suitable values of kV. and mA.s. to be selected, the values so selected often being shown also on meters.

The uniform beam of X-rays (11) produced by the X-ray tube is directed on to the appropriate part of the patient. This is possible since the X-ray tube mounting is designed to allow the tube to be moved freely over the table (15) on which the patient lies, and since the tube may also be angled in any required direction. When the X-rays strike the patient some are stopped (absorbed), some are deflected from their original direction (scattered), and some pass through unaffected (transmitted). This results in a pattern of intensities being created in the beam which emerges from the patient, since X-rays travel in straight lines unless they are scattered. The sizes, shapes, and positions of the patterns are produced and controlled by the size, shape, and position of the anatomical structures in the patient through which the beam has passed. In addition, the varying degrees of blackness in the pattern will depend upon the thickness and kind of material through which the X-rays have passed.

Although this pattern, from which the radiologist is to make his deductions, is actually present in the X-ray beam emerging through the patient, it cannot, of course, be seen since the human eye is not visually* sensitive to X-radiation. It is necessary, therefore, to make the pattern visible and there are two main ways in which this is done.

1. *Radiography* (*Fig.* 95).—In this method the pattern of X-rays is allowed to fall on to a photographic film placed behind the patient. Since the film would be affected by visible light it is contained inside a light-tight box called a cassette (13) which is carried on the cassette tray (14) beneath the table. After being chemically processed (16) either manually or automatically, the film shows a visible, stable picture of the pattern which existed in the transmitted X-ray beam during the (brief) time of the exposure. For diagnosis the film (18) is held or supported in front of a uniformly illuminated viewing screen (17). The regions of the film corresponding to places in the patient where a lot of X-rays were transmitted appear black (little light reaching the radiologist's eyes). Those regions corresponding to where few X-rays were transmitted appear relatively bright (a lot of light reaching his eyes). The final film is therefore in the form of a **negative**: dark where there is little X-ray shadow and bright where there is a shadow.

   The amount of radiation needed to produce a film of convenient blackness may be reduced by using a pair of intensifying screens, one in intimate contact with each side of the film, within the cassette. The deleterious effects of scattered radiation can be reduced by putting a grid (12) between the patient and the film.

2. *Fluoroscopy* (*Fig.* 96).—Here the X-ray tube (20) is usually situated beneath the table (21) upon which the patient lies, or against which he

---

* The lens is easily damaged by ionizing radiations and it is important that no attempt is ever made to 'see' the X-rays directly.

stands when the table is tilted as in *Fig*. 96. This tube is usually called the under-couch tube. The beam of X-rays transmitted through the patient, and containing the pattern of intensities of interest, is allowed

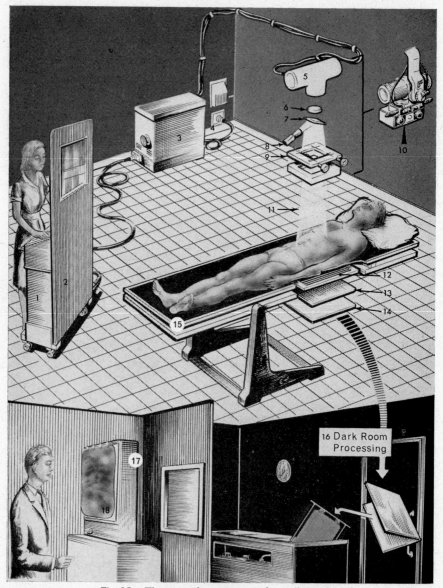

Fig. 95.—The general arrangement for radiography.

to fall on to the fluorescent screen (23) placed immediately above the patient. This results in an immediately visible picture of the pattern in the X-ray beam. The action of the X-rays on the screen is to produce an emission of visible light photons in amount proportional to the incident

X-ray intensity. The screen is bright where there are a lot of X-rays and comparatively dark where there are few X-rays. The picture is therefore a **positive** one and it exists for as long as the X-ray beam is switched on.

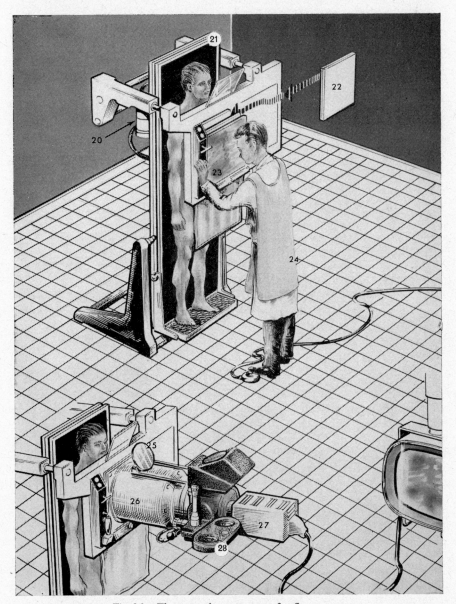

Fig. 96.—The general arrangement for fluoroscopy.

Furthermore, any movement of or in the patient is immediately seen. The picture is therefore instantaneous, ephemeral, and dynamic, as distinct from the radiograph which gives a permanent, static record of the situation existing at the moment of the X-ray exposure. The two techniques, radiography and fluoroscopy, are therefore complementary. If it is required to have a permanent record from which more detailed information can be obtained, then a cassette (22) is moved into position between the patient and the screen and a radiograph taken at the appropriate instant.

The brightness of the screen is not high, which leads to practical difficulties, but it may be made brighter, and the exposure kept small, by means of an *image intensifier* (26), the output screen of which may be observed either directly by means of a mirror system (25) or via a television system (27).

A static photograph of a fluoroscopic screen may be taken, usually on a reduced scale. This is photo-fluorography and is more commonly encountered in 'mass miniature' techniques using specially designed apparatus. In some circumstances a 'moving' film may be required. This is called cine-radiography and is nowadays usually effected by photographing (28) the output screen of the image intensifier. In this way the radiation dose to the patient is kept low.

However, no matter what device is employed, the final stage always consists of a radiologist looking at a pattern of various lights and darknesses and from them making a diagnosis of the patient responsible for its formation.

Since radiation always causes biological damage to any cells by which it may be absorbed it is important to ensure that no cells are irradiated either unnecessarily or excessively. There are two equally important aspects to this subject of 'Radiation Protection':

    a. The protection of the patient; and
    b. The protection of the X-ray worker.

To protect the patient the size of the X-ray beam is kept as small as possible consistent with examining fully the site of interest. In both radiography and fluoroscopy the beam size is restricted by a cone or a diaphragm (9) fixed to the unit between the X-ray tube and the patient. The area of the patient included in the beam may be visualized by means of a light beam diaphragm system in which a beam of light from a lamp (8) is directed by a mirror (7) through the diaphragm (9). The various items attached to the X-ray tube, shown in exploded view, in reality appear as on the right (10). The use of a small beam has an incidental but important effect on the quality of the final picture. Restriction of the beam minimizes the production of scattered radiation which would otherwise tend to spoil the film. The use of a filter (6) between the tube and the patient serves to remove the radiation which is not sufficiently penetrating to contribute significantly to the pattern in the transmitted beam and which would unnecessarily damage the patient.

The X-ray worker is primarily protected from radiation hazard by arranging that he is never exposed to the direct beam, even though it may already have been attenuated by the patient. This means that he must never sit or stand or place any part of himself behind or in front of the patient unless suitably protected—for example, by the lead glass backing the fluoroscopic screen (23), and the lead rubber apron (24) worn by the radiologist. It is also important to avoid exposure by radiation scattered from the patient or from other objects in the X-ray beam. This is achieved by suitable siting of the X-ray control desk (1), with respect to the tube and patient, and by the use of protective barriers (2). The reduction in beam size mentioned previously helps to reduce the amount of scattered radiation produced. In addition to radiation safety, proper attention must be given to electrical safety in view of the very large, and therefore dangerous, voltages employed.

In order to be able to produce a satisfactory picture without unnecessary exposure to the patient, the radiographer must know many things about the operation of his equipment. In particular, he must know about the amount of, and penetrating power of, the radiation being produced by the equipment, and that the equipment is functioning correctly. To this end various measuring devices are incorporated in the apparatus. These include instruments to measure the mains voltage, the kilovoltage, the tube current, and the exposure time. In addition, the amount of radiation leaving the tube is sometimes measured by means of an ionization chamber monitor incorporated in the light beam diaphragm unit or that reaching the film by some form of photo-timer.

This, then, is a brief, very superficial description of the general arrangement used in clinical radiology. In the next few chapters, we shall examine the various steps in the process, commencing with the film.

CHAPTER XV

THE X-RAY FILM AND ITS PROCESSING

ALTHOUGH the exposed* and processed film is the end-point in the making of the radiograph, it is convenient to describe its behaviour and properties immediately.

Construction of the Film.—The most commonly used type of X-ray film is built up in the way indicated diagrammatically, on a very much magnified scale, in *Fig.* 97. This shows a section through what is known as a *double-coated film*, so named because

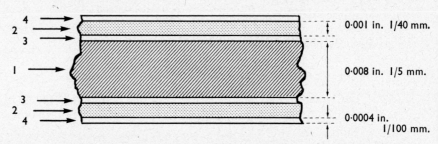

Fig. 97.—A greatly magnified cross-section of a double-coated X-ray film showing: 1, the film base; 2, the layers of emulsion; 3, the 'subbing' layers which make the emulsion adhere firmly to the base; and 4, the protective supercoatings.

it has two layers of *emulsion* (2). It is in these layers that all the changes occur which result in the eventual production of the visible pattern. The emulsion layers consist of gelatin in which is suspended a very large number of tiny flat triangular crystals, mostly of silver bromide, though small amounts of other silver halides may also be present. In order that the film should be equally sensitive over its whole area it is necessary that the crystals should be distributed uniformly throughout the gelatin layer. Careful investigation has shown that these crystals, which lie parallel to the film surface and are about 1/1000 mm. across, are not perfect in structure nor are they chemically pure. As will be described in more detail later, the photographic effect in the crystals arises from these faults and impurities which, along with the precise size and number of crystals present, govern the detailed photographic properties of the emulsion. By varying these parameters the manufacturers are able to produce films of different types and properties.

In between the two layers of emulsion is a comparatively thick, and transparent, layer known as the *film base* (1). Usually this is made of cellulose tri-acetate although recently manufacturers have started to use 'polyester'. A small amount of blue dye is added to the base and this helps in the ultimate viewing of the radiograph. The

---

* It was indicated in CHAPTER IX that there are general and special meanings to the word 'exposure'. In this and immediately following chapters the word will tend to be used in its general sense, and the phrase 'X-ray tube exposure' will be used to refer to the amount of radiation produced by the tube, whilst the words 'exposure' or 'exposed' will have the meaning of 'being or having been subjected to X-radiation'. When the word is used in the special defined sense of the amount of radiation received by the film measured in roentgens (R) or milliroentgens (mR) the expression 'Exposure (mR)' will be used.

film base serves as the support for the very fragile emulsion layers. It is moderately flexible and, of course, has not and does not acquire any visible pattern. Unlike the proverbial good child, it is there to do its job of supporting the emulsion but is not to be seen. This type of film base is referred to as 'safety film' since, unlike cellulose nitrate which was used in earlier days, it is comparatively non-inflammable, although it will burn if held in a flame. During chemical processing, as will be described later, the emulsion layer swells to many times its previous thickness and then contracts during the drying process. This change in the emulsion takes place almost entirely in the direction perpendicular to the film surface, since the base itself does not change in size. There is, therefore, no lateral movement of the pattern over the film surface, which is very important since it is essential that the various parts of the pattern shall be seen in exactly the same place as they were produced. The fact that the film base neither contracts nor shrinks in area is therefore essential. Cellulose tri-acetate is chosen since it has sufficient dimensional stability, although it is stated that the newer 'polyester' base is even better. It is also vital, of course, that the emulsion layer shall be firmly attached to this inert base. The very thin layers (3), which consist of gelatin plus a solvent for cellulose acetate, ensure that this is so. Finally, there are the layers (4) known as the supercoating, and which consist of clear gelatin. These layers serve to protect the emulsion layer from mechanical damage since the sensitive silver bromide crystals can be affected by such things as pressure, scratching or friction, as well as by X-rays and light. In addition, the supercoating forms a protective layer for the finished, processed radiograph, so that extreme care in handling is not of paramount importance.

The Production of the Pattern.—As a result of the various absorptions in the patient there is a pattern in the beam of X-rays which is incident upon the film. By this is meant that over some regions of the film there are a lot of X-ray photons, in other regions very few photons and elsewhere various intermediate values. The extent to which a particular small area of the film is affected by the X-rays depends upon the number of photons incident upon that area and hence the pattern contained in the X-ray beam will be impressed on the film. If it were possible to examine the film at this stage we would find that no *visible* change has yet occurred and the appearance of the film (and in particular of each silver bromide crystal) is exactly as it was before the X-ray exposure. However, a very important change has actually occurred and it is said that a **latent image*** exists. The pattern of the X-ray beam is there on the film but it cannot yet be seen. Before the results of the X-ray exposure are visible, the film must undergo chemical processing. The first stage of this is called **development**, during which the silver bromide crystals, which have been sufficiently affected during the exposure, are converted into tiny, opaque, black silver specks, whilst those which have not been sufficiently affected remain in their previous yellowish translucent state. The X-ray pattern is now 'visible': where there were a lot of X-rays there is a lot of opaque silver specks, which make these regions look black, whereas in those regions subjected to smaller amounts of X-rays there are proportionally small amounts of black silver specks and the film looks less black, i.e., grey. Unfortunately, the film cannot be left in this state for if it were, then the visible light (with which the film is being examined) would gradually convert the unaffected but still remaining silver bromide crystals into opaque silver, so that the whole film would become black. It is therefore necessary to **fix** the image and this is the next stage in

---

* 'Latent image' refers to the latent effect in the single crystal as distinct from the 'latent pattern' existing on the film as a whole.

the chemical processing. During fixation the unaffected silver bromide crystals are dissolved away, leaving only the record of the X-ray pattern in the form of a corresponding pattern of black silver specks embedded in gelatin. It often comes as somewhat of a surprise to learn that the usual experience of silver being a bright shiny material arises only because the surface of the metal has been made very smooth. The visual effect of a small blob of silver deposited from a solution is of a black spot. This is because its surface is very rough and, of course, the speck is opaque.

Although it has not yet been stated, it is to be understood that, from the moment of manufacture up to the time when fixation is completed, the film must not be exposed to visible light, to which the film is also sensitive. To achieve this the film is handled in a dark room and exposed to X-rays whilst in a light-tight container called a **cassette**. It is also important that the unprocessed film should not be unintentionally irradiated nor stored under bad atmospheric conditions such as high temperature or dampness. All these can result in unwanted blackening of the film which can be bad enough to impair seriously the usefulness of the desired radiograph.

After fixation all that remains is to wash the film thoroughly to remove all the various chemicals used for the processing, as well as the products of the various chemical reactions which have taken place during processing. The final step is to dry the film so that it can easily be viewed for diagnostic or other purposes.

After this brief and very superficial survey it is now necessary to examine in more detail exactly what happens at each stage. The whole process of exposure and chemical processing is, in fact, very complicated and it is only within the last decade that some of the details have been clarified.

The Structure of Silver Bromide.—A crystal of silver bromide consists of an orderly array of silver and bromine in what is known as a cubical structure. *Fig.* 98 illustrates this structure in which the silver and bromine are seen to be at the corners of (imaginary) cubes. It must be noted that these are silver and bromine ions and not atoms. When the atoms combine to form silver bromide the electron from the outer shell of the silver atom moves over to the bromine and so gives it an overall negative charge ($-e$). The loss of the electron from the silver makes it have an overall positive charge ($+e$). Even in such a tiny crystal as occurs in the emulsion, this regular pattern of ions is repeated many, many times to produce the already-mentioned overall crystal shape. This description is of a perfect crystal which would be, in fact, of no use photographically. Fortunately, during the manufacture of the silver bromide, and in the subsequent preparation of the emulsion, faults of various kinds arise in the crystals. These faults may be either of structure or due to the presence of a chemical contaminant. There have been many different suggestions about the exact identity of the contaminant responsible for the photographic property of silver bromide, but it is now commonly accepted that it is due to the sulphur compound, allyl thiocarbamide. Whatever it may be, the presence of this substance results in there being, on the surface of the crystal, a small region (*Fig.* 99 A) to which the name **sensitivity speck** is given. This region has the property that it is able to trap extra electrons and it is here that the black speck of silver will ultimately form. Apart from this small region the remainder of the surface of the crystal is composed of negatively charged bromine ions (*Fig.* 99 B). This does not mean, however, that the crystal as a whole is electrically charged, any more than the fact that there are electrons on the outside of atoms means that atoms are charged. Any excess of negative charge appearing on the crystal surface is exactly balanced by the presence of *extra* silver ions lying within (not at the corners of) the crystal lattice. These silver ions are called **interstitial** ions.

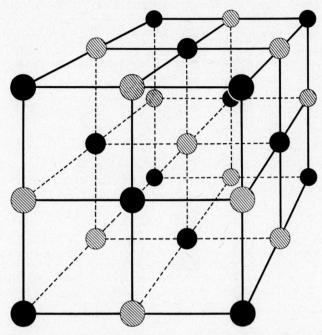

Fig. 98.—Part of a silver bromide crystal lattice. ⬤ Silver ion +, ◉ Bromine ion —

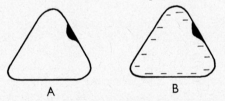

A   B

Fig. 99.—A single crystal of photographically active silver bromide showing: A, the sensitivity speck, and B, the negatively charged bromine barrier.

Exposure to X-rays.—It is now possible to describe the effects which exposure to X-radiation (and visible light) has on such a crystal. Although this description will take some time, the actual effects in the film resulting from the radiation take place almost instantaneously: certainly in a time very much shorter than the smallest contemplated X-ray exposure time. The sequence of events is illustrated schematically in *Fig.* 100, and the various steps are:

   a. Of the total number of photons passing through a particular crystal, imagine that one is absorbed. (If not even one is absorbed, as is often the case, then, of course, there is no effect and therefore nothing to describe!) This photon will probably have been absorbed by the photo-electric process, since bromine and silver have comparatively large atomic numbers ($Z = 35$ and 47 respectively) and in the diagnostic radiology range of qualities the photon energy is not particularly high. Alternatively, energy may have been absorbed by the Compton effect, but in either case the immediate result is the production of a fast-moving electron which has acquired its kinetic energy at the expense of the photon (*Fig.* 100 A).

b. As it moves through the crystal this photo- or Compton electron will gradually lose its energy by releasing other electrons which also move through the crystal. Some, if not all, of these electrons will pass close to the sensitivity speck and will be trapped there. The sensitivity speck

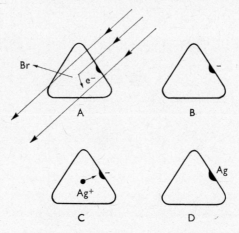

Fig. 100.—The formation of a latent image.

thus acquires a negative charge (*Fig.* 100 B). During this process negatively charged bromine ions are converted into neutral bromine atoms which leave the crystal and are taken up by the surrounding gelatin. The gelatin is thus seen to have an active role as well as the passive one of supporting the crystals, etc. If the bromine atoms were not removed into the gelatin, then the subsequent events would be quite different.

c. The negative charge at the sensitivity speck will exert an electrical attraction on the interstitial silver ions (*Fig.* 100 C) which are positively charged and are capable of moving through the crystal. This will result in one of these ions moving to the sensitivity speck where the charges neutralize each other; the silver ion becoming a neutral silver atom.

d. At the sensitivity speck there is now an extra neutral silver atom. Since many electrons were liberated by the original photo- (or Compton) electron, the process just described will occur many times and the final result of the absorption of one photon of X-rays by the crystal will be the congregation at the sensitivity speck of a small number of silver atoms (*Fig.* 100 D). This now constitutes the latent image. It is not known for certain how many atoms of silver are needed to create a developable latent image and, in any case, it depends upon the development method used. The number is between 10 and 100 and it is therefore not surprising that it is not detectable either visually or chemically. If the emulsion is sufficiently exposed to radiation then eventually there will be enough silver at the sensitivity speck to make it visible under the microscope. This, however, requires enormous amounts of radiation, the latent image being produced by exposures minute in comparison.

The absorption of just one X-ray photon by a crystal is thus seen to result in a latent image being formed in that crystal. With visible light whose quantum energy (and therefore the total number of electrons released per photon) is so very much smaller, it is found that many photons must be absorbed by a crystal before there are sufficient atoms of silver at the sensitivity speck to constitute a latent image.

Development.—The action of the developer is to convert the crystals containing a latent image into black specks of silver, and to leave unchanged those crystals not having a latent image. The conversion of silver bromide into silver occurs if the developing solution is able to donate electrons to the crystal since this results in the conversion of silver ions into silver atoms. Chemicals which are able to donate electrons are called *reducing agents* and the chemical action which they cause is called *reduction*. In this case silver bromide is said to be *reduced* to silver.

The conversion of each silver ion is accompanied by the liberation of a bromine ion which is first taken up by the gelatin (as in the exposure of the film) and eventually goes into solution in the developer. It is for this reason that the bromine concentration of a developing solution increases with use. The chemical action which the silver undergoes may be summarized as:

$$Ag^+ \quad + \quad e^- \quad \longrightarrow \quad Ag.$$

Silver ion	Electron	Silver
in crystal	from	atom
containing	developer	
latent		
image		

Clearly a chemical which is to be suitable as a developer is one which will easily donate electrons to latent-image-containing crystals but which is unable to donate electrons to those not having a latent image. This selectivity results from a correct choice of developing agent and emulsion manufacturing techniques. As has already been described, the exterior of the crystal is composed of negative bromine ions, with the positively charged silver ions (together with a lot more bromine ions) lying within this *bromine barrier*.

This barrier is represented diagrammatically in *Fig*. 101 A for an unexposed silver bromide crystal or for—what amounts to the same thing—one which has not yet acquired a latent image. In such a situation any attempt by the developer to donate an electron to the crystal will be opposed because of the electrical repulsion between the negative charge lying on the outside of the crystal and the negative electron (*Fig*. 101 B). The developer is thus not able to reduce this crystal of silver bromide to silver.

Now consider a silver bromide crystal which contains a latent image (*Fig*. 101 C). Here there is a congregation of silver atoms at the surface of the crystal and this constitutes a break in the barrier. At this point electrons from the developer are able to penetrate into the crystal and effect the reduction of the silver ions. This process will continue until all the silver ions have been converted into silver and all the bromine ions have passed into solution in the developer. The 'latent-image-containing silver bromide crystal' has been converted from its original yellowish, translucent form into a speck of black, opaque silver. Because of a rather complex transfer process the atoms of silver build up successively at the sensitivity speck, until the whole of the silver is built up into a single black speck at this point, and this is illustrated in the remaining steps of *Fig*. 101. It is important to realize that the final black speck of silver is situated in the emulsion in exactly the same place as was the irradiated silver bromide crystal in which the original photon was absorbed.

This description is a rather simplified version of the actual happenings in the development process but it nevertheless leads to the explanation of one or two important practical facts.

The Effect of the Developer.—The power of the developer will determine just how large the break in the bromine barrier, resulting from the presence of the latent image, must be before the crystal can be reduced. An extremely powerful reducing agent could, in fact, overcome the barrier even in the absence of a latent image. Such a strongly acting chemical is clearly no use as a photographic developer, since it would

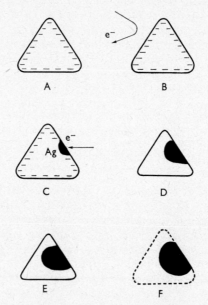

Fig. 101.—The development process. A and B, No effect without a latent image.
C–F, Formation of a silver 'grain'.

not be able to differentiate between the latent-image and non-latent-image crystals. At the other end of the scale the agent could be so weak as to require either an un-reasonably large latent image or a very protracted development. Again this would be an unsatisfactory developing agent.

By considering these extremes it is easy to appreciate that the exact character of the developing solution has a great bearing on the final image produced on the film. The practical importance of this is that, for a given type of film, the developer to be used will contribute to the determination of the correct exposure which must be given to the film. Conversely the kind of final picture produced will depend not only on the type of film used and exposure given but also on the development employed.

There is another type of development which can occur. Some of the silver bromide is dissolved by the developing solution and the reduction to silver takes place in the solution. This silver is then deposited at the latent image by a process not unlike electro-plating. The extent to which this type of development occurs in X-ray work is very small indeed and, in any case, leads to the same final result: a black opaque speck of silver, at the position of the latent image.

The Presence of Fog.—The way in which the absorption of radiation by a silver bromide crystal can result in the production of a latent image which makes the crystal developable has been described. Crystals can, however, be made developable in many other ways. Such effects as pressure (such as is produced by writing on a film), exposure to certain types of chemical fumes, and storage at elevated temperatures are some of the more usual causes met with in practice. In addition to these effects, it is found that the developer may well develop some unexposed, unaffected in any way, silver bromide crystals.

Although the developing agent will have been chosen for its ability to differentiate between those crystals having a latent image and those which do not, the situation in practice is not quite the 'all or none' phenomenon implied in the foregoing simple explanations. The optimum developer is one which readily reduces those crystals having a latent image and which experiences extreme difficulty in reducing those which do not have a latent image. This means that almost all those crystals with a latent image will be reduced to silver, but also that a few of those which have not been affected by radiation or any other agent will also be converted to silver.

Hence if a completely unexposed film is developed there will be a certain amount of blackening on the processed film. The amount of this blackening will depend upon the type of film, upon how it has been stored and handled, and upon the development to which it was subjected. This blackening is referred to as **fog** and, on a film which has been exposed to radiation, it exists in addition to the blackening produced by the radiation.

Blackening of the film can also result from accidental exposure to radiation during storage. This will also be observed as a general 'fog' on the film but it is clearly of a different nature from the usual fog blackening.

Fixation and Hardening.—The process of fixation is more simple than that of development since it is really just a question of dissolving, and so removing, the remaining unaffected silver bromide from the film. What happens, however, is still somewhat complex, the silver bromide first forming a complex molecule with the fixing agent, after which this complex molecule is itself dissolved in further fixing solution. This is the reason why there has to be an 'excess of fixer' present. Fixation is carried out in a weakly acid solution which, because development requires an alkaline solution, has the effect of terminating promptly the development process which might otherwise continue through developer soaked into the film. In photographic work, though seldom with X-ray films, development may be ended by washing the film in a simple acidic solution before it is placed in the fixing solution.

Simultaneously with the fixation process the emulsion of the film is hardened. Chemicals are included which serve to convert the flaccid, mobile gelatin into a hard layer. (This process is very similar to that used to harden or 'tan' leather.) Such hardening helps in the subsequent drying of the film since the water is more easily removed. The main purpose of hardening, however, is the protection of the film from damage during subsequent handling.

By way of summary the various stages in the production of the final processed radiograph, together with a brief description of what happens at each stage, are set out in *Table XVIII*.

The description of the photographic process given here has deliberately been in general terms only, no detailed information being presented, for example, about the various solutions used. This is because it is desired to emphasize the fundamental purpose and action of each stage. Details of the characteristics and composition of the various chemical solutions can be found in more specialist literature should they

Table XVIII.—THE STAGES IN THE PRODUCTION OF THE RADIOGRAPH

PROCESS	APPROXIMATE TIME	WHAT HAPPENS	
1. Manufacture		Crystals of AgBr of suitable size, and having sensitivity specks, are made and are suspended in gelatin	
2. Exposure	0·01–10 sec.	Latent image created	
3. Wetting	10 sec.	Wet the film so that subsequent development is uniform	In darkness
4. Development	3–10 min.	Convert latent image to silver	
5. (Acid) Wash	1 min.	Stop development and remove excess developer	
6. Fixing and hardening	10–30 min.	Dissolve out remaining silver bromide and harden gelatin	
7. Washing	30 min.	Remove products of development and fixing	
8. Dry	30 min.	Remove water	

Notes: (1) Stage 3 is often omitted, a wetting agent being incorporated in the developer.
(2) Stage 5 is sometimes omitted, and may be in plain water although the interaction of developer and fixing chemicals can cause staining.

be needed. The present state of the technology of the subject is that each manufacturer produces either completely or partially made-up developing and fixing solutions suitable for use with the various types of film commonly employed. These are accompanied by carefully thought-out recommendations for use. Although there may be special circumstances in which better results can be obtained by using modified techniques, it is doubtful whether any but the most experienced radiographer will be able to improve on these recommendations. It is therefore either a very clever or experienced, or a very foolish radiographer, who dares not accept the recommendations as instructions.

Automatic Processing.—It is becoming increasingly common to use automatic processing units in which the film is passed, successively, through the various stages either by rollers or by being attached to hangers which are moved on by a chain mechanism. The exposed film is inserted into the 'dark room' side of the unit and some few minutes later the completely processed, washed, and dried film is delivered at the 'light room' end of the unit.

The chemical reactions involved in automatic processing are very similar to those already described, the main differences being that the concentration of the solutions used tends to be greater, and the temperature at which the reactions take place is higher than for manual processing. In order to protect the emulsion during this processing it is partially hardened at the beginning of development, and hardening is completed during the final fixing stage. Even more than in manual processing, it is necessary to adhere to the manufacturer's recommendations on solutions and temperatures. The time of development is, of course, constant for all films once they have been placed in the machine.

CHAPTER XVI

THE PROPERTIES OF THE X-RAY FILM

THE important property of the films which we wish to use in radiography is the ability of X-radiation to produce a pattern of varying depths of blackness in the film. The film is held up against a uniformly illuminated screen and the varying amounts of visible light transmitted are observed by the radiologist. The important question now is: What is the relationship between the observed amount of blackening and the amount of X-radiation which was the original cause of the blackening? This information is contained in what is known as the 'characteristic curve' of the film in which, as shown in *Fig*. 102, the amount of blackening is plotted against the amount

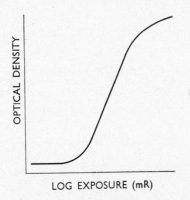

LOG EXPOSURE (mR)

Fig. 102.—A typical characteristic curve
for an X-ray film.

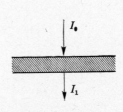

$$\text{DENSITY} = \log_{10} \frac{I_0}{I_1}$$

Fig. 103.—The meaning of
optical density.

of X-rays which produced it. The blackening is measured by means of a quantity known as the *optical density*, or more commonly just **density.**

Density.—Optical density is defined by the equation:

$$\text{Density} = \log_{10} \frac{I_0}{I_1},^{\star}$$

where I_0 is the intensity of visible light incident upon a small area of the film and I_1 is the intensity of light transmitted by that region of the film (*Fig*. 103).

For example, if the incident light intensity is 1000 units and the transmitted intensity is 1/100 of this, viz., 10 units, then the density is given by:

$$\text{Density} = \log \frac{1000}{10} = \log 100 = 2.$$

---

* Two sorts of logarithm are used. They are the 'common' logarithms, based on the number 10, and 'natural' or Naperian logarithms, based on the exponential number e, which is approximately 2·718. 'Logs to the base 10', of which the above is an example, will, henceforth, be written as 'log' whilst 'logs to the base e' will be written as '$\log_e$'.

This is a fairly high density and corresponds to the density of the fairly black region of a diagnostic film. If the transmitted intensity had been 1/10, viz., 100 units, then the density would have been:

$$\text{Density} = \log \frac{1000}{100} = \log 10 = 1.$$

Some idea of what this medium density means may be obtained from the fact that if a film uniformly blackened to a density of 1 is placed over a printed page in a fairly well-illuminated room, then it is just possible to read the print.

It must be noted that the density is independent of the actual intensity of the light used for the measurement (or for viewing the radiograph). If, in the first example, the light intensity had been reduced from 1000 to 100 units, then the transmitted intensity would have fallen from 100 to 1 unit and the density would remain equal to 2 since:

$$\text{Density} = \log \frac{100}{1} = \log 100 = 2.$$

This is another example of exponential absorption which was discussed in CHAPTER VI where it was pointed out that *fractions* of the incident radiation are absorbed or removed from the beam.

Table XIX.—OPTICAL DENSITY AND TRANSMISSION

Density	Fraction of Light transmitted	
0	1	= 1
0·3	0·5	
0·5	0·32	
0·6	0·25	
1·0	0·1	= 1/10
1·3	0·05	
1·5	0·032	
1·6	0·025	
2·0	0·01	= 1/100
2·3	0·005	
2·5	0·0032	
3·0	0·001	= 1/1000
3·3	0·0005	
3·5	0·00032	
4·0	0·0001	= 1/10000

The range of densities which is encountered in radiography runs from about 0·25 up to about 2·5. The fractions of the incident intensity transmitted by various densities are listed in *Table XIX*. When exact data are needed of the density existing at any part on a radiograph, it may be measured by means of an instrument known as a densitometer. In this instrument the fraction of light transmitted is measured by a photo-cell, the output of which is read on a suitably scaled and calibrated meter.

Addition or Superimposition of Densities.—Because density is measured in terms of the fractional transmission of light, if two or more densities are superimposed then the total effect is of a density equal to the sum of the separate densities. For example, if a film of density equal to 2 is laid over one of density equal to 1, then the total effect is of a density equal to 3. This can be seen to be so by reference to

Fig. 104, where the initial intensity of 1000 units is reduced to 10 units by the density of 2, and this intensity is itself reduced to 1 unit by the extra density 1. As can be seen from *Table XIX*, a reduction from 1000 to 1 is precisely the reduction effected by a density of 3.

Visual Effect of Density.—In addition to the convenience of being able to add them together, the use of density as a measure of film blackening has a further important aspect. It so happens that the physiological response of the eye to visible light of different intensities is also logarithmic. This means that the objective measurement

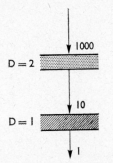

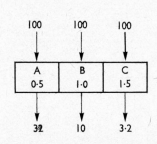

Fig. 104.—The successive reduction in intensity by two overlying attenuating layers.

Fig. 105.—The reduction in intensity by three attenuators having densities of 0·5, 1·0, and 1·5 respectively.

(density) agrees with the subjective appearance of a film. Consider the situation illustrated in *Fig.* 105, where three regions of a piece of film have densities of 0·5, 1·0, and 1·5 respectively. If the incident light intensity is uniform and equal to 100 units, then reference to *Table XIX* shows that the transmitted intensities are 32, 10, and 3·2 respectively. It can be seen that the difference in the light intensity transmitted by areas *A* and *B* $(32 - 10 = 22)$ is more than three times greater than the difference in light intensity transmitted by areas *B* and *C* $(10 - 3·2 = 6·8)$. In spite of this, area *A* will appear to be exactly that much more bright than area *B*, as area *B* appears to be brighter than area *C*. In other words, the eye 'sees' the equal differences in density rather than the very unequal differences in light intensity.

What the radiologist sees, therefore, when he looks at a radiograph is a pattern of densities and in particular he takes note of the difference in density existing between the various regions of the film. This difference in density is very important and is given the special name of **contrast**. The contrast (*C*) between two points on a radiograph is very simply defined as being equal to the difference in the densities $(D_1$ and $D_2)$ at these points:

$$\text{Contrast, } C = D_2 - D_1.$$

The importance of contrast in radiology cannot be stressed too much, since it is only when the contrast between two areas on the film is sufficiently large to be appreciated by the radiologist that it can be used for making a diagnosis. The minimum contrast (difference in density) which can be detected visually under the best conditions is about 0·02.

Variation in Density with Radiation Exposure.—The density of a processed radiograph is controlled by the amount of silver present and it can be shown that, for not too large densities, the density is proportional to the mass of silver present. This in its turn is controlled by and is proportional to the radiation Exposure (mR) to the film. It is therefore to be expected that the density is proportional to the Exposure. *Fig.* 106 A shows that, for a film used without an intensifying screen, this is so; the density being proportional to Exposure up to a density value of nearly 2. For a film exposed in conjunction with an intensifying screen, the fact that the latent image is then produced principally by visible light leads to a slightly different behaviour. From *Fig.* 106 B it can be seen that the initial exposure produces very little density (the curved part of the graph) but that higher exposure results in densities which are proportional to the exposure.

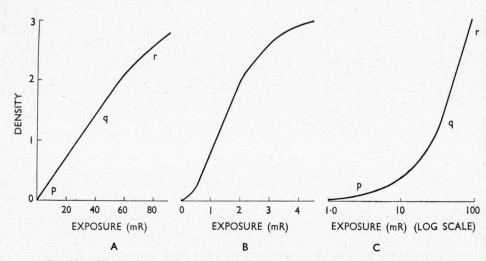

Fig. 106.—The variation of density with Exposure (mR) for A, a non-screen film and B, a screen film. Curve C repeats the information of curve A with the Exposure plotted on a logarithmic scale.

At densities above about 2, the graph of density against Exposure curves away from the straight line. This occurs with both screen and non-screen films. It arises because the number of silver specks has become large and they will therefore overlap each other to an increasing extent and because much of the silver halide has been used up. This means that some of them are wasted from the point of view of density since even one speck is sufficient to absorb completely all visible light photons incident upon it. The net result is that, at higher densities, the density does not increase as rapidly with increase in Exposure, as was the case for lower densities.

In *Fig.* 106 C the line *pqr* of *Fig.* 106 A has been replotted but now with a logarithmic scale for the Exposure. It can be seen that although the facts (of *Figs.* 106 A and C) are the same, the whole shape of the graph is changed by this choice of a different Exposure scale. The reason for choosing such a scale is so as to be able to include a very wide range of exposures within a single graph. It should be noted that this way of plotting the graph spreads out the low-Exposure region and compresses the higher-Exposure region of the curve. In *Fig.* 106 C the Exposure range 1–10 occupies as much space as does the much larger range of 10–100.

The Characteristic Curve.—The graph of density against the logarithm of the X-ray exposure is called the **characteristic curve** and a typical example is shown in moderate detail in *Fig.* 107. The actual shape of the curve is controlled by the detailed way the film was made, stored, and processed. It is, therefore, not to be expected that all films will have the same characteristic curve. However, it so happens that the general shape of all characteristic curves is more or less the same. For purposes of discussion it is convenient to divide the curve into four different regions, as indicated in *Fig*. 107, and these will now be discussed.

The Fog Level (*ab*).—In the first part (*ab*) of the curve there is a region of low density, the value of which is almost independent of Exposure. This is to be expected since, as already described, a large part of this blackening arises for reasons unconnected with Exposure. A contributor to this low density, in addition to those already mentioned, is the inevitable absorption of light by the various layers of the film, principally the film base.

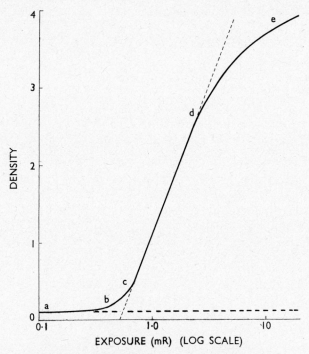

Fig. 107.—The regions of the characteristic curve.

This background density is always present even in film which has been exposed to significant amounts of radiation, and is added to the density resulting from the exposure. The omnipresence of this background density (usually lumped together under the name of 'fog') is emphasized in the characteristic curve of *Fig*. 107 by the broken horizontal line running across the graph. Densities measured from this line as a baseline are referred to as 'densities above fog' and are the densities caused by exposure to radiation. In practice, with good, well-stored, and correctly processed films, the fog level is sufficiently small to be unimportant in radiography.

The Straight-line Portion (*cd*).—The region of the film between the two points *c* and *d* (*Fig*. 107) is probably the most important region of the film. With most emulsions this part of the curve is more or less (although never exactly) a straight line. In this range of Exposures the density is approximately proportional to the logarithm of the Exposure, which means that multiplication of the Exposure by equal factors will increase the density by equal amounts. For example, if Exposures of 10 and 20 units produce densities of 1 and 1·5 respectively, then an Exposure of 40 units will produce a density of 2·0; in this example, increase of the Exposure by a factor of 2 in each case increases the density by an amount 0·5.

Although the curve is not exactly a straight line it is very nearly so, and it is always possible to draw a straight line which is almost coincident with the curve over a very wide range of Exposure values. Since the eye responds to contrasts (that is, difference in density) it is important to consider the difference in density brought about by different Exposures. The slope of this curve measures the maximum density difference resulting from two chosen Exposures, and is given the special name of **gamma** (γ).

The Film Gamma.—The gamma (γ) of a film is defined as the maximum slope of the characteristic curve and is measured by:

$$\text{Gamma, } \gamma = \frac{D_2 - D_1}{\log E_2 - \log E_1},$$

where, as is shown in *Fig.* 108, D_2 and D_1 are the densities which result from Exposures of E_2 and E_1 respectively.

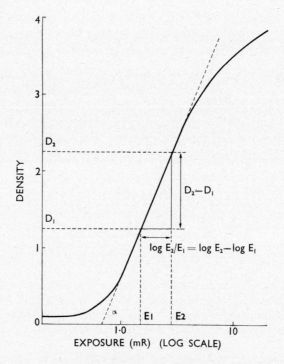

Fig. 108.—The gamma (γ) of a film.

It is often stated that $\gamma = \tan \alpha$, where α is the angle between the projected straight-line portion of the characteristic curve and the abscissa (horizontal axis). This is so if, and only if, the ordinate (vertical axis) and abscissa are drawn to the same scale. Alteration in either scale would alter α, but clearly cannot alter the film characteristics. Therefore, $\gamma = \tan \alpha$ is not recommended as a definition, since it does not emphasize the important facts about the curve which are expressed in the correct definition.

The equation, for γ, can be rewritten in the form:

$$\text{Contrast, } C = D_2 - D_1 = \gamma(\log E_2 - \log E_1)$$
$$= \gamma \log (E_2/E_1).$$

As will be described in a later chapter, the relative value of the Exposures E_2 and E_1 (that is E_2/E_1) are determined by the composition of the patient and the radiographic technique employed. It is therefore obvious that there are two distinct and separate factors which contribute to the observed contrast in the film:

1. The patient and the irradiation conditions which determine the value of $\log E_2/E_1$; and
2. The slope of the characteristic curve.

It cannot be overemphasized that γ is a property of the film and its processing only. In view of the importance of γ in determining the final contrast, it is important to state the factors which control it. Fortunately this is easily done, for the γ of film is determined, in practice, almost entirely by how it was made. During manufacture the size of the silver bromide crystals can be controlled. If they all have more or less the same size then the γ is high, whereas if there is a wide range of crystal sizes present the γ is lower. As will be described later in this chapter, the development also has an effect on γ. For films in common radiographic use, the value of γ is usually about 4.

In this straight-line portion of the curve the contrast (differences in density) caused by two Exposures such as E_2 and E_1 is a maximum, since the slope of the curve is here greatest. For this reason this region (cd) of the curve is referred to as the 'Region of Correct Exposure'. There is, in fact, nothing 'correct' about it except that in this range the contrast produced is maximal, which (other things being equal) is usually desirable.

The 'Toe' and 'Shoulder' of the Curve.—The curved regions of the characteristic curve (bc and de of Fig. 107) are called the 'toe' and 'shoulder' respectively. At a point such as b (Fig. 107) the density is just measurably greater than the fog level and reflects the detectable effect of the X-ray Exposure. The actual exposure at b is called the 'threshold Exposure'. In this region the density rises slowly from about 0·1 at b to about 0·4 at c. This range of densities represents the 'bright' regions of the radiograph, such as are obtained in the region of a bone shadow.

At a point such as d the region known as the 'shoulder' commences. The density at d is usually in the range 3–4, although it can be more for films specially chosen for use over a very wide range of densities. This region corresponds to the very black part of a radiograph, such as might occur in the shadow of a well-aerated lung or round the outside of a patient exposed to an over-large beam.

In both the 'toe' and 'shoulder' regions the contrast produced by a certain ratio of Exposures (E_2/E_1) is much less than that produced in the straight-line portion of the curve since the slope of the curve is less. For this reason the exposures are chosen so as to avoid these regions if maximum contrast is required, and they are therefore often referred to as the regions of under-exposure ('toe') and over-exposure ('shoulder'). However, most radiographs have on them areas which include these regions of the curve, particularly the 'toe', and useful information is often obtainable in spite of the reduced contrast resulting from the smaller slope of the curve.

As has been said, the γ of a film measures the slope of the characteristic curve in its straight-line part. When the rest of the curve is considered as well it is obvious that the slope changes, being small in the 'toe' region (bc), reaching a maximum in the straight-line portion (cd), and becoming small again in the 'shoulder' region (de). The term **film contrast** is used to measure the slope of the characteristic curve at any point, and clearly therefore film contrast varies with density. It is measured by drawing a tangent to the curve at the point of interest, as in *Fig.* 109, and calculating:

$$\text{Film contrast (at density } D) = \frac{D_a - D_b}{\log E_a - \log E_b},$$

where D_a and D_b are the densities, on this tangent, corresponding to the Exposures E_a and E_b.

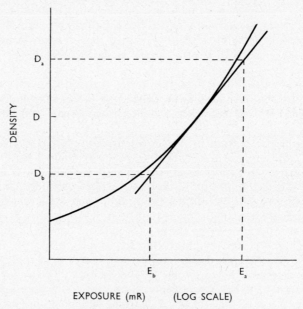

Fig. 109.—Film contrast at any selected density is measured by the slope of the tangent to the characteristic curve.

By comparing this expression with that already given for the γ it can be seen that γ is a special case of film contrast, viz., the film contrast of the straight-line portion of the curve.

The importance of film contrast is that it measures the average slope of the characteristic curve over a small region. When the contrast between two not very different densities is being considered, the film contrast is a measure of the contribution of the film to this contrast. The contrast visible at a particular point of the film is given by:

$$\text{Contrast, } C = D_2 - D_1 = m(\log E_2 - \log E_1),$$

where E_1 and E_2 are the Exposures which result in densities D_1 and D_2 and m is the film contrast, or mean slope, over the density range D_1 to D_2.

The 'Speed' of a Film.—The Exposure which is needed to produce a chosen density (usually $D = 1$) depends upon the type of film. If only a small Exposure is needed, then the film is described as 'fast', whereas if a large Exposure is needed the film is described as being 'slow'. These terms are obviously only relative but it is not usual to quote a numerical value for the 'speed' of a film in radiography. All that is usually done is to say that one film is, say, 'three times as fast' as another, by which is meant

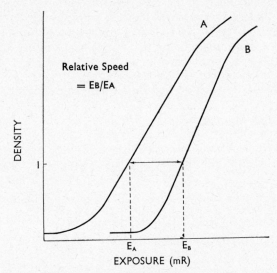

Fig. 110.—The characteristic curves of two films. Film **A** is 'faster' than Film **B**, i.e., needs a smaller Exposure for the same density.

that the first film requires only one-third the Exposure required by the second film to produce a certain density. The characteristic curves of two such films are shown in *Fig.* 110.

If for any reason a numerical value of film 'speed' is wanted the reciprocal of the Exposure, in roentgens, needed to produce a stated density may be used. For the types of film being considered it is convenient to use the formula:

Speed $= 100/$milliroentgens to produce a density of 1.

As with γ, the 'speed' of a film is determined principally by the way in which that film was made. The faster film has a greater number of larger, and therefore more sensitive, silver bromide crystals in its emulsion. Since a wide range of crystal sizes accompanies the larger crystals, this will lead to the faster film having a smaller γ than a slower film would have. This will be seen in *Fig.* 110. Since the γ of the faster film (A) is lower than that of the slower film (B), the ratio of the exposures required to produce a certain density in each film will be different at different densities. In other words, their relative speeds depend upon the density, and tend to fall as density increases. It is for this reason that the density ($D = 1$) is specified when relative speeds are quoted.

Effects of Development on Film Characteristics.—In the discussion of development in the last chapter, brief mention was made of the effects which could result from a change in development. The important factors in development are:

a. The chemical composition of the solution;

   b. The temperature at which it is used;

   c. The time for which it is allowed to act;

   d. The degree of agitation of the film in the solution during development.

All these affect the 'degree of development' in the sense that increases in the reducing power of the chemical, increases in time and temperature of development or in the amount of agitation, all produce increases in film density for a given exposure. To a very limited extent each can be used to compensate for change in the others and for errors in exposure. However, it must be pointed out that the manufacturer will have taken a lot of trouble to match the developing solution to the film and will have determined the optimum conditions of time, temperature, and agitation. As stated previously, these recommendations should be adhered to.

The overall effect of increases in development are:

   a. Increased density for a given Exposure, i.e., increased speed;

   b. Increased γ;

   c. Increased fog level.

The characteristic curves for an excessive range of development times are shown in *Fig.* 111 A, from which it can be seen that the whole shape and position of the curve are changed. *Fig.* 111 B shows the way in which the fog level, γ, and speed change

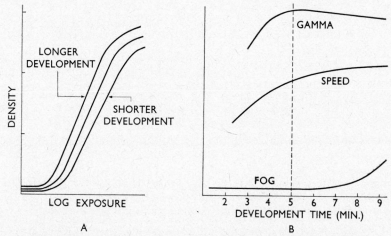

Fig. 111.—The influence of development on: **A**, The characteristic curve; and **B**, the film gamma, speed, and fog level. The dotted line indicates the optimal development.

with development time. The degree of development indicated by the dotted line is optimal in the sense that the γ is almost as high as it can be for this film and developer, whilst the fog level has not yet become significant. A further increase will lead to excessive fog without any appreciable increase in γ, whereas a reduction would lead to a marked deterioration in γ, the fog level remaining much the same.

Changes in development temperature lead to similar changes. Temperature and time of development can be used to compensate for each other, and for a typical situation the following pairs of values will produce the same degree of development, that is, the same characteristic curve:

75° F. (24° C.)	$2\frac{1}{2}$ min.
65° F. (18° C.)	5 min.
55° F. (13° C.)	10 min.

Film and Exposure Latitude.—The expression **latitude** refers to the range of Exposures (roentgens) which can be given to a film and yet have acceptable density values (that is, densities between 0·4 and 2·0, say). There are two aspects to latitude. Firstly, consider a certain X-ray pattern incident upon a film. This pattern will comprise low Exposure (E_B) in the bone shadows, high Exposure (E_L) in the lung shadows, together with the whole range of intermediate values. For film A of *Fig.* 112, all these Exposures will produce a density within the acceptable range and on the straight part of the characteristic curve. For film B, however, the lung shadows will be too

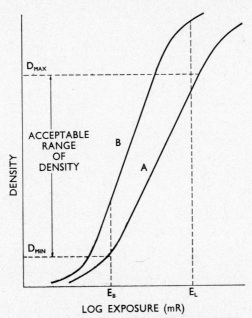

Fig. 112.—Film **A** has a greater latitude than film **B**, in that it is able to produce densities within the acceptable range for a wider range of Exposure values than can film **B**.

black and therefore unacceptable. A reduction in X-ray tube exposure (mA.s., say) would reduce these high densities to acceptable values but then the bone-shadow densities would be too low. It is not possible to fit this wide range of Exposures into the acceptable density range and the range which can be accepted is referred to as the **film latitude.** The greater the γ, the smaller is the latitude.

The second aspect concerns the situation illustrated in *Fig.* 113, where the range of Exposures incident on the film may be either $E_B - E_L$ for a small X-ray tube exposure or $E_B' - E_L'$ for a greater X-ray tube exposure. Both these ranges are produced by the same patient, an identical X-ray tube kV. being used. This being so,

$$\frac{E_L}{E_B} = \frac{E_L'}{E_B'}.$$

Clearly the use of either the lower or the higher X-ray tube exposure results in an acceptable radiograph since all the densities lie within the acceptable range. The difference between the largest and the smallest X-ray tube exposure for which this is true is regarded as the **exposure latitude.** In *Fig.* 113 lines A and B measure this latitude, which can be regarded as the 'margin for error' in the choice of radiographic exposure technique. There are two factors which control the exposure latitude: the first is the range of Exposures presented to the films ($E_L - E_B$ and $E'_L - E'_B$) and the second is the film γ. Increase in either or both of these will reduce this latitude.

The Effect of Visible Light.—X-ray film is sensitive not only to X-rays but also to visible light. In fact, it is more sensitive to visible light than it is to X-rays. This is so in spite of the fact that many more photons of visible light have to be absorbed for the formation of each latent image than in the case of X-rays, where each photon absorbed results in a latent image, simply because the incident visible light energy

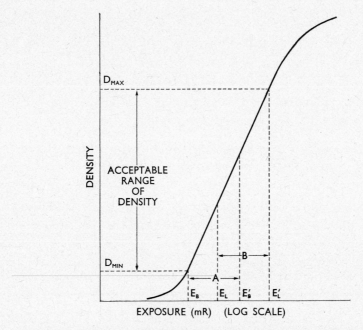

Fig. 113.—A given ratio of Exposures ($E_L/E_B = E'_L/E'_B$) can be accommodated with the range of acceptable values for both a smaller and a larger Exposure if the film has enough latitude.

is completely absorbed by the film whereas a very high fraction of the X-ray energy passes through the film without being absorbed. It is for this reason that film must be handled and exposed in the dark or at least in low levels of light intensity of a suitable colour—a 'safe light'.

In general the behaviour of films exposed to visible light is the same as when exposed to X-rays. There is, however, one important exception. This concerns what is known as the **reciprocity law**. The Exposure (E) given to a film is actually the product of the intensity (I) and the time (t) for which it acts:

$$E = I.t,$$

where E = Exposure in roentgens,
$\quad\ I$ = intensity in roentgens/sec.,
$\quad\ t$ = exposure time in sec.

For X-rays it is found that the same Exposure (E) produces the same density (D) on the film no matter what the individual values of intensity (I) and exposure time (*t*) are. For instance, an intensity of 1000 units acting for 1 sec. results in the same exposure and the same density as an intensity of 1 unit acting for 1000 sec., etc. For this reason X-rays are said to obey the reciprocity law.

For exposure by visible light, however, it is found that this law does not always hold. Exposures resulting from either very short or very long exposure times produce smaller densities on the films than would the *same Exposure* given at an intermediate time. The explanation of this effect is to be found in the actual mechanism of the build-up of the latent image during the exposure. Although the details are of no importance, the failure of this law has a practical aspect. When intensifying screens are used, the effect on the film is almost entirely produced by visible light so that in such a circumstance the effects of reciprocity law failure may be observed. Fortunately, the effect is not large and it occurs only when the exposure is outside the approximate range 0·01–10 sec.

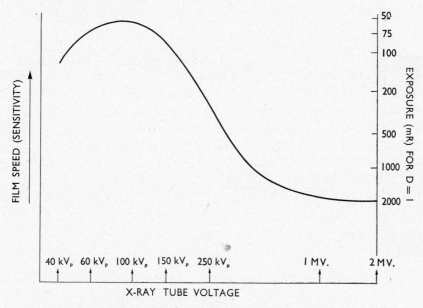

Fig. 114.—The variation of film sensitivity (or 'speed') with radiation quality.

Variation in Film Sensitivity with Radiation Quality.—The amount of blackening produced on a film is found to be dependent upon the quality of the radiation used. This variation is shown in *Fig.* 114 in which relative film sensitivity (i.e., speed) is plotted against photon energy.

It is to be expected that the amount of blackening will be determined by the amount of energy absorbed by the silver bromide and the shape of the curve shown arises from the fact that the *absorption* coefficient of silver bromide changes with radiation quality.

The increase in sensitivity (blackening) which occurs as the photon energy is decreased is to be expected since the absorption coefficients generally increase as photon energy decreases. However, the flattening off of the curve, and then the fall in sensitivity for energies of less than about 40 keV., are more difficult to explain until it is recalled that silver and bromine have (K) absorption 'edges', at 26 and

13 keV. respectively. The presence of these has the effect that although the *attenuation* of the radiation continues to increase rapidly as the radiation photon energy is decreased towards the edge, the bulk of the energy so removed from the beam is reradiated as characteristic radiation and is therefore not absorbed. Most of this characteristic radiation is able to escape from the silver bromide crystal (because a substance is relatively transparent to its own characteristic radiation) and is either absorbed by the gelatin (where it causes no photographic effect) or even escapes from the film.

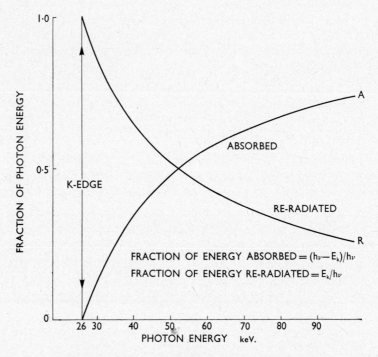

Fig. 115.—The relative absorption and reradiation of energy in the vicinity of the K-edge for silver.

Fig. 115 shows how the fraction of the energy removed from the beam which is actually absorbed falls to zero as the (silver) edge is approached. Since it is only the energy which is actually *absorbed* by the silver bromide which can produce subsequent film blackening, the result is a falling-off of blackening as the radiation quality is decreased.

In practice the beam of radiation is not monochromatic and a very wide range of photon energies is present. This, together with the fact that there are the two edges (bromine and silver) each of which has its effect, leads to the film sensitivity being almost constant over a fairly wide range of X-ray tube voltages. In fact, in practice, for tube kVp ranging from about 40–120 kVp, the variation in film sensitivity is small enough to be neglected for many purposes.

Doubled-coated Film.—There are two independent, very good reasons why it is usual to have a double-coated film. The first is the practical one that if the emulsion were to be put on one side only, then the various changes which occur during the processing would result in the flat film curling itself up into a tight spring-like roll.

The presence of identical emulsion on both sides of the film base prevents this happening.

The second reason is also important but applies only when the film is used in conjunction with intensifying screens. Here, as will be described in detail in the next chapter, the image on the film is actually caused by visible light which is emitted

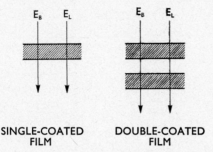

SINGLE-COATED   DOUBLE-COATED
FILM   FILM

Fig. 116.—The irradiation of a single-coated or a double-coated film by the same two Exposure values.

from the screen as a result of X-rays being absorbed by the screen. This light is very easily absorbed by the emulsion and thus only the outer layer of the emulsion is affected (in practice only thin emulsions are therefore used).

Consider the effect of irradiating a single- and a double-coated film in the manner indicated by *Fig.* 116. The emulsion layers are assumed to be identical and each

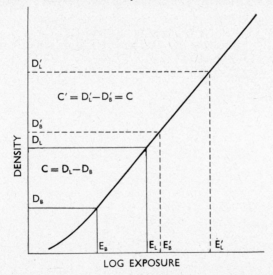

Fig. 117.—The identical contrasts (*C* and *C'*) produced on a single-coated film by the same ratio of Exposures at a lower and a higher X-ray Exposure.

may be assumed to receive the same two X-ray exposures E_B and E_L. The result of these two different exposures will be a contrast on the film, which in the case of the single-coated film will be $C = D_L - D_B$ (*Fig.* 117).

In the case of the double-coated film the contrast will be twice this. Each of the two emulsion layers will have the same densities as for the single emulsion, so that when the film is viewed the densities seen will be $D_L + D_L = 2D_L$ and $D_B + D_B = 2D_B$ respectively. This is because, as stated on p. 167, the superimposition of two densities produces a density equal to the sum of the separate densities. The contrast seen will therefore be:

$$C = 2D_L - 2D_B = 2(D_L - D_B),$$

which is twice the value obtained with the single-coated film.

Of course the overall blackness of the double-coated film will be twice as great as for the single-coated film. It might be thought that by giving an increased exposure to the single-coated film both its density and its contrast could be increased to equal those of the double-coated film. This is not so. Increase in exposure will equalize the general density level but the contrast of the single-coated film will remain half that of the double-coated film. Why this is so can be explained by reference to *Fig.* 117. The dotted lines refer to the situation when the exposure to the single-coated film has been increased so as to obtain an increased density. The ratio of the two new exposures E'_B and E'_L will remain exactly as before (since both will have been increased by the same factor) so that the contrast C' remains equal to the previous contrast C; assuming the characteristic curve to be a straight line.

The same result as is obtained with a double-coated film could be obtained with a single-coated film of twice the thickness. Such a thick emulsion would be useless, however, since it would not be accessible to the light from the intensifying screen. The only use of a thick emulsion would be for non-screen work but here the anti-curl property alone is sufficient to make the use of single-coated film rare.

The use of a double-coated film, then, has the following advantages:

1. Prevents the film curling.
2. Doubles the contrast (when screens are used).
3. Gives greater blackening for the same exposure, that is, increases the film speed (when screens are used).

CHAPTER XVII

INTENSIFYING AND FLUORESCENT SCREENS
AND XERORADIOGRAPHY

MENTION has already been made of the use of *intensifying screens* in radiography, and of *fluorescent screens* in fluoroscopy. Although these two techniques are very different, the physical phenomenon involved is the same in both cases. This is, very simply, that some materials are able to absorb X-rays and re-emit, in the form of visible light photons, the energy so extracted from the X-ray beam. The amount of light emitted is strictly proportional to the amount of X-ray energy absorbed which is, in turn, proportional to the X-ray Exposure (mR) to which the screen is subjected. Hence any pattern (of intensities and Exposures) in the X-ray beam will be converted into an identical but *visible* pattern.

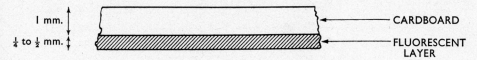

Fig. 118.—A greatly magnified cross-section of an intensifying screen.

INTENSIFYING SCREENS

In practice the intensifying screen (*Fig.* 118) consists of a stiff sheet of cardboard (about 1 mm. thick) over which is spread a uniform layer of the chosen luminescent material in the form of small crystals. These crystals are suspended in and held on to

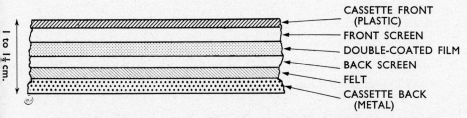

Fig. 119.—A double-coated film sandwiched between two intensifying screens contained in a cassette.

the carboard by means of an inert binding material. Between the cardboard and the fluorescent layer proper there is usually a thin layer of a very white material (e.g., magnesium oxide or titanium dioxide) which serves to redirect to the film a large fraction of the emitted visible light which is moving away from the film and which would therefore otherwise be lost. It is also usual to protect the actual layer of the screen from scratching, etc., by means of a very thin but tough layer of waterproof material.

Intensifying screens are used in pairs, being held in close contact with the emulsion on each side of the double-coated X-ray film. The sandwich of screen–film–screen is contained in a light-tight envelope called a cassette. A sectional diagram of a loaded cassette is shown in *Fig.* 119. The felt pad ensures that the screen and film emulsion are in close contact over their whole surface. The metal backing to the cassette reduces the amount of radiation scattered back to the film sandwich. The presence of large amounts of such back-scattered radiation would result in the production of an inferior radiograph because of the reduction in contrast (*see* CHAPTER XX).

The effect of using intensifying screens is to increase the resulting density on the film or, as is more usual in practice, it allows a smaller X-ray exposure (mA.s.) to be used than would be necessary to give the same density without the screen.

Intensifying Action of the Screens.—The intensifying action of the screen arises because of the much greater amount of energy absorbed from the X-ray beam by the screen than is the case for the film alone. This results in the production of a very large number of visible light photons; so many, in fact, that although many visible light photons are required to produce each latent image, the final total number of latent images produced is much greater when screens are used. How this is so may be more clearly described by reference to a numerical example, in which the values are chosen for purposes of illustration only.

Fig. 120 shows a film and a screen-film pair both irradiated by 500 X-ray photons. Of these 500 photons the screen will absorb 100 and the film only 5, say, because of their very different absorption coefficients and thicknesses. In the film

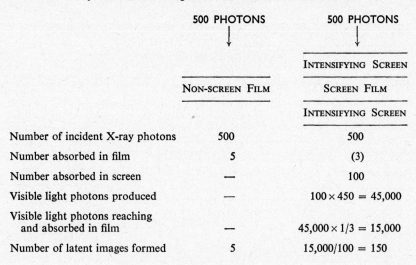

	NON-SCREEN FILM	INTENSIFYING SCREEN SCREEN FILM INTENSIFYING SCREEN
Number of incident X-ray photons	500	500
Number absorbed in film	5	(3)
Number absorbed in screen	—	100
Visible light photons produced	—	$100 \times 450 = 45{,}000$
Visible light photons reaching and absorbed in film	—	$45{,}000 \times 1/3 = 15{,}000$
Number of latent images formed	5	$15{,}000/100 = 150$

RELATIVE EFFECT $= 150/5 = 30 : 1$

Fig. 120.—The latent images produced in a non-screen film and by a film-intensifying screen combination.

the 5 absorbed photons will lead to 5 latent images and to 5 silver specks in the processed film. In the screen the 100 absorbed X-ray photons (of high energy) will each release a large number (450, say) of visible light photons (of low energy), a third of which, say, will reach the film. The remainder are either absorbed in the screen or are moving away from the film. If it is assumed that 100 photons of visible light are required to produce each latent image, the final number of black silver specks produced will be 150. Some X-rays will be absorbed by the film directly and produce latent images, just as is the case in the absence of the screen. The number of latent images so produced will not be very great and will certainly be less than 5, since the intensity of X-rays reaching the film is reduced by the absorption in the screen. In the present example, it is unlikely to be more than 3 or 4 and so can be neglected. The total number of latent images formed can therefore reasonably be taken as 150. This is to be compared with the 5 produced in the film in the absence of the screen, so that the amount of blackening produced is 30 times greater in the case of the screen film. This is more usually expressed by saying that an exposure (mA.s.) 30 times smaller can be used to achieve the same density, when the screen is employed.

It should be noted that although the screen increases the efficiency of production of the radiograph, the actual efficiency of the screen is still quite low. Each of the visible light photons has an energy of between 2 and 3 eV., so that the 450 produced by each X-ray photon accounts for only 1·0–1·5 keV. The energy of the X-ray photon could well be 30 keV., so that less than 5 per cent of the X-ray energy actually absorbed eventually appears as visible light.

Practical Fluorescent Materials.—The main requirements for a material which is suitable for use in X-ray screens may be summarized as:

1. The material should be able to absorb X-rays to a high degree. In other words, it should have a high absorption coefficient and it is for this reason that most luminescent materials used have a moderately high atomic number (Z).
2. The material should emit a large amount of light of a suitable energy and colour.
3. There should be no significant afterglow.

The materials which have these properties, and which are commonly encountered in radiological work, are calcium tungstate, zinc sulphide, zinc cadmium sulphide, and barium lead sulphate, all of which may be described chemically as 'salts'—and hence the name 'salt screen'. Calcium tungstate (or, as it is usually called, 'tungstate') is the material most commonly used for intensifying screens whereas zinc cadmium sulphide is the choice for fluoroscopic screens. Until quite recently barium lead sulphate screens were preferred for use at the higher diagnostic kilovoltages (80–120 kV.), where they were superior to calcium tungstate screens. Recent developments and improvements of calcium tungstate screens have changed this situation and barium lead sulphate is now no longer preferred. Zinc sulphide is also no longer used in intensifying screens but is sometimes used in screens employed in mass miniature radiography (photofluorography).

As has already been stated, the colour of the light emitted is a property of the intensifying screen and is controlled by the exact position of the energy level (T) above the filled band (*see Fig.* 51). In other words, it depends upon how the crystals are made and exactly what kind of chemical 'impurity' is added by the manufacturers. To a limited extent the colour of the emitted light can therefore be controlled by the manufacturer and he does this so as to match the use to which the material is to be put. For radiographic intensifying screens the colour is usually in the ultraviolet-blue end of the spectrum, to which light the film is very sensitive. For fluoroscopy the colour is chosen to be in that part of the spectrum to which the eye is most sensitive, viz., the yellow-green. For photofluorography and cine work, where ortho- and panchromatic film is used, the colour can be adjusted to extend more into the

7

red part of the spectrum. *Fig.* 121 shows how the spectral pattern of the light emitted by the screen matches the film-sensitivity pattern and the eye-sensitivity pattern and *Table XX* lists the wavelengths of the emitted light for some typical screens. The wavelength of the emitted light, it will be remembered, depends on the screen only and not on the X-ray quality (kVp).

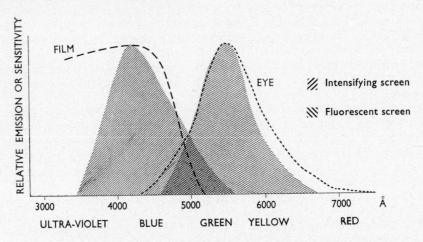

Fig. 121.—The spectral emission of an intensifying screen and of a fluorescent screen is adjusted to lie within the range of maximum sensitivity of the film and the eye respectively.

Table XX.—WAVELENGTH OF EMITTED LIGHT

Material	Minimum	Maximum	Peak	Colour
Calcium tungstate	3500	5800	4200	Violet
Zinc sulphide	3900	5500	4300	Violet
Barium lead sulphate (10 per cent Pb)	2600	4000	3000	Ultra-violet
Zinc cadmium sulphide	4500	6800	5500	Yellow-green

Intensification Factors.—The result of using an intensifying screen is that the X-ray Exposure needed to produce a chosen film density is much reduced. The extent to which this is so is measured by the **intensification factor** (I.F.) which is defined by:

$$\text{I.F.} = \frac{\text{Exposure required when screens are not used}}{\text{Exposure required when screens are used}} \text{ for the same film density.}$$

A screen with a high-value I.F. is referred to as a **fast screen.**

Fig. 122 shows the characteristic curve for a certain film exposed without (*A*) and with (*B*) screens. The intensification factor for this combination of film and screen, at a density = 1, is given by:

$$\text{I.F.} = \frac{E_A}{E_B}.$$

The value of the intensification factor can be quite large, which means that considerable reduction in Exposure results from the use of intensifying screens.

It will be noted also (*Fig.* 122) that not only is the exposure required to produce a certain density reduced but also that the γ is increased by the use of intensifying screens. This arises because the actual exposure to the film is by visible light when screens are used, but by direct X-irradiation in the absence of screens. The change in γ is quite large; in the example given it is from $\gamma = 3$ to $\gamma = 4$. Because there is a change in γ, the value of the I.F. increases as the density at which it is calculated increases. It is for this reason that it is usual to quote the I.F. at a density $= 1$. Non-screen films (i.e., those designed for use without screens) have a higher γ than screen films (which are designed to be used with screens) used without screens. However, when used in the intended fashion, i.e., screen films with screens and non-screen films without, the screen films have the higher γ.

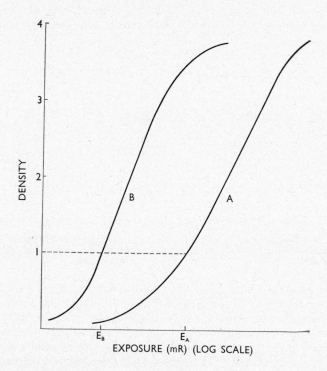

Fig. 122.—The characteristic curve of a film exposed (**A**) without, and (**B**) with, intensifying screens.

Factors Controlling Intensification Factor.—The intensification factor is determined by a number of factors, by far the most important of which are associated with the material structure of the screen and film. Intensification obviously depends upon:

1. The amount of X-ray energy absorbed by the screen;
2. The efficiency of its conversion to visible light;
3. How much of this light reaches the film and its effect on the film.

Screen Thickness.—Clearly the more material there is in the screen (i.e., the thicker and more heavily loaded with crystals the screen is) then the greater is the X-ray absorption. But although there is more light produced, that produced in regions of the screen away from the film will be absorbed by the screen itself, and so prevented from reaching the film. This is shown in *Fig*. 123, for a screen placed behind the film (a so-called **back screen**) where the intensity of light emitted from the screen is plotted against screen thickness for a constant X-ray exposure. Initially there is an almost linear rise in light output as more and more X-rays are absorbed by the thicker screen. Eventually, however, the graph curves over as the light intensity emitted becomes almost constant. Although more and more X-rays are being absorbed and therefore more and more light is being produced, the light from the lower levels in the screen is reabsorbed by the screen and so does not reach the film. The saturation occurs when light is no longer able to pass through the screen from the lower levels to the film.

For the front screen the behaviour is a little different, as is shown in *Fig*. 124. Initially the curve rises, just as for the back screen, as more X-rays are absorbed.

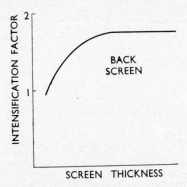

Fig. 123.—The variation in intensification factor with screen thickness for a back screen.

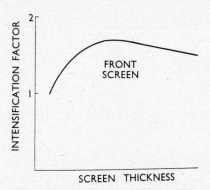

Fig. 124.—The variation in intensification factor with screen thickness for a front screen.

Instead of becoming constant, however, the curve flattens off and then falls progressively as the screen thickness is increased. This fall occurs because the upper layers of the screen are attenuating the X-ray beam so that the X-ray intensity at the layers of the screen closer to the film is reduced. It is these layers which contribute the light to the film. It can be seen that in the case of the front screen an excessive thickness results in a reduction in light emission and, therefore, in intensification factor, whereas for a back screen an unnecessarily great thickness is not harmful.

Thus there is an optimum thickness for the front screen, which depends on the kV. range in which the screen is to be used. Although the density on the front emulsion (caused by light from the front screen) is usually greater than that on the back emulsion (caused by light from the back screen), especially at low kV., the effect can be minimized by using different thicknesses for the two screens. The thickness of the back screen is not critical but is thicker than the front one. For this reason it is important not to interchange the two screens: if it is done a pale film may result. Typical values for the thicknesses of the fluorescent layers are about 0·2 mm. and 0·5 mm. for the front and back screens respectively.

In practice the advantage of using different thicknesses for the front and back screens is small and, for reasons of simplicity and economy, it is now quite usual for the front and back screens to be identical.

Screen Material.—The absorption of X-ray energy and its conversion into visible light depend upon the screen material and in particular on the minute amounts of added impurities. The size of the crystal is said to have an effect, the larger crystal giving a greater intensification factor. However, recent work has tended to indicate that the magnitude of this effect, if it exists, is probably small. Much more important is the absorption of the visible light in the screen layer which is controlled by the inclusion therein of absorbing dyes. Such dyes limit the extent to which light can pass through and leave the screen layer and so reach the film. The presence of a dye, therefore, leads to a reduction in the intensifying factor.

As has already been described, the colour of the emitted visible light is also controlled by the character of the screen material used, and the added impurities. The sensitivity of the film to the colour of light emitted is clearly important.

It can be seen, therefore, that just as with a photographic film, the major properties of an intensifying screen are under the control of the manufacturer. Many different

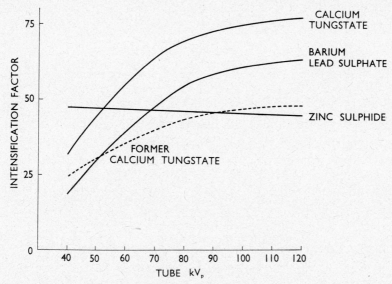

Fig. 125.—The variation of intensification factor with radiation quality for various intensifying-screen materials.

combinations of material, impurity, screen thickness, and dye inclusion are possible, but, in fact, only three main types of intensifying screen are manufactured. Each manufacturer uses his own special name but the three main types are usually identified by names such as 'High Speed', 'Normal', and 'High Definition', which have intensification factors of about 100, 50, and 35 respectively, at 70 kV.

Although, as has just been described, the actual constitution of the screen is the most important item in determining its intensification factor, there are others which are under the radiographer's control and these are:

Radiation Quality.—The variation in intensification factor with X-ray quality is shown in *Fig.* 125 for calcium tungstate, barium lead sulphate, and zinc sulphide. It can be seen that both calcium tungstate and, especially, barium lead sulphate show a very great increase in intensification factor with increase in kV. Zinc sulphide, on the other hand, shows very little variation in intensification factor with quality and is clearly more efficient at the lower kV. It is not often used, however, because it tends to cause an unnecessarily large blurring of the radiograph.

Until recently the curve for calcium tungstate would have been as shown dotted, which explains why barium lead sulphate was preferred for use at the higher kV. (80–120 kV.). Recent improvements in calcium tungstate have, however, removed this advantage.

The increase in intensification factor with increase in kV. may appear to be contradictory to the known fact that as kV. increases the X-ray absorption of all material falls and tends to become more nearly equal, so that the enhanced absorption of the screen compared with that of the film should decrease and tend to become the same as the kV. increases. The diagrammatic graphs of *Fig.* 126 show how the absorption in the three materials of interest varies with photon energy (kV.). This is the same type of variation which has already been discussed for the photographic film in CHAPTER XVI. In the range of kV. of interest, the absorption in silver bromide

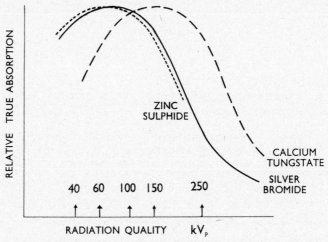

Fig. 126.—The variation with radiation quality of radiation absorption in some fluorescent materials.

is almost constant whereas that in the higher atomic numbered 'tungstate' is still increasing with increased kV. because of the influence of the tungsten absorption 'edge' at 70 keV. This leads to an increase in intensification factor with kV. For the lower atomic numbered zinc sulphide (the zinc absorption 'edge' is at 10 kV.), however, the absorption curve is falling similarly to the curve for silver bromide so that the intensification factor is almost constant over this range of kV.

It follows also from these considerations that the intensification effect of 'salt screens' will become small at very high kV. (500 kV. and above) although their intensification factor always remains greater than that of metal screens (*see* p. 203).

New Intensifying Materials.—Over the past few years intensifying screens in which the suitably activated oxysulphide of the rare-earth elements lanthanum or gadolinium is used have been developed. The original versions of these new screens emitted light in the green part of the spectrum and therefore normal (ultra-violet, blue-sensitive) X-ray film was unsuitable and special (green-sensitive) film had to be used. This was very inconvenient and fortunately many of the currently available rare-earth screens (as they are called) have their light emission in the blue part of the spectrum. They can therefore be used with normal X-ray film.

Rare-earth screens have sensitivities which are greater than those of the more usual calcium tungstate screens by a factor of between 2 and 8. They therefore permit a reduction in exposure—and patient dose—by the same factor. The higher sensitivity arises because first, a higher fraction of the incident X-ray beam is absorbed by the screen, and secondly, compared with tungstate screens, a higher fraction of the X-ray energy so absorbed is converted to visible light.

The higher X-ray absorption arises, in the case of gadolinium for example, because it has its photo-electric K absorption edge at about 50 keV. whereas that for tungsten is at about 70 keV. For this reason photons in the energy range 50–70 keV. are more strongly absorbed in gadolinium than in tungsten. Although, because it has a higher atomic number than gadolinium, tungsten generally has a higher absorption than does gadolinium, in this particular energy range the situation is reversed. In *Fig.* 127 the

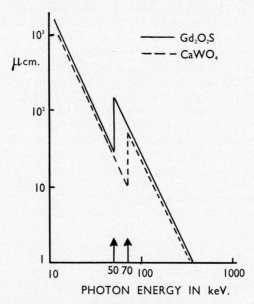

Fig. 127.—Variation of absorption coefficient, with photon energy for calcium tungstate and gadolinium oxysulphide.

variation of absorption coefficient for the relevant materials (calcium tungstate and gadolinium oxysulphide) are plotted over the photon energy range of interest.

Clearly, the statement concerning the high absorption in rare-earth screens compared with that in calcium tungstate screens is true only for specified quantities of the two materials, i.e., for specified screen 'thicknesses'. A fair comparison would be between two types of screen producing approximately the same amount of screen blurring. It is for this situation that the factors quoted above refer.

The importance of and interest shown in rare-earth screens arise because a large fraction of radiographic examinations are done using photon energies in the range 50–70 keV. Remembering that it is the photons penetrating the patient which are of interest, and assuming that there is not too much scattered radiation reaching the film, this range of energies corresponds to a range of operating kilovoltages of approximately 60–90 kV. At a significantly higher and lower operating kV, the newer screens do not offer any substantial advantage over the very much cheaper calcium tungstate screens.

The increased efficiency of conversion of absorbed X-ray energy into emitted visible light (15 per cent compared with approximately 3 per cent) is a bonus but may be of doubtful value. In so far as it reduces exposure it helps to minimize dose to the patient. On the other hand, it will tend to increase quantum mottle (*see* p. 203) since fewer X-ray photons are contributing to the final picture. The increased X-ray absorption in the screens, however, results in both reduced patient dose and reduction of quantum mottle.

Although reduction of patient dose is an important feature of the use of these new screens, it should also be noted that the general reduction in exposure that they permit also leads to other benefits associated with the possible use of decreased size of focal spot, tube current and exposure time.

The Degree of Film Development.—In a film exposed in conjunction with screens the image tends to be near the surface of the film emulsion since the visible light is only able to penetrate a short distance into the emulsion. Complete development of the affected silver bromide crystal is, therefore, effected by very modest amounts of development, since the superficial layer of the film is very accessible to the developer. For films exposed in the absence of screens the affected silver bromide crystals are distributed throughout the whole thickness of the emulsion and longer development is required if all these are to be converted into silver. From this it follows that the intensification factor will fall as the amount of development is increased. This is not because of any effect in the screen–film combination but because of an increase in density on the film exposed without screens. Although the change in intensification factor can be quite large, this is not an important effect in practice, since the degree of development is selected for other reasons. The fact that only the region of the emulsion close to the screen is utilized in a screen film means that the emulsion in a screen film can be very much thinner than it is in films designed for use without screens.

The Type of Film.—From what has already been described, it is obvious that the screen and film operate, and have been designed to operate, as a matched system. The intensification factor refers not to the type of screen but to the screen and film combination. When used with different types of film a given type of intensifying screen will produce different intensification factors from those with its normal film.

The Exposure Times.—It is found that the density produced by a chosen exposure (mA.s., say) depends upon the duration (sec.) of the exposure. For example, an irradiation for 0·05 sec. at 1000 mA. produces a different blackening to that produced by an irradiation for 1 sec. at 50 mA., in spite of the fact that in both irradiations the amount of X-radiation reaching the screen–film combination is identical (or proportional to 50 mA.s.). The magnitude of this difference is significant only when the exposure times are either very long (over 10 sec.) or very short (less than 0·01 sec.). A smaller density results from such long or short exposures than from the intermediate times. In the commonly used range of diagnostic exposure times the effect is not noticeable, but may be so in some of the newer techniques which employ millisecond exposure times.

This effect, called reciprocity law failure, arises because the blackening of the film is due to visible light. It does not occur when the film is irradiated in the absence of screens where the blackening is produced directly by X-rays, because for X-rays the reciprocity law (which essentially says that the blackening is dependent on the product of mA. and seconds and not on their individual values) holds.

Some clues as to why the law fails for visible light but holds for X-rays have already been given in CHAPTER XVI, where it was mentioned that the absorption of several photons of visible light by the same crystal is necessary to produce a latent image. It would appear that for very short exposure times the rate of production of electrons in the silver bromide crystal by the light photons is too rapid and that some are lost and do not therefore contribute to the production of a latent image. For the very long exposure times the rate of build-up of the latent image is slow, due to the interval between the absorption of the several visible light photons necessary for the production of the latent image. It so happens that this rate of build-up may be too slow for stability and the partial latent image may leak away, thus requiring a large number of visible light photons to be absorbed before the latent image is completed and stable. The result in both cases, long and short exposure time, is that a smaller number of latent images, and therefore a smaller blackening, is produced by a given X-ray exposure (mA.s.).

The Effect of Screens on Image Sharpness.—So far it would appear that the use of an intensifying screen with the highest intensification factor is desirable since this will lead to the greatest reduction in X-ray tube exposure (mA.s.) and patient Exposure (roentgens). Unfortunately, the use of any screen, and in particular of one with a high intensification factor, leads to a deterioration in the sharpness of the pattern on the film. How this arises can be seen by reference to *Fig.* 128. This illustrates how an X-ray photon, absorbed at some depth inside the active layer of the screen, results in the emission, in all directions, of many light photons. Not all these photons will reach the film but those which do will contribute to the formation of latent images over the region of the film indicated. In practice the situation will be worse than this on account of the scattering of the light which takes place in the screen. The inclusion of a dye in the screen helps to minimize this scattering. This is to be compared with the situation where an X-ray is absorbed directly by the emulsion. In this case the image is produced at the point where the silver bromide crystal is located.

The effect of the screen is therefore to blur the pattern which exists in the beam of X-rays incident upon the film. For instance, consider the very simple pattern illustrated in *Fig.* 129, which consists of a lot of X-rays on one side of the line *AA*, and very few on the other side. If such a pattern were directed on to a non-screen film then the pattern of density shown by line *a* in the lower part of the diagram would be obtained, i.e., a high density to the left of the line *AA* and a lower one to the right, with a sharp change at the position *AA*. In other words, the sharp edge in the X-ray pattern would show up as a sharp change in density on the film. If screens are used, however, the pattern will be as shown by line *b*. The extra density to the right of the line *AA* is caused by the spread of the light photons generated by the larger number of X-ray photons to the left of *AA*. In this case the sharp edge in the X-ray pattern has been blurred and the pattern on the film will appear fuzzy and unsharp. This effect is called *screen unsharpness* and is one of the causes of unsharpness on a radiograph. The extent to which screen unsharpness occurs increases with increasing screen thickness, increased transparency of the luminescent layer to the visible light photons, and increased crystal size. It will be recalled that the first two of these are the factors which also control the intensification factor and it is unfortunate that a screen with higher intensification factors produces also larger unsharpness.

In making his screen, the manufacturer controls the screen thickness, crystal size, and amount of dye included in order to produce the optimum combination of intensification factor and screen unsharpness. As has already been stated, there are three main types of screen: 'High Definition', 'Normal', and 'High Speed'. It is not possible to give precise numerical values to unsharpness produced by screens but it ranges from about 0·15 mm. for the so-called 'High Definition' screen to about 0·45 mm. for a so-called 'High Speed' screen. It is important to notice that the use of any screen produces an additional amount of image blurring over what would occur if a non-screen film were used and that this extra blurring is greater for screens with a higher intensification factor.

This is not the whole story, however. The reduction in X-ray exposure, which results from the use of screens, will usually lead to a reduction in the amount of the

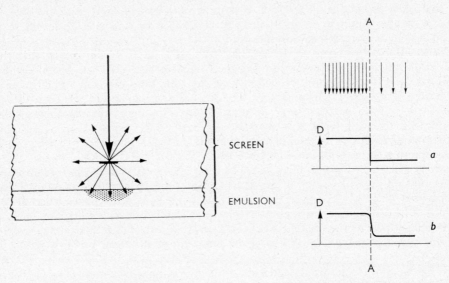

Fig. 128.—The production of 'screen unsharpness'.

Fig. 129.—A sharp pattern in the X-ray beam produces a sharp image on the film when (a) screens are not used but a blurred (unsharp) image when (b) screens are used.

other types of unsharpness. The overall result, therefore, is that the *total* unsharpness may be (and often is) smaller when screens are used than when they are not—in spite of the extra blurring caused by the screen. This point will be discussed more fully in CHAPTER XXI after the other types of unsharpness have been described.

Screen Mottle.—There is another type of effect which can be visible on a radiograph produced by the use of intensifying screens. This is called *mottle* since it consists of a faint irregular pattern of density variations, which is not present in the X-ray beam. Mottle can arise for two different reasons. Firstly, any non-uniformity in the fluorescent layer may show up on the radiograph since the intensification factor will vary over the surface of the screen. Although this type of mottle has been observed, with good modern screens it is not significant.

The second reason is rather more complex and is concerned with the actual number of X-ray photons which arrive at the cassette. With modern fast films and screens the actual number of X-ray photons, which reach the cassette and so cause the pattern on the radiograph, is comparatively small. The density on a film represents the average effect of the silver specks in that region of the film. Now the emission of X-rays is a random process so that even in a 'uniform' beam the average number of X-ray photons directed at any part of the screen will not be the same unless the number of X-ray photons involved is large. As has already been stated, with fast modern screens and films this number can be small so that random variations in X-ray intensity over the surface of the screen are apparent. This variation in intensity is not the same kind as that due to absorption in the beam, heat effect, etc., since it is quite random and is never in the same place and of the same pattern on different occasions.

The existence of this second effect, which is called *quantum mottle*, points a limit to the possibilities of using faster films and screens and consequently lower X-ray Exposures. In simple language, there will always have to be some X-rays reaching the cassette to form the radiograph and unless there are a reasonably large number of X-ray photons, the radiograph will show mottle. Fortunately, this stage is not yet reached in practice and further reduction in X-ray Exposure is still possible without introducing excessive mottle.

Care and Use of Screens.—If there is any gap between the screen and the film then the blurring will be increased because of the greater area of the film over which the light can be spread. It is, therefore, most important that close contact should be maintained between screen and film. The felt in the cassette has this function, but when a cassette has become buckled or bent by misuse (e.g., dropping) it may not be possible to achieve the required close contact. Whether this is so can be tested by placing a wire mesh on top of the cassette and making an exposure at a large focus-film distance. Any fuzziness on the processed film image indicates a lack of screen–film contact.

The presence of scratches, dust, or grease (from finger marks, for example) on the screen will also prevent the light photons passing from the screen to the film and their presence will therefore show up as clear pattern on the film. Screens should therefore be dusted and cleaned from time to time, and handled with great care so as to avoid scratching and soiling.

A simple test to show whether there is any afterglow from the screen (which is very unlikely) may be made by placing an opaque object on the cassette (e.g., a coin or piece of lead), make an exposure, and then very quickly insert a film into the cassette (in the dark, of course). After leaving for a few minutes the film is processed. Any suspicion of a pattern on the film will indicate the existence of afterglow.

Lead Intensifying Screens.—Lead intensifying screens are used only for high kV. radiography. They are never used below about 120 kV. and are best used with 250-kV. X-rays or cobalt-60 gamma rays. Their intensification factor is quite small, about 2–3, and their mode of action is completely different from that of 'salt screens'.

The absorption of X-rays by the screen results in the production of fast-moving electrons (photo-electric or Compton) and it is these electrons which—in the case of lead screens—produce the latent image and intensification. Clearly, metal intensifying screens can only be usefully employed at kV. sufficiently high to produce electrons capable of leaving the screen and reaching the emulsion. As with 'salt screens', lead screens are used in pairs but they are considerably thinner. The front screens is usually about 0·1 mm. (0·004 in.) and the back screen 0·15 mm. (0·006 in.) thick.

Because of their thinness lead screens introduce no additional screen blurring; neither do they suffer from reciprocity law failure.

THE FLUOROSCOPIC SCREEN

In simple fluoroscopy the pattern of visible light emitted by the screen is viewed directly by the radiologist. Since the intensity of light emitted by each part of the screen is exactly proportional to the intensity of X-rays incident upon that part of the screen, the visible light pattern corresponds exactly with the X-ray pattern. The fluorescent screen thus enables the radiologist to 'see' the X-ray pattern.

The main difficulty in fluoroscopy is that unless the patient is irradiated by a very intense X-ray beam, the intensity of the light emitted by the screen is very low, and therefore difficult to see. At these low levels of light intensity the eye is most sensitive to the green part of the spectrum, and therefore the fluorescent material chosen for this work is one whose light emission is in this part of the spectrum. The material usually chosen is zinc cadmium sulphide. By changing the relative proportions of zinc and cadmium, the colour of the emitted light can be adjusted to that required. In addition, the light emission from zinc cadmium sulphide is very much greater than that from calcium tungstate. So as to obtain as much light as possible from the fluoroscopic screen, the thickness tends to be rather larger than for intensifying

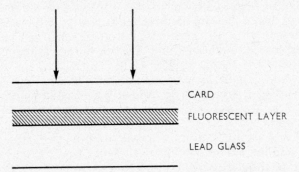

Fig. 130.—A greatly magnified cross-section of a fluorescent screen.

screens and the net result is that the blurring of a fluoroscopic screen is much greater than that of an intensifying screen. Although it may be as much as 0·45–0·65 mm., this is still acceptable since the eye is not very good at perceiving sharpness at the low light intensity level involved, i.e., the eye does not appreciate the blurring although it is there. The character and visibility of the fluoroscopic image will be discussed in a little more detail later, after the formation of the X-ray pattern has been described.

The structure of the fluoroscopic screen is illustrated in Fig. 130. The fluorescent layer of zinc cadmium sulphide in a suitable binding material is mounted on a card. Between the card and the zinc sulphide layer there is a reflecting layer of white magnesium oxide which reflects back towards the radiologist any light emitted in a direction away from him. Between the radiologist and the fluoroscopic screen there is a sheet of what is known as 'lead glass'. This is a special type of glass which contains a large proportion of lead (about 60 per cent by weight). Such glass is transparent to visible light but effectively absorbs all the X-radiation transmitted by the fluoroscopic screen, and it thus protects the radiologist from this X-radiation.

The protective power of a radiation barrier such as this is measured by what is known as the *lead equivalent*. This is the thickness of lead (in mm.) which absorbs radiation to the same extent as the barrier in question (in this case a sheet of lead glass) at the same radiation quality (kV.). The lead equivalent of lead glass in a fluoroscopic unit is 1·5 mm. of lead for kilovoltages up to 75 kV.; 2·0 mm. of lead for kilovoltages up to 100 kV., and 2·5 mm. of lead for kilovoltages up to 150 kVp.

Since the active layer is permanently protected on both sides, a fluoroscopic screen does not require the same kind of care and attention as does an intensifying screen. It is stated, however, that if a fluoroscopic screen is left uncovered for long periods in a lighted room, then its efficiency gradually falls. It is for this reason that fluoroscopic screens are covered when not in use, although modern screens have usually been treated to minimize this deterioration. There is no evidence of reduction in efficiency with use for either fluoroscopic or intensifying screens.

Photofluorography.—Brief mention must be made of the type of screen used in photofluorography or mass miniature radiography (as it is now usually called). In this technique the visible light emission from a fluorescent screen is photographed on a reduced scale (usually 35-, 70-, or 100-mm. film). Clearly the photographic film used must be sensitive to the light of the colour emitted by the screen.

Two types of screen are used. Zinc sulphide activated by silver which has an emission in the blue region of the spectrum is used in conjunction with ordinary blue-sensitive type of photographic film. Such a combination has the advantage that the film can be handled in the same 'dark room' safelight as is used for X-rays. Zinc cadmium sulphide, which has its emission in the green-yellow region of the spectrum, is preferred by some workers. With this type of screen an orthochromatic type of film which is sensitive to the yellow-green light must be used and such film requires to be handled under more stringent dark-room conditions.

XERORADIOGRAPHY

Xerography (which is made up from two Greek works 'xeros' and 'graphein' meaning 'dry' and 'to write') is based on the photo-conductive properties of some semi-conductors, such as vitreous selenium. Whilst it is kept in the dark, selenium is a good insulator so that an electrical charge placed on its surface will remain there for several hours. Any regions of a flat sheet of selenium which are exposed to light or to X-rays will become conducting, so that any charge previously placed on the surface will leak away leaving unexposed regions still charged. Thus a 'latent image' of charge pattern, corresponding with the pattern of the incident radiation, is produced. The invisible image is then made visible by exposing the material, in the dark, to a powder aerosol.

This process has been used for document copying for many years but it was not until about 1965 that much progress was made towards its exploitation in radiography. Since 1971 equipment for xeroradiography has been commercially available. How it works is probably best understood by following, step by step, the procedures leading to the desired xeroradiograph.

The central element in the system is the photo-receptor plate, which is the counterpart of the film in conventional radiography. It consists of a thin layer of vitreous selenium held on a rigid metal backing plate and, in use, is housed in a lightproof cassette. Externally, at least, the cassette is similar to the conventional film cassette. In particular it has a front which is uniformly 'transparent' to X-rays.

Since xerography is a physical process, no wet chemical or associated washing and drying facilities are needed. All the operations on the plate must, however, be carried out in the dark and for this purpose automatic equipment is now available. It consists of two units, a conditioner and a processor, each of which is about 1 m. high, 1 m. deep and 0·5 m. wide. No conventional dark-room is needed.

In the conditioner is a store (1) for a dozen or so photo-receptor plates. (The numbers in parentheses refer to items in *Fig.* 131.) When a radiograph is to be taken an empty cassette (3) is inserted into the machine, which thereupon transfers a plate, through the charging unit (2), into the cassette. This charging unit contains some fine wires running across and close to the path of movement of the plate. They are at a voltage high enough to ionize the air by a corona discharge and since they are biased positively, positive ions are drawn on to the selenium surface. As the plate is drawn under these wires it receives a uniform positive charge which raises its surface potential to about 1500 V. relative to the backing plate. Thus charged, it passes into a light-proof cassette (3) and is ready for use.

After exposure (4), the cassette is inserted into the processer, where the photo-receptor plate is removed from the cassette (5) and passed into the development chamber (6). This chamber contains a cloud of very fine blue powder, each particle of which is electrically charged. Assuming that the powder is negatively charged it will be attracted to any positive charges remaining on the plate. The amount of powder attracted to any particular region of the plate will, to some extent, be proportional to the magnitude of the residual charge. (A more detailed discussion of the pattern of powder deposition and, in particular, of the valuable feature called 'edge enhancement' will be given later.) The resultant image is analogous to a photographic 'positive'—light areas corresponding to those most irradiated, dark (or heavily powdered) areas where little radiation reached the plate. Provision can, however, be made for the use of positively charged powder, if desired, and this will tend to collect on areas from which the original charge has been removed, the resulting picture being comparable to the conventional X-ray film, i.e., dark areas corresponding to irradiation, light areas where no radiation has fallen.

As for the 'unfixed' photographic image, arrangements must be made for viewing and retaining the xero-image. It is usual practice to transfer it from the selenium plate on to a sheet of suitable paper. There are electrostatic forces strongly binding the developer powder to the photo-receptor plate, and these forces must be neutralized before attempting to transfer the powder image on to the paper on which the final image will be produced. Therefore, after development is complete, the plate is passed over another ion-emitting device (7) which sprays it with ions to neutralize existing charges and so 'loosens' the powder for easier transfer. At the next stage a sheet of plastic-coated white paper is brought into contact with the plate (8) and at the same time the back of the paper is charged to a polarity opposite to that used to 'loosen' the powder. The charging ensures close contact between paper and plate and hence efficient powder transfer to the paper.

At the end of the short transfer period the paper and plate go their separate ways. If not treated further the powder image on the paper would smudge if touched. Therefore, to make the image durable, the paper is briefly heated (9) to soften the plastic coating into which the powder becomes incorporated. On passing out of this 'fixing' section of the processer the paper cools and is pushed, through a light trap, into the output tray (10) for ultimate collection and inspection. The process from insertion into the processer to the ultimate emergence of the finished picture is about 90 sec.

The used photo-receptor plate is transferred to the cleaning section (11), where any untransferred powder is brushed off before the plate passes into a storage bin (12) which usually holds half a dozen plates. When full, this bin is automatically released for manual transfer to the conditioner unit. Then the plates are automatically passed from the bin (12) into an oven (13) where they are heated for a short time to remove any residual charge or 'ghost' of the picture just taken. Finally, the plates are returned to the original store (1) ready for re-use.

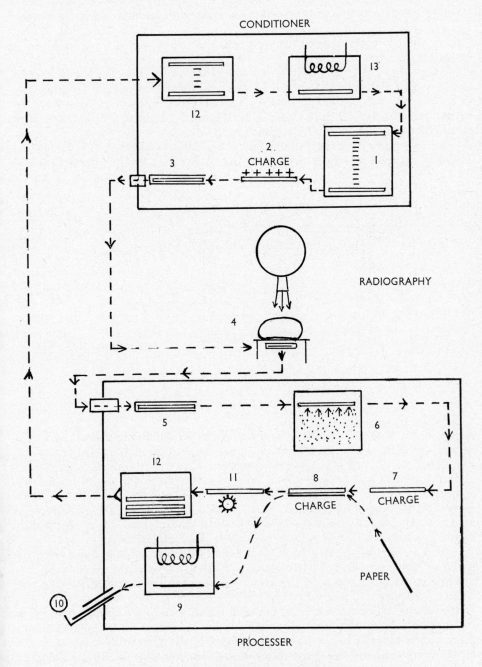

Fig. 131.—Xeroradiography processing unit.

Features of the Xeroradiograph.—The sensitivity of the xeroradiograph system depends, in a complex way, upon the quality of the radiation being used, the thickness of the selenium layer (usually of the order of 0·1 mm.) and the development process. Even under the best conditions, however, it is considerably less sensitive than a standard film-intensifying screen combination, though it is faster than a non-screen film. On the other hand xeroradiography has the important advantages of very high resolution, high exposure latitude and, the feature already mentioned, edge enhancement.

Resolution as high as 200 lines per millimetre has been claimed under special circumstances, though under normal radiographic conditions patient movement and focal spot size will considerably reduce the attainable resolution. The two other advantages stem from features of the development system to which rather more detailed consideration must now be given.

Fig. 132 shows the main features of the development chamber ((6) in *Fig.* 131). The photo-receptor plate is clamped on to the top with the positively charged selenium

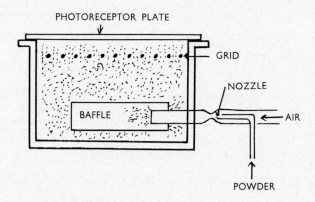

Fig. 132.—Xeroradiography development chamber.

surface inside, whilst the aerosol of fine blue powder is produced by a device very like a commercial paint spray. In this the powder is sprayed through a fine nozzle using compressed air as the carrier. A suitably orientated and designed baffle produces a uniform powder 'atmosphere' within the box. Friction in the nozzle charges the powder electrostatically, the size of the charge depending upon the materials of the powder and of the nozzle. The grid, placed a few millimetres from the photo-receptor plate, by being held at the appropriate potential controls the size of the charged powder reaching the plate and hence the nature of the final picture.

The charged particles eddy and float around in the box and only those very close to the photo-receptor plate will be affected by its electric field and stream in towards it. Since there is a uniform powder density to within one or two millimetres of the plate surface, the amounts of powder reaching lightly and heavily charged areas (except near their edges, as will be discussed below) will not differ greatly *provided the development period is brief*. In other words, the overall contrast is low (but *see below*) and hence a much greater range of Exposures can be received by the plate without the acceptable range of densities in the final image being exceeded (cf. the situation for the film p. 185 and *Fig.* 112): the xeroradiograph has a high Exposure latitude.

However, wherever there is a marked change in charge density on the plate surface, i.e., wherever there was a marked change in the amount of radiation reaching the plate (an 'edge'), there is a small zone of distortion of the electric field which directs powder away from one side of the 'edge' and piles it up on the other, under-emphasizing one side and over-emphasizing the other. Because of this, fine detail of 'edges' (thanks also to the high resolving power of the system) can be recorded even through quite thick layers of tissue.

Fig. 133 illustrates both the latitude and 'edge enhancement'. Part of a photoreceptor plate is exposed to a direct beam, part of it is exposed to the beam which has passed through a block of material two half-value layers thick and yet another part is unexposed.

The relative Exposures and residual voltages are shown and the variation of powder blackness is indicated, though it must be stressed that the thickness scale is a gross exaggeration. The build-up of powder on the high-charge side of the 'edges' and the depletion on the low-charge sides are shown, as is the fact that the powder thicknesses

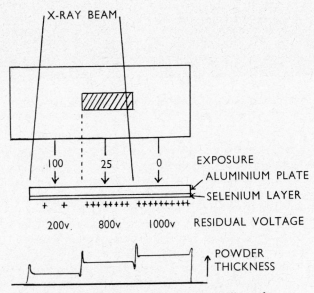

Fig. 133.—Edge enhancement in xeroradiography.

over the main areas differ much less than the residual charges or the radiation Exposures.

Finally one other important feature of the xeroradiograph must be mentioned. No special illumination or viewing equipment is needed for its inspection and interpretation. Normal room lighting is adequate.

Clinical Applications of Xeroradiography.—Because of its slower speed compared with that attainable with a conventional film-intensifying screen combination, up to the present, xeroradiography has been mainly used where non-screen film techniques (which are slower) would otherwise have been used and especially when 'edge enhancement' is advantageous. Some examples of its use are given below, but it must be stressed that the technique is still relatively new so that faster speeds and new applications are to be expected.

Mammography.—It is in this relatively new field of radiography that xeroradiography has received most attention recently. This is mainly because there are small but sharply defined contrasts between blood vessels, ducts, skin, and any cysts or tumours, and these are especially suitable for exploiting contrast edge enhancement of xeroradiography. *Fig.* 134 A shows the type of radiograph obtained using this technique. It should be noted that since the overall contrast is low the latitude is correspondingly high, and an important advantage of the method is its ability to make visible structures in both the thicker parts of the breasts and in the thinner subcutaneous layers. In spite of this low overall contrast, individual structures, even those of inherently low contrast, are nevertheless very clearly seen because of the contrast enhancement of their edges.

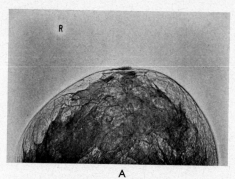 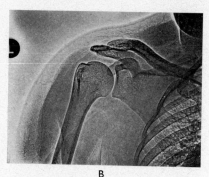

A   B

Fig. 134.—Typical xeroradiographs. A, A supine lateral mammogram; B, A shoulder, illustrating the latitude and detail available with the xeroradiographic process. (*By courtesy of Dr. J. D. Spencer, Royal Marsden Hospital, London.*)

Bones and Joints.—It is claimed that the diagnostic quality of xeroradiographs of bones and joints is superior to that obtained with film; fine fractures, in particular, benefiting from 'edge enhancement'. As *Fig.* 134 B shows the greater latitude enables soft tissues and bone detail to be obtained on the same film and edges can be clearly distinguished even when lying behind thick bones.

Arteriography and Venography.—Arteries and veins passing through muscle tissue cannot be radiographically revealed without the injection of some artificial contrast material (*see* CHAPTER XIX for further detail). Using conventional film techniques a considerable quantity of high concentration material may have to be injected and this can be painful. With xeroradiography the amount or concentration of the injection can be reduced by about 50 per cent with a very significant reduction of the pain suffered by the patient. Furthermore, better definition of the vessels is achieved and especially where they cross behind or in front of bones.

The Future.—Although xeroradiography had been used to a limited extent for many years, in the early 1970s, an increased interest started to be taken in it. There is little doubt that, over the next few years, there will be significant technical improvements in this and similar techniques (e.g., ionography). If for no other reason, this will be because, although the processing equipment and plates are costly, the running costs are quite small. As has been described, the plates are re-used and there is no consumption of costly and potentially scarce materials such as silver, as is the case in photographic radiography. In addition, there are the added benefits of high resolution, high effective local contrast arising from the edge enhancement effect and high exposure latitude. The present higher patient dose will, it is expected, be reduced by the development of faster systems.

CHAPTER XVIII

GEOMETRIC FACTORS WHICH INFLUENCE THE RADIOGRAPHIC IMAGE

THE pattern of intensities in the X-ray beam which reaches the film or fluoroscopic screen, and which contains the 'picture' from which the radiologist will ultimately make his diagnosis, arises because of two important properties of X-radiation. These are:

1. X-rays travel in straight lines.
2. X-rays are attenuated (and transmitted) to different extents by different kinds and/or thicknesses of material.

Both these properties have been described in previous chapters. In this and the next chapter the practical implications of these properties in diagnostic radiology will be described in a little more detail.

The fact that X-rays travel in straight lines controls the size, shape, and position on the X-ray film or screen of the image of the various anatomical structures of the body. Although the pattern is usually referred to as an *image* it is more accurately described as a *shadow*. In this chapter it will be assumed that the patient (object or body) is composed of two kinds of material only; one kind being completely transparent, the other kind being completely opaque to X-rays, and that there is a sharp boundary between them.

In such a circumstance the body will cast a shadow into an X-ray beam in the same way as a shadow is cast when a hand is held between a source of visible light (a lamp) and a screen (e.g., a wall). As is known (and can easily be demonstrated) the size of the shadow is different from that of the object (e.g., the hand) casting the shadow and, in radiology, it is important to know the relationship between the size of the shadow and that of the object.

MAGNIFICATION AND DISTORTION

Shape and Size of the Image.—*Fig.* 135 illustrates the formation of the shadow where a thin disk of an opaque material is placed parallel to the film and between it and the source of X-rays. In this simple situation the X-rays are assumed to come from a point source, T (i.e., an infinitely small focal spot). Of the large beam of X-rays produced those inside the cone bounded by TA and TB will be prevented from reaching the film. After processing, the film will show a clear circular region of diameter AB (since no X-rays reached this region) surrounded by a blackened film, with a sharp boundary between these two regions.

The ratio of the size of the image (AB) to that of the object (ab) is called the 'magnification' since, for an object parallel to the film, the image size is always greater than the object size.

$$\text{Magnification, } m = \frac{AB}{ab}.$$

The value of the magnification can be calculated by considering the geometry of the two triangles TAB and Tab, in *Fig.* 135. These two triangles are similar and hence:

$$\text{Magnification, } m = \frac{AB}{ab} = \frac{f}{h} = \frac{f}{f-d},$$

where f is the focus–film distance (F.F.D.); h is the focus–object distance; and d is the object–film distance (O.F.D.).

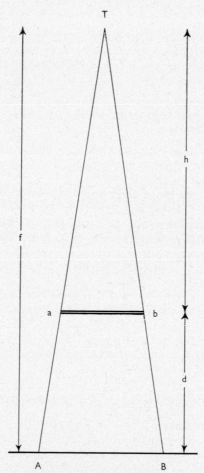

Fig. 135.—Simple magnification.

It can thus be seen that the magnification *increases*:
1. As the object–film distance (d) is increased and
2. As the focus–film distance (f) is decreased.

Hence, if a small magnification is required, and it usually is, then the object should be placed as close to the film as possible and as large an F.F.D. as practicable used. *Fig.* 136 shows how magnification depends upon these two factors (F.F.D. and O.F.D.).

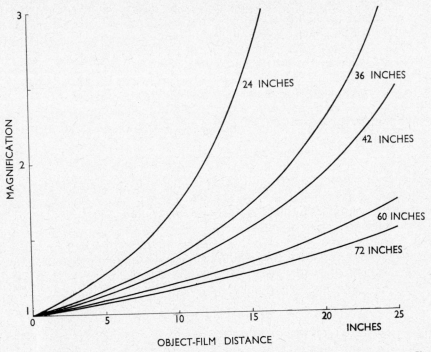

Fig. 136.—The variation of magnification with object–film distance for a range of focus–film distances.

Although this calculation has been done for only the one diameter of the disk which happens to be in the plane of the drawing, it is obvious that the same calculation applies to all the diameters. The shadow of the circular disk is therefore also a circle. In other words, although the image is larger in size than the object, it is exactly

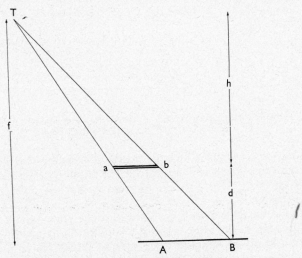

Fig. 137.—Magnification by oblique rays.

the same *shape*. This is true not only for circular objects but also for all shapes of object since every dimension of the object is magnified to the same extent.

The Effect of the Oblique Rays.—In the situation described by *Fig.* 135 the central ray of the X-ray beam passes through the centre of the object or, in other words, the beam is 'square on' or perpendicular to the film and object. Now consider what happens when this is not so and the object is placed to one side of the central X-ray The shadow is now cast by what are known as *oblique rays*. This situation is shown, geometrically, in *Fig.* 137. Again, it can be shown by considering similar triangles that the magnitude is given by:

$$\text{Magnification, } m = \frac{AB}{ab} = \frac{f}{f-d},$$

which is exactly the same as was obtained for the situation illustrated by *Fig.* 135. The magnification is thus seen to be the same whether central or oblique rays are used and thus magnification is controlled only by the perpendicular distances from the film of the object and tube focus. That this is really so can easily be tested by taking a radiograph of three coins arranged as in *Fig.* 138. It will be found that, provided they are parallel to the film, each coin will cast a *circular* shadow and, provided they are all at the same perpendicular distance from the film, all three shadows will be the same size.

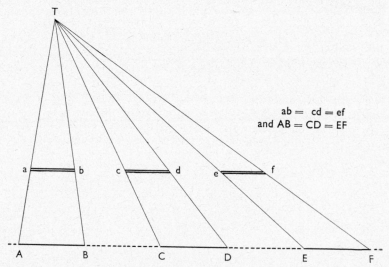

Fig. 138.—Three coins, placed parallel to the film and at the same distance from it, give equal circular shadows wherever placed.

Thus, if an object is placed parallel to the film then a magnified image (shadow) of exactly the same shape will be cast on the film. This is true whether central or oblique rays are used—the only requirement is that the object shall be parallel to the film.

The Effect of the Object being not Parallel to the Film.—In all the previous discussion the object has been in the form of a thin flat body placed parallel to the film. *Fig.* 139 illustrates what happens when such a body is placed at an angle (θ) to the film. It can be seen that the shadow (AB) of the object (ab) is smaller than the shadow

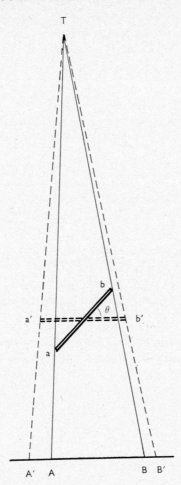

Fig. 139.—The reduced shadow size of an inclined object.

($A'B'$) which would have been cast if the object ($a'b' = ab$) had been parallel to the film and at the same average distance from it. The image is said to be **foreshortened** and clearly the amount of this foreshortening, and reduction in image size, depends upon the angle θ. When θ is large the foreshortening is large and the image size is reduced and may, in fact, be smaller than the real object size.

In a circumstance such as this the shape of the shadow cast by a circular disk will be an ellipse, the precise shape and size of which will depend on the inclination (θ) of the circular object to the film. The size and shape will also depend on whether oblique or central rays are used. *Fig.* 140 shows how the size of the shadows of three identical and equally inclined objects differs when central and oblique rays are used. It is obvious that the situation can be complex and that, in general, no certain deductions about the shape of an object can be made from the shape of its shadow unless either it is placed parallel to the film or its orientation with respect to the film and the beam central axis is known.

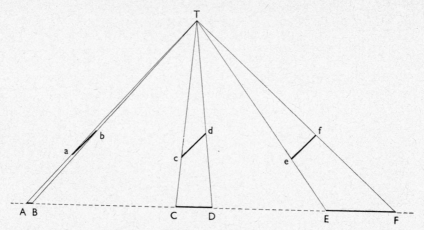

Fig. 140.—The size and shape of the image of an inclined object depend upon its lateral position in the X-ray beam.

The change of shape brought about in this way is often referred to as *distortion*.

Distortion of Position.—The relative position of the shadows of two objects can be different from the true relative positions if the objects are at different distances from the film. This is shown in *Fig.* 141, where the object *p* casts its shadow at a greater distance from *A* than does another object *q*, although *p* is, in fact, closer to the central

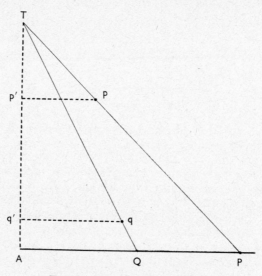

Fig. 141.—Distortion of position.

axis *TA* than is *q*. In other words, the object *p appears* to be much more laterally placed than object *q*, although it is in fact slightly less laterally placed. What has happened is that the distances *pp'* and *qq'* have been magnified to a very different extent because of their very different distances from the film.

Solid Objects.—If the object being radiographed is a thin flat plate, as has been assumed, then it is possible to place it parallel, or at any chosen angle, to the film. This is not so with a solid object. In such an object each part of it will be magnified by a different amount, depending on its distance from the film, so that both its overall shape and the relative positions of its various parts from the central axis will be distorted. Only the section of the object which happens to be parallel to the film will be undistorted and merely magnified. If the experiment involving three coins is repeated, but this time using three solid spheres (for example, large ball bearings) as indicated in *Fig.* 142, then three different shapes will be seen on the film.

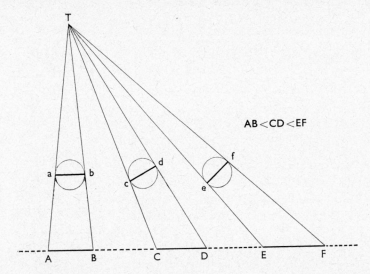

Fig. 142.—The relative sizes and shapes of the shadows of three spherical objects placed parallel to the film depend upon their relative lateral positions. The more laterally placed have the more elongated elliptical shadows.

The sphere on the central axis will show up as a circle, but the two laterally placed spheres will show up as elongated ellipses.

Practical Positioning.—In practice every situation is a complicated one, but it can readily be seen from the above discussion that in order to see the correct outline or shape of some anatomical or pathological object, care must be taken to have the section of interest of the object parallel to the film. Also, if it is desired that the various parts of an object (or objects) lying at different distances from the film are to be seen in their (approximate) correct spatial relationship, then that portion of the X-ray beam which is perpendicular to the film should be directed at the region of particular interest. Distortion of shape and position can be minimized by reducing the magnification which, as is shown in *Fig.* 136, is done by using a large F.F.D. and small O.F.D.

It is the correct orientation of the patient with respect to the film (and vice versa) and the choice of F.F.D., O.F.D., and beam direction which form the major part of 'Radiographic Positioning'. Unless the patient is in the 'correct' position the film may not show all it is intended to. When these things cannot be done, then it is necessary to consider carefully the actual arrangement used in taking the radiograph before any deductions of relative position and shape are made.

IMAGE UNSHARPNESS (OR BLURRING)

So far it has been assumed that the source of X-rays is a point and, as has been shown, this produces a sharp shadow of a definite size. In practice the X-rays originate at a small, but finite-sized, area on the target. This area is called the *focal spot*. As will be described later in more detail, it is advantageous to have a sloping target surface since this reduces the effective size of the focal spot. The formation of an X-ray shadow in such a circumstance is illustrated in *Fig.* 143. X-rays are produced at all points on the area of the actual focal spot (*b*) and the rays from each point moving in the direction of the film cast their own shadows of the object *pq*. The

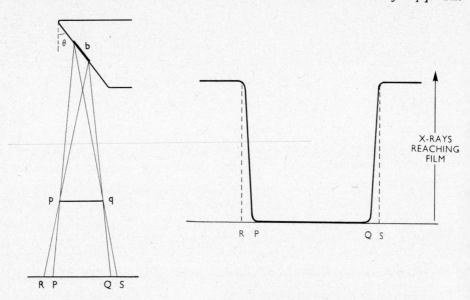

Fig. 143.—Geometric unsharpness—RP and QS—at the edge of a shadow due to the finite size of the focal spot.

Fig. 144.—Geometric unsharpness. The change of density at the edge of the shadow is not sharp but occurs over a finite distance, RP and QS.

shadows caused by the two points at the extreme edge of the focal spot are shown in *Fig.* 143, in which, for purposes of illustration, the size of the focal spot has been exaggerated. Over the region *PQ* no X-rays can reach the film and this is therefore the region of the full shadow or **umbra.** To the left of *R* and to the right of *S*, rays can reach all parts of the film from all parts of the focal spot, so that the film is blackened. Between *R* and *P* and between *Q* and *S*, X-rays can reach the film from only some points on the focal spot, so that there is here a partial shadow or **penumbra** and the film is less heavily blackened. A graph of optical density along the line *RPQS* of the film would be as shown in *Fig.* 144.* The visual appearance of the film is of a central transparent region (*PQ*) surrounded by a fuzzy edge (*RP, QS*). This fuzzy edge is called *geometric unsharpness* since it arises from geometric reasons.

---

* The actual shape in the penumbra of *Fig.* 144 is controlled by the uniformity of emission from the focal spot, the shape of the focal spot, and the characteristic curve of the film. Although often difficult to identify, the points *R* and *P*, *Q* and *S* are still used to define the limit of the unsharpness.

The geometry of the situation has been redrawn in *Fig.* 145, where the line *a* represents the effective (or apparent) focal spot, which is the size of the focal spot as seen in the direction of the central X-ray. It is the projection of the actual focal spot (*b*) and is smaller than it. In fact:

$$a = b \sin \theta,\star$$

where θ is the angle of inclination of the target surface to the central ray (*Fig.* 143). In practice θ is about 17°, so that for an actual focal spot size (*b*) of 4 mm. the effective

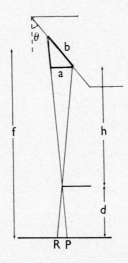

Fig. 145.—Geometric unsharpness. The focal spot size and the relative object–film and target–object distance determine the magnitude of geometric unsharpness.

size (*a*) is only 4 sin 17 mm. = 1·2 mm. Using *Fig.* 145, the size of the penumbra *RP* can be calculated, again using similar images.

$$\frac{RP}{a} = \frac{d}{h} = \frac{d}{f-d}.$$

As already stated, this penumbra is called the geometric unsharpness and is usually given the symbol U_g. So that:

$$\text{Geometric unsharpness} = U_g = a . \frac{d}{f-d}.$$

The unsharpness increases (gets worse) as:
1. The effective focal spot size increases.
2. The focus–film distance decreases.
3. The object–film distance increases.

$\star$ As can be seen from *Fig.* 145, this equation is not perfectly true, but because the F.F.D. is large and *a* is small, it is almost exactly true and is certainly sufficiently accurate for this purpose.

Thus, in order to have a sharp edge (small U_g) to the image, as large an F.F.D., as small a focal spot, and as small an O.F.D. as circumstances allow must be employed.

Effects of Focal Spot Size on Image Size.—In discussing magnification it was assumed that the X-rays were produced at a point focal spot. In practice (*Fig.* 146), because of the finite size (*a*) of the effective focal spot, the shadow (umbra) will be slightly smaller than that (*I*) calculated by the simple formula already given. Similarly, the total shadow will be slightly greater than that calculated. It must be

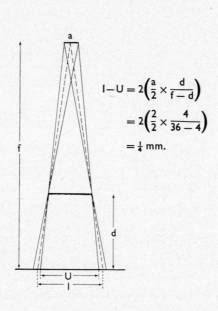

$$I - U = 2\left(\frac{a}{2} \times \frac{d}{f - d}\right)$$

$$= 2\left(\frac{2}{2} \times \frac{4}{36 - 4}\right)$$

$$= \tfrac{1}{4} \text{ mm.}$$

Fig. 146.—The effect of focal spot size on image size is usually negligibly small.

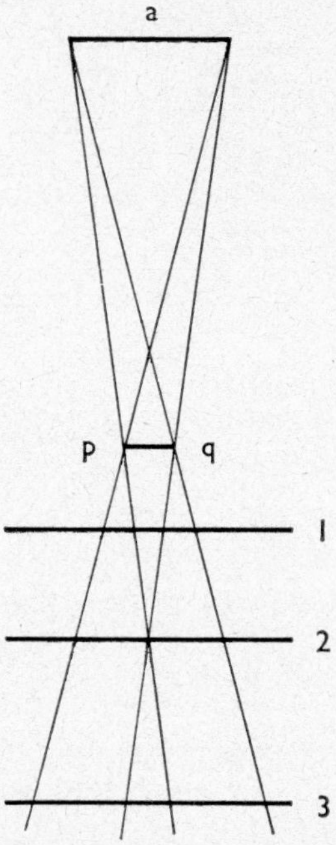

Fig. 147.—The appearance of the shadow caused by an object which is small compared with the focal spot size.

emphasized, however, that it is only in some rare and unusual circumstances that these differences are significant. As the example in *Fig.* 146 shows, with an effective focal spot of 2 mm., an object–film distance of 4 in. and a focus–film distance of 36 in. the reduction in size ('ideal' umbra) is only $\tfrac{1}{4}$ mm.

Fig. 147 depicts such a circumstance on a very exaggerated scale. A small object *pq* is being radiographed using a (comparatively) large effective focal spot (*a*). A film placed at the level (1) will show the usual central umbra surrounded by a wide penumbra: the image will appear very fuzzy. If the film is placed at level (2) the umbra will have disappeared, the penumbras from each edge *pq* of the object just meeting, in the centre. In these circumstances the shadow proper (umbra) has disappeared and all that is left is a relatively large, indistinct area of penumbra. The situation is even more unusual if the film is placed at the level (3). Here the shadow fails to reach the film but the penumbras associated with the two edges of the object overlap over the region where the shadow should be. A so-called *pseudo-image* is formed by these overlapping penumbras.

This is a very fuzzy shadow which is not distinctly visible. Its actual shape and size, and also its density, compared with the surroundings, are very dependent upon the exact circumstances. The film density of the pseudo-image is less than that of the immediately surrounding single penumbra region but not as low as in the full shadow. The formation of a shadow of this type is a very rare occurrence but it can occur in some fine detail bone work, when a large object–film distance is unavoidable.

Movement Unsharpness.—Additional image unsharpness can arise if there is any relative movement, during the exposure time, of the X-ray tube, film, or object being radiographed. In some techniques (e.g., tomography) deliberate movement is introduced to blur out some of the shadows. This must be done very carefully in a very special way, so as to avoid blurring those shadows which it is wished to see. How this is achieved is described in a later chapter.

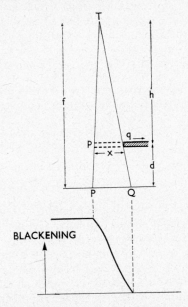

Fig. 148.—Movement unsharpness. The edge of the object moves from p to q during the exposure and produces the gradual change in density between P and Q.

In the normal radiography of an object (e.g., a patient) there may be an unwanted movement during the exposure and, as has already been said, this leads to a blurring of the image. How this occurs is shown in *Fig.* 148. At the start of the exposure the edge of the object is at *p* and a shadow starts to form at *P*. As the exposure progresses the edge of the object moves and by the end of the exposure has reached *q*. The edge of the shadow is thus moved progressively over the region of the film *PQ* and the density so produced is as shown. The full shadow exists to the right of *Q* with a fuzzy edge extending over the region *PQ*. As with geometric unsharpness, the exact shape of the density curve in this region depends on the exact circumstances. The size of this movement blurring, or *movement unsharpness* (U_m) as it is called, is calculated, again by the geometry of similar triangles.

$$U_m = PQ = \frac{f}{f-d}.x = \frac{f}{f-d}.vt,$$

where f and d are the F.F.D. and O.F.D. respectively, x is the amount of object movement, t is the exposure time, and v is the velocity of object movement. In practice it is required to keep this unsharpness to a minimum, which is achieved by using, as far as circumstances allow,

1. Small O.F.D. (d);
2. Large F.F.D. (f);
3. Small exposure time (t);
4. Small velocity of movement (v).

Velocity of Movement and Exposure Time.—It is clear that it is the product of velocity of movement and exposure time which controls movement unsharpness rather than their separate values. In some circumstances it is possible, by the use of suitable devices perhaps, to restrict movement sufficiently to allow quite long exposure times to be used. For instance, when a hand or leg is being radiographed the amount of movement can be kept quite small so that comparatively long exposure times may be used. In other circumstances, especially where involuntary movement is involved, the exposure time must be curtailed if movement blurring is to be kept sufficiently small. *Table XXI* sets out the *maximum* exposure times which it is

Table XXI.—MAXIMUM EXPOSURE TIMES FOR VARIOUS SITES. LONGER EXPOSURES
WOULD PRODUCE MOVEMENT BLURRING WHICH IS LIKELY TO BE UNACCEPTABLE

Chest, heart	0·05 sec. ⎫	Involuntary movements
Stomach	0·5 sec. ⎬	over which no external
Colon	1·0 sec. ⎭	control is possible
Genito-urinary tract	2 sec. ⎫	Voluntary movements
Pelvis, spine	5 sec. ⎬	reduced by adequate
Extremities	10 sec. ⎭	immobilization

advisable to use for various types of examination. These times, taken with the probable velocity of movement of the particular region of the body, will result in an acceptably small movement blurring. The whole subject of choice of exposure conditions from the point of view of minimizing blurring will be discussed later in more detail, in CHAPTER XXI. But it is clear from what has been said above that the correct choice of exposure time will depend very much on the site being radiographed.

Obliteration.—As mentioned earlier, movement blurring may sometimes be used deliberately to blur out overlying shadows. The main example of this is tomography, which is discussed in CHAPTER XXVI. Another example of this is in the P.A. radiograph of the sternum, when the patient is held gently but firmly down on to the table by a compression band. The X-ray beam is angled slightly but sufficiently so that the shadow of the spine does not overlie that of the sternum and an exposure of about 20–25 sec. made (at a low mA. of course). During this time the patient breathes smoothly and fairly deeply, the result of which is to blur out the shadow of the overlying lung and the hilar shadow (because of their movement) but to leave a sharp shadow of the sternum, which does not move (and which incidentally also has a small geometric unsharpness because of its proximity to the film).

Similarly, geometric unsharpness and magnification may be used to aid the obliteration of overlying shadows. If, in a similar P.A. view of the chest, a short F.F.D. is used, the sternum will be seen sharply, whereas the posterior section of the ribs and the spine will be greatly enlarged and unsharp and therefore less noticeable.

Macroradiography.—In some instances it is desirable to obtain a radiograph on which the shadows of the object are deliberately magnified. This is done by making d/F large. Of course d/F can never be greater than 1 and is, in fact, usually less than $\frac{3}{4}$. *Fig.* 149 shows how the magnification varies with d/F, from which it can be seen that by making $d/F = \frac{1}{2}$, i.e., by putting the object half-way between focus and film, a magnification of 2 is achieved.

Macroradiography, as this approach is called, is usually done in order to see detailed structures, but unfortunately the use of such a large value of d/F leads to large movement and geometric unsharpness, which could blur out such details. It

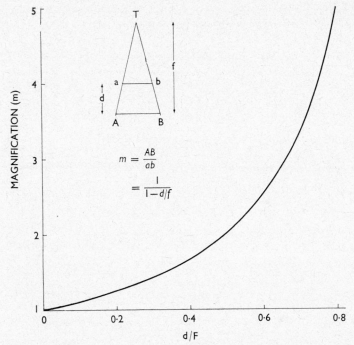

Fig. 149.—The relationship between magnification and the relative distances of the object and target from the film.

is therefore necessary to use a very small focal spot (usually 0.3×0.3 mm.²) and very short exposure times (unless the object can be kept very still, in which case longer times can be used).

Magnification and Unsharpness in Practice.—Although, as has been indicated, deliberate blurring (geometric or movement) and magnification are sometimes required, it is more usual to attempt to produce a radiograph on which the shadows (images) are sharp, and of the shape and in the same relative positions as the objects causing the shadow. The actual size of the images are of secondary importance but a film with minimum magnification seems to be preferred. All this is achieved, as has already been described in detail, by using:

1. Large focus–film distance.
2. Short exposure time.
3. Small object–film distance.
4. Object parallel to the film and in the centre of the beam if not thin.
5. Small movement.
6. Small focal spot.

Unfortunately, some of these requirements are contradictory from the point of view of X-ray tube loading (rating) and the optimum 'exposure factors' are, of necessity, a compromise.

Beam Size.—It is good radiographic practice to use a beam of X-rays whose size (cross-section) is the same as (or slightly smaller than) the film being used. Not only does this reduce the unwanted radiation dose to the patient, but, as will be described later, results in a better radiograph. The X-ray beam size is limited by a diaphragm which basically consists of a sheet of metal (opaque to the X-rays) with a hole of a suitable size through which the X-rays pass.

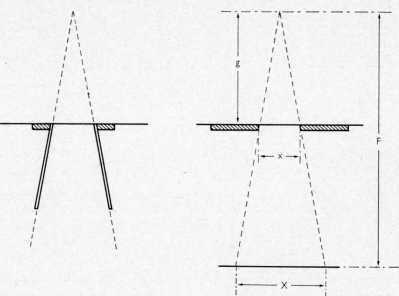

Fig. 150.—A cone used to delineate a beam to the desired size and shape.

Fig. 151.—Variable collimator. The relationship between the separation (x) of the beam-defining blades and the beam size at the film is determined by the relative distances of the blades and of the focus from the target.

In practice two alternative beam-defining systems (or collimators) are used. These are:

1. *Cones.*—A cone gives a fixed size of beam and, as is shown in *Fig.* 150, consists of a flat sheet of metal (steel) together with a conical metal tube, extending towards the patient.

   It is usual to have a set of cones of various sizes, each being so made as to be used in conjunction with a particular film size. Cones giving both rectangular and circular cross-section beams are available. The inconvenience of having to have such a set of cones and to interchange appropriately as different film sizes are used has led to the unpopularity of cones. For this reason it is nowadays more usual to employ the alternative type of collimator which is:

2. *The Diaphragm System.*—A diaphragm system consists of two movable pairs of sheets of metal, arranged as indicated in *Fig.* 151, where one of the pairs is shown. The other pair is at right-angles to the pair shown,

so that a rectangular beam is produced. Since these sheets of metal move in pairs, any size of shape of rectangular beam from zero up to a certain maximum may be produced. The size of the beam at the film clearly depends upon the size of the hole (x) and also the relative distance of the diaphragm and film from the tube focus. The knobs which control the position of the diaphragms are usually calibrated so as to show the size (X) of the beam at the film for a certain, or several, F.F.D.s.

The size of the hole (x) is calculated using the geometry of similar triangles from which it follows that:

$$\frac{x}{X} = \frac{g}{f}$$

or

$$x = Xg/f,$$

where g is the target to diaphragm distance and is fixed for any given piece of apparatus.

For example, if the diaphragms are placed at 12 cm. from the target and a focus–film distance of 100 cm. is used, then in order to cover a 30 × 25 cm. film the separation of the diaphragms must be:

$$30 \times \tfrac{12}{100} \quad \text{and} \quad 25 \times \tfrac{12}{100},$$

i.e., 3·6 and 3·0 cm. respectively.

Since the diaphragms are relatively close to the target, and distant from the film, the cut-off at the edge of the beam will not be very sharp. In other words, there is a comparatively large geometric unsharpness to the beam edge. In diagnostic work this is of no importance since there is no great interest in the beam edge. In therapeutic work, on the other hand, a sharp edge to the beam is desirable so that a specially designed collimating system has to be used. This is discussed in CHAPTER XXXV.

Light Beam Diaphragm System.—The moving diaphragm system just described usually has incorporated into it a visible light system so arranged that the size of the X-ray beam is demonstrated (on the patient) as a visible light patch. This is done by including a lamp and mirror as shown in *Fig.* 152. The lamp and mirror are positioned so that the light beam is in the same direction and of the same size as the X-ray beam. This can be achieved, as shown in the diagram, by placing the mirror at 45° to the beam and the lamp exactly as far in front of the mirror as the X-ray target is behind it, and in a line at 45° to the mirror surface. The mirror is of thin glass, silvered, or of polished metal, and the reduction in X-ray intensity which it causes is not very large.

Maximum Beam Size.—Even in the absence of a cone and light beam diaphragm system, the X-ray beam is not infinitely large—although it is usually far too big for actual use and it always needs to be reduced to the desired size by a collimating system.

In order to know the largest film which can be covered under any given conditions, it is necessary to consider what it is that limits the maximum beam size. The limitation arises for two reasons. Firstly, there is always a master diaphragm or collimator which consists fundamentally of a hole in the X-ray tube shield. The existence of such a fixed collimator makes it possible to manufacture a light beam diaphragm system which is reasonably small since it does not have to deal with an excessively large beam. This fixed collimator is shown diagrammatically in *Fig.* 153, in which the second limitation to beam size can also be seen. This is that on the anode side (right of the diagram) no radiation beyond the line *TA* can leave the target. The

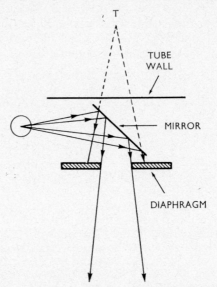

Fig. 152.—A variable collimator with light-beam indication.

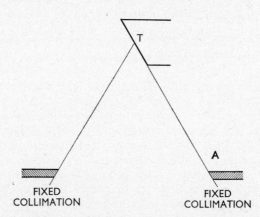

Fig. 153.—Fixed collimation. The beam size is determined at the anode side by 'anode cut-off'. A fixed hole in a sheet of lead limits the maximum size of the emerging X-ray beam.

greater the inclination of the target, the smaller is the possible beam of radiation. This is called *anode cut-off*. It can be seen that with the usual target angle of 17° and an F.F.D. of 100 cm., the distance from the central axis at which this occurs is 31 cm.

There is no similar cut-off at the cathode side, nor in the direction at right-angles to the plane of *Fig.* 153, but since it is required to place the film with its centre on the central ray, it is usual to arrange for the fixed master collimator to limit the beam in all directions to that determined by the anode cut-off. In this example, therefore, the maximum beam size at 90 cm. is a circle 56 cm. in diameter, which is just about big enough to cover a 43 × 36 cm. film. It should be emphasized (since it is a common error to state otherwise) that the focal spot *size* has no effect on the maximum beam size and that conversely the beam size has no effect on image sharpness.

Heel Effect.—Although there is an X-ray beam over the whole of the region covered by the maximum beam size which has just been discussed, the X-ray intensity

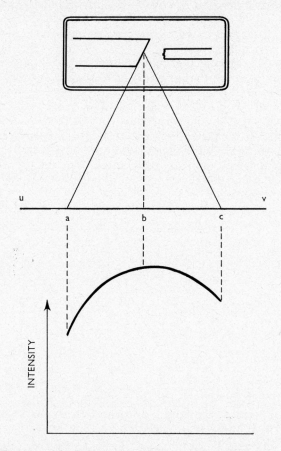

Fig. 154.—Distribution of radiation across an X-ray beam.

is not uniform over this area. The graph of *Fig.* 154 shows one example of how the intensity of X-rays may vary along the line *u–v*, which is at right-angles to the X-ray beam central axis.

There are several reasons why the intensity is not constant along this line (i.e., at the film):

1. Points *a* and *c* are further from the target than is point *b* so that the intensity is smaller at *a* and *c*. This is referred to as the Inverse Square Law (I.S.L.) fall-off and results in the intensity being decreased progressively at points away from the central axis.

2. The radiation passing to points such as *a* and *c* has passed obliquely through various absorbers such as the glass wall of the X-ray tube, the insulating oil, the filter, and anything else which happens to be in the beam. Again, this results in the intensity being decreased uniformly at points away from the central axis.

3. As has already been pointed out in CHAPTER V, X-rays are not emitted from the target uniformly in all directions, but rather the intensity in the direction of *a* (the anode side of the central ray) tends to be greater than that in the direction of *c* (cathode side) and also than that along the central ray, *b*. At diagnostic qualities (40–120 kV.) and for field sizes used in diagnostic work, the effect is not great, but it can be important in radiotherapy.

4. X-rays emitted in the direction between *a* and *b* tend to be more absorbed by the target than are those emitted in the direction between *c* and *b*, which results in the intensity at points such as *a* being further reduced compared with *c* and *b*. This effect, which is known as the **heel effect,** arises because the X-rays are generated at a small depth inside the target and also because the target surface is rough (on the microscopic scale). *Fig.* 154 shows how X-rays so produced have to pass through a greater thickness of tungsten and so are attenuated. The thickness of tungsten involved, and therefore the attenuation, is greater for the X-rays on the anode side of the beam.

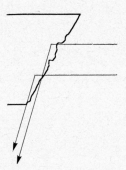

Fig. 155.—The heel effect. X-rays produced at a small depth inside the target and travel-ling in the direction shown are attenuated in the target. The intensity on the anode side of the beam is therefore reduced.

This effect exists (towards the edges of the maximum beam on the anode side) even with a new target whose surface is smooth. When a target has been in use for some time and especially if it has been misused by the use of excessive kV.–mA.s. combinations, the target surface becomes rough and the amount of heel effect increases. This shows up, of course, as a reduction in X-ray intensity (leading in practice to a pale or, as it is usually called, a 'thin' film) on the anode side of the beam.

The effects (1) and (2) result in a symmetrical reduction in intensity on all sides of the central ray, since they exist not only in the plane of the drawing (*Fig.* 154) but in all other directions as well. The heel effect is an asymmetric effect and occurs only on the anode side. To some extent this effect is counterbalanced by effect (3), but at these voltages the heel effect predominates and it is this which is responsible for the curve (*Fig.* 154) being asymmetric. As has already been stated, this asymmetry will increase with use of the tube.

Variation in Effective Focal Spot Size.—Effective focal spot, as defined on p. 219, and as quoted for any particular tube, refers to that in the direction of the central ray. In other directions the value is different and it is of interest to note how the effective focal spot size, and its effect on the image, vary along a line in the anode–cathode direction.

Fig. 156 shows on a very exaggerated scale the penumbra at the edge of the shadow cast by the objects *a*, *b*, or *c*, placed at the same level but to the anode and cathode sides and on the central axis of the beam respectively. It can be seen that the sharpness is much better on the anode side than it is at the centre and that it is better at the centre than it is on the cathode side. There is no significant similar effect in the direction at right-angles to the anode–cathode direction; the sharpness is the same on the two sides of the centre and slightly better (but not noticeably so) than in the centre.

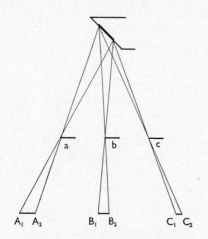

Fig. 156.—The variation in effective focal spot size for objects placed in the anode–cathode direction results in different values of geometric unsharpness.

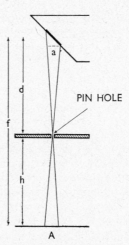

Fig. 157.—The pin-hole camera. An image (A) of the focal spot (a) is formed via a pin-hole in a sheet of lead.

This effect can be utilized if great sharpness is required by using the anode side of the beam—but it must then be remembered that the intensity will be reduced by heel effect, etc. Also, if the left-hand side of a radiograph is to be compared with the right-hand side, as for example in a chest film, then the anode–cathode axis of the tube should be parallel with the length of the patient so that the sharpness of both left and right lungs is identical.

Determination of Focal Spot Shape, Size and Position, and Condition.—As has been shown, the focal spot has an important bearing on the sharpness of a radiograph and it is often desirable to measure its size, to determine its exact position, or to examine the uniformity of the X-ray emission from it. This is equally useful to ensure either that the tube is operating correctly before being put into use, or that it is continuing to work correctly, or to find out why it is not working as well as it did! For instance, a cracked or pitted target will cause both a non-uniform beam and a reduced output, and a defocused or incorrectly focused electron beam will change the image sharpness.

The state and size of the focal spot may be determined by taking what is known as a *pin-hole picture*. The apparatus and its arrangement are shown in *Fig.* 157. A sheet of lead with a small (pin-) hole in it is placed approximately midway between the target and a film, with the hole as nearly as possible vertically below the target.

Another sheet of lead is placed below the film to reduce backscatter and a suitable exposure (mA.s.) made. After processing the film will show an image of the focal spot. The pattern of blackness will indicate the uniformity, or lack, of X-ray emission. For instance, a deep pit or crack will show as a clear area since no X-rays succeed in reaching the film from such a region. Even with a new tube it is usual for there to be a pattern on the focal spot picture and this takes the same form as the filament. The focused beam of electrons from the cathode strikes the anode and the pattern of X-ray emission is the same as the pattern in the electron beam, which is determined by the filament shape.

The size (A) of the image on the film is proportional to the size of the apparent focal spot (a) and, using the geometry of similar triangles, it is seen that:

$$\text{Apparent focal spot size } (a) = \text{Image size } (A) \times \frac{d}{h}$$

$$= A \times \frac{f-h}{h},$$

where f, h, and d are the dimensions shown on the figure. The quantity $(f-h)/h$ is the magnification and in particular if $h = d$, as it is when the sheet of lead is placed midway, then this is unity and the image is the same size as the apparent focal spot.

Any displacement of the image of the focal spot from the position of the central ray indicates a mis-centred focal spot, and a pin-hole picture can be used to assist the positioning of the X-ray tube correctly in the tube housing.

Although it is so very simple to obtain, the pin-hole focal spot picture gives a wealth of information about the focal spot and it is useful to make such a picture for each tube as it is installed, so that it can be compared with subsequent ones should any doubts arise about the continuing perfection of the focal spot.

Determination of Target Angle.—The angle of the target may be determined experimentally by means of a double pin-hole apparatus, and one way in which this can be done is described below. These details lie a little outside the interests of the majority of radiographers and it is not suggested that too much time should be spent on the following paragraphs, especially if the geometry proves uncongenial.

Fig. 158 shows the arrangement used. A sheet of lead is positioned so that the two pin-holes (P_1 and P_2) in it lie symmetrically on either side of the central ray. After exposure and processing, the film will show two pin-hole pictures of the focal spot. The one on the anode side (ef) will have a smaller size (S_2) than that on the cathode side (bc) whose size is S_1. This difference in size arises because the true focal spot (ad) is being viewed from two different directions and therefore the effective focal spot is different for these two images. In this example (*Fig.* 158) the effective focal spot in the direction P_1 is gd, and in the direction P_2 is hd. This effect has been mentioned previously when the variation in sharpness along the anode–cathode axis was discussed on p. 229. For example, if the quoted (i.e., central axis) effective focal spot size is 2×2 mm., then at the anode side the effective focal spot size could be

1×2 mm., and on the cathode side 3×2 mm. These figures, incidentally, indicate the magnitude of the changes in sharpness previously referred to. From the difference in the size of these two images (S_1 and S_2) the angle (θ) of the inclination of the target to the X-ray beam central axis may be determined in the following way.

Because triangle gdP_1 is similar to triangle P_1bc and triangle hdP_2 is similar to triangle P_2ef it follows that bc is proportional to gd and ef is proportional to hd.

Furthermore, the constant of proportionality is the same in both cases, and since $bc = S_1$, and $ef = S_2$, it follows that:

$$\frac{gd}{S_1} = \frac{hd}{S_2} = \frac{gd - hd}{S_1 - S_2} = \frac{gh}{S_1 - S_2}.$$

The separation (K) of the two images on the film can be measured and hence (knowing the focus–film distance, F.F.D.) a triangle of the *same shape* as triangle *acf* can be drawn at any convenient size. Such a triangle is shown in *Fig.* 159, where capital letters have been used to identify the similar vertices. In this triangle $CF \propto K$ and $AT \propto$ F.F.D.

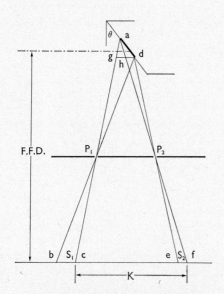

Fig. 158.—Determination of target angle. The relative sizes of the two pin-hole images (bc and ef) of the focal spot enable the target angle to be calculated.

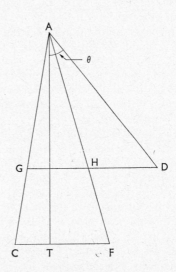

Fig. 159.—Determination of target angle. A greatly enlarged reconstruction of the focal spot region of Fig. 158.

A line GH is now drawn at any convenient level, and continued to a point D such that:

$$\frac{GD}{S_1} = \frac{HD}{S_2} = \frac{GH}{S_1 - S_2}.$$

For example, if $S_1 = 3$ cm. and $S_2 = 1$ cm. and *GH happens* to be 10 cm. then:

$$\frac{GH}{S_1 - S_2} = \frac{10}{3 - 1} = 5,$$

and therefore

$$HD = 5 \times S_2 = 5$$

and

$$GD = 5 \times S_1 = 15.$$

A line is now drawn joining the points A and D. The triangular array $AGHD$ now represents (on a very much larger scale, of course) exactly the same *shape* as the array *aghd* which exists close to the focal spot (*Fig.* 158) since the relationships between GD, HD, and GH have been drawn to be identical with those between *gd*, *hd*, and *gh*. A line AT is now drawn perpendicular to CF and the angle between AT and AD measured. This is the required angle of inclination of the target.

Modulation Transfer Function and Image Sharpness.—The distance over which the image of the edge of a structure is spread, whilst a major factor, is not the only one which determines the apparent sharpness of a shadow. The combined effects of contrast and unsharpness on the visibility of the fine detail of a radiograph (or fluorescent screen) is discussed in CHAPTER XXI, where it is pointed out that it is the overall shape of the variation of pattern of density with distance on the film which is the determining factor. Ideally, of course, the radiographic system as a whole should be capable of faithfully reproducing the pattern of the structures being radiographed.

The quality of pattern reproduction by a system can be tested by the use of such things as wire meshes of different wire thickness and spacing. Whilst this is useful, it is not completely satisfactory for the lower-contrast patterns of importance in medical radiology. It has become fashionable (and to a limited extent, useful) over the past decade or so to use as an index of faithfulness of reproduction the concept of 'Modulation Transfer Function'.

A detailed description of the difficult mathematical concepts and calculations involved in the use of this function is beyond the scope of this book. However, for those who wish to have some knowledge of it, a rather superficial and certainly simplified description, the aim of which is to point out the main features of the modulation transfer function and associated concepts, is given in APPENDIX III. Direct measurements of the function is not usually possible: a brief description of the usually employed indirect method using the 'line spread function' is also given in APPENDIX III. A concept similar to the modulation transfer function which is also sometimes used is the 'Contrast Frequency Response'. This is practically rather simpler than, but theoretically not quite as good as, the modulation transfer function.

It is important to realize that both the modulation transfer function and the contrast frequency response are objective measurements of the potential resolution of detail by a system: they say nothing about the subjective aspects referred to in CHAPTER XXI.

CHAPTER XIX

THE EFFECT OF X-RAY ABSORPTION ON THE
RADIOGRAPHIC IMAGE

In addition to being composed of sizes and shapes, the pattern on the X-ray film has differing degrees of greyness, ranging from almost clear film, corresponding to those regions of the patient where the X-rays were almost completely attenuated and so prevented from reaching the film, to almost black film, corresponding to those regions where large amounts of radiation passed through the patient and so reached the film. Similarly the fluoroscopic screen has brightnesses ranging from very dull areas, where few X-rays succeed in reaching the screen, to fairly bright areas where large amounts of X-rays reach it.

From these differing degrees of greyness or brightness the radiologist attempts to make deductions about the thickness and kind of material through which the X-rays have passed. It is upon these deductions that he bases his clinical diagnosis.

At the simplest level it can immediately be stated that where the fraction of X-rays transmitted through the patient is small, then that part of the patient is either very thick and dense or is composed of materials which are highly absorbing or, of course, both. Likewise, if a high fraction of X-rays is transmitted then that part of the

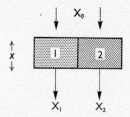

Fig. 160.—The relative transmission of X-rays by two different materials.

patient is either thin or composed of not very absorbing materials, or both. In this chapter the relationship between the structure and composition of the patient and the different degrees of greyness on the film (or brightness on the screen) will be described.

Consider first the radiography of the simple type of structure illustrated in *Fig.* 160. A uniform beam of X-rays is directed on to equal thicknesses of two different materials, bone and muscle, say. In passing through the bone (1) the intensity of the X-ray beam is reduced from X_0 to X_1, whilst in passing through the same thickness of muscle the intensity is not reduced so much and the transmitted intensity X_2 is greater than that transmitted by the bone. This difference in X-ray intensities X_1 and X_2, transmitted by the bone and muscle, constitutes the pattern in the X-ray beam which will eventually be seen.

Fluoroscopy.—In fluoroscopy this pattern of intensities transmitted by and caused by the 'patient' is directed on to a fluorescent screen. The brightness (L) of the light emitted from any point on the screen is proportional to the intensity (X)

233

of the X-rays incident upon that point of the screen. Hence any pattern of intensities in the X-ray beam is faithfully reproduced as a pattern of different brightnesses of visible light. Where there are a lot of X-rays there will be a lot of light, and vice versa. It can therefore be truthfully said that the fluoroscopic screen enables the radiologist to 'see' the X-ray pattern.

It is now necessary to consider how the pattern depends upon the exact conditions of the irradiation. The items which are important are:

1. The quality (kV.) of the X-rays.
2. The thickness of the absorbers (patient).
3. The nature (atomic number and density) of the different materials. (In the present example bone and muscle are referred to but clearly any two materials could be involved.)

At this point it is necessary to recall from CHAPTER VI that in passing through any material X-rays are reduced in intensity according to an *exponential* law. This means that the intensities (X_1 and X_2) of the transmitted X-ray beams are related to that (X_0) of the incident beam by the equations:

$$X_1 = X_0 e^{-\mu_1 x},$$
$$X_2 = X_0 e^{-\mu_2 x},$$

where μ_1 and μ_2 are the linear attenuation coefficients of the two materials (e.g., bone and muscle) and x is their thickness (*Fig.* 160).

These two equations may be rearranged to give:

$$X_0 = X_1 e^{+\mu_1 x} = X_2 e^{+\mu_2 x}$$

from which, by taking logarithms (to the base 10), we get:

$$\log X_1 + \mu_1 x \log e = \log X_2 + \mu_2 x \log e.$$

Hence, since $\log e = 0\cdot 4343$,

$$\log X_2 - \log X_1 = 0\cdot 4343(\mu_1 - \mu_2) x.$$

Now, as has already been stated, the intensity (L) of light emitted from the fluorescent screen is proportional to the intensity (X) of the X-rays responsible for it, so that:

$$L_1 = \rho X_1 \quad \text{and} \quad L_2 = \rho X_2,$$

where L_1 and L_2 are the light intensities (brightnesses) produced on the screen by the X-ray intensities X_1 and X_2 respectively, ρ is a constant which need not be known. It has also been stated in CHAPTER XVI that the physiological action of the eye is such that it 'sees' light logarithmically. In other words, intensities in the ratios 1 : 10 : 100 : 1000 are seen as equal steps in brightness. From this it follows that the contrast seen between two regions on a fluorescent screen depends upon the difference in the logarithms of the brightness of the two regions.* In the present example the contrast seen is therefore given by:

$$\text{Contrast, } C = \log L_2 - \log L_1$$

but

$$\log L_2 - \log L_1 = \log (\rho X_2) - \log (\rho X_1)$$
$$= \log \rho + \log X_2 - \log \rho - \log X_1$$
$$= \log X_2 - \log X_1.$$

---

* *N.B.* $\log 1 : \log 10 : \log 100 : \log 1000 = 0 : 1 : 2 : 3.$

If this result is now combined with the earlier equation (p. 234) relating X-ray intensities and linear attenuation coefficients, it is seen that the visible contrast (C) on the fluorescent screen is given by:

$$C = \log L_2 - \log L_1 = \log X_2 - \log X_1$$
$$= 0{\cdot}4343(\mu_1 - \mu_2)\,x.$$

This contrast pattern which is present in the X-ray beam incident upon the fluorescent screen and which is caused by the different X-ray attenuations in the various parts of the 'patient' (*Fig.* 160) is called the *patient contrast*, or more usually the *radiation contrast*.

The fact that the fluorescent screen brightness is proportional to the X-ray intensity means that the pattern of contrasts seen by the radiologist corresponds exactly to the pattern in the X-ray beam. In fluoroscopy the radiologist 'sees' the radiation contrast.

Radiography.—In radiography the pattern of X-ray intensities is directed on to the film (or film plus intensifying screen). After processing it is found that, although the shape and size in the visible pattern are the same as in fluoroscopy, the contrasts are now much greater, in spite of the fact that the X-ray intensity pattern is the same. This greater contrast seen on the radiograph compared with that seen on the fluorescent screen is most important in practice and arises partly from subjective and partly from objective reasons.

Some of the increase is due to the difference in viewing conditions. This will be considered in more detail later: suffice it to say, at this stage, that when viewing the radiographic image, the eye is able to appreciate (see) smaller contrast differences than it can in the smaller brightness of the fluorescent screen. So even if the contrast were the same in each, the contrast in the film would *appear* greater.

But more important, there is, in fact, greater contrast on the radiograph than on the fluorescent screen even though the conditions of irradiation of both are identical. The reason for this extra contrast is to be found in the properties of the X-ray film.

In CHAPTER XVI it was stated that the contrast on a radiograph is the difference in the densities,* i.e.,

$$\text{Contrast, } C = D_2 - D_1,$$

where D_2 and D_1 are the optical densities produced by the X-ray Exposures E_2 and E_1 respectively. In the straight-line portion of the characteristic curve the densities and Exposures are related by the following equation:

---

* It will be recalled that the density is measured by the logarithm of the ratio of the incident to the transmitted light intensities.

Hence

$$D_2 - D_1 = \log \frac{L_0}{L_2} - \log \frac{L_0}{L_1}$$
$$= \log L_0 - \log L_2 - \log L_0 + \log L_1$$
$$= -(\log L_2 - \log L_1),$$

i.e., the magnitude of the contrast equals the difference in the logarithm of the light intensities transmitted by the two regions of the radiograph. This is exactly the same as the fluoroscopic screen where the contrast seen is likewise equal to the difference in the logarithms of the two light intensities. The density is thus seen to be the correct way of measuring the blackness of a film since it corresponds with what the eye sees (both density and the eye being logarithmic). The minus sign indicates the fact that the radiograph is a negative (i.e., where there were few X-rays one sees a lot of light and vice versa) whereas the fluoroscopic screen is a positive.

$$\text{Gamma, } \gamma = \frac{D_2 - D_1}{\log E_2 - \log E_1}$$

or more usefully:

$$\text{Contrast, } C = D_2 - D_1 = \gamma(\log E_2 - \log E_1).$$

Now the X-ray Exposure (E) at the film is proportional to the intensity (X) of the X-ray beam at the film, i.e.,

$$X_1 = KE_1 \quad \text{and} \quad X_2 = KE_2,$$

where K is some constant which depends upon the exposure time and on the different units used for measuring X and E.

Substituting these values in the last equation, it follows that:

$$\text{Contrast, } C = D_2 - D_1 = \gamma(\log X_2 - \log X_1),$$

but it is already known (p. 235) that

$$\log X_2 - \log X_1 = 0.4343(\mu_1 - \mu_2)x.$$

Hence the contrast on a radiograph is given by:

$$\text{Contrast, } C = D_2 - D_1 = \gamma.0.4343(\mu_1 - \mu_2)x.$$

It can be seen that this expression is almost identical to that given previously for the contrast on the fluorescent screen; the only difference is the factor gamma (γ). The contrast on the radiograph is called the *radiographic contrast* and is seen to be equal to the product of the *radiation contrast* (i.e., the effect of the patient on the X-ray beam) and the film gamma* (i.e., the effect on the film of the X-ray intensities).

Radiographic contrast = Radiation contrast × film contrast.

For an X-ray film the value of γ is usually in the range 3–4, so that for otherwise identical circumstances, the contrast on the radiograph is three or four times that of the fluorescent screen.

Factors controlling Contrast.—The two equations given above for the contrast in fluoroscopy and radiography are very important and even if their derivation is forgotten, their meaning should be remembered. This is, that the visual contrast is controlled, and is proportional to:

1. The difference in linear attenuation coefficients of the materials creating the contrast.
2. The thickness of the material.
3. (In radiography.) The slope of the characteristic curve of the photographic film.

The greater the difference in attenuation coefficient and the greater the thickness, the greater will be the contrast. If the difference in attenuation coefficient is small then, in order to achieve a high contrast, the thickness must be large. Conversely, if the thickness is small, then there must be a large difference in attenuation coefficient

---

* If the X-ray exposure is such that not all the X-ray intensities lie within the straight-line portion of the curve, then the contrast on the film will not be enhanced so much. In general, the contrast on the radiograph is given by:

$$C = m.0.4343(\mu_1 - \mu_2)x,$$

where m is the slope of the characteristic curve over the exposure range employed. The maximum, and usual, value of m is, of course, γ.

if the contrast is to be seen. From this it is obvious that the linear attenuation co-efficients of the materials comprising the patient, and so creating the pattern in the X-ray beam, are the important factors in determining the contrast in the visual pattern.

Effect of Material on Contrast.—In CHAPTER VII the dependence of linear attenuation coefficient on density, atomic number, and radiation quality was discussed. *Fig.* 161 shows how the linear attenuation coefficients of bone, muscle (soft tissue), and fat vary with radiation quality. It will be recalled that the great change observed in the curve for bone is due to the rapid change ($\propto$ photon energy cubed) in the amount

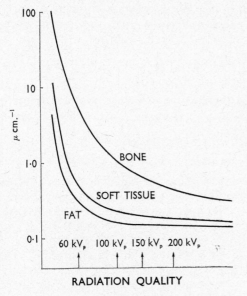

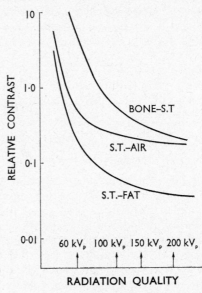

Fig. 161.—Variation, with radiation quality, of the linear attenuation coefficient for bone, muscle, and fatty tissue. (*Note*: μ is on log scale.)

Fig. 162.—Variation, with radiation quality, of the contrast caused by bone/muscle, muscle/fat, and muscle/air. (*Note*: Contrast is on log scale.)

of photo-electric effect, which is the major process of attenuation in the relatively high atomic numbered bone ($Z = \sim 13$). For fat ($Z = \sim 6$) and muscle ($Z = \sim 7.5$), although the linear attenuation coefficient decreases as the radiation quality is increased, the change is not so great since in these materials photo-electric effect is less important and the principal process of attenuation is the Compton effect, which is less dependent on photon energy and which is also almost independent of atomic number. The densities of the three materials are also different (bone = 1·8; muscle = 1·0; fat = 0·90) which results in a further difference in attenuation coefficient which persists even at high photon energies, where the difference in atomic number is unimportant.

The observed contrast on an X-ray film* is proportional to the *difference* in linear coefficients and this difference is plotted in *Fig.* 162 for bone and muscle and for muscle and fat. It can be seen that the contrast in both cases decreases with

---

* In this chapter, where film is referred to, the same comment applies to the fluorescent screen with the proviso that the contrast on the screen is less than that on the film by a factor, γ.

increase in radiation quality but that the change is much more marked for bone/muscle contrast than it is for muscle/fat contrast. It should be noted, however, that, for equal thicknesses, the bone/muscle contrast is always greater than the muscle/fat contrast because of the greater difference in density (g./c.c.).

The variation, with quality, of the muscle/air contrast is also shown in *Fig.* 162. In this range of X-ray quality the attenuation by air is negligibly small so that this contrast is determined by, and therefore follows exactly, the attenuation coefficient of muscle.

The contrast of muscle to lung varies in a similar way to that of muscle/air, except that the magnitude of the contrast is about 25 per cent less. Lung tissue has exactly the same atomic number as muscle (soft tissue) but has a density which is only about one-quarter as great. The linear attenuation coefficients are therefore related by the expression:

$$\mu_L = 0 \cdot 25 \mu_M,$$

where μ_L and μ_M are the linear attenuation coefficients of lung and muscle tissues respectively. The contrasts, being proportional to the difference in attenuation coefficients, are thus seen to be proportional to:

$$\text{Contrast: Muscle/air, } \mu_M - \mu_{air} = \mu_M;$$

$$\text{Contrast: Muscle/lung, } \mu_M - \mu_L = \mu_M - 0 \cdot 25 \mu_M = 0 \cdot 75 \mu_M.$$

It should be noted that both these contrasts fall as the radiation quality (kV.) is increased in spite of the fact that effectively only one material (muscle) is involved. The air, as has already been stated, has a negligibly small effect. This decrease in contrast with increase in radiation quality (kV.) is thus seen to arise because the linear attenuation coefficient always decreases as the quality is increased.

Fig. 162 shows how, at very soft qualities, the bone/muscle contrast is very much greater than the muscle/air and therefore muscle/lung contrast. This is because of the very great difference in the atomic numbers of bone and muscle, which matters in this quality range where photo-electric effect predominates. At the harder qualities (higher kV.) the difference is less marked and, in fact, above about 200 kV. (where Compton effect predominates) the muscle/air contrast is greater than the bone/muscle contrast. This is because the difference in atomic number is unimportant and the difference in density of muscle to air ($1 - 0 \cdot 001293 \approx 1$) is greater than the difference in density of bone to muscle ($1 \cdot 85 - 1 = 0 \cdot 85$).

Contrast due to Different Thickness.—Contrast may also arise because of a different thickness of the same material. Furthermore, an alternative way of regarding the contrast created between **tissue** and air (or any other gas) such as may occur with a gas-filled cavity is as a contrast brought about by a different thickness. This may arise naturally as in the case of a nasal sinus, or artificially as in pneumography.

The situations illustrated in *Fig.* 163 are identical radiographically and the contrast is caused by the attenuation in the extra thickness (x) of muscle compared with the negligible absorption in the equal thickness of air. In this situation the expression for the contrast in radiography is simplified to:

$$\text{Contrast} = 0 \cdot 4343 \gamma \mu x,$$

where μ is the attenuation coefficient of the tissue involved.

Contrast in General.—The more general situation of different thicknesses of different materials creating a contrast is illustrated in *Fig.* 164. There a material

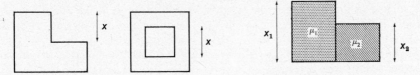

Fig. 163.—The creation of a contrast by different thicknesses of the same material.

Fig. 164.—The creation of a contrast by different thicknesses of different materials.

of attenuation coefficient μ_1 and thickness x_1 is adjacent to another material of attenuation coefficient μ_2 and thickness x_2. Using the same calculation methods as before, it can be shown that the radiographic contrast is given by:

$$C = 0.4343\gamma(\mu_1 x_1 - \mu_2 x_2).$$

This general expression can be simplified in particular circumstances to those already given earlier in this chapter. For convenience the various formulae are collected in *Table XXII*.

Table XXII.—THE MAGNITUDE IN VARIOUS CIRCUMSTANCES OF THE CONTRAST IN RADIOGRAPHY AND IN FLUOROSCOPY

CONDITIONS CAUSING CONTRAST				RADIOGRAPHY	FLUOROSCOPY
1. Different thickness	Same material	x_1		$C = k\gamma(x_1-x_2)\,\mu$	$C = k(x_1-x_2)\,\mu$
2. Different material	Equal thickness	x		$= k\gamma(\mu_1-\mu_2)\,x$	$= k(\mu_1-\mu_2)\,x$
3. Different thickness and material	General	x_1		$= k\gamma(\mu_1 x_1 - \mu_2 x_2)$	$= k(\mu_1 x_1 - \mu_2 x_2)$
4. Soft tissue/air	Equal thickness	x		$= k\gamma x \mu_{ST}$	$= kx\mu_{ST}$
5. Soft tissue/lung	Equal thickness	x		$= 0.75k\gamma x\mu_{ST}$	$= 0.75kx\mu_{ST}$

N.B.— $k = 0.4343$.

Practical Aspects.—The contrast pattern created in an X-ray beam by the patient is determined by the kind (atomic number and density) and thickness of the various materials present, and by the radiation quality. In general, the magnitude of the contrast decreases as the radiation quality (kV.) is increased. This decrease is very great over the quality range up to 60–80 kV. for contrasts involving bone, because of the rapid change in the attenuation coefficient of the relatively high atomic number of bone. The contrasts between soft tissue, fat, lung, and gas are much less variable but also fall as the kV. is increased. The contrasts between soft tissue and lung or between soft tissue and fat tend to be inherently small because of the relatively small differences in density and atomic number (i.e., in attenuation coefficient). For this reason it is very often necessary to use the lower range of kV. in order to obtain sufficient contrast. In other words, it is necessary to utilize the increase in contrast, albeit rather small, which results from decrease in kV. It is for this reason that soft-tissue radiography, and especially mammography, are performed with relatively low kV. Even with low kV. the contrast may be small unless large thicknesses are involved. For instance, the planes separating muscle (which are seen as a contrast between the muscle and the slightly lower density, loose intramuscular or areolar tissue) are only seen when the planes are orientated approximately at right-angles to the film.

For bone/soft tissue contrast, on the other hand, the large density of bone coupled with its high atomic number means that sufficient contrast can be obtained with even high kV.

Latitude versus Contrast.—If it is required to include within an acceptable range of densities on the same radiograph bone, soft tissue, and lung shadows it will, in general, be found impossible to do this at the lower kV. This is because the range of X-ray intensities reaching the film exceeds its latitude (CHAPTER XVI). If, on the other hand, a high kV. is used, the bone/soft tissue contrast will be reduced without impairing the soft tissue/lung contrast too much and it will then be found possible to accommodate both bone and lung shadows within the latitude of the film.

Control of Contrast.—For any particular radiographic examination the principal variable factor which controls contrast is the radiation quality (kV.), the contrast being greater at the lower kV. Although, in general, a high contrast is desirable, this is not always so. Furthermore, as will be described later, there are other considerations which make a higher kV. desirable. A compromise therefore has to be effected and the choice of the correct kV., so as to achieve the optimum result, is one of the major features of good radiology.

The Effect of Patient Thickness.—In the description so far it has been assumed (*Fig.* 160) that the single anatomical structure is isolated. In practice it will, of course, either be immersed in, or lie on the surface of, a patient. Such a situation can be illustrated, still in a simplified way, by *Fig.* 165, where the structure is inside a larger volume of a uniform material (water, say).

When such a large volume is irradiated a large amount of scattered radiation will be produced, principally by the Compton process. If this scattered radiation is able, and is allowed, to reach the film then the contrasts in the pattern created by the anatomical structure of interest will be reduced. This effect of scattered radiation on contrast will be discussed more fully in CHAPTER XX, and, although in practice it can be of major importance, for the present the effect will be ignored.

This being so, the general description and conclusions already given in this chapter about the contrast on the radiograph created by such a structure (*Fig.* 160) still apply when the structure is inside the patient (*Fig.* 165). That this is so can easily be demonstrated by reference to *Fig.* 166. Using the same type of calculation and symbols as before, it can be seen that:

$$X_1' = X_1 e^{-\mu r} \quad \text{and} \quad X_2' = X_2 e^{-\mu r},$$

where μ is the attenuation coefficient of the surrounding material and r is the thickness of material between the structure and the film. X_1 and X_2 are the different

X-ray intensities transmitted by the structure and X_1' and X_2' the reduced values which reach the film.

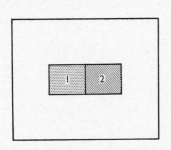

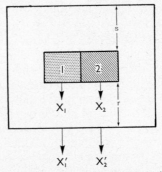

Fig. 165.—The structure of radiological interest within a large surrounding body.

Fig. 166.—The intensities X_1 and X_2 transmitted by the structure are identically attenuated in passing through the underlying tissue: $X_1/X_2 = X_1'/X_2'$.

The contrast on the film is proportional to the difference in the logarithms of the intensities at the film (p. 236), i.e.,

$$\text{Contrast, } C \propto \log X_1' - \log X_2'.$$

If the values given above for X_1' and X_2' are substituted in this equation then the contrast is seen to be given by:

$$\text{Contrast, } C \propto \log X_1' - \log X_2' = \log (X_1 e^{-\mu r}) - \log (X_2 e^{-\mu r}),$$

that is

$$C \propto \log X_1 - \log X_2,$$

which is exactly the same equation as given before for the isolated structure. The presence of the underlying absorbing material (of thickness r) is thus seen to have no effect on the contrast produced by the structure. It could similarly be shown that the presence of the overlying material (of thickness s) likewise has no effect on contrast.

This result is to be expected since it is not likely that the presence of a uniformly attenuating material could affect the pattern of contrast created.

Increase in Exposure.—Apart from the production of scattered radiation (which is being ignored at the moment) the principal effect of the over- and underlying tissue is to reduce the fraction of radiation transmitted through the patient to the film. This means that if the amounts of X-radiation reaching the film are to be kept the same as for the isolated structure (so as to maintain the desired range of densities on the film), then the amount of X-rays produced by the X-ray tube and directed on to the patient must be increased. In day-to-day language, the thicker the patient then the greater is the required X-ray tube exposure.

The extent to which this is necessary is determined, of course, by the attenuation by the over- and underlying thicknesses of tissue (s and r). Using the same type of calculation as before it is easily shown that the X-ray tube exposure has to be increased by a factor $e^{(r+s)\mu}$, which clearly depends upon the thickness of the patient ($r + s$) and the radiation quality (kV.) which determines the value of μ.

Theoretically this increase in radiation output of the X-ray tube could be brought about by an increase in the milliampere seconds (mA.s.), the kV. already having been selected in accordance with the contrast required. However, this is not always possible since the permissible tube rating may then be exceeded. Furthermore, if the increase in mA.s. is obtained by an increase in time then the amount of movement unsharpness may be undesirable. It is therefore often necessary to achieve the desired increase in X-ray output by an increase in kV. This has the added effect that the transmission through the patient (the 'penetration') is improved, so that a smaller increase in X-ray tube radiation output is needed in order to maintain the required amount of radiation at the film. Of course, the contrast will be reduced because of this increase in kV., and this is one of the factors in the compromise referred to on p. 224. The use of a higher kV. also leads to a reduction in the radiation dose to the patient, which is very desirable.

Filtration by the Patient.—Although it has been stated that the contrast produced by a certain anatomical detail is not affected by the presence of the surrounding tissues, this is not exactly true, even when the contrast-reducing effect of scattered radiation is ignored. The beam of X-rays directed on to the patient is heterogeneous so that (unless it has been very heavily filtered, which is not usually so) the patient will tend to filter the beam. This increases the radiation quality (even if the tube kV. is kept constant) and so reduces the contrast on the film. This effect is not very important in practice and is mentioned only for the sake of completeness.

It can be seen, therefore, that the contrast produced by any anatomical detail is fundamentally independent of the presence and size of the surrounding tissues; unfortunately, this is not so in practice. For several reasons the contrast is lowered on account of the presence of these surrounding tissues. These reasons are summarized here for convenience:

1. The production of scattered radiation (*see* CHAPTER XX).
2. A higher kV. tends to be used to 'penetrate' the patient.
3. The patient filters the beam.

The Effect of Overlying Structures.—Even the situation illustrated in *Fig.* 165 is simpler than an actual patient since the anatomical detail of interest is not surrounded by a characteristic, uniform medium (e.g., water) but by other anatomical structures. Each of these structures will, of course, cause its own contrast on the film or screen. This is obviously a very complicated situation since the contrasts caused by each overlying structure are not recorded separately but are successively added together to give the final picture on the film. The radiologist has to use his knowledge of both normal and pathological anatomy to try to sort out these overlying patterns. If this is not possible from a single film, different angled views or tomographic techniques must be resorted to.

Artificial Contrast.—In many circumstances the anatomical structure which it is wished to examine radiologically does not differ sufficiently in atomic number, density, or thickness from its surroundings for it to produce a visible contrast. Furthermore, a potential cavity may be collapsed so that it may not be possible to 'see' its wall radiographically. In both these circumstances it is sometimes possible to produce a contrast by means of what is known as an *artificial contrast medium*. There are two general types:

1. *Opaque.*—This is a material which contains elements having a higher atomic number. The material is introduced into the patient (e.g., orally or by injection) when it either surrounds, fills, or coats the surface of, the structure of interest. The result is that an artificial contrast, which it is possible to see, is produced on the film. Examples of this type are the use of barium compounds, for the examination of the oesophagus,

stomach, and colon, and iodine compounds for ureter and kidney investi-gations. The actual chemical composition of the particular compound used is selected to make it physiologically suitable for its particular usage.

Since the contrast is caused by a high atomic number material, the contrast can be very high and is, of course, very dependent upon kV.

2. *Transparent.*—With the transparent type of contrast medium the contrast is caused by a difference in density. A gas (usually air, oxygen, or carbon dioxide) is injected into the patient, so as to fill or create a cavity. There is thus a large difference in density between the 'hole' so formed and the surroundings which results in a visible contrast on the film or screen. In this case, since no large atomic number is involved, the contrast is not very dependent upon kV.

An example of this technique, which is called 'pneumography', is the examination of the ventricles in the brain by the injection of air.

CHAPTER XX

THE EFFECTS AND CONTROL OF SCATTERED RADIATION

The Effect of Scattered Radiation on Contrast.—In the discussion of contrast we have so far assumed that it is only those photons of the X-ray beam which are transmitted by the patient which affect the X-ray film and fluorescent screen. However, as was described in CHAPTER VI, not all photons which are removed from the beam are absorbed by the patient. Many of the photons are scattered so that some of the original photons are replaced by others travelling in different directions and with a

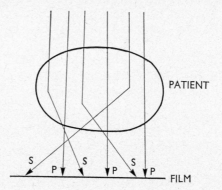

Fig. 167.—The radiation emerging from the patient, and incident upon the film, consists of primary photons (P) and obliquely moving scattered photons (S).

reduced energy and penetrating power. The film or screen is thus irradiated by two groups of photons (*Fig.* 167) which comprise:

1. The primary photons which have travelled from the X-ray tube and through the patient without being changed in any way except, of course, that they are reduced in number. It is this beam of primary photons which carries the pattern, in which we are interested, to the film.
2. Scattered photons which have been produced in the patient mainly as a result of Compton (or modified) scattering. This group of photons is, in general, patternless and irradiates the whole area of the film more or less uniformly, or, at least, with a slowly varying, characterless pattern.

The effect of this patternless, scattered radiation on the film is to reduce the contrast. It may be thought that since this scattered radiation is spread uniformly over the film it would cause no effect other than an overall increase in film density, which could easily be compensated by an increase in the brightness of the viewing screen. This is not so. As will be explained, the reduction in contrast brought about by the presence of scattered radiation can be very serious and of major importance in radiography.

Consider the situation illustrated in *Fig.* 168 A. As has been described previously, the radiation intensities in the shadow cast by the two absorbers will be different.

244

Their relative values will depend upon the exact circumstances but for purposes of illustration they are assumed to be 13 and 47 units respectively. The characteristic curve (*Fig.* 168 B) of the particular film/screen combination in use shows that these intensities will result in densities of 0·5 and 2·7 respectively and hence a contrast of $C = 2·7 - 0·5 = 2·2$.

Let it now be assumed that the two primary intensities have added to them an amount of scattered radiation equal to 13 units (*Fig.* 168 C). The two intensities striking the film are now $13 + 13 = 26$ and $13 + 47 = 60$, which will produce increased densities of 1·7 and 3·1, and hence a reduced contrast of 1·4 compared with the previous value of 2·2. It is thus seen that the scattered radiation not only brings about an overall increase in density but also a major reduction in contrast.

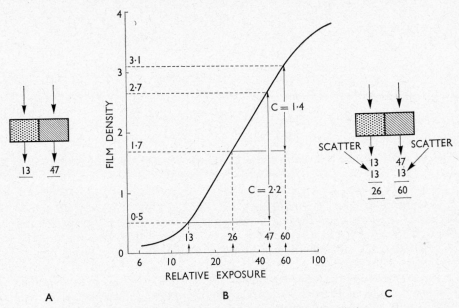

Fig. 168.—The reduction of contrast by scattered radiation.

The addition of an amount of scatter equal to the smaller primary intensity (13 units) may seem excessive but this is, in fact, most reasonable. Depending upon the exact circumstances, the amount of scattered radiation may well equal and often exceed the amount of primary radiation. In extreme circumstances there can be as much as ten times more scattered radiation than primary. The simple conclusion arrived at in an earlier chapter, that the contrast of an object is determined only by its thickness and relative linear attenuation coefficient, is now seen to be incorrect if scattered radiation is present.

A further consequence of this is that the contrast of an object is dependent upon its distance from the film. If a radiograph is taken of two identical objects suspended in a large tank of water at different distances from the film (*Fig.* 169) then it will be found that the contrasts of the two images on the film are different. The contrast of the object (1) nearest to the film will be almost exactly as it would be in the absence of the water, that is, in the absence of scattered radiation. On the other hand, the contrast of the object (2) furthest from the film will be considerably reduced because of the presence of large amounts of cross-moving scattered radiation which is able to undercut its shadow. In practice it could happen that the object close to the film could exhibit an increased contrast due to the formation of a shadow by the scattered radiation which is superimposed on top of that due to the primary. Since the scattered radiation is of a softer quality, the shadow will have an increased contrast although the sharpness of this shadow will be poor, arising from the fact that the scattered radiation is produced at a large source (the water) rather than at the more usual small focal spot. Unless the circumstances are known, the radiograph resulting from the arrangement of *Fig.* 169 would be erroneously interpreted as meaning that object 2 is either thinner or of a lower atomic number or less dense than object 1.

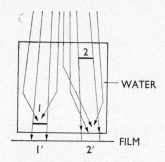

Fig. 169.—Contrast for object 2 is much less than for object 1 because of greater scatter reaching the film at its image.

It is therefore most important that the effects of scattered radiation should be taken into account when reading a radiograph. In practice the problems can be considerably simplified by arranging for these deleterious effects of scattered radiation to be substantially eliminated. Just how this is done forms the major part of the remainder of this chapter.

The Production of Scattered Radiation.—Although the process by which radiation is scattered has been discussed in some detail in CHAPTER VI it is worth while recalling those aspects which are important in this context.

The first fact is that the scattered photon has a lower energy than has the primary photon and is therefore less penetrating. (There is a certain amount of unmodified scattered radiation present but this is small and can be neglected.) Although the scattered radiation may travel in any direction, at least half of it is moving towards the film in the same general direction as the primary beam. It is, of course, this generally forward-moving scatter which constitutes the present nuisance. As the X-ray tube kV. is increased so is the fraction of the total scatter which is moving forwards.

However, it has already been stated in earlier chapters that as the X-ray tube kV. is *increased*, then the total amount of scattered radiation produced *decreases*. This is for two reasons. Firstly, the fraction of radiation which is scattered (measured by the linear attenuation coefficient for Compton effect σ) decreases as the radiation kV. is increased. Secondly, the higher kV. radiation penetrates the patient more easily so that the given amount of radiation required at the film to produce the chosen blackening demands a smaller amount of radiation to be directed at the patient from the X-ray tube. For purposes of the present discussion it can be safely assumed that the sensitivity of the film does not change significantly with radiation quality in this diagnostic range of tube kV., so that as the X-ray tube kV. is increased a decreased fraction of a decreased amount of radiation is scattered with the consequent reduction in the amount of scattered radiation produced.

In spite of this, it is a well-known practical fact that the deleterious effects of scattered radiation on contrast become much more important at the higher kV.: this apparent contradiction can be explained by reference to the situation illustrated in *Fig.* 170, where a fairly large tank of water (the physicist's favourite patient!) is irradiated by a large beam of X-rays.

Scattered radiation will be produced at all points of the water within the beam and a fraction of this will be moving towards a point such as O on the film. Consider first that produced in the thin layer of water P which is part of a sphere centred about O. The contribution of scattered radiation from P to O depends upon (*a*) the amount

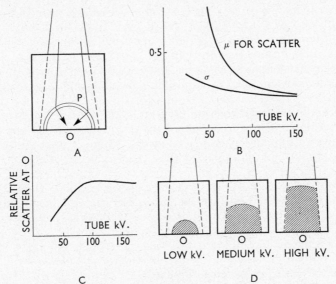

Fig. 170.—Why the scattered radiation emerging from the patient generally increases with increasing kV.

of scattered radiation produced in P and which is moving towards O and (*b*) the extent to which it is attenuated by the water between P and O. Although the amount of scattered radiation produced in P will decrease as the X-ray tube kV. is increased, the fraction of it which succeeds in reaching O will increase on account of the greater penetrating power of the scattered radiation produced by the higher energy primary photons. A complete analysis of the whole situation is very complex, especially in view of the possibility of multiple scattering and associated changes in photon energy. However, it can be seen from *Fig.* 170 B that whilst the scattering coefficient σ (upon which the amount of scatter produced depends) falls with increasing tube kV., the attenuation coefficient of this scattered radiation falls much more quickly, so that although the amount of scattered radiation being produced ($\propto \sigma$) falls as the kV. is increased, a greater fraction of it is able to reach the point O since it is less easily absorbed ($\propto \mu$ for the scattered radiation).

What is true for the layer P is also true for the whole of the irradiated water and the net result is that the higher fraction of the smaller amount of scattered radiation produced can result in a greater amount of scattered radiation reaching O as the tube kV. is increased.

Fig. 170 C shows the relative amount of scattered radiation which succeeds in reaching the point O (and all other points) on the film as the tube kV. is increased. The same information is given in *Fig.* 170 D in a rather different way. The shaded area represents the region from which significant amounts of scattered radiation can reach the film at O. The associated volumes increase much more rapidly than the amount of scattered radiation produced per unit volume decreases as the tube kV. is increased. Although much more scattered radiation is produced at the lower kV., its penetrating power is so small that little of it reaches O. At kV. in excess of 150 kV. the whole irradiated medium is able to contribute scatter to O so that the scatter at O falls progressively with further increase in kV. in accordance with the known fall in the scatter coefficient, σ.

This, then, is the reason why there is a rapid increase in the deleterious effect of scattered radiation as the tube kV. is raised from 50 kV. to 100 kV. It arises not from a real increase in scattered radiation but from an increase in the amount of scattered radiation able to reach the film. At higher kV. the proportion of obliquely moving scattered radiation reaching the film remains fairly constant but diminishes gradually as the kV. is raised to very high values. In the megavoltage range the effects of scattered radiation are fairly unimportant.

The Amount of Scattered Radiation Present.—The amount of scattered radiation present at the film is very dependent upon the exact circumstances of the irradiation and no simple quantitative data can be given. Suffice it to say that the amouut increases as the volume of irradiated tissue increases and as the X-ray tube kV. is increased from 50 kV. to 100 kV. In the worst circumstances there can be five or even ten times more scattered than primary radiation present. The successful elimination of the effects of this contrast-spoiling scatter is a very important, and indeed essential, task which is achieved by attention to the following complementary points:

1. Reduce the amount of scattered radiation produced.
2. Reduce the amount of scattered radiation reaching the film.
3. Reduce the effect of the scattered radiation on the film.

Reduction of Scattered Radiation Produced.—

Beam Size.—The major factor in determining the amount of scattered radiation produced is the volume of material which is irradiated. This material comprises mostly that part of the patient being radiographed but includes also the various structures behind the film which may be irradiated by the radiation transmitted through the cassette. Restriction of beam size (area) by means of a suitable *cone* or *light beam diaphragm* system is one of the most effective ways of improving radiographic contrast. There is an incidental but nevertheless important advantage in using a small beam, namely that the irradiation of the patient is kept to a minimum. The extent to which the beam size can be reduced is limited but certainly it should never be significantly greater than the film size being used: some radiologists prefer, in fact, to see evidence of the edges of the beam on each film. It is implied, of course, that the film itself is not excessively large for the part of the patient being examined. The use of an unnecessarily large film and beam size in order to be sure of 'getting it on the film' is evidence of a poor radiographer.

So-called *compression* of the patient can also be useful in reducing the amount of tissue being irradiated and therefore the amount of scatter produced. What happens when a compression cone or band is used is that tissue is pushed out of the way to the side of the beam. Compression *per se* has no effect on scattered radiation production, although it can have other clinical advantages to the radiologist, such as holding the patient steady.

Kilovoltage.—A suitable choice of kV. can also help in reducing scattered radiation. If the kV. is kept low then not only is contrast inherently greater but the deleterious effect of scatter is not so great as has already been discussed. Unfortunately, the use of a higher kV. is often preferred since there is then a greater latitude arising from the inherently smaller contrast and also a reduction in radiation dose to the patient.

Reduction in Scattered Radiation reaching the Film.—The main method by which scatter is prevented from reaching the film is by the use of a *grid*, the details of which will be discussed later in this chapter. The grid is a very important item of radiological equipment and is used in the majority of radiographic techniques, especially when the radiological examination involves a large volume of tissue, but even when

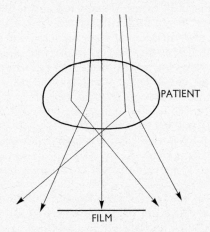

Fig. 171.—An air gap between the patient and the film reduces the amount of scattered radiation which reaches the film.

the volume has been reduced to a minimum, the grid is most effective in preventing a large fraction of the scattered radiation from reaching the film. Some small amount of primary radiation is absorbed by the grid and because of the removal of both this and the scattered radiation, the use of a grid calls for an increased X-ray tube exposure in order to maintain a suitable film density.

The metal backing of the film cassette attenuates the primary radiation transmitted by the film and thus reduces (*a*) the amount of stray radiation in the room and (*b*) the amount of scattered radiation which otherwise would have reached the film from structures beyond it, such as the floor. There is relatively little backscattered radiation from the backing. The amount of scattered radiation generated depends on the scatter coefficient (σ) whilst the fraction of that radiation absorbed in the backing depends on the total attenuation coefficient ($\mu = \sigma + \tau$). Since τ is very large for the lower energy scattered radiation in the high Z material, whilst σ is relatively independent of atomic number, the amount (proportional to $\sigma/\sigma + \tau$) of backscattered radiation reaching the film will be small for the higher Z backing material.

Filters.—The placing of suitable sheets of metal—filters—between the patient and the cassette has been suggested as a suitable means of selectively removing the scattered radiation. This is not usually a practical possibility since the discrimination between primary and secondary is not sufficiently great. However, both salt and lead intensifying screens do filter a little; in fact, below about 200 kV. this is all that a lead screen would do. The use of a filter between the X-ray tube and the patient, whilst very desirable for other reasons, is useless in reducing scatter to the film. Most of the radiation removed by the filter could not penetrate the patient, so clearly it could not produce scattered radiation capable of reaching the film.

A more effective method is to have a large *air gap* between the patient and the film (*Fig.* 171), in which circumstances the obliquely moving scatter will miss the film and so will not impair the contrast. Unless, of course, large focus–film distances are used, such a system results in a magnified, more blurred radiograph which may not be desired. Conversely, if magnification radiography is being carried out from choice, then there is often no need to use a grid and so the increase in tube exposure demanded by a grid is avoided.

Reduction in the Effect of Scattered Radiation on the Film.—There is little that can be done in this respect unless intensifying screens are being used, since the film itself is more or less equally sensitive to both scattered and primary photons. With an intensifying screen, however, the harder, primary photons are 'intensified' more than are the softer, scattered ones. This leads to a reduction in the relative effect of scattered radiation on the film so that the reduction in contrast is not so great when screens are being used. This results, in great part, from the filtration effected by the screens, which was mentioned above, but also from the inherently greater intensification of higher-energy photons (*see Fig.* 125).

In addition, because the γ of a film is greater when screens are used, the final visual contrast on the film is greater than when screens are not used. It is therefore possible to tolerate a little more reduction in contrast by the scattered radiation than would otherwise be the case.

It is for these reasons that intensifying screens are sometimes claimed as being 'able to reduce scattered radiation' or 'not sensitive to scattered radiation'. Whilst not strictly true, these claims do indicate that the objectionable effects of scattered radiation are reduced by the use of screens.

THE GRID

The *scatter grid* (or as it is usually called—the *grid*) is composed of a large number of long parallel *strips* of lead held apart and parallel to each other by an X-ray transparent *interspace* material (*Fig.* 172).

The way in which the grid is able to reduce the amount of scattered radiation reaching the film, whilst still allowing the pattern containing primary beams to reach the film placed immediately below the grid, is illustrated in *Fig.* 173. The scattered radiation will be moving obliquely because of the change in direction which occurs in the scattering process. The majority of this radiation will be unable to pass through to the film since it will be stopped by the lead of the grid. On the other hand, the majority of the primary radiation, which is moving forward, will pass through the interspace and reach the film upon which it will therefore impress the X-ray pattern.

Some scattered radiation will pass through to the film, as can be seen in *Fig.* 174. Scattered radiation produced in the part of the patient shown shaded, and which happens to be moving in the direction of O, is potentially able to reach the film at O.

Similar considerations apply to all other points of the film lying below the inter-spaces. In the absence of the grid there is the possibility of scattered radiation generated at any point in the patient reaching the film, so that clearly the presence of the grid results in a reduction in scatter at the film. Careful measurements have

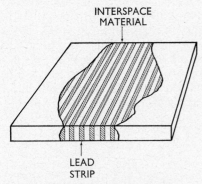

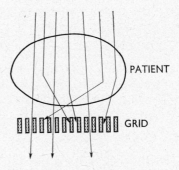

Fig. 172.—A grid, showing the long, thin, parallel lead strips separated by wider interspace material. The whole is enclosed in a metal outer covering.

Fig. 173.—Obliquely moving scattered radiation is stopped by the grid, whilst the forward-moving primary photons pass through to the film.

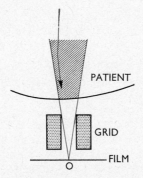

Fig. 174.—Scattered radiation produced within the shaded region of the patient and moving towards O is able to reach O unimpeded by the grid.

shown that a reasonable grid is able to remove as much as 80–90 per cent of the scattered radiation present. The removal of this scatter produces a very worth-while and large increase in the contrast. This improvement is measured by a quantity known as the 'contrast improvement factor' (K), where

$$K = \frac{\text{X-ray contrast with grid}}{\text{X-ray contrast without grid}}.$$

For the grid to be a good one, K should be large. It is found that practical grids have values varying from 1·5 to about 3·5, depending upon the exact construction of the grid and the exposure conditions. These values refer to situations where a reasonable amount of scatter is present since, of course, even an ideal grid cannot produce any contrast improvement if there is not any scatter present to be removed!

For instance, in the radiograph of a hand the amount of scattered radiation present is very small and a grid is not usually used.

Although the grid is able to remove the majority of unwanted scatter quite successfully, it unfortunately also removes some of the useful primary radiation. As can be seen from *Fig.* 175, those primary photons (*a*) which hit the lead strips will be absorbed and only those (*b*) incident on the interspace transmitted to the film. The proportion of primary radiation removed, usually about 10–15 per cent, is determined by the ratio $d/(D + d)$, where d is the thickness of the lead strip and D the separation between the strips (*Fig.* 176). This primary absorption creates on the film an overall pattern of thin parallel white (clear) lines which are in fact the shadows of the lead strips. These are known as *grid lines* and might distract the radiologist's attention from the anatomical detail or even spoil fine detail. It is usually arranged either for this pattern to be of sufficiently fine lines as to be not

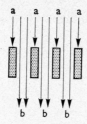

Fig. 175.—A fraction of the forward-moving primary radiation is stopped by the grid.

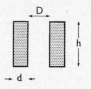

Fig. 176.—The controlling dimensions of a grid are the width (d) of the lead strips, the width (D) of the interspace, and the height (h) of the strips.

noticed or for the lines to be blurred by the use of a *moving* grid. Fortunately, provided the lines are fine and reasonably closely and uniformly spaced over the radiograph, the radiologist very quickly learns not to notice the grid lines and is able to make his diagnosis without distraction.

In the spaces between the lines the film density produced by the primary radiation is exactly the same as it would be in the absence of the grid (for the same X-ray tube exposure). However, the physiological effect in the radiologist's eye is such that he 'sees' the average density existing over a small region of the film. This region includes some of the clear grid lines as well as the blackened region so that the visual effect is of a reduced *average* density. The extent to which this averaging takes place depends upon the visibility of the lines, that is, their width and spacing. If the grid is a 'fine' one the averaging is almost complete; if it is a very coarse one, there may be very little averaging. This is the situation in a stationary grid. With a moving grid, where the grid lines are blurred out, the blackening is completely averaged out. All this means that the removal of some of the primary radiation requires the X-ray tube exposure to be increased if the film density is to be maintained at a satisfactory level.

In the absence of the grid, the scattered radiation which would have been removed by the grid would also contribute to film density so that tube exposure must be further increased on this account. The use of a grid, therefore, makes greater demands on the X-ray equipment and also results in a higher radiation dose to the patient. This increase in exposure is usually achieved by increasing the kV., which sacrifices a little of the extra contrast resulting from the use of the grid but minimizes the increase in patient dose.

The design and use of a grid involve, therefore, a compromise between achieving sufficient reduction in scattered radiation to produce the required contrast improvement without reducing the primary radiation so much that excessive demands are made on the X-ray equipment or an excessive dose given to the patient.

Grid Characteristics.—The construction of the grid is based on such considerations, and, as may be expected, the evaluation of the relative advantages and disadvantages of various grids is extremely complicated. In any case, the properties of scattered radiation present depend upon the exact circumstances of patient and beam size and of the tube kV., so that the optimum choice of grid may well vary with these circumstances.

Some of the relevant characteristics of a grid which have to be taken into account in the design of a grid are illustrated in *Fig.* 176 and discussed below.

The Number of Strips of Lead per cm. (N).—As has already been stated the grid consists of a parallel set of lead strips which cover the whole film. The length of each strip and the total width of the grid can therefore vary between about 20 cm. up to 43 cm. depending upon the film size with which it will be used. The total number of strips of lead in a grid varies from a few hundred up to a thousand or more. The greater the number (*N*) of *strips* (or as they are more usually called—*lines*) per cm. the less will the grid lines on the film be visible to the radiologist. But what is just as important as having a large number of lines per cm. is that this number must be the same over the whole film, and the lines must be straight and parallel. A uniform, yet more coarse pattern (smaller value of *N*) is *less* visible to the radiologist than a fine (larger value of *N*) but non-uniform pattern. The manufacture of a uniform grid with a large number of lines per cm. is very difficult and therefore very costly. The commonly used grids have between 20 and 28 lines per cm. although good grids having as many as 40 lines per cm. are now available.

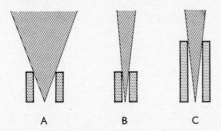

Fig. 177.—Grid A has a smaller ratio than grids B and C which have the same ratio. The volume of the patient from which scattered radiation can reach the film decreases as the grid ratio increases and is the same for grids of the same ratio (B and C).

The Grid Ratio (r).—The grid ratio measures the narrowness of the slit through which the primary radiation passes and also determines the extent to which oblique moving scatter is absorbed. Grid ratio (*r*) is defined by:

$$r = \frac{h}{D},$$

where, as shown in *Fig.* 176, *h* is the height of the lead strips and *D* is their separation or interspace. It can be seen from *Fig.* 177 that a higher ratio leads to a greater restriction in the volume from which scattered radiation can reach the film. From the point of view of restricting scattered radiation, a high ratio is therefore desirable.

Unfortunately, a high ratio means either a large value of h or a small value of D. It is very difficult, however, to manufacture a grid with large values of h, and/or small values of D, since the strips are thin and it is difficult to keep them flat and parallel. The increase in grid ratio also usually leads to an increase in the absorption of useful primary radiation by the grid. For these two reasons it is neither possible nor desirable to use an excessively high grid ratio. The usual values are from about 5 or 8 to about 10 or 12, although in some circumstances (e.g., high-kV. work) some radiologists prefer to use grids having ratios as high as 16.

The Lead Content (p).—The grid ratio has been traditionally regarded as the index of the grid's ability to remove scattered radiation and, as has just been discussed, it is a fact that it is the ratio which determines the fraction of scattered radiation arrested by the grid. There is, however, a further aspect relevant to the efficiency of a grid. Removal of scatter is important but then so is transmission of the primary beam, for it is after all this which contains the pattern of interest. The amount of primary radiation transmitted by a grid is not affected by the ratio *per se*. As described on p. 252, the fraction of primary radiation removed from the beam is determined by $d/(D + d)$. In so far as a small interspace value (D) often accompanies a high ratio, then the absorption of the primary tends to increase with grid ratio.

The selectivity of a grid is defined by:

$$\text{Selectivity} = \frac{\text{Transmitted primary radiation}}{\text{Transmitted scatter radiation}},$$

and obviously an efficient grid should have a high selectivity.

Recent work has shown that the actual lead content per unit area (measured as g. per cm.^{2}) is a determining factor for the efficiency of a grid. A 'heavy' grid, that is, one with a lot of lead per sq. cm., is more efficient than a 'light' one. Values of lead content in commonly used grids range from 0·2 g. per cm.^{2} to 0·9 g. per cm.^{2} Of course the presence of lead in itself is not enough—a plain sheet of lead would be a very poor grid! The lead must be arranged appropriately as a grid.

For two grids of the same ratio, the heavier one will remove the greater amount of scatter while still transmitting the greater amount of primary radiation. In fact, a heavier grid of a lower ratio can be better than a lighter grid of a higher ratio.

Grid Factors.—The 'grid factor' represents the extent to which the X-ray tube exposure must be increased to compensate for the loss of primary and scattered radiation reaching the film. It is expressed as the ratio of the exposure needed to achieve the same film blackening when the grid is used to that needed in the absence of the grid. Typical values of grid factor range between about 2 to about 6, the value depending, of course, on the type of grid used and how much scatter there is to remove.

The Interspace Material.—In order to protect the delicate thin strips of lead and interspace material from the effects of atmospheric conditions, such as humidity, and from mechanical damage, the grid structure is enveloped in a sealed aluminium container. The strips of lead which make up the grid are held apart and parallel by means of a thicker strip of some suitable material (the interspace material), and this separating is the principal function of the interspace material. However, both the interspace material and the outer aluminium container will absorb radiation to some extent. There has been much discussion about the relative merits of various interspace materials. Certainly it is to be expected that some useful filtration of the remaining scattered radiation could be effected by a suitable material in the interspace. However, most of this scatter will be travelling in much the same direction as the primary and will not, therefore, be very much softer. Any filtration effect is likely to be small and it would appear that any difference between the use of, say, aluminium and a plastic as the interspace material is trivially small compared with other factors which determine overall grid efficiency. On balance a plastic is preferred since the increase in exposure which would be required by the use of an aluminium interspace could be better utilized in conjunction with a heavier and higher ratio grid.

The Thickness of the Lead Strips.—It has been assumed so far that any scattered radiation which hits a lead strip is completely absorbed and so prevented from reaching

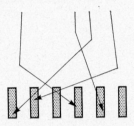

Fig. 178.—The number of lead strips through which obliquely moving scattered radiation has to be transmitted increases with the obliquity of the scatter.

the film. This is true only if the lead is of sufficient thickness (*d*). Fortunately, very obliquely moving scattered photons can encounter several lead strips, as is shown in *Fig.* 178. The extent to which this occurs increases as the grid ratio increases. The individual lead strips can therefore be rather thinner than would otherwise be necessary. The use of thick lead strips will result in coarse grid lines on the film and in a large absorption of the primary radiation. As usual a compromise has to be made between the choice of a strip thickness large enough to reduce the scattered radiation intensity sufficiently and one thin enough not to absorb a large amount of primary and to give the desirable fine lines on the film. The usual thickness employed is 0·005–0·008 cm.

TYPES OF GRID

The Linear Grid.—The grid which has so far been described is known as a linear grid since the strips of lead are strictly parallel to each other. The overall size of the grid may be quite large since it has completely to cover the whole film area. When the effect away from the centre of the beam is considered it is immediately obvious that, as illustrated in *Fig.* 179 A, a difficulty arises. The primary radiation is travelling radially from the X-ray tube focal spot to the film and will therefore encounter the lead strips obliquely. The width of the lines on the film, which are exposed to the primary radiation, will be reduced so as to be now smaller than the interspace thickness (*D*) (*Fig.* 179 B), and therefore the grid lines on the film will be wider and the apparent average density will be reduced. At a sufficiently large distance from the centre of the beam there can be complete cut-off of the primary. It can be seen from *Fig.* 179 C that the distance (*x*) out from the centre at which complete cut-off of the primary beam occurs is given by:

$$\tan \theta = \frac{D}{h} = \frac{x}{\text{F.F.D.}}$$

and hence

$$x = \frac{D}{h} \cdot \text{F.F.D.} = \frac{\text{F.F.D.}}{r}.$$

If the ratio is 10 and the focus–film distance (F.F.D.) is 90 cm. then $x = 9 \cdot 0$ cm. The maximum film width which can be used is therefore much less than 18 cm. With a 5 ratio grid the cut-off will occur at just over 18 cm. and for a 15 ratio grid at just over 5 cm. from the centre! With a linear grid, therefore, the average film density will fall progressively from centre to edge of film. The distance out from the centre at which noticeable reduction in density occurs will become smaller as the grid ratio is increased and as the F.F.D. is reduced. This means that a high ratio grid may be used only with small films or with large F.F.D.s.

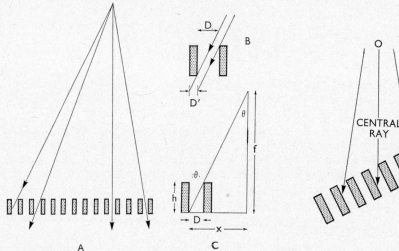

Fig. 179.—The decrease of effective interspace and the eventual 'cut-off' towards the edge of a uniform grid.

Fig. 180.—The cut-off of primary radiation due to the grid not being normal to the central ray.

Cut-off of the beam can occur even in the centre of the film if the grid is not exactly perpendicular to the beam central axis (*Fig.* 180). Again the magnitude of the effect is greater with the higher ratio grid which therefore demands great care in setting up. Cut-off occurs when the angulation error is only 6° in the case of a grid of ratio 10, whereas for a grid ratio of 5 the error can be 26°! These comments apply only to angulation across the grid strips. In the direction parallel to the strips there is no cut-off, neither towards the edge of the film nor with angulation of the beam. It is therefore of practical importance that, when a grid is in use, any angulation of the beam central axis should be only in a plane parallel with the grid lines and never across the grid. Such considerations arise in tomography and in angled views. A further practical point is that in those circumstances where the setting up of the grid and film perpendicular to the X-ray beam central axis is difficult, such as may occur in a theatre or a ward, the use of a high-ratio grid is to be avoided if possible.

The Focused Grid.—The difficulty of primary cut-off away from the beam centre can be avoided by the use of a focused grid. Here the strips of lead are angled progressively from centre to edge (*Fig.* 181) so that the interspaces point at the focal spot. There is now no reduction in the primary towards the edge. The comments made previously about the use of angled views still apply, with the additional limitation that the F.F.D. used must be that for which the grid was designed. The use of

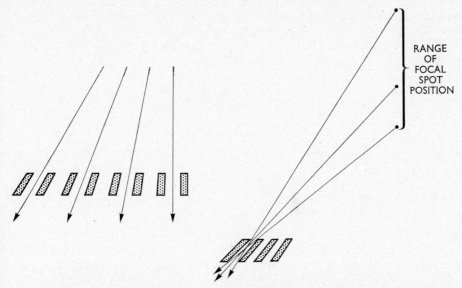

Fig. 181.—The principle of a focused grid.

Fig. 182.—A focused grid designed for use at a particular F.F.D. can be used over a limited but acceptably large range of F.F.D.s.

smaller or larger F.F.D.s will lead to a reduction in film density away from the film centre (*Fig.* 182). There is, fortunately, a range of F.F.D.s over which the grid can be used which, just as with angulation, is more restricted for grids of higher ratio, smaller focusing distance, and large beams. For instance, a grid of ratio 12, designed for use at a focusing distance of 60 cm., may be used for F.F.D.s in the range 55–65 cm., whereas one of ratio 6 designed for use at 120 cm. may be used over the range 75–200 cm. without noticeable decrease in density towards the edge. It should be noted that whenever a grid is used at a distance other than the focusing distance for which it is designed, then some reduction in film density away from the centre will always occur and this reduction will be greater as the grid ratio and beam size are increased and as the focusing distance is decreased. At the limit of the range quoted above there is a 50 per cent reduction in intensity 15 cm. from the beam centre.

A further limitation in the use of the focused grid is that the central X-ray must pass through the grid centre. Again there is some latitude and in the range already quoted the possibility of a 1-cm. miscentring has been included. It is, of course, of paramount importance to have the correct face of the focused grid towards the X-ray tube. If it is reversed the edge cut-off is far greater than for the unfocused grid.

Setting up of the patient, film, and grid for radiography has to be done more carefully and correctly from the point of view of F.F.D., angulation, and centring

9

when a high-ratio grid is used. Therefore it is making the execution of the technique unnecessarily critical to use a grid of higher ratio than the amount of scattered radiation present demands.

Pseudo-focused Grid.—The manufacture of a focused grid is extremely difficult and, as previously stated, failure to achieve a uniform grid pattern may seriously mar the visual appearance and usefulness of a radiograph. Some manufacturers prefer to concentrate on producing a perfectly uniform linear grid and to eliminate the extra reduction of primary radiation away from the centre of the beam in another way. This is by reducing the height of the strips progressively, as shown in *Fig.* 183, resulting in a reduction in grid ratio from centre to edge but, in spite of this, the over-all efficacy of such a grid is sometimes preferred.

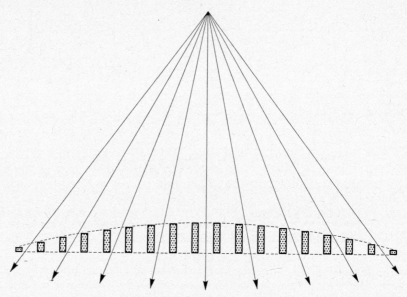

Fig. 183.—A pseudo-focused grid.

The Crossed Grid.—It has so far been assumed that all scattered radiation which is moving sufficiently obliquely is cut out by the grid. This is certainly so when the direction across the grid lines is considered. In the direction parallel to the lines, however, the scattered radiation is not impeded at all by the grid except for the very minor absorption in the interspace material. The amount of obliquely moving scattered radiation which is moving in planes sufficiently parallel to the grid lines to be transmitted by the grid is quite small and can usually be tolerated. If it cannot be tolerated, then two grids of the type already described, placed on top of each other and mutually at right-angles, may be used. Such a combination of grids is very efficient at removing scattered radiation. In fact, in those circumstances where a high grid ratio is needed, it is often better to use a crossed grid of smaller ratio. For instance, two crossed grids, each of ratio 7, can be better than a single grid of ratio 15.

When using crossed grids, the central axis of the X-ray beam must be perpendicular to the grids, as no large amount of angulation in any direction is permissible.

THE MOVING GRID

One of the disadvantages of using a grid is that a pattern of clear (white) lines is cast on to the film. This pattern of grid lines can be distracting to the radiologist, especially if the lines are thick and widely spaced (i.e., d large and N small). One solution to this problem is to move the grid sideways across the film during the exposure. The shadows of the grid strips are blurred out and are, therefore, not visible. Of course there is just as much reduction in scattered and primary radiation reaching the film, so that such a moving grid produces the same increase in contrast and demands the same increase in exposure as does an identical stationary grid. The only difference is that the grid lines have disappeared.

For the lines to be effectively blurred the grid must move a distance equal to at least 3 or 4 interspaces during the time of the exposure. If the grid speed is not sufficiently great then random variations in density are produced across the film due to the incomplete blurring out of the lines. The required minimum speed of movement is therefore determined by the exposure time and by the number of grid lines per inch. If the exposure is short or the number of lines per cm. small, then the speed must be high. For example, a grid having 12 lines per cm. must move at least $3 \times \frac{1}{12}$ cm. $= 0.25$ cm. during the exposure. If this is 0·04 sec. then the minimum grid speed is $0.25/0.04 = 6.25$ cm. per sec. If the exposure time is decreased to 0·004 sec. then the grid speed would have to be 62·5 cm. per sec. The use of a grid having 24 lines per cm. would demand speeds only half as great.

These speeds are quite high and it is important that they should be achieved without any movement being communicated to the film cassette or patient. If any movement is transmitted, then unnecessary and unwanted movement unsharpness will be produced.

Since the grid lines are blurred out there is not the same necessity of having a large number of lines per inch in the moving grid as there is for the stationary one. On the other hand, a small number of lines per inch necessitates a high-speed grid unless very long exposure times are being used. The amount of movement is usually about 1·25 cm. either side of the central position and this is an acceptable amount of off-centring provided the focusing distance is not too small and the grid ratio not too high. A good average installation would have a grid movement and grid with the characteristics in the range:

Ratio: 8–10.
Focusing distance: 90 cm.
Movement: 0·6–1·2 cm. either side of centre.
Lines per cm: 30–24.

The 'Stroboscopic' Effect.—There is another difficulty which can arise when grids are used in conjunction with X-ray equipment having 2- or 4-valve half- or full-wave rectification circuits. In such equipment the majority of the effective X-rays are emitted in the form of pulses of about 0·003 sec. duration at a frequency of either 50 (half-wave) or 100 (full-wave) cycles per second (*Fig.* 184). If it should happen that the grid moves a distance equal to exactly 1, 2, 3, etc., spaces in $\frac{1}{50}$ or $\frac{1}{100}$ sec. then the shadows of the grid strips will exactly overlie each other and the grid-line pattern will not be removed and the moving grid will appear to be stationary. This is called a 'stroboscopic effect'.

A similar type of explanation accounts for the spoked wheels of a wagon appearing stationary in some TV films. This occurs when the speed of rotation of the wheels is in synchronism with the frame speed of the film. In the X-ray case it arises if there is any synchronism between the grid movement and the X-ray emission. Partial or complete synchronism can thus result in the production of a pattern of density variation on the film, caused by the grid and not by the patient. It is clearly an effect to be avoided by suitable design of the grid-moving mechanism. This is the reason why such things as spring and oil dash-pots tend to be used in these mechanisms in preference to electrically driven motors, which, because they use the same (50 c.p.s.) electrical mains, could easily result in a synchronous grid movement. Of course, motors can be used but provision must be made to avoid any synchronism.

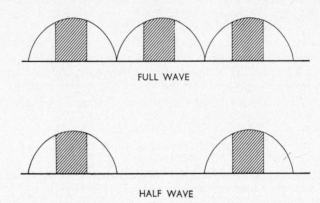

FULL WAVE

HALF WAVE

Fig. 184.—The majority of X-radiation which reaches the film is produced during the central period (shown shaded) of each pulse.

Since the introduction of the moving grid in 1920 by Dr. Potter* many different designs of moving mechanism have been suggested and used. The essential features of the mechanism are that the grid shall move fast enough for a sufficient distance without imparting any movement to either the patient or film and without there being any stroboscopic effect. The main types of movement employed are described briefly below.

Single Stroke.—In this type of mechanism a spring is used to pull the grid, at a uniform speed, across the film. The speed of the movement is controlled by an adjustable oil dash-pot. The overall movement is about 2·5 cm. (i.e., 1·25 cm. either side of centre) and the time which the grid takes to cover this distance can be adjusted from about 0·2 to 15 sec. With this type of mechanism it is therefore necessary before an exposure is made to 'cock' the grid spring and also to select a suitable movement time. This time is selected to be just a little larger than the exposure time so as to ensure that the grid continues to move throughout the whole of the exposure, and at a sufficiently high speed. When the 'exposure' button is pressed the grid is released and as soon as it is moving a subsidiary contact activates the main 'exposure' contactor and the exposure commences. Provided the 'grid time' has been correctly chosen, the grid will come to rest a short time after the X-ray exposure has been terminated by the X-ray timer.

---

* Although the moving grid system is often referred to as a 'Bucky' it was, in fact, Potter who first suggested the use of a *moving* grid. Bucky was responsible in 1913 for first suggesting the use of a grid which at that time was composed of comparatively thick lead strips. Subsequently the use of the stationary grid was revived by Lysholm who showed how the number of lines per inch could be increased and the lead thickness decreased.

One of the disadvantages of the single-stroke mechanism is that it has to be set manually before each exposure. This defect can be overcome by arranging for the grid to move at a variable speed during the exposure. In the so-called catapult system this is achieved by having the speed controlled by a motor-driven cam. The way in which the speed varies throughout the exposure time is shown in *Fig.* 185. Initially the grid moves very quickly (after a short time in which it is speeded up) and then slows down progressively. The total time taken for the grid to move across the film is large, 8–15 sec. The mechanism is fitted with a contact so that the exposure always starts at the instant S; the time at which the exposure terminates is controlled by the timer and may be any time after S, say at E_1 for a short exposure, or E_2 for a longer one. If the exposure is short (S–E_1) then the grid is moving at the

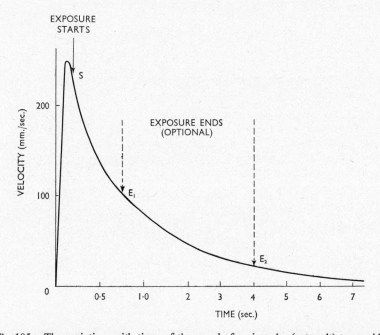

Fig. 185.—The variation, with time, of the speed of an impulse (catapult) type grid.

appropriate high speed. On the other hand, if the exposure is long (S–E_2), the high speed is not essential (but not detrimental) and the lower speed tail of the curve is utilized. With this type of mechanism no setting, on the occasion of each exposure, is required: the grid is always ready for use. If the exposure is very long indeed then the pattern can be repeated although this is fairly uncommon.

Oscillating and Reciprocating Movements.—Here the necessity of resetting the grid and adjusting the speed of movement for each different exposure is avoided by arranging for the grid always to be moving at a sufficiently high speed. The grid moves to and fro across the film repeatedly during the exposure time. As with the single-stroke grid the total movement is about 1·25 cm. either side of the centre. If the exposure time is very short then it takes place during part of one movement cycle of the grid, whereas for longer exposures several cycles are utilized. At the extreme of each cycle the grid is stationary for a very small time, but this is so small that no grid-line pattern is produced on the film. The main difference between the oscillating and reciprocating grid movement lies in the actual patterns of their speed. These are shown in *Fig.* 186. As is implied by its name, the oscillating grid has a pattern which is approximately sinusoidal. The time for one complete swing is usually about 0·5 sec. During each cycle the speed rises to a maximum in one direction and then falls slowly until it comes to rest, at which point the pattern is repeated with the grid moving now in the opposite direction. This movement can be achieved by simply mounting the grid on four leaf springs, one at each corner. When the exposure button is

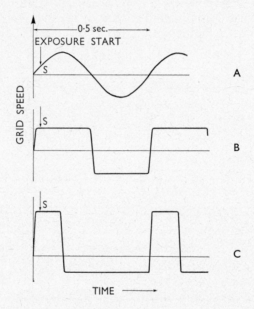

Fig. 186.—The variation, with time, of the speed for three types of moving grid. **A,** The harmonically oscillating grid. **B,** The reciprocating grid in which the forward and reverse movements are identical. **C,** The reciprocating grid in which the forward stroke is relatively fast and the reverse stroke relatively slow.

pressed the grid is pulled to one side by an electromagnet and then released. As soon as it is released the exposure is started and continues for a time determined, as usual, by the timer. During the whole of this time the grid continues to oscillate with a gradually diminishing speed and amplitude (i.e., the movement is damped) until finally it comes to rest—but after quite a long time and several seconds after the exposure has finished.

The reciprocating grid movement, whilst still a repeated to-and-fro one, is a driven one rather than a free oscillation. The movement may be a simple sinusoidal one, as in the case of the oscillating grid, but not now, of course, a damped oscillation. Such a movement can be achieved by using a simple motor. However, because the movement is a driven one, it is possible to modify the speed pattern to that shown in *Fig.* 186 B. The grid is accelerated to its maximum speed very quickly and this speed maintained throughout the forward movement. After reversal the same pattern is repeated, but in the opposite direction. The whole cycle of events continues for as long as the exposure time demands. In most reciprocating movements the time (and speed) of the forward stroke is different from the time (and speed) of the return stroke (*Fig.* 186 C). This arises because in most mechanisms the grid is pushed over quite quickly and then allowed to return more slowly, the speed of the movement being under the control of an oil dash-pot.

At the present time all these various types of movement (and some others which are modifications and combinations of these basic movements) are in use. The choice of the best movement is to a certain extent a personal one and the degree of preference is often dependent on both manufacturer and installation, as well as the use to which it is to be put. The important point to which attention must be given is that the grid shall move fast enough during the exposure time, and that it shall do this without any synchronism and without imparting any movement to the patient or film. For a great proportion of cases the simple types of mechanism, although not mechanically perfect, have much to commend them from the practical point of view.

Although successful blurring out of the grid lines can be achieved it is worth while remembering that since good stationary grids, having fine lines and a large number of lines per inch, are now available, the need for movement of the grid is reduced. The almost invisible and certainly unnoticed pattern of grid lines produced by such grids makes it hardly worth while risking the difficulties and expense associated with the movement mechanism.

The moving grid suffers from a further disadvantage. This is that a space of about 5 cm. is required between the patient and the film in order to accommodate the movement. This extra distance brings about an unwanted increase in magnification and in movement and geometric unsharpness. The stationary grid is usually only about 6 mm. thick and can be brought into close contact with the patient and film.

CHAPTER XXI

THE RADIOGRAPHIC EXPOSURE

CLEARLY, the radiologist can make his diagnosis only in so far as he can 'see' the shadows cast by the various structures of the patient which are relevant to the diagnosis. It is therefore quite essential that these shadows shall produce, on the radiograph, patterns which are sufficiently sharp, are of densities sufficiently different from

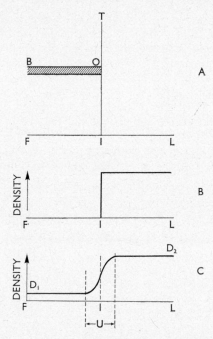

Fig. 187.—The objective contrast and unsharpness at the edge of the shadow of an object.

those of the immediately surrounding film for them to be seen, and which have an acceptable overall density range. The extent to which this is possible will depend upon:

1. The character of the structure in the patient.
2. The 'exposure factors' (i.e., kV., mA.s., type of film, etc.).
3. The conditions under which the radiograph is viewed.

In previous chapters, the factors which determine the pattern and nature of contrasts in the transmitted beam and, consequently on the film, have been described. In this chapter the physical aspects involved in the selection of the exposure factors and viewing conditions appropriate to the particular structures under investigation will be discussed.

Image Contrast and Sharpness.—Let us consider the very simple situation illustrated in *Fig.* 187 A where there is a point source of X-rays (*T*), a completely X-ray opaque and stationary object (*BO*), and a film (*FIL*). In such a circumstance the shadow will have a perfectly sharp edge and there will be a high contrast on the film. This arises because X-rays are not able to penetrate the object (*BO*) and so reach the region of the film *FI*, whereas the full amount of X-rays is able to reach the region of the film *IL*. At *I* there is a perfectly sharp boundary between the two regions. If the film density along the line *FIL* is measured and plotted on a graph the result shown in *Fig.* 187 B will be obtained. In practice, of course, no such ideal situation is encountered and the usual pattern of density in the region of the edge of the shadow is more like that shown in *Fig.* 187 C. There is some radiation transmitted by the object, resulting in the density D_1, and the sharp transition at the point *I* is replaced by a mere gradual one extending over a certain distance, *U*. The contrast, $C = D_2 - D_1$ is called the *objective contrast* since it is this which is measured by an (objective) instrument. The distance over which the transition from D_1 to D_2 occurs is called the *objective sharpness* (*U*).

Interdependence of Contrast and Sharpness.—At the edge of each shadow on the radiograph there is an objective contrast and an objective sharpness and these are quite distinct and separate things which are completely independent of each other. When viewed by the radiologist, however, their appearance can be quite different from the objective facts. The contrast appears to depend upon the unsharpness and vice versa. We therefore refer to the *subjective contrast* and the *subjective sharpness* as being the apparent contrast and sharpness as seen by the eye. It turns out that

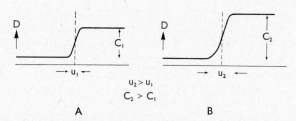

Fig. 188.—Different combinations of objective sharpness and contrast can produce similar subjective appearances.

if the contrast is high then the edge of the shadow appears to be sharper than it really is and when the shadow is sharp (small unsharpness) then the contrast appears greater than it really is, and vice versa, in each case. Hence the inherently unsharp image may be visually acceptable if the contrast is high enough, or a structure which produces little contrast may be perfectly visible provided its shadow is sharp. This idea is illustrated in *Fig.* 188 where the density in the vicinity of the edge of the shadow is plotted. In *Fig.* 188 A the contrast is low but the unsharpness small whereas in *Fig.* 188 B the contrast is greater but so is the unsharpness. The observed contrast and sharpness can, however, appear very similar in these two cases.

There is a certain visual interplay between sharpness and contrast and to a limited extent the one can be used to compensate for deficiencies in the other. The amount of the interplay depends upon the size of the image detail at which the radiologist is looking and upon the conditions under which he is looking. If the size is large compared with the unsharpness then there is very little interplay and the subjective appearance is very similar to the objective facts. On the other hand, if the detail and the unsharpness are of comparable size then there can be considerable inter-dependence of contrast and sharpness. As a necessary prerequisite for the discussion of the selection of the exposure factors which follows, the three important aspects of the successful radiograph, viz., the sharpness, the contrast, and the viewing conditions, are each to be considered in turn.

The Causes of Unsharpness.—The several causes of unsharpness (or blurring as it is often called) have been discussed in earlier chapters and it is sufficient to recall that they are:

1. *Geometric Unsharpness, U_g* (p. 218).—The magnitude of geometric unsharpness is minimized by having a small focal spot size and/or a small value for the ratio object–film distance/focus–film distance.

2. *Movement Unsharpness, U_m* (p. 221).—The prime factor controlling the movement unsharpness is, of course, the actual movement of the structure which occurs during the exposure. It is minimized by having a small value for the ratio object–film distance/focus–film distance and by choosing a small exposure time. What is meant by a small exposure time depends upon the amount of movement which is likely to occur. For extremities which can easily be immobilized the time can be long (even a few seconds), whereas for the radiography of internal structures which are subject to involuntary movement, which cannot be immobilized, the time must be appropriately short.

3. *Screen Unsharpness, U_s* (p. 201).—For a given type of screen this blurring is constant, but it varies from type to type. Very fast screens have unsharpness values of about 0·3 mm., whereas so-called high-definition screens will have values of half this. These values of screen blurring, which are independent of other conditions, are, of course, dependent upon having a good contact between film and screen. For screens which are being misused the value can be considerably in excess of these values quoted. The blurring of the type of screen encountered in fluoroscopy is in the region of 0·5 mm. or even more.

    Although geometric, movement, and screen blurrings are the ones of principal importance, there are in fact two other sources of unsharpness which should be mentioned.

4. *Parallax Unsharpness, U_p.*—Parallax blurring is rather different from the blurring already described. It arises only with doubly coated film and is caused by the fact that the observer is really looking at two patterns rather than at a single one.

    Since the two images are separated from each other by the thickness of the film base, it is never possible to look 'straight on' to both images simultaneously. The result is that the edges of the shadow do not properly overlie each other and unsharpness results.

    For the dry film the magnitude of the effect is negligibly small. For a wet film, however, when the separation of the two images is considerably increased by the expansion of the gelatin, the unsharpness can be noticeable. It is for this reason that the detail observable in a dry radiograph is greater than that on a wet one. For some of the newer, thinner emulsions which in addition do not expand much during processing, this effect is considerably reduced.

5. *Film Unsharpness, U_f.*—X-rays and visible light photons entering the film can be scattered so that their effects are spread over a small region. This also leads to unsharpness but to an extent which, in radiology, is completely negligible.

Inherent Unsharpness.—In this discussion of unsharpness it has been assumed that unsharpness arises because of various defects in the system being used to make the radiograph, and that the object at which we are looking has a perfectly sharp edge. In other words, we assume that if movement, geometric, and screen blurrings were all absent then the image on the radiograph would be perfectly sharp. To a certain extent this is so, but in addition it must be remembered that the patient is not composed of objects of uniform thickness with nice sharp edges. Almost all anatomical structures have a rounded edge so that, even in the complete absence of unsharpness, we would expect that the density pattern in the vicinity of the edge of such a structure will be like that shown in *Fig.* 189 A rather than that for the ideal structure shown in *Fig.* 189 B.

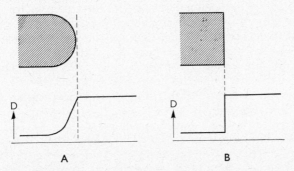

Fig. 189.—Inherent unsharpness. The varying transmission at the edge of a rounded object produces a density pattern similar to, but different from, true unsharpness.

This pattern arises since the radiation passes through varying thicknesses of material and is therefore attenuated less and less as the edge is approached. To the unsharpness arising from defects in the system must therefore be added this extra one which, for want of a better name, has been called 'inherent unsharpness'. In truth, although it has the appearance of unsharpness, it is not unsharpness at all but a varying contrast. However, in view of the visual interplay between contrast and unsharpness previously referred to, the distinction is of academic interest only.

Combined Unsharpness.—In any radiograph most, or all, of these types of unsharpness are present simultaneously. The question now is, What is their combined effect? Fortunately, it is not as bad as might be imagined. The various unsharpnesses overlap each other so that the total unsharpness is bigger than the biggest single unsharpness but smaller than the sum of the separate values. Why this should be so can be illustrated as follows. Imagine that an attempt is being made to drop three pieces of sheet metal on to a spot on the floor and assume that the experimenter is fairly skilful! Each of the three different sheets is intended to represent the size of one of the unsharpnesses. After they have been dropped the three pieces will not exactly overlie each other nor will they lie side by side. They will lie somewhere between these two extremes. The area of the floor covered will be greater than the area of the largest sheet (but not much greater, if the largest sheet is much larger than the other two) but less than their added area. So it is with unsharpness.

The mathematics involved in assessing total unsharpness is very complicated but a good empiric approximation is given by:

$$\text{Total unsharpness, } U = \sqrt[3]{(U_g{}^3 + U_m{}^3 + U_s{}^3)},$$

where U_g, U_m, and U_s are the geometric, movement, and screen unsharpnesses respectively, it being assumed, as is the case in practice, that the other unsharpnesses are negligibly small.

Clearly the total unsharpness is small if the separate unsharpnesses are also small. Since it is desirable that the total unsharpness shall be sufficiently small that it does not impair perception of detail it is imperative to make the separate unsharpnesses as small as possible. This is done by choosing appropriate exposure factors and the basis of this choice is discussed later in this chapter. Unfortunately, the different types of unsharpness are not independent of each other because any attempt to decrease one of them tends to produce an increase in one or more of the others. For example, if geometric unsharpness is decreased by increasing the focus–film distance then, in order to compensate for the accompanying reduction in radiation intensity at the film, the exposure time may have to be increased. This would lead to an increase in movement unsharpness. Alternatively, faster screens could have been used, which would lead to an increase in screen unsharpness. Nevertheless, the increase in movement or screen unsharpness in our example may well be less than the decrease in geometric unsharpness which occasioned it so that the total unsharpness will be reduced.

Now it can be shown that if minimum possible total unsharpness is achieved then the separate unsharpnesses are equal to each other. If any unsharpness is significantly greater than the others then it is theoretically possible to select other exposure conditions (kV., time, F.F.D., focal spot size, screen, etc.) which will lead to a reduction in the total unsharpness. Likewise it is not worth while trying to make the other unsharpnesses significantly smaller than the inherent unsharpness, over which the radiographer has no control.

The exact value of minimum unsharpness is, of course, dependent upon the radiological examination being undertaken. It is not always essential to achieve the ideal state of affairs of minimum unsharpness since even if the unsharpness is greater than the minimum possible value the eye may not be able to detect any difference. Furthermore, it may not even be desirable, since the factors which control unsharpness also have effects on contrast which may be made less acceptable. As always, a compromise must be made and in this case it is between unsharpness and contrast.

Factors affecting Contrast.—Although the factors which control contrast have also been discussed in earlier chapters it is useful to summarize them here. There are three broad groups of relevant factors.

1. *The Patient.*—The atomic number, density, and thickness of the structure creating the contrast are the prime factors which determine the contrast. All the other factors must be chosen, appropriate to each circumstance, so as to render the structure of interest visible on the radiograph as a contrast.

2. *The Radiation.*—The quality of the primary radiation (as determined by the kV. and filtration employed) is the variable which the radiographer has at her disposal in her attempt to achieve the contrast required.

The presence of scattered radiation has a marked effect on contrast. The amount of scattered radiation effective at the film is determined principally by the kV., the volume of tissue radiated (beam size, patient thickness), and the nature of any grid present.

3. *The Recording Medium.*—The type of film, screen, and processing used determines the film contrast and hence have their effect on radiographic contrast. The actual exposure used (kV., mA.s.) also has its effect since the amount of radiation reaching the film determines the region of the characteristic curve in use. The exposure factors are usually so selected that the straight-line portion (region of maximum contrast = gamma) is used.

Viewing the Radiograph.—The subjective appearance of the radiograph brought about by the interplay between objective contrast and unsharpness depends on the viewing conditions. In particular, the appreciation of contrast is very much affected by these conditions, the important features of which are:

1. It is important to use a viewing screen which is *uniformly* illuminated over its whole surface with light of an acceptable *colour*. This is easily achieved nowadays by means of fluorescent tubes which emit a blue-white light. The blue tint of the film base is a hangover from the days when ordinary incandescent lights were used, the blue of the film base complementing the reddish light from the filament lamps. It is conjectural whether it is still necessary to have blue-base film—but in so far as it is subjectively acceptable perhaps it had better be retained.

2. The viewing light must be of a suitable *intensity*. This arises because the eye functions best over quite a small range of light intensities. If the light is either too bright or too dim then the eye is not able to see small contrasts, even though they exist (objectively) on the radiograph. An example of this is when a portion of a radiograph is grossly overexposed and appears very black and no contrast pattern is visible. Even so, the latitude (i.e., straight-line portion) of the film may be such that the objective contrast on the radiograph is just as great as if the film had received a smaller exposure needed to produce an acceptable density.

This is illustrated in *Fig.* 190 where two examples of the same, 10 : 1, range of exposure (viz., 1 to 10 and 100 to 1000) are shown to produce the same contrast (viz., $1.5 - 0.5 = 1$ and $4 - 3 = 1$). On the usual viewing screen contrasts in the density range $0.5-1.5$ will be visible whereas those in the range 3–4 will not. The remedy is to increase the intensity of the viewing illumination so as to bring the level of light intensity transmitted by the density range 3–4 into the range acceptable to the eye. When this is done then the contrasts will become visible. It is for this reason that most radiologists insist on having a viewing screen whose intensity can be varied over a wide range or, at least, a small supplementary high-intensity light with which to view any small areas of the radiograph which are of high density.

At the other end of the scale, not only are the underexposed parts of the radiograph likely to be lacking in objective contrast because of the curvature of the characteristic curve, but even this reduced contrast may well not be fully appreciated if the level of light intensity is too bright. A little help can be obtained by dimming the light somewhat but, of course, nothing can change the low level of objective contrast: the only real remedy is a fresh, more heavily exposed radiograph.

3. The level of light intensity in the regions surrounding the area of the film of immediate interest is also very important. For instance, when viewing a radiograph of the chest the high level of light transmitted by the mediastinal region of the film can obscure lung detail. If these brighter portions of the radiograph are covered over then the detail in the denser region will become more apparent. This effect is most marked,

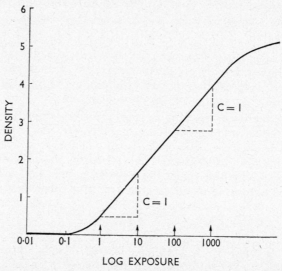

Fig. 190.—Subjective contrast. Although having the same objective contrast, identical relative exposures can produce different apparent contrasts depending upon the general level of density.

of course, when a radiograph consists of areas of both high and low density but it always exists to some extent. It also exists in large measure when the film size is smaller than the viewing screen: the glare from the surrounding edge often completely masking detail which would otherwise very easily be seen.

The remedy is to mask off these brighter areas and it is therefore important to have blinds fitted to the viewing screen which enable this to be done. Alternatively, a series of opaque masks with various viewing apertures can be used.

In a smaller way the level of light intensity in the room is also important. It may not be necessary to have a completely blacked-out room, but a rather low light level and a complete absence of local bright sources of light such as reading lamps or shafts of sunlight are conducive to contrast appreciation.

4. In addition to these external factors the ability of the radiologist to see small contrasts depends upon the techniques of viewing. This will, of course, vary from radiologist to radiologist, each will find his own best method. There are, however, some common features. Absence of visual fatigue is important and the apparent extravagance of a pleasant, well-ventilated, and comfortable (but not too!) room is more than justified.

The screening off of all but the small areas of immediate interest has already been mentioned and this should be coupled with the adoption of different viewpoints. These comprise using a scanning technique, i.e., not keeping the eyes fixed on one spot; standing back to see objects of rather low contrast which are not too sharp and using a magnifying glass to see small, high-contrast detail.

Patient Dose.—In addition to radiographic density, sharpness, and contrast, there is another item which must be remembered when selecting exposure factors. This is the radiation dose given, of necessity, to the patient. As far as possible, this dose must be kept low so as to minimize any possible harm to the patient and it is the professional responsibility of the radiographer to ensure this. On the other hand, it must be stressed that for most radiographic examinations the likelihood of benefit to the patient resulting from a high-class radiograph is very, very much greater than the likelihood of significant damage being done to the patient. In fact the patient may suffer more harm (because of incomplete or inadequate diagnosis, and need to repeat the radiographic exposure) from a poor film than he is ever likely to suffer from the Exposure associated with a good radiograph. It is not possible to make a good radiograph without the use of radiations even though some workers seem to be attempting and recommending it!

In general, patient dose is reduced when higher kV. larger focus–film distances, smaller beam sizes, faster films, and faster screens are used. The use of a grid always leads to an increase in the patient dose, but when the grid is needed this must be accepted for without the grid the radiograph may well be almost useless. The use of a filter between the tube and patient always reduces the patient dose.

For most diagnostic X-ray apparatus the Exposure (mR) at the surface of the patient towards the X-ray tube can be calculated to a reasonable approximation by the formula:

$$\text{Exposure} = P \times \frac{\text{kV.}^2 \times \text{mA.s.}}{D^2} \text{ milliroentgen,}$$

where D is the focus–skin distance in cm.; kV. is the kilovoltage applied to the tube; and mA.s. is the milliampere-seconds used.

P is a factor equal to about 15. Its exact value depends upon the voltage waveform, the filtration, and beam size used. It is usually in the range 10–30 and is unlikely to be outside the range 5–50. For example, an exposure of 5 mA.s. at 80 kV. will produce an Exposure on the skin of the patient 100 cm. distant from the target of:

$$15 \times \frac{80^2 \times 5}{100^2} = 48 \text{ milliroentgens.}$$

Practical Aspects of Radiographic Exposure.—The ideal radiograph is thus one which has the desired range of densities, the desired contrast, and maximum sharpness. What is meant by 'desired' will, of course, vary from radiologist to radiologist and from circumstance to circumstance. Nevertheless, there is, for each particular radiographic exposure, an optimum set of exposure factors which will result in a radiograph from which the particular radiologist concerned is most likely easily and successfully to make his diagnosis. It is the prime task of the radiographer to select his techniques in such a way that this radiograph is achieved. The various variable factors which are at his disposal are set out in the first column of *Table XXIII*. This table summarizes facts which have been discussed in detail in earlier chapters and shows which of the items of interest on the radiograph (viz., sharpness,

Table XXIII.—FACTORS AFFECTING THE RADIOGRAPH

	Unsharpness			Contrast	Density	Patient Dose	Magnification
	Geometric	Movement	Screen				
Kilovoltage Wave form Filter				+	+	+	
Milliamperes Time (sec.)		+			+ +	+ +	
F.F.D. O.F.D. Focal spot size	+ + +	+ +			+	+	+ +
Grid Beam size				+ +*	+ +*	+*	
Film type Screen type Processing			+	+ + +	+ + +		
Patient	+	+			+	+	+

* Because of scatter.

contrast, etc.) are affected by the various exposure factors. Where there is a cross then there is an effect (for example, focus–film distance affects geometric and movement unsharpness and also film density). Where there is no cross then there is no effect (for example, neither focus–film distance nor focal spot size has any direct effect on contrast). Of course, in so far as a change in the value of one factor may necessitate the change in value of another factor there are endless possibilities for indirect effects. (For example, although focal spot size has no direct effect on movement blurring, if the use of a smaller focal spot necessitates the use of a longer exposure time, as it probably will, then, since this will increase movement blurring, so *indirectly* the focal spot size influences movement blurring.)

Although it is not really an exposure factor, chemical processing is included in the table since its detailed effects must be known and borne in mind when selecting the other exposure factors. In the same way the patient, being the fundamental cause of the radiographic pattern, is included in the table.

Selection of Exposure Factors.—Since each exposure factor affects more than one aspect of the radiograph and since each aspect is affected by more than one exposure factor, the situation is rather complex and the selection of the optimum set of exposure factors is far from simple. Any change in exposure factor that is made in order to modify one radiographic aspect will simultaneously change some other radiographic aspect, which will therefore necessitate a change in one or more of the other exposure factors in order to preserve the latter aspect. For example, a change in kV. made to change the contrast will also affect the film density which may be restored to its original value by, say, a change either in mA. or exposure time or both.

Fortunately few modern radiographers have to start from scratch since the same or, at least, a similar type of examination and X-ray unit will have been used before and hence the appropriate factors already known. It is not without interest, however, to consider, in fairly general terms, how the optimum factors may be selected.

Processing.—Nowadays the chemical processing is hardly a factor of choice since it is quite likely that it will be done automatically or at least will be standardized. The processing will, however, have been originally arranged to be appropriate to the type of film used and the radiographic result required by the radiologist. As already mentioned, the details of the processing used will affect the values of the other factors selected.

Films and Screens.—Similarly with films and screens the choice is limited since it would be most inadvisable, if only from the point of view of avoiding confusion, to have more than one or two types of each available in any one department. Again the original choice will have been made in such a way as to produce a radiograph of acceptable characteristics. Usually a fairly fast film and screen combination is used since this will minimize patient dose, as well as geometric and movement unsharpnesses. In some circumstances the associated screen unsharpness will be unacceptably high so that slower screens may be used. These, although reducing screen unsharpness, will probably lead to an increase in the other unsharpnesses, but the total unsharpness will almost certainly be improved in these circumstances.

If extreme detail is required a non-screen film may be used, provided that the mA.s. can be sufficiently small that movement or geometric unsharpness is not too great. The most common circumstance in which this arises is in the radiography of bony extremities.

Beam Size.—The beam size must be large enough to include all the region of the patient of interest but it should be kept as small as possible consistent with this, in order to minimize both the dose to the patient and the production of scattered radiation.

Grid.—A grid must be used whenever there would be a significant reduction of contrast due to excessive scattered radiation. This arises mainly when large volumes are being irradiated or when high kV. is used. The use of a grid and/or the reduction in beam size will also decrease the blackening on the film and may therefore necessitate an increase of mA.s.

Focus–film and Object–film Distance.—The focus–film distance selected will be sufficiently large to reduce geometric blurring, magnification, and distortion to acceptable levels (unless any of these are specially required) without using such a large distance that the amount of radiation reaching the film is ridiculously small. Changing the F.F.D. affects the Exposure at the film according to the inverse square law since the focal spot size is tiny compared to the distance and, although there is attenuation in the patient, this remains the same whatever the F.F.D. Most radiography is done using a focus–film distance of about 100 cm. since this is a reasonable compromise for a wide range of anatomical sites. For the more easily penetrated chest where sharpness as well as low magnification and distortion are needed, a better compromise is obtained by using a distance of 180 cm.

The object–film distance is not really under the control of the radiographer since it is determined by the position of the structure in the patient. Some control of its effect on geometric and movement blurring and on magnification, however, can be effected by the orientation of the patient (AP or PA) and by the position of the cassette (immediately next to the patient or in the tray below the table). It is the relative value of focus–film distance and object–film distance which really controls these aspects of the radiograph.

Choice of Focal Spot Size.—The primary effect of focal spot size is on geometric blurring. Obviously an infinitely small focal spot size would give the greatest freedom from geometric blurring but this is not possible or even advisable, since its use would lead to an excessive concentration of heat production at the target which could lead to a disastrous rise in temperature. The larger the focal spot size, the easier it is to avoid too great a rise in temperature at the target. The minimum size of focal spot is determined by the value of kV., mA., and exposure time being used (since these control the production of heat): a subject which is returned to later when 'rating' is discussed. Suffice it to say here that for most work an effective focal spot size of about 1 × 1 mm. is used. If the exposure is particularly heavy a size of 2 × 2 mm. may be used and if it is sufficiently light a size of 0·3 × 0·3 mm. may be used.

Choice of Kilovoltage.—Although the various factors discussed above can be varied it is not usual to do so in the day-to-day application of any particular technique. The values used will, of course, affect the values chosen for the remaining factors. These latter factors (kV., mA., time) which are usually regarded as the truly variable ones are discussed below.

The kilovoltage is important from the point of view of both contrast and film density. As discussed in CHAPTER XIX, it is the kilovoltage which determines for a particular set of anatomical structures the radiation (patient) contrast and, hence, the radiographic contrast. The kilovoltage is therefore selected, primarily, in accordance with the desired contrast (and latitude). If a low contrast (large latitude) is needed then a high kV. is chosen and vice versa. The actual value of kV. necessary is, of course, dependent upon the particular structure creating the contrast. It is also dependent on the voltage wave form since the average photon energy from a smooth (i.e., constant-potential or three-phase generator) wave form is greater than that from a pulsating wave form of the same nominal kV.

In addition to controlling the quality of the radiation the kilovoltage affects, in large measure, the intensity of the radiation emitted from the target. As will be recalled from CHAPTER V, intensity is approximately proportional to the square of the kilovoltage. The actual effect of change in kilovoltage on film blackening is, however, rather greater than this since the fraction of radiation transmitted by the patient is also increased by increase in kV. A complicating factor is the change in response with change in kV. of the film-screen combination. As an approximate guide for average circumstances it may be assumed that the overall effect is roughly proportional to the fourth power of the kV., i.e., kV.[4] Thus if the kV. is increased from 50 to 60 kV. for example, then in order to keep the density on the film more or less constant, the mA. may be reduced by a factor equal to:

$$(\tfrac{50}{60})^4 = 0.48.$$

This is the basis for the working rule that an increase of 10 kV. allows the current (mA.) to be halved. There is, incidentally, nothing magical about reducing the mA. to one-half—we could have, alternatively, reduced the exposure time to one-half the former value, since radiation output is directly proportional to both time and current.

This working rule is valid only over a limited range of kilovoltages since a change of 10 kV. at, say, 100 kV. is a smaller fraction and therefore causes less effect. This is easily seen if the effect of a change from 85 to 100 kV. is calculated, viz.,

$$(\tfrac{85}{100})^4 = 0.52.$$

Thus in this range of generating voltage a change of 15 kV. leads to a halving of time or mA.

Choice of Time.—The primary effects of exposure time on the radiograph are on its density and on movement unsharpness. Depending upon whether any patient movement can be immobilized or not, and whether it is involuntary, the exposure time is chosen so that the resulting movement unsharpness is commensurate with

THE RADIOGRAPHIC EXPOSURE

the other unsharpnesses. For instance, a hand can usually be made completely stationary so that there is no significant movement either voluntary or involuntary. In such a case the exposure time may be quite long. It is, of course, an advantage from the movement unsharpness point of view to use a short exposure time even in these circumstances, but, of course, an unnecessarily short exposure time may well compromise the optimum selection of other exposure factors. For the radiography of internal structures when involuntary movement exists, such as say of the colon, the exposure time selected must be appropriately short.

Choice of Tube Current (mA.).—The mA. affects only the amount of radiation leaving the X-ray tube (and therefore reaching the film) and has no effect on any other aspect of the film. In a simple, ideal situation all the other factors would be selected first, in accordance with the various requirements discussed above, and finally the mA. selected so as to produce a range of Exposures (mR) at the film such that the resultant densities lie within the desired range (usually 0·5–1·5 approximately). Sometimes this is possible but usually the mA. so required is impossibly large, since, for the size of the focal spot, kV., and exposure time selected, the target may become too hot: in other words, the 'tube rating' is exceeded. What must be done in order to make the exposure permissible? There are many possibilities, all of which include some degree of compromise of the factors already selected. For example, a larger focal spot size may be selected; this has no effect on the radiation output but it may allow the required large mA. to be used (i.e., it is within the rating of this larger focal spot). Such a course will increase the geometric unsharpness but this may be acceptable or may have to be accepted. Alternatively, a faster film-screen combination could be used. This would enable the same film blackening to be achieved with a smaller amount of radiation; in other words, a smaller mA. could be used. The use of a faster screen will increase screen blurring but again this must be accepted. Another possibility is to increase the exposure time (and hence movement unsharpness) which will mean that a smaller mA. will be needed. This does not exhaust the list of possibilities, and of course more than one factor may be changed simultaneously, but it does indicate the way in which the compromise is made—the underlying thought being that the optimum is to be sought, within the rating of the tube, where the various unsharpnesses are approximately equal and the total unsharpness sufficiently, but not unnecessarily, small.

Even after such an attempt at a suitable compromise the required mA. may remain impossibly large. In such a circumstance it is usual to increase the kV., since as will be remembered this has a large effect on the amount of radiation reaching the film ($\propto$ kV.^{4}). The contrast will, of course, be decreased but this must be accepted. In everyday language the kV. has to be chosen sufficiently large to 'penetrate' the patient but not so large as to seriously diminish contrast. Because the change in intensity at the film is large for small changes in kV. whereas the associated change in contrast is quite small, it is common practice to compensate for patient-to-patient differences by changes in kV.

Although in the above discussion the mA. and the seconds have been discussed separately the amount of radiation reaching the film and hence the film density is controlled by their product (mA.s.) rather than by their individual values. For example 100 mA. for 1 sec., 10 mA. for 10 sec., or 1000 mA. for 0·1 sec. will all yield the same film density since all correspond to an exposure of 100 mA.s.* On many

---

* This assumes that the reciprocity law holds (CHAPTER XVI) which is true over much of the likely range of exposure values in day-to-day radiography. For very long and very short times a slight increase in mA.s. may be required when using screen films.

present-day units it is usual to select first the kV. and then the mA.s. appropriate to the contrast and film density required. The mA. is then adjusted to be equal to the maximum that the X-ray tube rating will allow (and to some fraction, say 80 per cent, of this); the exposure time will then be the minimum possible under the circumstances. If the time is too large then a higher kV. is chosen and the mA.s. decreased accordingly. Such a method of working ensures that the full potentialities of the unit are being utilized.

Although the various exposure factors have been discussed in what the authors, at least, think is a logical way, it must be quite obvious that the problem is a circular one in so far as each change of factor either directly or indirectly affects one or more of the others. The whole set of factors are chosen to be compatible and to give a good radiograph. Fortunately, the selection is not as critical as might be imagined, since differences of up to about 25 per cent in radiation Exposure (mR) reaching the film are only just detectable and can therefore be accepted. Just how the compromise between the various opposing requirements is effected in any particular case will depend upon what is regarded by the radiologist involved as the optimum radiograph for the particular examination being done. In any case the exact values will vary from X-ray unit to X-ray unit. The many published sets of 'Exposure Tables' are, however, a useful starting point for the tyro.

Calculation of Changed Factors.—The question of determining the change in one factor necessitated by a change in another factor is sometimes encountered in both practice and in examination questions; it is therefore useful to consider one such example.

It is found that an exposure of 12 mA.s. at 90 kVp produces a radiograph of acceptable density when the focus–film distance is 90 cm. What exposure (mA.s.) would be required to produce a radiograph of the same overall density if the F.F.D. were to be changed to 105 cm. and the kilovoltage to 75 kVp?

In doing the calculation the two changes, of F.F.D. and kV., are considered separately since their effects are quite independent. If the kV. is kept at 90 kVp and the F.F.D. changed from 90 cm. to 105 cm., the mA.s. value will have to be increased so as to compensate for the extra inverse-square-law effect. The new value will be:

$$12 \times (\tfrac{105}{90})^2 = 16\tfrac{1}{3} \text{ mA.s.}$$

In this calculation it has been assumed that the inverse square law holds and this is the case since (1) the focal spot size is small compared with the distance, (2) the absorption in air is negligible, and (3) the absorption in the patient is constant.

The effect of the change in kV. may now be estimated. It has already been stated that here the effect is dependent on kV.[4] (approximately). The decrease in the kVp from 90 to 75 kVp will necessitate an increase in mA.s., the new value being given by:

$$16\tfrac{1}{3} \times (\tfrac{90}{75})^4 = 33 \cdot 8_6 \text{ mA.s.}$$

In fact the dependence on kV. is not quite so much as this. If the dependence was according to kV.[3] the value would have been:

$$16\tfrac{1}{3} \times (\tfrac{90}{75})^3 = 29 \cdot 5 \text{ mA.s.}$$

In practice a value of about 30–32 mA.s. would be chosen and this would probably be quite satisfactory.

CHAPTER XXII

THE DIAGNOSTIC X-RAY TUBE AND SHIELD

A SIMPLE description of the basic tube used for the production of X-rays has already been given in CHAPTER V. In this chapter a rather more detailed description will be given, although it is not intended to enter into an elaborate account of the finer points of detail involved in the many different makes of tube available. For such a description the student must refer to the more specialized texts; here it is the relevant physics which is presented.

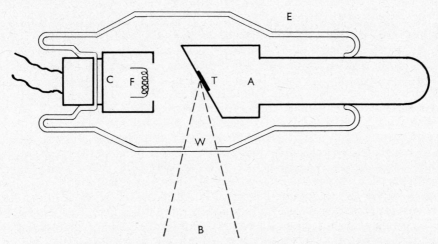

Fig. 191.—A stationary anode X-ray tube. A, Anode structure; B, Useful beam; C, Cathode assembly; E, Glass envelope; F, Filament; T, Tungsten target; W, X-ray window.

The X-ray tube illustrated in *Fig.* 191 shows, in a stylized way, the basic features of a stationary anode tube such as may be fitted in a low-power or a mobile unit. It consists of a filament (*F*), mounted inside a cathode assembly (*C*), which is supported opposite the anode structure (*A*), in the centre of which is a tungsten target (*T*). The whole structure is contained within an evacuated glass envelope (*E*). The useful beam (*B*) of X-rays is in the direction shown in *Fig.* 191 and the glass of the envelope is usually made thinner in the region shown and constitutes the *X-ray window* (*W*). The thinner glass absorbs less radiation, of course, and so results in a larger X-ray output than would be obtained were the glass not thinned. The filament is heated by passing a current (*the filament current*) through it, and as a result electrons are thermionically emitted from the filament into the surrounding space. These electrons are then directed and accelerated towards the target because of the electric field which exists between the filament and the target. The velocity with which the electrons finally hit the target is determined by the voltage which exists between the target and filament. On arrival at the target the electrons are rapidly

277

slowed down and in doing so their *kinetic energy* is converted into (a small amount of) *X-radiation* and (a large amount of) *heat*. Since the X-ray tube is evacuated the electrons are not impeded in their passage from filament to target.

The magnitude of the filament current determines the temperature of the filament which, in its turn, controls the number of electrons emitted per second from the filament. Since these emitted electrons constitute the current flowing through the X-ray tube to the target (*the tube current*), it is the filament current which is used to control the tube current and hence the X-ray output. It should be noted, however, that whereas the tube current is usually in the range 1–500 mA. (and, rarely, as much as 1000 mA., i.e., 1 amp.) the filament heating current is usually in the range of 4–5 amp. The voltage applied between the filament and target of the X-ray tube (usually referred to as the *tube kilovoltage* or *kV*. since its value is usually in the range 40–120 kV.) affects both the kind of (quality or energy) and the amount of (quantity or output) X-rays emitted from the tube.

THE FILAMENT

The X-ray tube filament is almost invariably made of a small coil of fairly thick tungsten wire (*Fig.* 192). The diameter of the wire is typically about $\frac{1}{5}$ mm. and the coil $\frac{1}{2}$–1 mm. in diameter and 1–1$\frac{1}{2}$ cm. long. Tungsten is used in preference to other material since it can provide, when necessary, a copious thermionic emission (i.e., a high tube current), both because the emission from tungsten is inherently high compared with many other materials and also because tungsten can be raised to a high temperature without detriment; its melting-point being 3380° C. (It will be remembered that the amount of thermionic emission rises very rapidly as the temperature is raised.) Furthermore, the evaporation of tungsten from the filament at these high temperatures is not excessive. This is important for two reasons. Firstly, if significant evaporation takes place, the filament must become thinner, which leads to a change in temperature (and therefore tube current) for a given filament current and to eventual failure of the filament and therefore of the X-ray tube. With tungsten this type of tube failure is rare. It can happen, of course, that due to manufacturing defects a filament breaks during the early life of a tube but once this time is passed it is not too common for filament failure to occur. The second reason for not wanting to have significant evaporation is because this vaporized tungsten will be deposited (at least partly) on the inside of the glass envelope. That portion which falls on the glass window of the X-ray tube will serve as an additional filter and will reduce the intensity (output) of X-rays emerging from the tube. This is one of the reasons why the output of an X-ray tube falls with years of use. The presence of the tungsten on the walls of the tube also disturbs the electrical insulation properties of the glass and so enables the glass to act as another electrode to which some of the electrons in the tube may be attracted. Such electron bombardment of the walls liberates gas, so reducing the degree of vacuum inside the tube. This in its turn facilitates further electron bombardment of the walls and, through an ever-increasing circle of such events, leads, eventually, to loss of the vacuum and the demise of the X-ray tube. It is thought that this, rather unspectacular, chain of events is the most common cause of ultimate X-ray tube failure. Another cause of X-ray tube failure arises from the damage done to the target in the manner described later in this chapter (p. 280). It is worth emphasizing, however, that in spite of these comments on the reasons for ultimate tube failure, such failure is a rare event. The manufacture of X-ray tubes is now very well controlled and, although initial failures can and do occur, once a tube has run for several hours it will usually continue to do so, giving several years of service before it gradually dies, unspectacularly, of old age in the ways described above.

The Filament Assembly.—Not only must the desired number of electrons (mA.s.) reach the target with the appropriate kinetic energy (keV.) but also they must impinge upon a sufficiently small area of the target surface. This small area constitutes the region over which the X-rays are produced and, as was shown in CHAPTER XVIII,

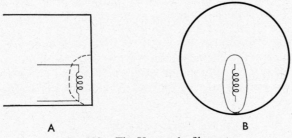

Fig. 192.—The X-ray tube filament.

p. 219, it is important for it to be small. In practice the size of the filament is larger than the real focal spot size and this together with the mutual repulsion of the electrons naturally leads to a spreading out of the electrons over a large area of the target surface. In order to have the desired small focal spot it is, therefore, necessary to incorporate some focusing device which will narrow down the electron beam appropriately. Examination of an X-ray filament (which every student should endeavour to do, there being few departments which do not have a demonstration tube available) will show that the filament is set into a shaped slot, called the 'focusing cup', cut into the surrounding metal housing. *Fig.* 192 A is a diagrammatic, sectional drawing of such a filament, while *Fig.* 192 B attempts to give an impression

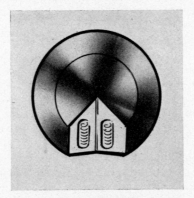

Fig. 193.—A dual-filament assembly.

of the cathode assembly as seen from the front. The electrical potential of the surrounding metal is kept at a different value from that of the filament by connecting one end of the filament to the surrounding housing. Thus if the voltage across the filament is 12 V. then the potential difference between the centre of the filament and the housing is about 6 V. This simple device, together with very careful design and construction, results in the production of an electric field in the neighbourhood of the filament which serves to bring the beam of electrons, thermionically emitted from the filament, to a focus having the required size on the surface of the target.

As described earlier (CHAPTER XVIII, p. 219), the target surface is inclined at an angle (usually about 17°) to the central axis of the X-ray beam so that the actual area in the target surface is larger than the effective (apparent) focal spot size. In practice, the true focal spot size is chosen in the range 6×2 mm. to 1×0.3 mm. which corresponds to a range from 2×2 mm. to 0.3×0.3 mm. for the apparent focal spot size.

Most diagnostic X-ray tubes have two focal spots of different sizes and these are obtained by having two filaments, each in its own focusing cup, side by side in the filament assembly. By appropriate external switching either one or the other of the filaments (not both) is selected for use. A dual-filament arrangement is shown in *Fig.* 193.

THE TARGET

Almost invariably the target of a diagnostic X-ray tube is made of tungsten. In CHAPTER V it was mentioned that the efficiency of X-ray production is increased by using high atomic number material for the target. Although there are other materials which have higher atomic numbers than tungsten, their other properties are not so suitable. Because of the large amount of heat which accompanies the production of X-rays the temperature of the target will rise. It is clearly important that it shall not tend to melt, for not only would this roughen the target face (the smoothness of which is important for reasons already set out in CHAPTER XVIII), but in extreme cases the whole anode structure could become distorted and useless. A high melting-point is therefore called for, and tungsten (m.p. 3380° C.) has one of the highest.

For a given exposure (kV. $\times$ mA.s.) the rise in temperature depends upon the thermal capacity of the target and the ease with which it can transfer heat through itself to the surrounding supporting material. The specific heat and thermal conductivity of the target material are therefore important. Those for tungsten whilst not particularly large are acceptable.

Even well below its boiling-point there is considerable evaporation from a material like water, as is shown by the normal drying of wet clothes, for example. The same is true, though to a different extent, for all materials, even solids. A very important feature of a target material is that it should not readily evaporate, for reasons that have already been given in the case of the filament, even at fairly high temperatures. The vapour pressure of tungsten is low and this is another reason for this material's use for targets.

The Anode Structure.—Although a material (tungsten) with a high melting-point has been chosen, it is still important to remove the heat from the target and so avoid a build-up of temperature due to subsequent exposures or to allow the continuance of one which takes a comparatively long time. In the stationary anode tube the tungsten target is in the form of a circular (or sometimes rectangular) disk about 1 mm. thick and about 1 cm. in diameter, which is embedded in a large block of copper which itself passes through the glass envelope (*Figs.* 191 and 194). Since the copper is at a lower temperature than the tungsten, which has been heated by the impinging electron beam, heat will pass from the tungsten to the copper and will be distributed throughout the copper by conduction. The rate of heat conduction, i.e.,

rate of passage of heat through the copper, is determined by the temperature difference, by the thermal conductivity of the copper and of the tungsten, and by the cross-
section of the copper block. This passage of heat from the hotter tungsten to the
cooler copper serves to cool the tungsten and prevent its temperature rising too much.
Of course, if a very heavy exposure (viz., large kV., mA.s.) is made the rate of
production of heat may be too great and the temperature of the tungsten may exceed
an acceptable value before the heat has time to be conducted into the copper. This
fact imposes a limitation on the magnitude of the X-ray exposure which can be
made, a point which will be discussed more fully in CHAPTER XXIV.

It is also important to remove the heat so given to the copper in order that there
can be continuing transference of heat from the hot tungsten to the cooler copper.
As the temperature of the two materials becomes more equal the rate of heat transfer
will progressively diminish. The route by which heat is transferred from the copper
is by further conduction into the cooler oil which surrounds the glass envelope and
into which the copper anode stem protrudes (*Fig.* 194). Obviously this oil itself

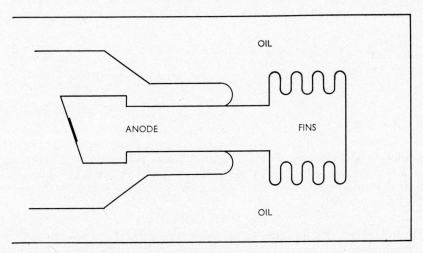

Fig. 194.—The anode protrudes into the surrounding oil. The rate of heat transfer is
increased by increasing the area of contact by means of fins.

becomes hotter, the heat being distributed throughout it by convection, just as
heat is distributed through the water in a heated kettle. Contact between the oil
and the metal casing allows heat to pass from one to the other whilst in its turn the
casing transfers the heat to the surrounding air, so that the heat is eventually distributed throughout the whole room by convection. In some cases where large amounts
of heat are being produced, a fan is used to blow air over the surface of the casing
in order to improve the rate of cooling and, therefore, permit greater X-ray exposures.
Loss of heat from the X-ray tube casing to the surroundings is almost entirely by air
convection (either natural or forced). Loss of heat from the outer casing by radiation
is very small, although for many years it was said that the sombre black colour of the
X-ray tube housing was chosen in order to improve removal of heat in this way. This
is incorrect and more pastel (feminine!) shades are now permitted.

Fig. 195 summarizes the processes of passage of heat from target to surroundings. It should be noted that the rise in temperature produced in the copper, oil,

and air is much smaller than that produced in the tungsten since the mass of copper, oil, and air heated is much greater than the mass of tungsten heated. Hence the relatively large amount of heat produced in the tungsten is gradually spread around over a large amount of material, the temperature of which only rises slightly. In the final event the 'cooling' of the X-ray tube has been achieved by heating up the room!

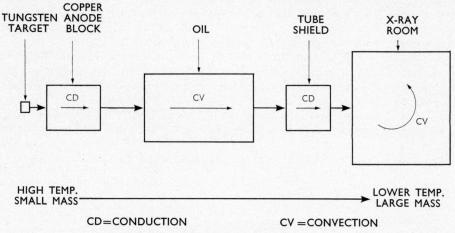

Fig. 195.—The steps in the cooling of the target.

From the above description it is obvious that during the life of the tube the various structures within the evacuated glass envelope are heated to varying extents. Any gas molecules absorbed on or occluded in them could be released by this heating and the vacuum so spoiled. It is practice therefore to use 'outgassed' materials and to heat up the tube and its contents during the evacuation and so remove as much of this gas as possible.

THE TUBE HOUSING

Oil Insulation.—The presence of oil surrounding the glass envelope has already been mentioned in connexion with its role in the cooling of the target. The oil has another, equally important, role, namely that of an electrical insulator. It must be remembered that there may be anything from about 40 up to 150 kV. between the filament and target of a diagnostic X-ray tube (and even more in a therapy tube) and therefore considerable care has to be taken to ensure that there is sufficient electrical insulation between these two structures. Inside the glass envelope their physical separation and the absence of gas ensure this. The glass of the envelope is also able to withstand the voltage although the distance along the glass surface is often increased by suitable choice of shape (*Fig.* 196) in order to improve the insulation. It is worth noting, in passing, that the external separation of the filament and target connexion has to be increased when higher kV. are being used and this, of course, leads to larger tubes being needed at higher kV. even though the internal separation of filament–target is not much different.* For instance, a dental tube

---

* It is worth noting that the internal separation between filament and target has no effect on the energy acquired by the electrons. It is often, incorrectly, stated that at higher kV. the separation has to be great in order to give the electrons a chance to speed up. This is not so. The electron will gain the full energy appropriate to the kV. no matter how small the separation. The size of the separation is chosen appropriate to the required insulation and focusing conditions.

capable of working up to 70 kV. is only 15 cm. long whereas a tube for use up to 150 kV. may be 45 cm. long.

The surrounding oil both maintains the insulation properties of the glass envelope and also insulates the tube from the metal shield. The X-ray tube is, of course, supported in the centre of the metal shield by insulating columns. These columns carry the insulated supply leads which bring the appropriate voltage and current supplies to the filament and the target.

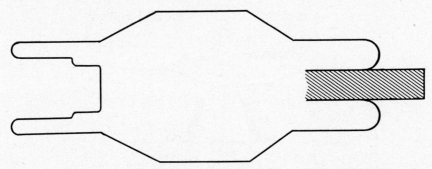

Fig. 196.—The re-entrant glass envelope giving a longer path, and therefore better insulation between the electrodes.

It is important that the oil should not become too hot (and remember that it does become heated as a consequence of the exposure) since insulators progressively lose their insulating properties as their temperature rises. It is, therefore, necessary to have some form of device which will prevent the tube being used if the oil temperature rises too high. This usually takes the form of a metal bellows which extends as the heated oil expands (and which, therefore, simultaneously acts as a safety device preventing the increasing oil pressure from damaging the tube and/or shield). If the bellows expand beyond a certain amount (i.e., the oil has exceeded a certain temperature) then they operate a micro-switch which prevents operation of the tube until the oil has cooled sufficiently.

The Tube Shield.—In addition to the obvious function of containing and supporting the X-ray tube and oil, and protecting them from external damage, the metal tube shield has two other very important functions to perform.

Firstly, it provides a completely encircling metallic shield which, because it is (and must be) firmly connected electrically to earth potential, protects the user from any possibility of electrical shock. The filament and target of a diagnostic tube may well be at an electrical potential, with respect to the radiographer (earth), of anything up to 70 kV. (say). Contact with such a high potential could well be lethal. It is for this reason that safety regulations demand that all components of an X-ray unit (e.g., transformer, valves, cables, tube, etc.) shall be contained within closed metallic coverings and that these latter shall be firmly and directly connected to the thick metal earthing strip which accompanies the power input cable.

The second purpose of the tube shield is to afford protection to the radiographer and patient against unwanted X-radiation. It is arranged that any X-rays (both primary and secondary) which are not within the wanted beam are attenuated by the shield. This is usually achieved by lining the steel shield with appropriate thicknesses of lead, the actual thickness depending upon the likely intensity of radiation reaching that portion of the shield. There is, of course, an aperture opposite the target through which the maximum size of useful beam can emerge. This beam is reduced to the size required, i.e., that needed to just cover the film size in use, by a set of collimating diaphragms (*Fig.* 197), or by a cone. It is nowadays common practice for all X-ray tube shields to be carefully tested after manufacture to ensure that the prevailing protection requirements are met.

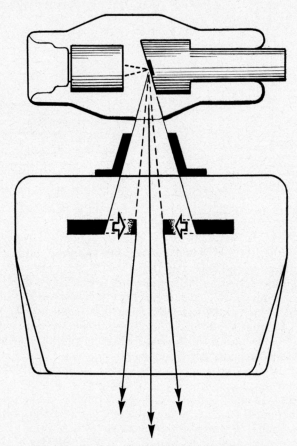

Fig. 197.—Beam collimation by moving diaphragms.

It has already been mentioned that the tube shield forms part of the chain involved in the removal of heat from the target and the dissipating of it to the surroundings. Heat loss is increased by having a large surface area and fins are sometimes fitted to the casing to increase its surface area. For ease of movement and convenience, on the other hand, a small, light-weight shield is desirable and a compromise has to be made between this and one large enough to tolerate a large production and dissipation of heat.

The High-tension Cables.—In some low-power X-ray units the transformer which supplies the high tension is also contained within the tube shield and the oil serves to provide cooling and insulation for the transformer as well as for the tube. More usually, however, the transformer (and rectifying valves, etc.) are contained in a separate, oil-filled box. Connexion between this (usually called the generator) and the tube is by means of two specially constructed high-tension cables, one connected to the filament side and one to the anode side of the tube. The construction of these cables is in the form shown in *Fig.* 198. The central conductor is insulated from the inner metallic braid by 1–2 mm. of rubber. Surrounding this inner braid there is a multiple insulating layer of rubber and fabric which totals about 6–7 mm. in thickness. Outside this there is the outer metallic braid and finally an outer cover of cotton or plastic. In some modern cables insulating materials other than rubber are used although the flexibility of rubber-insulated cables is often preferred.

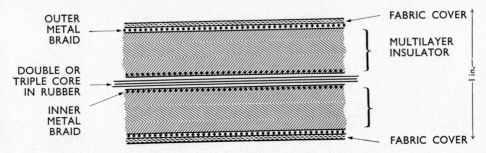

OUTER METAL BRAID

FABRIC COVER

MULTILAYER INSULATOR

DOUBLE OR TRIPLE CORE IN RUBBER

INNER METAL BRAID

FABRIC COVER

Fig. 198.—Cross-section of a shockproof high-tension cable.

The inner conductor is in the form of a dual or triple cable (rather like ordinary twin- or three-core electric light cable). The insulation between these members of the inner conductor is sufficient for the few tens of volts to be applied between them. In the case of the anode high-tension cable these inner conductors are all connected together and form the connexion between the target (anode) and the positive side of the generator. The insulation between these inner conductors and the outer metallic braid, which is connected to earth, must be sufficient to withstand more than the maximum voltage supplied by the generator. The fact that the outer braid of the cable is connected to earth means that anyone who happens to touch the cables whilst the unit is energized is fully protected against electric shock; for this reason such cables are called 'shockproof'.

The cable which goes to the filament uses the inner conductors to provide the filament-heating current. In other words, they form the connexion between the filament transformer (in the generator tank) and the filament. One of these inner conductors also forms the connexion from the filament to the negative potential side of the generator. In most X-ray tubes, as already stated, there is a choice of two possible filaments so that the three inner conductors are required to supply these separately, and to provide the connexion from the negative side of the generator to the filament (cathode). The use of the same type of cable for both the anode and cathode side is done for economy. It is cheaper and more convenient to have only one type even though the anode cable does not require the multiple inners.

At each end of both high-tension cables specially constructed terminations are used to connect the cable to the X-ray tube and generator tank. *Fig.* 199 shows diagrammatically such a termination together with the socket into which it fits.

The pins at the end form the connexion for the centre of the cable to the anode (or cathode). The flange to which the outer braid is soldered bolts on to the metal of the tube shield (or of the generator tank) so that the whole of the external, accessible part of the unit (tube shield, cables, and generator) forms a continuous, safely earthed, protective barrier. The whole system can thus be said to be 'shock-proof'.

Although modern cables are very substantial and fairly flexible they should, nevertheless, be handled with great care and moved about as little as possible. Cables must be inspected regularly for damage and wear since any break in the earthed outer braid could be potentially dangerous.

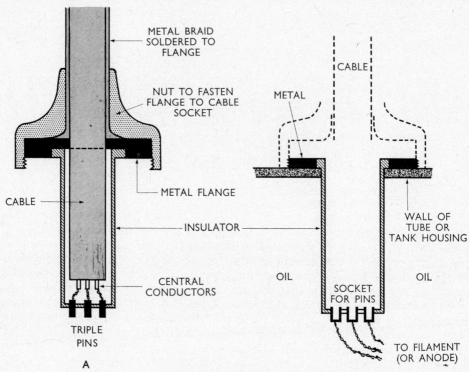

Fig. 199.—A, H.T. cable termination. B, The socket into which it fits.

TYPES OF TUBE

The Stationary Anode X-ray Tube.—The stationary anode X-ray tube so far described in this chapter and illustrated in *Fig*. 200 is limited in range of application because of the comparatively low X-ray intensity obtainable from it. When the exposure time is small, as it is in radiography, then very little of the heat generated at the target can be dissipated during the exposure time, in spite of the high thermal conductivity of the anode structure. The rise in temperature of the target will depend upon the size of the area over which the electrons bombard it (that is, on the real focal spot size). For a given focal spot size and exposure time there is, therefore, a maximum to the amount of electrical energy (equal to kV. × mA.s.) which can be used without raising the target to an excessively high temperature. It turns out that, for a reasonably effective focal spot size (2 × 2 mm. say), the accompanying X-ray emission allows only a limited range of application and is not sufficient, for example, for a good pelvic radiograph. Alternatively, if a large enough emission of X-rays is to be attained then the focal spot size must be increased so as to distribute over a larger area the larger amount of heat resulting from the use of increased kV. and/or mA.s. Unfortunately, such an increase in focal spot size leads to increased, and usually unacceptable, geometric blurring on the radiograph.

Another course of action is to increase the exposure time so that the required large amount of X-rays are produced in a longer time. This means that the heat is also produced more slowly, thus making it possible for some heat, at least, to be

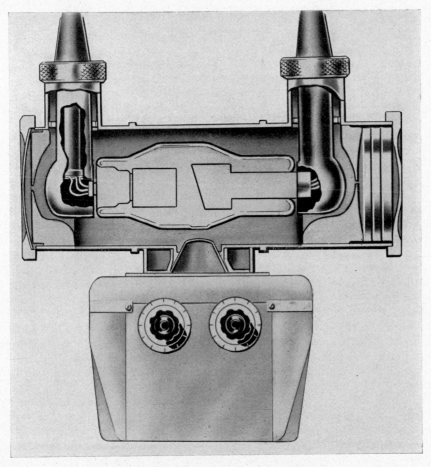

Fig. 200.—A stationary anode X-ray tube head.

conducted away from the target during the course of the exposure and so, in this way, to avoid the target temperature rising too high. Providing the accompanying increase in movement blurring occasioned by the increased exposure time is not unacceptable, this is a way out of the difficulty. In those examinations, however, where a small focal spot size, a short exposure time, and a large quantity of X-rays are required simultaneously the stationary anode tube cannot cope. Unfortunately, such circumstances seem to form a large fraction of the total. It is nowadays almost universal to use a rotating anode tube, which does not have the same stringent limitations, for most radiographic work and to retain the stationary anode tube for a restricted range of work such as is done by a portable or mobile unit: although even here rotating anodes are now sometimes used.

The Rotating Anode Tube.—The construction of the rotating anode tube is illustrated in *Fig.* 201. It is similar to the stationary anode tube in that it has a filament (usually dual) mounted in a focusing filament assembly and positioned opposite to the anode structure. The whole is contained in an evacuated glass envelope which is itself contained in an oil-filled, metallic, shockproof tube shield, the function of all these being exactly the same as in the case of the stationary anode tube.

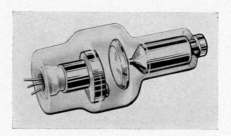

Fig. 201.—A rotating anode X-ray tube.

The difference between the two types of tube lies in the structure of the anode. In the rotating anode tube it consists of a disk of tungsten (usually about 7·5–10 cm. in diameter and 6 mm. thick) which is capable of being rotated at a high speed. This rotation is achieved by means of an electric motor which must have a rather special construction since the moving parts are inside the evacuated envelope. It is virtually impossible to make a reliable vacuum-tight seal capable of being rotated. The arrangement usually adopted is shown in *Fig.* 202. The central shaft (S) on which the disk of tungsten (T) is mounted is attached to the rotor (R) of the electric motor, and is constrained to rotate about the fixed shaft (F) by means of the ball races (X). The whole system is very carefully constructed and balanced so that the rotation of this anode structure is very free and once set running will continue to do so for many minutes (as anyone who cares to listen in an X-ray department may check). Furthermore, the accuracy of the alinement is so good that no matter how the tube shield is oriented there is absolutely no wobble of the rotating anode, which therefore appears to be stationary even though it is rotating. Being in a vacuum, oil cannot be used to lubricate the bearings nor can they be further lubricated once the tube is evacuated. A special metallic (lead or silver) lubricant is therefore used. The life of these bearings is not unlimited and once it becomes difficult to rotate the anode sufficiently quickly (or at all!), due to their wear, complete failure of the tube is imminent. It is therefore important to rotate the anode only when necessary, i.e., during the actual exposure, in order to extend tube life.

The stator coils of the electric motor are outside the vacuum as shown in *Fig.* 202 and are therefore freely accessible. The motor is usually of an induction type and produces a rotation of 3000 revolutions per minute.

The edge of the tungsten disk is bevelled as shown in *Fig.* 203 and this bevelled edge forms the target surface on to which the electron beam is focused. As in the case of the stationary anode tube the electrons are focused so as to give an apparent focal spot size of small dimensions ($0·3 \times 0·3$–2×2 mm.^{2}). The important difference is that, since the disk is rotating at high speed during the exposure, the particular area of tungsten being bombarded by electrons, and therefore heated, is continuously being changed. The heat is, therefore, spread out over a much larger mass of tungsten and the rise in temperature is therefore much smaller than would be the case with a stationary target. For example, if the radius of the track over which the heat is

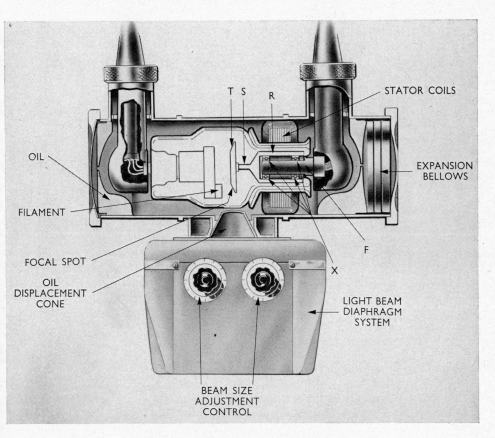

Fig. 202.—A rotating anode X-ray tube head.

spread (*Fig.* 203) is 40 mm., which is a typical value, then the length of the track is $2\pi \times 40 = 250$ mm. If the target angle is 20° and the apparent focal spot size is 1×1 mm. then it is easily calculated that the size of the area on the tungsten surface which is bombarded is 1×3 mm.² = 3 mm.² (which is exactly the same as the true focal spot size of a stationary anode tube). The area over which the heat is spread out, however, is 250×3 mm.² = 750 mm.²

It can be seen therefore that the use of a rotating anode tube leads to a huge difference between the apparent focal spot size and the area over which the heat is spread. For a stationary anode the ratio of these two areas is about 1 : 3 whereas for a rotating anode tube it is more like 1 : 750. It is therefore possible to use much greater values of mA.s. and kV. without causing an excessive rise in anode temperature, and therefore to achieve much larger X-ray outputs with a rotating anode tube than is possible with a stationary target.

10

Provided that the anode is rotating quickly enough the actual speed of rotation is not particularly important. However, as will be discussed later, if the exposure time is very short, speeds higher than 3000 r.p.m. may be needed. As a general rule it is desirable that the anode should rotate through at least 5 revolutions during the actual exposure time.

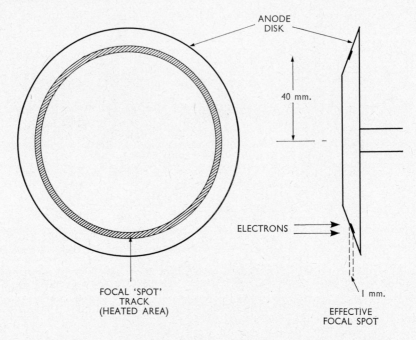

Fig. 203.—The rotating anode showing the area over which the heat is spread.

Electrical Connexion to the Anode.—The fact that the anode is rotating means that no firm, permanent connexion can be made between the positive high-tension cable and the anode. How then is the tube current (mA.) able to pass through the tube? Fortunately the currents used are not unduly large although they can be as much as 1 amp. (1000 mA.) in some modern equipment. The area of contact of the bearings is sufficient for the current to pass and the electrical connexion is thus made via the fixed central shaft (*Fig.* 201).

The Cooling of the Rotating Anode Tube.—The method of heat dissipation from the rotating target is very different from that of the stationary one. Since the whole structure is rotating on a set of bearings there is little possibility of transfer of heat via the anode stem to the surrounding oil. Conduction depends, amongst other things, on the area of cross-section of the conducting path and clearly in a bearings system this is tiny, and therefore conduction is minimal. Convection of heat is not possible either since in the evacuated tube there is nothing to convect the heat. Only the third mode of heat transfer, radiation, remains and it is on this that the removal of heat from the rotating target depends.

It will be remembered that any hot (i.e., above the temperature of the surroundings) object will radiate to its surroundings more heat than it receives from the surroundings and that therefore it will gradually cool. The radiation referred to here, of course, is infra-red, visible, and ultra-violet radiation which, as we know, pass easily through the vacuum which isolates the anode from the surrounding glass envelope and oil. The rate of heat loss depends upon the difference in the fourth power of the absolute temperatures, that is:

$$(T_{\text{anode}})^4 - (T_{\text{oil}})^4.$$

This means that at low temperature differences the rate of heat loss is very small but that at high temperature differences it is very high. Doubling the temperature difference increases the rate of heat loss by a factor of 16. It is therefore only after the anode has reached a fairly high temperature that any rapid loss of heat occurs. For this reason the anode of a rotating anode tube becomes red, and even white hot, in use. One very important consequence of this is that a self-rectified circuit can never be used and a rectified voltage must always be provided for a rotating anode tube. (*See* CHAPTER XXIII.)

It has already been stated that no significant heat transfer takes place through the rotation bearings. Furthermore, it is very important that the bearings should not become hot. If they were to do so then their running could be impaired (due to thermal expansion) and rotation could be slowed down and even stopped. Both these could lead to eventual anode failure since the heat would not be spread over as large an area as intended and therefore the anode temperature could become too high. Heat must therefore be kept away from the bearings and this is achieved by using a long, thin (i.e., small area of cross-section) shaft between the anode disk and the rotor and by making it of a low-conductivity metal such as molybdenum. In some designs of tube a heat shield behind the target has also been fitted so as to prevent radiation of heat towards the rotor.

CHAPTER XXIII

THE ELECTRICAL CIRCUITS OF THE X-RAY UNIT

IT has already been described in CHAPTER V how X-radiation is produced when electrons, thermionically emitted from the heated filament, are accelerated across the evacuated tube by the application of a high voltage between the filament and the target, and are allowed to strike the target. In this chapter some details will be given of the electric circuits associated with the X-ray tube. As always, the emphasis will be upon the reason for the presence of the various components and their basic function rather than on the detailed description of circuits actually employed. In fact, it is worth stating quite clearly at the outset that modern units have extremely complicated circuits, the detailed description of which is unnecessary to the radiographer and beyond the capabilities of the present authors. In any case each manufacturer uses different methods to achieve the required features of the finished unit. The rather simple circuits suggested in this chapter are intended only to illustrate what needs to be done and to indicate briefly the type of solution adopted. What is imperative, however, is that, no matter how it is done in practice, the various aspects of the complete circuit described in the chapter have to be taken into account in some way or other by the manufacturer.

The basic requirement of an X-ray unit is that it shall be possible to choose, independently, the kilovoltage (kV.) and the milliamperage (mA.) at which the tube operates. It is perhaps not realized by modern radiographers how important is this independence of choice of kV. and mA., although older workers, who remember the gas-filled tube in which kV. and mA. were very interdependent, fully realize its merits. As indicated in CHAPTER XXI the kV. is selected according to the required contrast and penetration whilst the product of mA. and exposure time is chosen so as to achieve the desired film density. Although it appears trivial, it is worth remembering that the accurate timing of the exposure (i.e., the ability to switch on and then, after the desired interval, to switch off) is a further important necessity. In addition to being able to adjust the values of the kV. and mA. it is also important to know what are their values, or, more accurately, it is important to know, before the exposure starts, what their values will be. The simple circuit shown in *Fig.* 204 enables these various requirements to be met.

THE BASIC ELECTRICAL SUPPLIES

High-tension Transformer and kV. Supply.—The X-ray tube kilovoltage is provided by the high-tension transformer (2)* which is a step-up transformer having a large number of turns in its secondary winding and comparatively few turns in its primary winding. Since this transformer may be required to produce voltages which range up to as high as 150 kV. in modern diagnostic equipment, it is important that it shall have adequate electrical insulation. The centre of the secondary winding is commonly earthed so that the target and filament are both at a high potential. In this circuit the X-ray tube is being operated as, what is known as, a 'self-rectified'

---

* The bracketed numbers in this section refer to the numbered items in *Fig.* 204.

tube. The H.T. alternating voltage provided by the H.T. transformer is applied directly to the X-ray tube (4). The filament is therefore positive and the target negative during one half-cycle and vice versa during the second half-cycle. Provided the target is sufficiently cool (so that no electrons are emitted thermionically from it) there can be no passage of current during the half-cycle when it is negative. Current can flow through the X-ray tube only when the target is positive, since it is only in this half-cycle that the negative electrons, thermionically emitted from the filament,

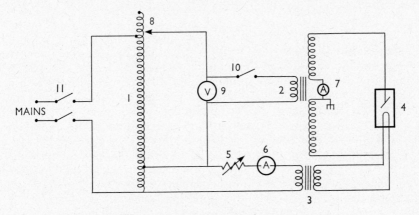

Fig. 204.—Basic circuit of an X-ray generator.

are able to pass to the target. The X-ray tube here is acting as its own rectifying valve. Later in this chapter circuits will be described which convert the alternating voltage provided by the H.T. transformer into a unidirectional voltage which is then applied to the X-ray tube. In such circuits the tube is not acting as its own rectifier. The interposition of a rectifying circuit in the H.T. circuit makes very little difference to the remainder of the circuit and what follows may be taken as applying equally to self-rectified and rectified circuits.

Control of kV.—The insulation required by the H.T. transformer makes it necessary to mount it within an oil-filled tank. The high degree of insulation makes it impossible to have a variable turns ratio which could be used to obtain a variable high voltage (kV.). The only way, therefore, by which the kV. applied to the X-ray tube may be varied is by varying the input voltage to the H.T. transformer. The autotransformer (1) is used to provide this variable voltage. The fraction of the supply mains voltage which is applied to the primary coil of the H.T. transformer is changed by changing the position of the upper contact (8) in the autotransformer. This voltage is measured by the A.C. voltmeter (9) but, since the X-ray tube kV. is a fixed multiple of it, it is convenient to calibrate the scale of this voltmeter in terms of the X-ray tube kV. It is called the **prereading voltmeter** (P.R.V.) and indicates, before the exposure 'on' switch (10) is closed, the kV. which will be across the X-ray tube during the exposure. This voltmeter is, of course, one suitable for A.C. and will be either a moving iron meter or a moving coil meter incorporated into a rectifying circuit. Since the peak kV. across the tube is the value of interest, as far as X-ray production is concerned, the scale of the instrument will be scaled to indicate the peak value which, it will be remembered, is 1·414 times the R.M.S. value. For example, if the primary H.T. voltage (V_p) is 150 volts (R.M.S.) and the turns ratio (T) is 400 : 1 then the H.T. transformer secondary voltage (V_s) will be given by:

$$\frac{V_s}{V_p} = T,$$

i.e.,

$$V_s = 150 \times 400 = 60 \text{ kV. (R.M.S.).}$$

The peak voltage (V_{peak}) across the X-ray tube is, therefore.

$$V_{peak} = 60 \times 1 \cdot 414 = 85 \text{ kVp.}$$

Filament Supply.—The filament of the X-ray tube is heated, so as to produce the desired thermionic emission of electrons, by passing a current through it. The current is provided by the filament transformer (3). This transformer is usually a step-down transformer which, typically, provides a filament heating current of about 4–5 A. at a voltage of 10–12 V. Such a current could, of course, be obtained directly from the autotransformer but the filament transformer is essential for another reason. In this type of circuit, the filament of the X-ray tube will sometimes, if not always, be at a very high electrical potential (say 50 kV.) and the filament transformer is necessary to provide sufficient insulation between the filament and the autotrans-former. The filament transformer must therefore be capable of withstanding the same magnitudes of kV. as does the H.T. transformer. The filament and H.T. transformer are usually contained, separately, in the same oil-filled tank. Although in principle it is possible to adjust the value of the filament current and so control the tube current by means of a variable tapping on the autotransformer, just as for the kV. adjustment, it is more normal to employ a series resistance (5) for this purpose. By changing the value of this resistance the temperature of the filament is controlled and hence control of the tube current (mA.) effected. Although the meter (6) measures the filament transformer primary current, since this is directly related to the tube mA. this meter can be used to indicate what the mA. will be during the exposure. The actual tube current which flows during the exposure can be measured directly by means of the meter (7) which is in series with the secondary winding of the H.T. transformer. Since this meter is at earth potential it can, like both the other meters, be positioned with safety on the X-ray unit control desk.

Making an Exposure.—By way of summary it is useful to consider the sequence of events involved in making a radiographic exposure:

1. Close the mains switch (11) which results in electric power being available at the autotransformer. In this simple circuit closing this switch also results in the filament being heated.

2. Adjust the filament control resistance (5) so that the meter (6) indicates that the required value of tube mA. will be obtained.

3. Adjust the kV. control (8) on the autotransformer until the P.R.V. meter (9) indicates that the required tube kV. will be obtained.

4. Close the switch (10). This connects the voltage supply through the H.T. transformer to the X-ray tube, and the production of X-rays starts. The actual value of the mA. passing is shown on the meter (7).

5. After the required time open the switch (10). This terminates the exposure.

6. Open the switch (11), which switches the unit off, in particular the tube filament.

Although the descriptions given in this chapter are those relevant to a diagnostic X-ray unit, in principle the above circuit and sequence of events apply equally to a therapy unit.

RECTIFICATION OF THE HIGH VOLTAGE

As indicated above, the X-ray tube is perfectly capable of acting as its own rectifier. However, it is usually only satisfactory to allow it to do so for low power units such as small mobile, dental, and portable units. The limitation is that if the X-ray tube is to act also as a rectifier, then its target must be kept at a comparatively low temperature and must not be allowed to rise to such a level that thermionic emission of electrons can occur from the target. This, clearly, limits the exposure (kV., mA.s.) which can be used and it is therefore usual to incorporate some extra system of rectification.

Half-wave Rectification—Circuit Description.—The simplest type of rectification is achieved by using the circuit illustrated in *Fig.* 205, and in which a rectifying valve

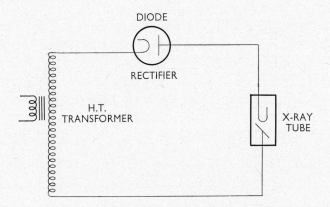

Fig. 205.—Basic half-wave rectification circuit.

is placed between the H.T. transformer and the tube to suppress the half of the voltage cycle which would make the filament the anode and the target the cathode. To understand how this comes about it will be helpful first to consider the way in which a diode valve functions.

The Diode Valve.—This device, shown diagrammatically in *Fig.* 206, consists of two electrodes—a filament and a 'plate'—sealed into an evacuated tube. When the filament is heated electrons are produced and, if the filament is the cathode of the circuit, these electrons will cross the valve to the plate, so that a current flows through the valve. On the other hand, if the polarity is reversed, and the filament becomes the anode, no current can flow across the valve so long *as no electrons are emitted by the plate*. The diode valve thus passes current in one direction only and can be used as a rectifier.

The pattern of the current flowing through the valve is shown in *Fig.* 207. The shape of this curve arises as follows. If the filament is heated, electrons are emitted and, if there is no field to remove them (no voltage across the valve), they form a cloud—or a 'space charge'—around the filament. When a voltage is applied across the valve so that the plate is the anode, some of the electrons from the space charge will be pulled across the valve, and therefore a current flows. The higher the voltage

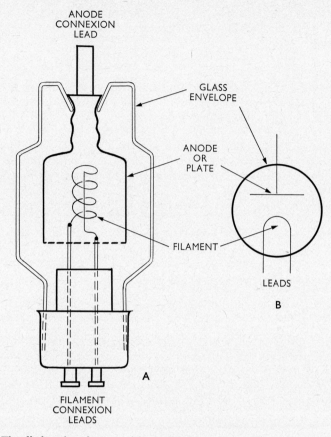

Fig. 206.—The diode valve, **A**, as used in an X-ray generator; **B**, as it appears in a circuit diagram.

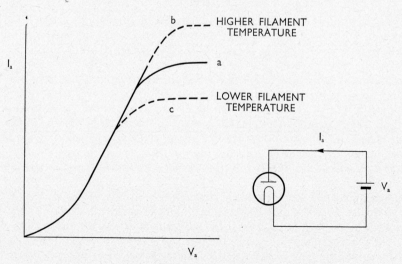

Fig. 207.—The variation of anode current with anode voltage.

the more electrons will be pulled over—the higher the current. In the rising part of the curve (a) the current is said to be 'space-charge limited'. Ultimately, however, the rate of removal of electrons is as great as the rate at which they are being produced from the filament, and no increase in the voltage across the tube will produce more. The current therefore reaches a maximum and the valve is said to be 'saturated'. The magnitude of the current in this region does not depend on the voltage across the valve but on the heating of the filament, i.e., the supply of electrons. (Curves for a lower (c) and higher (b) filament temperature are also shown in *Fig.* 207.) Therefore the current is said to be 'emission controlled' or 'temperature controlled'. The voltage at which saturation occurs increases as the filament temperature (tube saturation current) increases.

The Rectifying Valve and the X-ray Tube.—From the above it will be realized that the X-ray tube, as well as the rectifying valve, is a diode valve, but their operation as well as their function is quite different. For the X-ray tube high voltage is required to give the electrons a high energy for X-ray production. The rectifying valve is merely a one-way street, passing the current in one (appropriate) direction but passing none in the other.

The current through the X-ray tube (and hence the filament heating) must be exactly that needed to give the required X-ray output, no more, no less. The valve, on the other hand, must have emission much greater than is needed for this current. *Fig.* 208 shows the difference in characteristic curves of the tube and valve, and it

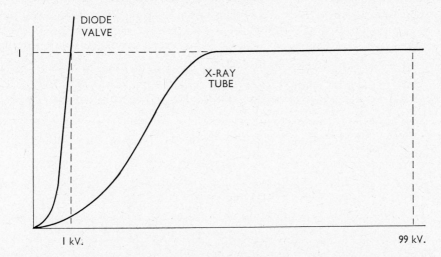

Fig. 208.—The characteristic curves of an X-ray tube and a valve, showing the currents at different voltages.

will be seen that the tube is working in the saturation or emission-controlled part of the curve whereas the valve is far from saturated. For example, if H.T. secondary voltage is 100 kV. the voltage across the valve will be about 1 kV. only, whereas that across the tube will be the remainder, namely 99 kV. During this forward half-cycle, therefore, the action of the circuit is almost completely independent of the presence of the valve.

On the reverse half-cycle the valve must pass no current in order to protect the tube whose inevitably warmed target may emit electrons and so allow a current to flow in the wrong direction. It is imperative that there should be no heating of the valve plate, which therefore has a large area (often blackened to encourage radiation heat loss) over which the electrons are allowed to spread as widely as possible, thus avoiding local heating. In any case, since the voltage across the valve in the forward half-cycle is low, the energy acquired by the electrons will be low and little heat will be produced. In the inverse half-cycle the sharing of the H.T. voltage is such that almost all the voltage is across the valve. The reason for this is that since the anode of the tube is warm during use there will be a small amount of thermionic emission from it. If there were a large voltage across the X-ray tube then an inverse current would start to flow. But since the anode of the valve is not heated there can be no passage of current through the valve. The bulk of the available voltage will therefore exist across the valve in an attempt to force a reverse current. This results in there being only a comparatively small voltage across the X-ray tube through which the inverse current does not, therefore, flow.

The desirable features of the valve are achieved by its having a large and adequately heated filament to provide a copious supply of electrons. If the filament emission in the valve is too small for any reason (such as inadequate filament size or insufficient heating) then the share of the voltage taken by the valve will be too great and that to the tube decreased accordingly. In addition, the electrons crossing the valve will gain more energy, produce more heat (and, in extreme cases, X-rays) at the anode, and thus cause the valve to fail as an efficient rectifier. Adequate emission in rectifier valves is an essential to the proper functioning of an X-ray set.

Voltage Wave Form.—In the self-rectified circuit current flows through the tube only during the forward half-cycle. *Fig.* 209 shows how the current and voltages vary with them. The voltage across the tube is the same as that across the transformer

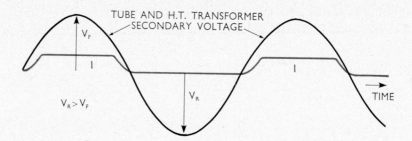

Fig. 209.—The voltage and current wave forms for a self-rectified circuit.

secondary coil. During the inverse half-cycle the voltage is greater than that in the forward half-cycle. The reduction in the forward cycle is due to transformer regulation which reduces the voltage to an extent depending upon the current flowing. This is zero in the inverse half-cycle.

In the case of the half-wave rectified circuit, the voltage across the X-ray tube during the forward half-cycle is slightly less than that across the transformer secondary due to the small voltage across the valve. This difference is negligible. In the inverse half-cycle the voltage across the tube is much less than that across the valve, which is almost equal to that across the secondary of the H.T. transformer. As for the self-rectified circuit the inverse transformer voltage is a little greater than the forward voltage. The inverse voltage across the valve is therefore usually greater than the forward voltage across the X-ray tube. *Fig.* 210 shows how the voltage across and current through the tube vary with time.

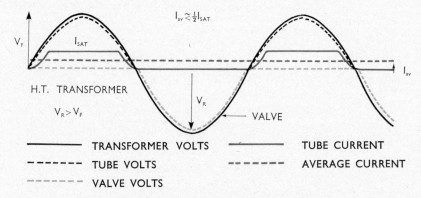

Fig. 210.—The wave forms with half-wave rectification.

For simplicity the shape of the current (I) curve has been idealized a little. At first as the voltage across the tube rises the tube current is space charge limited and is therefore much less than the saturation value. In the central portion of the half-cycle, when the voltage is high, the current is at the steady, saturation value, determined by the filament temperature.

The horizontal dotted line in *Fig.* 210 indicates the value read by the moving-coil meter connected at the centre point of the H.T. transformer secondary coil. Since this coil and the X-ray tube are in series the same current—the tube current—flows through both. The meter reads the *average* value of the current flowing over the whole cycle and can be seen to be less than the maximum current value. It is this average value which is referred to when tube current or mA. is quoted.

In some half-wave rectified circuits two valves are used, one on either side of the X-ray tube. The operation and function of this circuit are identical to the single-valve circuit. The only difference is that the inverse voltage is shared between the two valves, each of which therefore has only approximately half the total inverse voltage.

Full-wave Rectification.—The half-wave rectified circuit is inefficient both in the sense that some inverse voltage can exist across the X-ray tube but more especially because current flows and X-rays are produced during approximately only half the overall exposure time. The use of the full-wave rectifying circuit shown in *Fig.* 211 A eliminates some of these objections. Such a circuit is sometimes called a 'bridge' rectifier or Graetz circuit and is identical in operation with the circuit used to enable a moving-coil meter to be used for the measurement of alternating currents or voltages. This use is illustrated in *Fig.* 211 B, in which the common convention of drawing the rectifiers as thick arrows showing the direction of positive current flow is used.

The mode of operation of this four-valve circuit is as follows. During the half-cycle when the lower end of the transformer is positive, current flows through the valves (a) and (b) and through the X-ray tube. In this half-cycle the circuit is just like that of the two-valve half-wave circuit described above, almost all the transformer voltage being across the X-ray tube. Whilst valves (a) and (b) are conducting, valves (c) and (d) are not conducting, both of these having an inverse voltage equal to that of the X-ray tube forward voltage. During the next half-cycle when the lower end of the transformer is negative the roles of the valves are reversed: (c) and

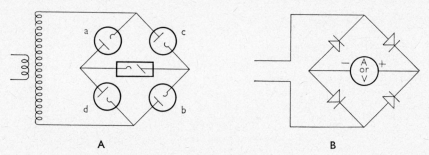

A

B

Fig. 211.—The full-wave rectification circuit, A, for an X-ray generator; B, for an A.C. meter.

(d) conduct whilst (a) and (b) are subjected to the full inverse voltage. The important feature is that the current flows through the X-ray tube in the same direction during both half-cycles, the *electron* current path during each half-cycle being shown in *Fig.* 212.

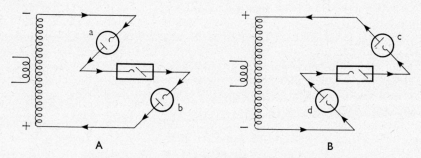

A

B

Fig. 212.—The electron paths in the four-valve circuit.

The operation and function of the valves and X-ray tube are exactly the same in this circuit as in the half-wave rectified circuit. The voltage and current wave forms associated with this circuit are shown in *Fig.* 213. They are much the same as for the self- and half-wave rectified circuit except that, of course, current flows and X-rays

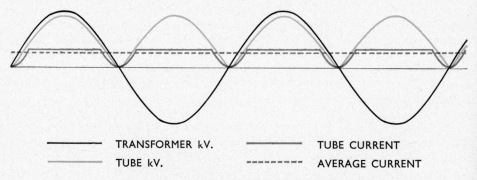

| ——————— | TRANSFORMER kV. | ——————— | TUBE CURRENT |
| ——————— | TUBE kV. | - - - - - - - | AVERAGE CURRENT |

Fig. 213.—The wave forms with full-wave rectification.

are produced during both half-cycles. The average current in this case is more nearly equal to the maximum current value. Since current flows during both half-cycles in different directions through the transformer the meter which registers this average current must be an A.C. meter. It is almost invariably a moving-coil meter, fitted with its own bridge rectifier circuit, as just described.

Three-phase Circuits.—In many modern units a three-phase electrical supply is used instead of the single-phase system so far assumed. The operation of such circuits is identical to those already described except that, since there are three phases rather than one, the circuits are at least three times more complicated!

A very simple version of a three-phase full-wave rectified circuit is shown in *Fig.* 214. The coils A, B, and C are, in fact, the three separate secondary windings

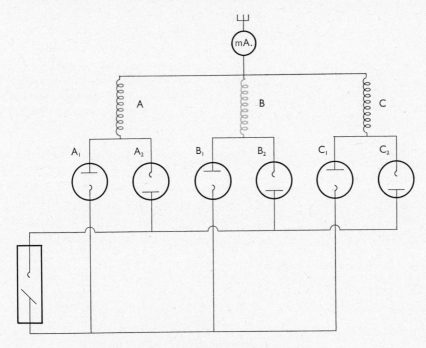

Fig. 214.—The three-phase circuit.

of the H.T. transformer which are required in a three-phase unit. There are also three primary windings but they are omitted from the diagram to avoid complicating it. The voltages existing in these windings A, B, and C are as shown in *Fig.* 215 and it can be seen that they are each out of phase with each other.

Consider that part of the cycle when the lower end of A is the most negative. During this part of the cycle the valve A_2 will conduct and so the voltage at the X-ray tube filament will be the same as that of the lower end of A. The same argument can be applied to those parts of the cycle when the lower ends of B and C are successively the most negative. The voltage of the X-ray filament is therefore given by the lower envelope of the three wave forms and is as shown in *Fig.* 216. Now consider that part of the cycle when the lower end of A is the most positive. During this part of the cycle when the valve A_1 will conduct, the voltage at the X-ray tube target will be the same as that of the lower end of A and similarly for those parts of the cycle in which the lower ends of B and C are most positive. The upper envelope of the wave forms (also shown in *Fig.* 216) thus gives the voltage at the target of the tube. The voltage between the filament and target is therefore given

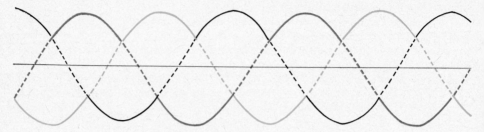

Fig. 215.—Voltage wave forms from a three-phase circuit.

by the separation of these two envelopes, i.e., by the separation along such lines as P_1, P_2, etc. The lower curve of *Fig.* 216 shows the wave form of this voltage between filament and target. It can be seen that the voltage is almost constant, having only a small ripple of frequency six times that of the input. The peak voltage is 1·732

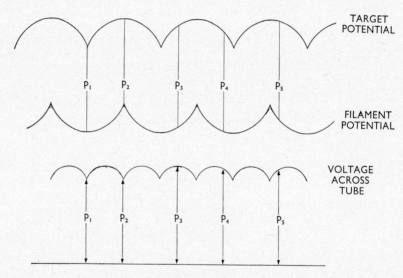

Fig. 216.—The wave forms of the target and filament potential and of the voltage across the X-ray tube.

(or $\sqrt{3}$) times as high as the peak voltage from the individual coils of the transformer. This is no real advantage since the peak inverse voltage across each valve, and which each valve has to withstand, is in turn also equal to this value.

Unlike the single-phase circuit the current through the X-ray tube is almost constant and the mean value measured by a moving-coil mA. meter is equal to this value. The meter is positioned in the circuit at the common end of the windings A, B, and C, which is earthed. It, of course, has to have its own three-phase rectifier circuit, which, to avoid complexity, is omitted from the circuit drawing.

Solid-state Rectifier.—Over the last decade thermionic diode valves have been gradually replaced by solid-state rectifiers. These consist of a multiple sandwich of two different, very pure materials, to which has been added a definite, but minute, amount of an 'impurity'. Such a sandwich behaves as a diode valve, in that it is easy for current to pass in one direction but very difficult for it to pass in the other direction. The material used was originally selenium but more recently silicon, a single sandwich of which can withstand about 300–400 V., has been employed.

It is now possible to produce a multiple sandwich in the form of a cylinder 1 cm. in diameter and 25 cm. long which can pass a forward current of 1000 mA. but which will withstand an inverse voltage of 150 kV. These solid-state rectifiers are much more robust than vacuum valves and are rather smaller. They do not need a filament heating supply and this is a real advantage since, as can be seen in *Figs.* 205 and 211, the valve filament can be at a high voltage, so that the valve filament transformer has to be able to withstand the full X-ray tube voltage. Since there is no filament to heat there is no power loss and the transformer tank is therefore cooler. There is a small amount of heat production in these rectifiers which leads to a limitation in the mA.s. which can be employed but this is not serious in practice.

For lower voltage (e.g., 230 V.) rectification, copper oxide has been in use for many years. It is this type which is used in the rectifier circuit for the moving-coil milliammeter referred to earlier in this chapter.

THE CONTROL OF VOLTAGE AND CURRENT SUPPLIES

Preselection of Tube Current.—Although the system of controlling the tube current (mA.) by adjusting a series resistance, until the primary filament current has the appropriate value, is a perfectly good one, it is not used in practice. The reason is that the variation in thermionic emission, and hence tube current, with change in filament temperature is very great, as shown by *Fig.* 217.

Because of this, the adjustment of filament current is very critical and must be done most carefully if radiographic exposures are to be comparable from occasion to occasion. It has been found preferable, and certainly more acceptable to most radiographers, to use a preset control for the tube current. The type used is illustrated in *Fig.* 218 and consists of a set of fixed resistors and a selector switch. The values of the resistors are chosen so that by selecting the appropriate position of the switch the required tube current will result. It is therefore possible to label the various positions of this switch with the tube current (mA.) which will result. This control is called the tube current selector. It can also be arranged for one of these selected positions to connect in a variable resistor and it is in this way that the 'free' control of the small tube current used in fluoroscopy is obtained, the control being adjusted until the direct-reading milliammeter (*Fig.* 204, Item 7) shows the desired value. Each of the resistors in the mA. selector can be adjusted (but not by the radiographer!) and in this way the manufacturer is able to ensure that the actual tube currents are what the selector switch dial indicates they should be. Since resistance values and/or the value of filament heating current required for a certain tube current are likely to change as the unit ages, a further resistance, R_6 (*Fig.* 218), is incorporated, which can be adjusted to compensate for such changes. It is also usual to insert a further special resistance in the circuit. This has a negative temperature coefficient and is there to compensate for any changes in the resistance value of the selected resistor which occurs as the temperature in the control desk changes.

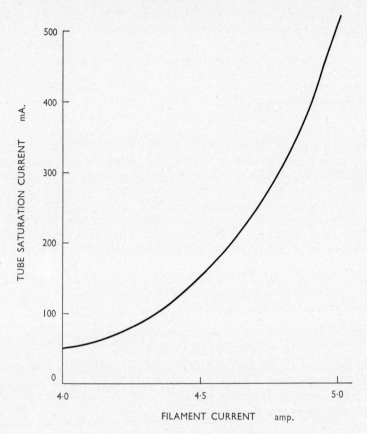

Fig. 217.—The variation of tube current (mA.) with filament heating current.

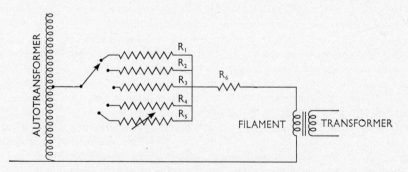

Fig. 218.—The tube current (mA.) selector circuit.

Filament Boost.—The evaporation of tungsten from the filament can be reduced and the tube life prolonged by keeping as small as possible the time during which the filament is fully heated. However, the filament takes a little while after the heating current has been switched on before it reaches its operating temperature, so that the heating current must be flowing before the exposure commences. A compromise solution is achieved by having an extra resistance in the filament circuit. When the unit is switched on this resistance restricts the current and the filament is only partially heated. As soon as the exposure 'prepare' button is pressed, this resistance is short-circuited and the filament quickly rises to full temperature. The exposure is then made.

The filament often continues to be fully heated until the exposure button is released. It is therefore important that there should be adequate but not undue delay between 'prepare' and 'expose' and that the exposure button be released immediately the exposure terminates. In this way the time for which the filament is at a very high temperature is minimized.

Preselection of Tube Kilovoltage.—Although continuously variable control of tube kV. is often available, the value of kV. obtained being read off a pre-reading meter, it is common practice to use a kV. selector. This consists of a multiposition switch, the terminals of which are connected to definite points in the autotransformer winding. This is illustrated in *Fig.* 219. The switch must be arranged so that it is

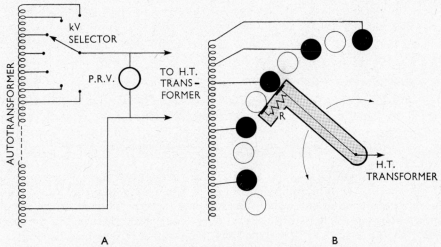

Fig. 219.—A, The kV. selector circuit. B, Detail of the anti-arcing contactor. The subsidiary contact maintains the circuit via the high resistance R as the main contact moves from one stud to the next.

not possible for it to be in contact with two adjacent studs at any one time otherwise a few turns of the autotransformer winding would be short-circuited, with disastrous results. Further, it is usually arranged for the circuit to be not broken completely as the switch is moved from one contact to another. One way of doing this is by means of the high resistance shown in *Fig.* 219, which is not functional when the switch is stationary on one of the contacts but which acts as a by-pass when the contact is being changed. A similar system is used in the filament selector. The voltage selector switch should not be changed during an exposure since it is not designed to switch on and off the huge currents which may be flowing. Fortunately such adjustment is not necessary.

Non-ideal Operation.—The description given so far in this chapter would be adequate if all the components operated in an ideal way. Unfortunately this is not the case and various, more or less complicated, circuit modifications have to be made to deal with departures from ideal operation. The features which have to be

11

dealt with fall into two groups. The first are associated with the X-ray unit itself and are conveniently called 'internal effects'. The others are associated with the fact that the electrical mains supply can vary and are referred to as 'external effects'.

Internal Effects.—There are two internal effects, the first due to the fact that the X-ray tube is not actually 'saturated' and the second to transformer 'regulation'.

1. *The X-ray Tube is not Fully Saturated.*—It has been stated that, in an X-ray tube, the current flowing is independent of the applied kV. and that the characteristic curve takes the form already shown in *Fig.* 208.

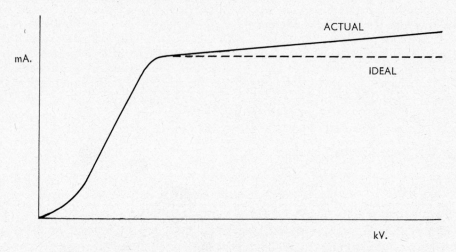

Fig. 220.—The ideal, and actual, variations of tube current with kV.

In practice there is always a slope on the 'saturation' part of the curve. As *Fig.* 220 shows, the tube current continues to rise a little as the kV. is increased. This is especially so at the higher values of mA., where, far from being 'emission limited', the X-ray tube is often space-charge controlled. This occurs to such an extent that at lower kV. it is sometimes not possible to obtain the higher mA. values which are possible at higher kV. Hence, although the mA. selector is set at a particular value, the actual tube current flowing will depend upon the applied kV. It is important to notice that the incorporation of a filament current meter is of no advantage here since this defect arises in spite of the fact that the filament heating current (and therefore filament temperature) is correct. It is a function of the X-ray tube construction.

The difficulty is solved by arranging, by suitable additions to the circuitry, for the filament temperature (current) to be increased at the lower kV. and decreased at the higher kV. A simple circuit for achieving this is shown in *Fig.* 221.★

Depending upon the position of the kV. selector a small voltage is inserted into the filament circuit via the transformer T_1. If a high kV. is selected the extra voltage opposes the existing current and so reduces the filament temperature and vice versa. The net effect, provided the transformer (T_1) ratio is properly chosen, is that the tube current remains constant as the kV. is changed. For example, the X-ray tube

---

★ In order to avoid undue complication the circuits used to overcome the various defects will be shown separately, as they would fit into the circuit of *Fig.* 204. In practice, of course, they become very intermingled.

changes from operation at point *A* (*Fig.* 222) to point *B* by a simultaneous increase in filament current when a smaller kV. is selected. The actual tube current remains constant at the desired value.

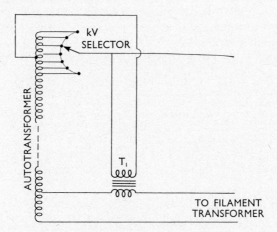

Fig. 221.—The saturation compensation circuit.

2. *The High-tension Transformer is not an Ideal One.*—Although the simple theory of the transformer shows the ratio of the output to input voltage to be determined by the turns ratio only, and, in particular, to be completely independent of

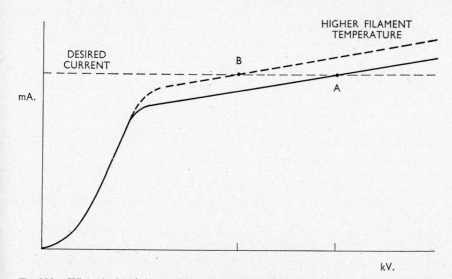

Fig. 222.—When the kV. is lowered, the filament heating has to be increased to allow the same mA. to be maintained.

the current flowing, this is not so in practice. Because of the resistance of the wires which constitute its windings the transformer suffers from inherent 'regulation'. This means that the value of the secondary voltage produced by the transformer depends to some extent upon the current flowing in the secondary, i.e., upon the tube current (mA.). As the current taken from the transformer is increased, then (even though the input voltage remains constant and the turns ratio is fixed) the secondary voltage will fall in value to an extent depending upon the current value.

The result of this is that, for a certain selected kV. (i.e., position of the selector switch at the autotransformer and therefore value of H.T. transformer input voltage), the actual kV. obtaining across the X-ray tube will depend upon the tube current (mA.). This is undesirable and a circuit of the type shown in *Fig.* 223 is used to

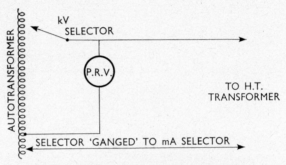

Fig. 223.—The 'regulation' compensation circuit.

combat the effect. The supply to the primary of the H.T. transformer is obtained by means of two tapped contacts to the autotransformer. The upper contact (*Fig.* 223) is the kV. selector previously described whilst the lower one is coupled, mechanically, to the mA. selector control. If a high mA. is selected then the primary voltage to the H.T. transformer obtained from the autotransformer is increased sufficiently to compensate for the transformer regulation, so that the desired secondary high tension is produced. If a low mA. is selected, the regulation effect will be less, and a corresponding lower voltage is obtained from the autotransformer. In this way the actual tube kV. is kept constant as different values of mA. are selected, in spite of the transformer regulation.

If a pre-reading kV. meter is used then it is connected as shown in *Fig.* 223, its reading being, as is desirable, independent of the mA. value selected.

In addition to transformer regulation there is a similar effect in the other components of the H.T. transformer primary and secondary circuits. For example, the voltage drop across any valves used to rectify the high tension will increase as the mA. increases. The same is true for any and all resistance components in the circuit. The solution illustrated in *Fig.* 223 can be used to compensate for all these 'regulation' type effects.

External Effects.—The external effects are all associated, in one way or another, with the fact that the various cables which connect the X-ray unit to the generator at the power station all have a finite resistance. This results in the voltage supply at the X-ray unit being variable due to a variable voltage loss in the cables brought about by the variable currents flowing in them. For example, assume that the total cable resistance is 0·5 ohm and that the generator produces a voltage of 240 V. If no current is flowing in the cables then the voltage at the X-ray unit will, of course, also be 240 V. But if a current of 100 A. is flowing, and this is quite a common occurrence, then the situation will be as illustrated in *Fig.* 224.

The voltage (Vg) at the generator is 240 V. but the voltage drop (Vd) in the cables will be given by the product of their resistance (r) and the current (I) flowing in them:

$$Vd = rI = 0.5 \times 100 = 50 \text{ V.}$$

The voltage Vm at the X-ray unit is, therefore,

$$240 - 50 = 190 \text{ V. only.}$$

If the current changes to 50 A. then the voltage at the X-ray unit will be 215 V., since only 25 V. will now be 'dropped' in the cables. Therefore it is quite obvious that

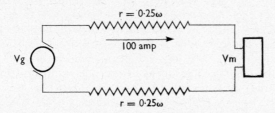

Fig. 224.—Cable voltage 'drop'.

changing current in the mains supply cables leads to changing voltages at the X-ray unit. There are two types of voltage changes, slow ones and rapid ones, and it is convenient to discuss them separately.

Slow Changes of Voltage Input.—The X-ray unit under consideration is not the only electrical equipment which is connected to the power station through the same substation and cables, so that the amount of electricity being used, and therefore current flowing, will vary throughout the day and from season to season. Most people are aware of the change in voltage which is likely to occur during the day as both domestic and industrial users change their demands. From their very nature these changes occur slowly and continuously and can therefore be noted and dealt with before the X-ray exposure commences. The most convenient way of dealing with this type of mains voltage variation is shown in *Fig.* 225.

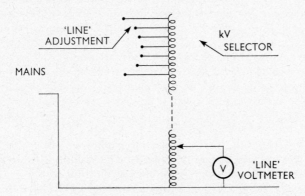

Fig. 225.—Manual 'line-voltage' compensation circuit.

One of the supply leads to the autotransformer is capable of adjustment and a meter is connected across a fixed number of turns. The basic need is that across each turn of the autotransformer there shall be a fixed voltage because, only in this way, can a selected number of turns (variable for the kV. circuit and fixed for the mA. circuit) give the correct voltage. The fundamental fact of a transformer is that the voltage across each and every turn is the same, and hence all that is required in order to achieve a constant voltage per turn is to adjust the number of turns across which the mains supply voltage is fed in. The moving contact enables this to be done. If the mains voltage is high then the number of turns selected must also be high and vice versa. The meter indicates when the adjustment has been made correctly. Since all that is required is that the meter shall measure a constant voltage across a fixed number of turns, this meter usually does not have a scale; it has only a single line (sometimes edged by a line on either side). This control is called the *line-voltage control* and the meter the *line voltmeter*. Before the exposure is made the control is adjusted until the meter pointer is on the line (or between the two lines). It is then known that the input voltages to the H.T. primary and the filament transformer are those intended.

In some units this manual adjustment of the line-voltage control by the radiographer is not required. In such units the control is effected automatically. The line voltmeter is replaced by an electrical or electronic unit which detects the departure of this voltage from what it should be and on the basis of this operates a motor which moves the line-voltage control to the correct position.

Rapid Changes of Voltage Input.—In addition to these slow changes of mains voltage, more sudden ones can occur. The example usually quoted is of a lift in the hospital, the operator of which takes a perverse delight in using the lift just as the radiographer starts her exposure! Like many other types of equipment, a lift takes a very large current especially when starting from rest and if such a piece of apparatus is connected to the same supply cable and is used during exposure, clearly, a large fall in supply voltage to the X-ray unit will result. The type of compensator referred to above is useless in this case since neither the manual compensation by the radiographer nor the automatic compensation can be done quickly enough, especially if the exposure time is small. In any case the radiographer should be observing the patient not the line voltmeter during the exposure.

Although a fall in supply voltage will result in a fall of both kV. and mA., it is particularly important for the mA. As has already been shown in *Fig.* 217 a small change in filament current (and therefore filament temperature) causes a disproportionate change in tube current, whereas for the kV. the change is exactly proportional to any change in supply voltage. It is therefore normal practice to accept the (unfortunate but not disastrous) change in kV. which results from any sudden change in supply voltage but to provide a special circuit which will maintain the filament current at its correct value in spite of such changes. The filament current is said to be stabilized. The device used is called a 'filament current stabilizer' and there are two common types:

  a. *The Static Stabilizer.*—This, as its name implies, is a device without any moving parts which is able to operate almost instantaneously and so effect compensation for very rapid changes in input voltage. It consists of a specially designed transformer circuit which has the very useful property that its output voltage remains constant even when the input voltage to it is changed over quite a wide range of values. Its other name is a 'constant-voltage transformer' and it is incorporated into the filament current supply circuit between the autotransformer and the filament current selector.

Although the static stabilizer automatically compensates for changes in input voltage it, unfortunately, makes the system frequency dependent. In other words, unlike the ordinary transformer, the constant-voltage transformer has an output voltage which depends upon the frequency of the electrical supply. In practice frequency changes are not common, but some units are fitted with a manually operated frequency compensator which works rather like the line-voltage compensator described above. Alternatively, a second static device (which uses a resonant circuit) is used to effect frequency compensation automatically. It must be emphasized that the necessity for frequency compensation in X-ray units arises only because the static stabilizer is frequency dependent.

b. *The Electronic Stabilizer.*—In this type of filament current stabilizer the filament voltage is used to control an electronic system which automatically adjusts the filament voltage (if not correct) to the correct value. Such a system is not frequency dependent and so no frequency compensation circuit is required.

The On-load Effect.—Even if all the external mains supply voltage variations have been eliminated, or compensated for, there is still the effect which results from the very large current drawn by the X-ray unit itself during the actual exposure. This results in a reduction in the supply voltage to the X-ray unit so that even if everything else is satisfactory before the exposure, it will not be during the exposure! It is useful to consider an actual example. Consider the case when the X-ray unit is being used to make an exposure at 80 kVp and 250 mA.

The H.T. transformer turns ratio is therefore given by:

$$\text{Turns ratio} = \frac{\text{Output voltage (R.M.S.)}}{\text{Input voltage (R.M.S.)}} = \frac{80,000 \div \sqrt{2}}{240} = 236.$$

The current in the primary is therefore given by:

$$\text{Primary current} = \text{secondary current} \times \text{turns ratio}$$

$$= (250/1000) \times 236$$

$$= 59 \text{ A., approximately.}$$

If the mains cable resistance is 0·5 ohm, such a current would cause a reduction of about 30 V. in the supply voltage. Such a reduction will, clearly, result in the kilovoltage and tube current (particularly the latter) being much smaller than intended.

The manufacturer realizes that it is impossible to have a mains supply of zero resistance so he assumes that it will be, say, 0·5 ohm. The apparatus is then designed on this basis. For example, the kV. selector position is set so that when used with this mains resistance the kV. will be as stated on the control. This can be done accurately for one particular setting of kV. and current only, but by slight compromise and by modification of the transformer regulation compensator it can be arranged that, for all current (mA.) settings, the kV. value is as selected. If an installation has a mains resistance less than 0·5 ohm a resistor is added to bring the total to the assumed value of 0·5 ohm. It is for this reason that the manufacturer states the maximum acceptable mains resistance, since should the resistance exceed the assumed value nothing can be done about it in the unit.

Some units are in fact fitted with selector switches to allow for changing the value of the added resistor. This is useful for, say, a mobile unit, which is to be used in a ward where the total mains resistance can be much greater than in the main department. In such an event a suitably smaller added resistance, appropriate to the individual ward, can be selected.

Filament Current Changes.—Although such compensation is satisfactory for the kV. circuit it is unsuitable for the valve filament circuit. Clearly, if the settings are made so that they will be correct during the exposures when the voltage drop exists, then before or after the exposure the filament current, and therefore the filament temperature, will be too high. This puts an unnecessary strain on the filament and therefore for the filament circuit a different method is used.

A supplementary transformer is added in series with that part of the autotransformer which supplies the filament current. The action of this added transformer is to boost the voltage to an extent which depends on the current flowing through the X-ray tube. By suitable design this boost can be arranged to exactly compensate the 'on-load' fall in voltage.

The tube filament current is maintained constant, in spite of the 'on-load' input voltage drop, by either the static or electronic stabilizers mentioned above.

Stabilization of Tube Current.—It has been described above how great effort is made in order to keep the filament current constant in spite of changes in voltage supply. This is being done in order that the tube mA. shall be accurately that selected. Such stabilization has to be very good in view of the great dependence of thermionic emission on filament temperature. Even when perfect stabilization is achieved the tube current is not necessarily as required because of the non-saturation effect and, hence, dependence of mA. on kV. All these difficulties can be overcome by stabilization of the tube current directly. If the actual value of tube current is fed into an electronic system, the output of which is used to control the filament current (rather like the electronic filament stabilizer mentioned above), then the tube current would be that selected, no matter whether any main voltage change occurs or not, or whether the kV. selection is changed or not. Such a system is not without its own difficulties. For instance, at very short exposure times, the system hardly has time to act before the exposure is over. Fairly recent developments have shown that it is possible to effect direct stabilization of tube current in this way even down to quite small exposure times, especially if the unit is also fitted with an automatic mains voltage compensator which ensures that the filament is correctly heated at the start of the exposure.

Which system is used to obtain correctly the required mA. depends upon the manufacturer, many of whom still prefer to use the indirect method of filament current stabilization.

TIMING THE EXPOSURE

The successful use of circuits of the type described above means that during the exposure the kilovoltage across the X-ray tube, and the current flowing through it, will have the values selected. All that remains now is to ensure that suitable switches are included in the circuit which enable the exposure to be started and then terminated after the required time. There are several types of timer used and these will now be described briefly. The simplest type is that which operates by clockwork. The setting of the required time on the dial of the timer simultaneously winds up a spring. When the exposure switch on the timer is pressed a contact is closed and the exposure starts. Under the action of the spring the timer dial rotates from its original setting back towards zero, reaching the latter position when the set time has expired. A second pair of contacts which terminate the exposure are operated as the timer reaches zero and in this way the desired exposure time is achieved. Such a simple timer is often found on mobile or portable sets which, because of their low output, are usually operated at long exposure times. Such a simple timer is not capable of operating with sufficient accuracy at low exposure times, so for this and other reasons it is not suitable for use in the high-power units used in X-ray departments.

The Synchronous Timer.—The synchronous timer was, until recently, the most common type of timer used. In action it is very similar to the simple spring timer already described and, in principle, works as follows. It consists of an electric motor (*M*) which rotates at a constant speed determined by the frequency of the electric mains (50 cycles per second in Great Britain). Such a motor is called a synchronous motor (*Fig.* 226). Attached to the motor shaft through a system of gears (*G*) there

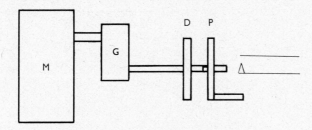

Fig. 226.—The synchronous timer.

is a disk (*D*) which is revolving continuously at the rate of about 1 revolution in 10 sec. Opposite to this disk there is a second one (*P*) which is also capable of rotation. Fastened to this second disk there is an arm, which, when the disk is at the zero position, closes a switch which operates the contact which terminates the exposure. The setting of the exposure time on the timer dial results in this second disk (*P*) and therefore the arm being rotated back through an angle proportional to the time set. When the exposure button is pressed the contact which starts the exposure is closed and simultaneously the two disks (*D* and *P*) are brought into contact (usually by one of them sliding along its shaft under the action of an electro-magnet which is omitted from the diagram). The second disk is hence rotated at the same speed as that of the first disk. As soon as the zero time position is reached (i.e., after a time equal to the exposure time) the arm on the disk activates the contactor which terminates the exposure and also uncouples the two disks. Such a timer can be used quite satisfactorily down to about 0·04 or 0·02 sec. but, of course, since it has to be reset after each exposure, it is not very convenient if rapid, serial exposures are to be made.

The Electronic Timer.—The simple circuit shown in *Fig.* 227 A forms the basis of the usual electronic timer. Initially the condenser is completely uncharged because the switch is closed. On opening the switch current flows through the resistance and charges up the condenser. The voltage across the condenser therefore increases with the passage of time in the way shown in *Fig.* 227 B which, incidentally, is an example of an exponentially rising quantity rather than the more familiar exponential fall. The three different curves, which are all of the same shape, are for different values of resistance and/or capacitance. It can be seen that in all three cases the final voltage achieved is equal to the voltage of the battery but that the time taken to reach both this voltage or any other voltage (V_o) depends upon the choice of resistance and capacitance values. The rate of the rise is, in fact, controlled by the product $R \times C$. For example, curve 1, which refers to a small value of RC, shows

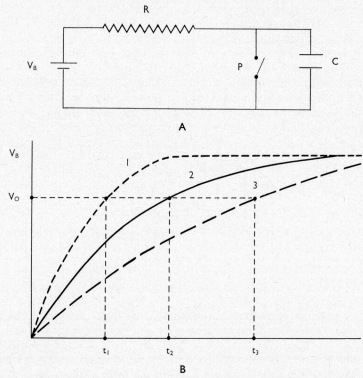

Fig. 227.—The electronic timer. A, Basic circuit; B, Exponential rise of voltage in it.

the chosen voltage V_o to be achieved in a small time t_1 whereas curve 3 shows how a much longer time t_3 is required when the value of RC is high.

Clearly if it can be arranged that the condenser is allowed to start to charge up (i.e., the switch opened) at the start of the exposure and the exposure is terminated as soon as the condenser reaches the voltage V_o, then such a circuit can be used to control the radiographic exposure time. A simple version of the circuit used is shown in *Fig.* 228.

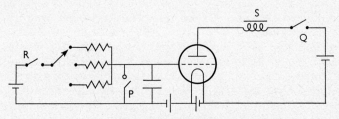

Fig. 228.—An electronic timer circuit.

The valve is what is known as a gas-filled triode, or thyratron, and is chosen because it is able to act as a switch. Whilst the grid is sufficiently negative no current is able to flow through the valve, in spite of the fact that there is a voltage between its cathode and anode. If, however, the grid is progressively made less negative then, suddenly, at one particular voltage, the valve will start to pass current. This current will continue to flow, no matter how the grid voltage is now changed, until the anode voltage is removed. The circuit works in the following way. Before the exposure starts the condenser is uncharged (because the switch P is closed) and the grid is negative. In this state no current flows through the valve. When the exposure button is pressed the switch P is opened and simultaneously switches Q and R are closed. The condenser therefore starts to charge up at a rate controlled by the resistance selected. The voltage so produced across the condenser is such as to make the grid progressively less negative. After the selected time the voltage on the grid will be such as suddenly to allow the valve to pass current. The passage of this current through its coil operates the relay (S) and terminates the exposure. When the exposure button is released, the switch P is closed and Q and R opened, thus automatically resetting the timer ready for the next exposure. Such a timer can obviously therefore be used in rapid serial work.

In the circuit three alternative values of resistance are shown which will therefore allow one of three different exposure times to be selected. In practice, of course, a very large range of different resistance values is available and what happens when the timer is set at a particular value is that a resistance is selected so that the product RC corresponds to the exposure time desired.

The Milliampere-second (mA.s.) Timer.—Although much effort is put into achieving the desired mA. and exposure time separately this is not, in truth, really necessary. For any particular X-ray tube and kV. the radiation exposure is controlled by the product of the tube current and time, viz. the 'mA.s.'. Hence, if the mA. is not quite that intended the error can be compensated by a slight change in exposure time. The mA.s. timer does this automatically and in fact terminates the exposure as soon as the desired mA.s. has passed through the tube. The circuit used is very similar to that used in the electronic timer already described. In this case the current which charges up the condenser is the actual tube current, the exposure being terminated as soon as the chosen charge (mA.s.) has passed through the X-ray tube and into the condenser.

A simple version of the circuit used is shown in *Fig.* 229. The valve conducts as soon as the positive voltage generated across the condenser is sufficient to oppose the negative voltage set on the potentiometer *PT*. Clearly the mA.s. value at which this occurs and the exposure terminated can be varied by changing the setting of the potentiometer *PT*; if it is set towards the point *a*, then the mA.s. will be small and if set towards *b*, the mA.s. will be large. This potentiometer is the *mA.s. selector*.

The Photo-timer.—In this type of timer the actual amount of radiation transmitted through the patient to the film is measured, and used to terminate the exposure. In the timers previously described the radiographer has to consider what values of kV. and mA.s. to use in order to achieve the film density desired. The selection clearly depends upon the site and size of the patient. If, however, the radiation transmitted through to the film is measured then a single setting of the 'timer' should be sufficient for all patients irrespective of size and site. The electronic circuit is exactly as for the mA.s. timer but the current which charges up the condenser is, in this case, obtained in the manner shown in *Fig.* 230.

Behind (or in front of) the cassette there is a small fluorescent screen from which light proportional to the incident X-ray intensity is emitted. This light then generates, in the photo-cell, a current which is fed to the timer. The total charge which passes is directly proportional to the dose of X-rays falling on the fluorescent screen and can therefore be used to terminate the exposure as soon as the exposure is sufficient.

This type of timer is in common use in mass miniature radiography.

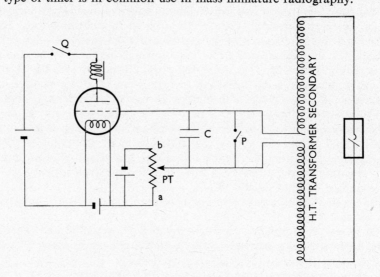

Fig. 229.—The milliampere-second (mA.s.) timer.

The Ionization Chamber Timer.—This timer differs from the photo-timer only in that the X-ray exposure is monitored by means of an ionization chamber. A thin, uniform, parallel plate ionization chamber is built into the cassette tray system so

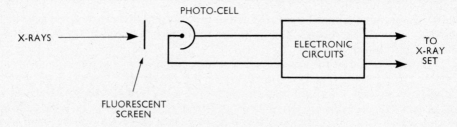

Fig. 230.—The basic photo-timer circuit.

that it is between the film and the pateint. As previously, the charge which passes from the chamber to the timer condenser is proportional to the X-ray dose. It is usual to have two or three alternative chambers positioned in different parts of the X-ray field for use in different types of radiographic technique.

When either the photo or the ionization chamber type of timer is being used then it should not be necessary to change the settings. Since the exposure is controlled by the radiation reaching the film a single setting should suffice for all patients and techniques. In practice it is found preferable to have a small range of different settings available for different techniques, sites, film sensitivities, and film densities that have to be dealt with. With the mA.s. timer, of course, an individual setting must be made for each occasion because of the variation in the patient. With all these timers (mA.s., photo, and ionization) variations in mA. which may occur during the exposure, or departures, for any reason whatever, from the selected mA., will have no effect on the final film density.

Starting and Stopping the Exposure.—The exposure is almost invariably started and stopped by switching on, and then off, the kilovoltage at the X-ray tube. The one exception to this is that some modern X-ray tubes have a grid which can be used to control the flow of current through the tube. In most equipment mechanically acting switches are used to make and break the primary circuit of the H.T. transformer. Separate switches are used for the 'make' (ON) and 'break' (OFF).

The 'break' switch is normally closed and the 'make' switch is normally open. When the exposure button is pressed the 'make' switch closes, H.T. is supplied to the tube, and the exposure starts. The filament of the tube is already at the required temperature since it is boosted at the 'prepare' position of the exposure button.

After the desired time (determined by the timer) the 'break' switch is opened, the kV. is removed from the tube, and the exposure stops. Simultaneously the filament boost circuit switch opens and the filament temperature falls to the standby value.

The switches referred to above are in fact contacts operated via relays which are themselves activated by the various buttons and switches on the control unit. There are several reasons for using relays for this work.

1. The value of the current flowing is very high (typically 50 or 100 A.) and the switch contacts have to be suitably designed to be able to switch on and off such large currents. It is usual to arrange for the contact to close (or open) at that time in the A.C. cycle when the current flowing is at zero. Such switching is called zero phase switching.

2. It can easily be arranged for one relay to open (or close) several different, isolated contacts either simultaneously or in a precise predetermined order. For example, the relay operated by the 'prepare' button boosts the filament and also sets the anode rotating at full speed.

3. The relay (and the contacts) can be positioned in the most convenient or appropriate place and not necessarily in the control unit. For example, the actual switches which start and terminate the exposure are usually in the H.T. transformer tank, remote from the control unit and operating buttons.

CHAPTER XXIV

THE RATING OF THE X-RAY TUBE

As described in earlier chapters, the optimum radiograph results from the correct choice of the various exposure factors and, in particular, the choice of kilovoltage, tube current (mA.), exposure time, and focal spot size. Unfortunately, this choice is not completely free and there are restrictions set by the detailed properties of the X-ray tube and its associated generator. As far as the generator is concerned there is little to be described. It will have been designed to work over a stated range of kilovoltage, up to a maximum value which is usually about 100 kV. for a small or mobile unit and between 125 and 150 kV. for a major unit. The generator will also be capable of delivering up to a certain maximum current (mA.) usually somewhere between 500 to 1000 mA. (viz., one-half to one amp.!). These maximum values are fixed by the detailed design of the voltage generator unit and, apart from needing to make sure at the time of the initial purchase of the X-ray unit that they are adequate (but not unnecessarily excessive) for the envisaged usage, they need be of no further concern to the radiographer.

The restrictions which arise because of the X-ray tube are, however, very much the daily concern of the radiographer and, in theory at least, due attention must be paid to them when each and every exposure is made.

Depending upon the kilovoltage, exposure time, and focal spot size selected there is an upper limit to the value of tube current (mA.) which may be then used.

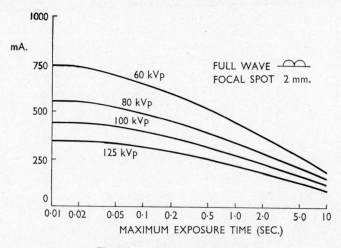

Fig. 231.—A typical rating chart.

This is referred to as the 'rating'. In addition, there is a limitation to the rate at which exposures may be repeated. Information about these restrictions is contained in what is known as the rating chart (*Fig.* 231) together with various associated

318

graphs (*Figs*. 243 and 246), all of which are supplied for each tube by the manufacturer. Although these charts are based upon fundamental physical aspects of X-ray tube function and design, it must be clearly understood that, in the end, the charts are empirical. The various values contained in them are the values which the manufacturers have found, from years of experience, to yield safe and satisfactory operating conditions.

In general terms 'rating' is concerned with the maximum rate at which radiation can be obtained from an X-ray tube and for how long it can be continued at this rate. This chapter will explain, though not in very great detail, the physical basis of the rating charts and indicate briefly how they should be used. There are two features from which the restrictions arise,

    a. Electrical,
    b. Thermal (or heating),
and both are taken into account in the rating chart.

ELECTRICAL RATING

The electrical limitations are fairly straightforward but, although they are implicit in the rating charts supplied with each tube, they are not often mentioned specifically. They must not, however, be forgotten.

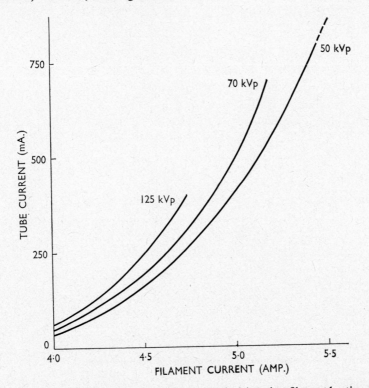

Fig. 232.—Characteristic curves for X-ray tube current (mA.) against filament heating current.

1. Maximum Kilovoltage.—The insulation of the X-ray tube and its oil-filled shield will have been designed to be adequate up to a specified maximum voltage, which should not be exceeded. This maximum value will usually be rather less than the full voltage of which the generator is capable although it is common practice to limit the maximum setting of the kV. control to the maximum permissible kV. for the tube.

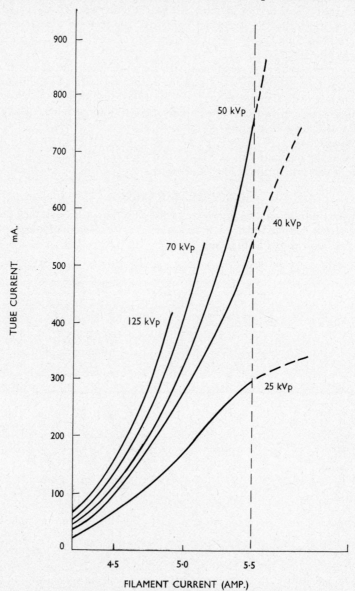

Fig. 233.—Characteristic curves showing limitation of tube current due to there being a maximum permissible filament heating current.

2. Maximum mA.—Although for any particular exposure there is a maximum permissible tube current set by conditions to be discussed later, there is an additional limitation arising from the nature of the voltage-current (saturation curve) characteristic of the tube. As described in CHAPTER XXIII the X-ray tube does not, in practice, operate under simple saturation conditions, which means that the tube current is controlled by both the filament heating current (filament temperature) and the tube kilovoltage (*Fig.* 232). The magnitude of this dependence of tube current on kV. increases markedly at low kV. and high mA. As was described in CHAPTER XXIII the lack of saturation is compensated for, and the tube current kept at the selected value, by increasing the filament heating at the lower kV. There is, however, an upper limit to the filament heating current since if the filament is heated to too high a temperature unacceptable evaporation of tungsten, filament distortion and, in the limit, melting will occur. There is therefore a maximum tube current (determined by this maximum permitted filament current), the value of which becomes smaller as the tube kV. is reduced (*Fig.* 233). It is for this reason that the rating chart (*Fig.* 234) shows maximum currents of about 550 mA. and 300 mA. at 40 and 25 kV. respectively whereas at 60 kV. more than 700 mA. is permitted. This effect, being

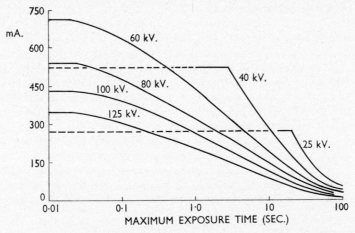

Fig. 234.—Rating chart showing low maximum current at low kV.

due to the voltage-current characteristic, is determined by the detailed structure and construction of the tube filament, the larger filament having the larger maximum mA. Larger filaments are, of course, associated with larger focal spot sizes (and vice versa), and it would thus appear from the rating charts that this maximum mA. depends upon the focal spot size. This is not true since the focal spot size, as such, has nothing to do with this effect. There is a dependence of maximum mA. on focal spot size which arises because of target heating and which is discussed later. The present limitation is, however, an overriding one and leads to the type of situation illustrated in *Fig.* 234.

3. Maximum Power.—It will also be noted in *Fig.* 232 that each curve stops at a certain value of tube current and that this value decreases as the kV. increases. In fact, the product of the kV. and the maximum mA. is approximately constant for any given tube and focal spot size. This product is, of course, proportional to the power (since power is proportional to kV. × mA.) and this restriction in tube current is thus seen to be really a restriction of power. Its value represents the maximum power which can be directed on to the anode, even for the shortest time without it melting. It is not a specific filament limitation although it is shown on the filament characteristic curves and is, in fact, a thermal limitation. In practice this restriction is of no great importance since, as is described below, other thermal considerations restrict the tube to smaller power values than this.

THERMAL RATING

As has already been stated, the generation of X-rays involves the simultaneous production of a considerable amount of heat and it is this heat which constitutes the most important limitation encountered in day-to-day radiography. Before considering how the limitation arises and the factors upon which it depends it is worth while recalling the principal factors involved in the making of a successful exposure and, therefore, radiograph. They are:

1. An exposure of sufficient magnitude and penetration so that the desired film blackening is produced.
2. An exposure time sufficiently small so that movement unsharpness is acceptable.
3. An effective focal spot size which is small enough to make the geometric unsharpness acceptable.

It has been stated in earlier chapters that, in selecting the exposure factors based on these requirements, a compromise is sometimes necessary because of the production of heat at the target. The circumstances in which a compromise must be made can be identified, for any given situation, from the rating charts (*see* example on p. 338).

Heat Produced.—The first of the requirements stated above dictates the milliampereseconds and kilovoltage which have to be used, since both control the Exposure (mR), and the kilovoltage also controls the penetrating power of the radiation. This requirement therefore dictates the energy passing to the X-ray target since energy $\propto$ kV. $\times$ mA. $\times$ seconds. Because only less than 1 per cent of this energy is converted into X-radiation, it also represents the amount of heat produced at the target. In order to understand the problem presented by the heating, it is interesting to calculate how much heat is produced in a typical exposure. If the kilovoltage is 100 kVp and the current 200 mA. the power dissipated, in full-wave operation, is:

$$\text{Power} = \text{volts} \times \text{amps} = \frac{1}{\sqrt{2}} (100 \times 1000) \times (200/1000)$$

$$= 14{,}200 \text{ watts} = 14 \cdot 2 \text{ kW.,}$$

the kilovoltage being assumed sinusoidal and the current constant. This means that heat is being generated at the X-ray tube target at the same rate as by fourteen single-bar electric fires! Fortunately the time for which this happens is small but even so the heat generated is considerable. If, for instance, the exposure time is 0·1 sec., the total heat produced is:

$$14{,}200 \times 0 \cdot 1 = 1420 \text{ joules} \quad \text{or} \quad \text{approximately 350 calories,}$$

which is enough to bring to the boil $3\frac{1}{2}$ ml. of water (in one-tenth of a second!).

If an exposure time shorter than 0·1 sec. is needed because of the second requirement then the mA. would have to be increased in proportion, the total mA.s. remaining constant. The same amount of heat would thus be produced but more quickly.

Temperature Rise.—If the third requirement calls for a small focal spot, then the heat will be produced over a small part of the target and the temperature rise will be greater than if the same heat were spread over a larger area. If this rise is excessive, then the target surface will be damaged and function of the tube impaired as described in CHAPTER XXII. If the temperature rises very high it may exceed the melting point of tungsten and considerable roughening of the target surface will occur. This means that for subsequent exposures the radiation output will be reduced.

Furthermore, excessive increase in temperature can lead to distortion of the rotating anode (either of the disk or of the shaft or bearing) which would result in a wobbling focal spot, giving the radiographic appearance of a focal spot very much larger than that intended. Even if the temperature does not exceed the melting point some general roughening of the target surface can be produced, in addition to evaporation of tungsten from the target.

It should be pointed out that these effects do not usually happen suddenly and spectacularly (except in the case of an extreme excessive overloading of the tube), but progressively over long periods of time (months or even years). Even when used correctly, all X-ray tubes slowly deteriorate in this way and what is observed, if it is looked for, is a slow and steady decrease in radiation output coupled with a deterioration in radiograph sharpness.

Cooling of the Target.—Clearly, if these effects are to be avoided or, at least, minimized, there is an upper limit to the rise in temperature which can be permitted. If no cooling of the target occurs then, irrespective of exposure time, the permitted mA.s. would depend only on the focal spot size and the kV. This means that the maximum mA.s. would be higher for large focal spots and lower for small ones: the maximum mA.s. would also be lower for high kV. and higher for low kV. If the exposure time were large the mA. would need to be correspondingly small and for short times the currents would be larger. The maximum amount of radiation produced during an exposure would therefore be the same for all exposure times and the rating chart would have the form shown in *Fig.* 235 A. In such circumstances there would, clearly, be no advantage in using long exposure times.

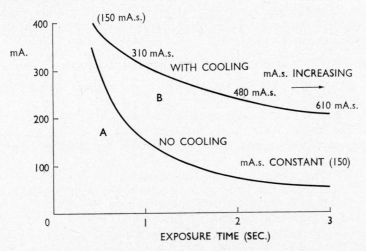

Fig. 235.—Idealized rating chart: (A) with no cooling of target, (B) with cooling.

Fortunately, even at the very small exposure times sometimes used, there is, as described in CHAPTER XXII, some cooling of the focal spot area by conduction into other regions of the target and by radiation. There is thus a flow of heat away from the target surface simultaneously with the production of heat in it. This means that, for the same rise in temperature, there can be a greater amount of heat production (i.e., larger mA.s.) than could be tolerated if no simultaneous cooling were to occur. The amount of cooling which can occur during the exposure is clearly greater

if the exposure time is greater and the net result is that, for the same rise in temperature of the target surface, the maximum mA.s. is greater at the larger exposure
times (*Fig.* 236). The maximum mA. still decreases as the exposure time increases

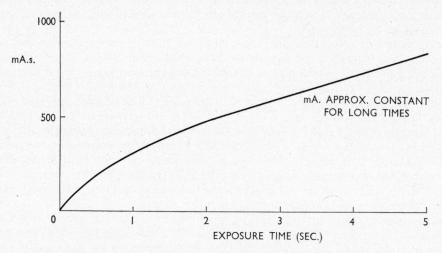

Fig. 236.—Increase of the maximum permitted mA.s. with exposure time.

but to a smaller extent than would be the case in the absence of cooling. The difference, as shown in *Fig.* 235, is very large and is the reason why a progressively much
greater amount of X-rays can be obtained from an X-ray tube if increasingly larger
exposure times are used.

FACTORS WHICH CONTROL RATING

Although, strictly speaking, the kilovoltage and milliampereseconds are both
involved in the problem of the loading of the X-ray tube, 'rating' is usually taken
to be synonymous with the maximum tube current, in mA., that can be used under
the stated conditions. What factors influence rating? Exposure time has already
been discussed to some extent, and will be returned to after some of the other factors
have been considered.

Tube Kilovoltage.—It has already been indicated that it is the product of kV.
and mA.s. which determines the rating. Thus if the kV. is increased the maximum
mA. must be proportionately decreased. For example, for a particular tube, focal
spot size, and exposure time the ratings at 100 kV. and at 60 kV. are 300 and 500 mA.
respectively. This linear relationship holds for all exposure times and focal spot sizes.

It must be remembered, however, that, since radiation output from the target is
proportional to the square of the kV., and the effect of the radiation at the film proportional to the cube (or even fourth power) of the kV., even though any increase
in kV. will necessitate an exactly proportional decrease in mA. the radiation output
and effect at the film will be greater for the increased kV.–decreased mA. combination.
For example, although exposures of 55 kV., 100 mA.s., and 65 kV., 85 mA.s.
are both at the maximum rating for a particular X-ray tube, focal spot size, and
exposure time the latter will result in a much greater blackening of the film. In this
sense, therefore, it can be said that the rating (although not the mA.) is greater at
the higher kV.

Focal Spot Size.—The focal spot is the area over which the heat is produced so that the larger the focal spot the greater is the tube current which can be used without producing an unacceptable temperature rise. It is commonly stated that the maximum power is 200 W. per square millimetre of *actual* focal spot area. This corresponds to about 6 kW. for a 3 × 3 mm. effective focal spot stationary anode tube. Such a tube is referred to as a 6-kW. tube. The value of 200 W. per sq.mm. is only approximate and depends upon the actual size and shape of the focal spot area: in any case it applies only to exposure times shorter than about 1 sec.

It has already been pointed out in CHAPTER XXII that the rating of a rotating anode tube is much greater than that of a stationary anode tube, since, for the same effective focal spot size, the area actually bombarded by electrons (the actual focal spot) is much greater in the rotating than in the stationary anode tube.*

Since the heat is spread over the focal spot area it might be expected that the maximum current would be proportional to that area, but in fact it is more approximately proportional to the linear size. For example, the maximum current at 90 kV., 0·1 sec. exposure is 370 mA. for a 1·2-mm.-square focal spot and 640 mA. for a 2-mm.-square spot. This is because some cooling takes place sideways from the heated area and the extent of this depends on the periphery of the area, which in its turn depends on the linear dimensions. For very small focal spots the size of the periphery and therefore the extent of the sideways cooling are small so that the maximum mA. is now more controlled by the area than by the linear dimensions. Thus, when a very small focal spot is chosen, there is an apparently disproportionately large reduction in maximum permissible current. For example, with a 0·3-mm.-square focal spot the rating corresponding to those quoted for the 1·2- or 2-mm. spots is only 36 mA., whereas direct application of a linear law would suggest about 90 mA. It is for this reason that one pays dearly, as shown in *Table XXIV*, in increased exposure time if a 0·3-mm. focal spot is used rather than a 1·2-mm. one, whereas the gain in changing to a 2-mm. one is not very great.

Table XXIV.—EXPOSURE AT 90 KV., 37 MA.S.

Focal Spot Size	Maximum mA.	Minimum Exposure Time
2·0 mm. square	695 mA.	0·055 sec.
1·2 mm. square	370 mA.	0·1 sec.
0·3 mm. square	29·5 mA.	1·25 sec.

Wave Form.—For any given wave form of the X-ray tube voltage the maximum mA. is inversely proportional to the kV. value as indicated above but the rating will have different values for different types of wave form. The wave forms in common use are:

1. Self-rectified.
2. Half-wave.
3. Full wave.
4. Three-phase full-wave rectified (which is practically equivalent to constant potential).

---

* It is interesting to note that at 3000° C., which is close to the maximum permitted temperature for the anode, the rate of loss by radiation (infra-red, visible, and ultra-violet) is about 1·6 W. per sq.mm. which is very much less than the 200 W. per sq.mm. heat input rate. In the stationary anode tube therefore there is no significant cooling by radiation. In the rotating anode tube, where the ratio of the size of the area available for cooling to that actually bombarded by electrons is very much greater (∼250 times) than for a stationary anode tube of the same effective focal spot size, cooling by radiation is the principal mechanism.

It will be noticed (*Fig.* 237) that the rating for a full-wave-rectified wave form is substantially greater than that for a half-wave one. For example, a stationary anode tube working at 60 kV., 0·5 sec. with a 1·5-mm. focal spot has a rating of 45 mA. for full-wave and 34 mA. for half-wave operation. (It is, incidentally, interesting to note how very much lower these values are than those quoted earlier for the rotating anode tube.) The reason for this difference in rating can be seen by

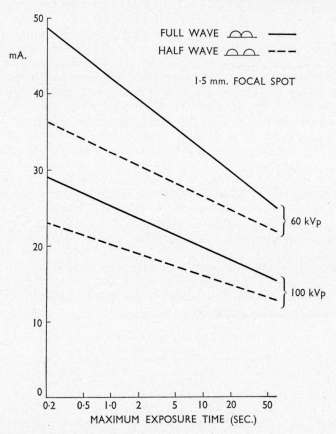

Fig. 237.—Comparison of rating for full-wave and half-wave rectifications. Stationary anode tube with 1·5-mm. focal spot.

referring to *Fig.* 238. This shows the idealized current wave form in the two cases for the same mean current, which is the value referred to in the rating charts. It is clear that the peak current is much greater for the half-wave operation than it is for the full-wave situation. Now it is the peak current, rather than the mean current, value which will determine the maximum anode surface temperature. Hence, if the anode temperature is to be kept at or below the maximum permitted value (which is the same for both half- and full-wave operation) the mean current in half-wave operation must be less than that for full-wave operation.

Since the voltage wave form during each operative half-cycle can be considered to be the same for half- and full-wave operation, it would be expected that the maximum mean mA. for the former would be half of that for the latter. In practice the difference is not quite so great because a different amount of cooling occurs between the 'heating' periods for the two wave forms. In full-wave operation this cooling is quite small but for half-wave (where there is a complete half-cycle for cooling between each heating half-cycle) the cooling can be considerable. The maximum instantaneous and mean currents which can be used in half-wave operation are, therefore, greater

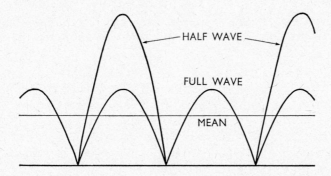

Fig. 238.—Current wave-form in full-wave and half-wave operation. Each gives the same mean current.

than expected compared with those for the full wave. Using the above figures, for the stationary anode, the ratio is approximately 3/4 (viz. 34/45). For a rotating anode, where different parts of the anode are heated during the exposure, the difference in cooling is less marked for the two wave forms and the maximum mean current ratio more nearly corresponds to a half. For the longer exposures it is about two-thirds, tending towards the limiting value of one-half for very short exposures.

The corresponding rating for self-rectified operation is only 22 mA. The wave form here is just the same as the half-wave rectification but in this case the maximum permitted temperature is less than for either full- or half-wave operation. This is because the X-ray tube is acting as its own rectifier and therefore its anode must be kept sufficiently cool if inverse current is to be avoided.

The efficiency of X-ray production and the quality of the radiation can be improved by a deliberate restriction of the current to that part of the cycle when the kV. is highest. For instance, the two wave forms shown in *Fig.* 239 both represent the same mean current, but the amount and quality of the X-rays produced by the restricted wave form (B) will be greater than those for the more normal wave form (A). This is because a larger fraction of the electrons is accelerated when the kV. is in the region of the voltage wave form peak and since output is proportional to the square of the kV. and quality increases with kV. The permitted rating (maximum *mean* current) for the wave form shown at (B) will be less than that for the normal wave form shown at (A) for the reasons just discussed, but nevertheless the radiation quality and output obtained using the restricted wave form (B) at its maximum rating will be better than those obtained using the normal wave form at its 'higher' maximum rating.

This desirable effect is obtained by suitable design of the filament and filament surroundings and is one of the considerations entering into the design of the focusing cup described in CHAPTER XXII.

The rating of three-phase operation, expressed in terms of radiation output at a specified kV., exposure time, and focal spot size, is greater than it is for full-wave operation. Some of the explanation for this follows the arguments set out above but there are a few complicating factors which can be the cause of confusion. It is convenient to leave further discussion of this subject until later (p. 330).

Longer and Shorter Exposure Times.—It has already been described how the maximum mA. falls as the exposure time is increased but to a less than proportional extent, with the result that the available amount of X-radiation is greater at the longer exposure times. This is always true, as is the fact that the rating for full-wave operation is greater than that for half-wave operation, which in its turn is greater than that for self-rectified operation. At very long exposure times, however, the difference in

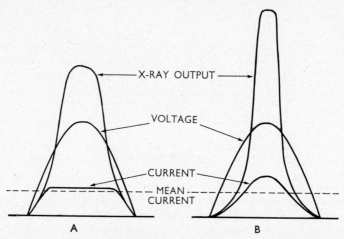

Fig. 239.—Increased X-ray production can be obtained by restriction of the current. A, Normal, and B, Restricted wave form.

rating between these three different operating conditions is very small and their ratings can be regarded as identical. So far, only the temperature at the focal spot has been discussed but this is not the only consideration. As described in CHAPTER XXII the heat produced at the focal spot gradually spreads through the anode structure and the remainder of the tube, all of which therefore become heated. There are, of course, limitations to the temperature to which these various structures can be raised and this has its effect upon the rating, especially at the longer exposure times or if the tube is being used continuously as in fluoroscopy. The rate of heat production at the target must not exceed the rate at which heat can be stored or dissipated by the tube shield into the surrounding air. Under such conditions it is the latter which determines the rating. The target surface temperature is no longer the restricting factor and the wave form or focal spot size therefore does not influence the rating. This is the reason why, for fluoroscopy, there is no need to rotate the anode (or at least only to rotate it slowly), the much reduced actual focal spot area of the stationary anode being sufficiently large for the permitted rate of heat production.

The previous discussion in which target surface temperature was regarded as the controlling factor applies strictly to very small exposure times only, and the present discussion to very long exposure times only. In the intermediate time range there is obviously a changeover from one to the other, and the temperatures of the anode structure as a whole, of the oil, and of the tube shield, each of which has its own maximum safe temperature, are the controlling features. The rise in temperature of the structures is, of course, brought about by the heat which flows from the cooling target surface and this rise is governed by their various heat capacities as well as by the amount of heat generated at the target. The basic need is that the exposure (mA., etc.) must be restricted so that none of the various components (i.e., target surface, anode structure, oil, etc.) rises to a temperature greater than can be allowed. For very short exposure times the anode surface region effects the major control, for medium–short times it is the temperature of the anode as a whole that matters, whereas for very long times it is the general heat dissipation to the surroundings. It is for this reason that for longer times the difference in rating between half- and full-wave operation becomes smaller than for the short (0·5 sec.) time referred to on p. 319. For example, at 60 kV., 80 sec. the ratings are 25 and 20 mA. respectively, which is a ratio of 1·2 compared with the previous ratio of 1·33. This is because the temperature of the anode as a whole is controlling the restriction: the different wave forms and the possibility of cooling in alternate half-cycles are of little importance.

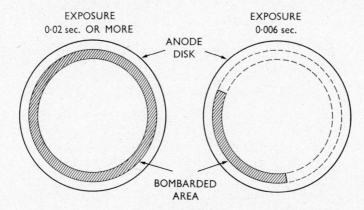

Fig. 240.—There is incomplete use of the available focal spot area of a rotating anode for exposure times less than 0·02 sec.

For very short exposure times there is a further item which affects the rating of a rotating anode tube. The speed of rotation is usually about 3000 rev./min., i.e., 1 rev. in 0·02 sec. For times longer than this the heating is spread out over the complete circle of the focal spot area as described on p. 290. For times smaller than 0·02 sec., however, only a fraction of the complete circle is used; in other words, the actual focal spot area is reduced (*Fig*. 240) and therefore the rating clearly will be affected. What happens is that for times less than for about 0·02 sec. current rating remains constant, since as far as each part of the target surface is concerned the heat input rate remains constant even though the exposure time is reduced, and therefore rating is independent of exposure time (below 0·02 sec.). Even at times longer than 0·02 sec. the same thing is happening to an extent since each part of the target has some time to cool between each instant at which it is acting as the focal spot. It is for this reason that the increase in current rating with decrease in exposure time rises less, for example, between 0·1 and 0·05 sec. than it does between 1 and 0·5 sec. and this leads (*Fig*. 241) to a gradual flattening off in the rating curve, with a complete flattening below 0·02 sec. For the stationary anode tube, of course, no such flattening off occurs.

Clearly, for times less than about 0·05 sec. the rating can be improved by using an anode rotating at a higher speed. In some modern equipment this is possible and is especially useful if a small focal spot size is also needed. Rating is always increased if high speeds of rotation are used but the increase is significant only at the shorter times. The constructional difficulties are large if a long life (years) is to be obtained and such high speeds are only of real value if these very short times

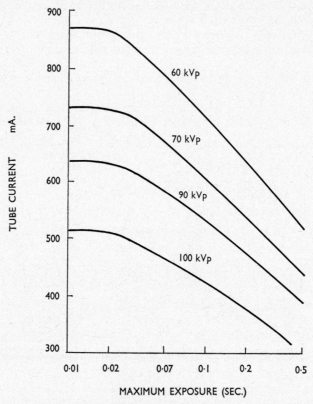

Fig. 241.—Rating chart for rotating anode tube showing constant maximum current for short (<0·02 sec.) exposure times.

are to be used. Conversely, as has already been pointed out, at longer times (e.g., fluoroscopy) it is common practice to use a more slowly rotating anode or even not to rotate it at all. It is advantageous not to rotate the anode since the heat generated by the flow of current in the stator coils helps to heat the tube as a whole, which is to be avoided.

Three-phase Operation.—The rating of an X-ray tube in full-wave-rectified three-phase operation is best described by comparing it with the rating of the same tube when used in single-phase full-wave-rectified operation, and considering first the relative rating at fairly long exposure times. Here, it will be recalled it is the tempera-ture of the anode as a whole which determines the rating and that this temperature is itself determined by the total electrical energy of the exposure. Energy is usually measured in joules but in this branch of X-ray technology a unit of energy called the **heat unit** is preferred. For a single-phase full-wave-rectified wave form, the number of heat units involved in an exposure is given by:

$$\text{Heat unit (H.U.)} = kV. \times mA. \times sec.,$$

whereas for the three-phase wave form the expression is:

$$\text{Heat units} = 1.35 \times \text{kV.} \times \text{mA.} \times \text{sec.}$$

The 35 per cent increase in heat units (for the same *mean* current, kV., and exposure time) arises because of the difference in wave form, the three-phase being more efficient. For convenience the relationships between electrical energy and heat units for the two wave forms are summarized in *Table XXV*. Since there is a constant ratio between the number of heat units and the number of joules (electrical energy) it can be seen that any temperature rise will be proportional to the number of heat units involved in an exposure.

Table XXV.—THE RELATIONSHIP, FOR SINGLE-PHASE AND THREE-PHASE FULL-WAVE RECTIFICATION, BETWEEN ENERGY, HEAT UNITS, KV., AND MA.S.

	Single-phase	Three-phase	
Energy	$\begin{cases} \text{kV.} \times \text{mA.s.} \times 0.71 \\ \text{Heat units} \times 0.71 \end{cases}$	$\begin{cases} \text{kV.} \times \text{mA.s.} \times 0.96 \\ \text{Heat units} \times 0.71 \end{cases}$	joules
Heat units	$\begin{cases} \text{kV.} \times \text{mA.s.} \\ \text{Energy} \times 1.4 \end{cases}$	$\begin{cases} \text{kV.} \times \text{mA.s.} \times 1.35 \\ \text{Energy} \times 1.4 \end{cases}$	

Still considering the longer exposure times, if exposures involving the same amount of electrical energy (and therefore heat units) are made using single-phase and three-phase wave forms then the rises in temperature of the anode structure will be the same for both wave forms. It therefore follows that, for the same X-ray tube, focal spot size, and (long) exposure time, the maximum mean current (i.e., the rating) for the three-phase operation will be 35 per cent less than for the single-phase operation. This is because a single-phase current of, for example, 135 mA.

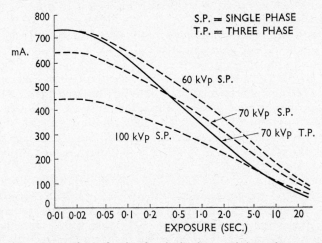

Fig. 242.—Comparison of rating for single-phase and three-phase operation.

will produce the same number of heat units (and therefore anode temperature rise) as will a three-phase current of 100 mA. This difference in rating is apparent from *Fig.* 242 in which some of the rating curves for both single- and three-phase operation are shown. It can be seen that for 70 kV., 20 sec. the single-phase rating is just over 100 mA. whilst that for three-phase is a little under 70 mA.

It is important to realize that since the tube kilovoltage is constant in three-phase operation and X-ray emission is proportional to the square of kilovoltage, the X-ray output is greater for the three-phase operation than for the full wave in spite of the fact that the mean current, mA., is smaller. Furthermore, the penetrating power (H.V.L.) of the radiation is greater in the three-phase case since all the radiation is produced by electrons having energy equivalent to the stated kV. whereas in full-wave-rectified operation the voltage varies from zero to the stated value (peak) during each half-cycle.

Considering now the rating at short exposure times, it will be recalled that the anode surface temperature is determined not by the mean electrical power but by the peak value. At short exposure times therefore, where anode surface temperature controls the rating, it is necessary to take into account the fact that the relationship between the peak and mean values is very different for a sinusoidal (single-phase) wave form than it is for an effectively constant (three-phase) wave form.

In three-phase the current and voltage values are almost constant so that there is very little difference between the peak and mean values whereas for single-phase the peak values are significantly greater than the mean values. Using the argument employed earlier (p. 326) when explaining the difference between the full- and half-wave-rectified wave-form ratings, it can be seen that, for short exposure times, the maximum permitted mean current is greater for three-phase operation than it is for single-phase operation. That this is so can be seen from the curves of *Fig.* 242.

At intermediate times both factors (i.e., mean and peak energy) play their parts and, as is shown in *Fig.* 242, the rating curves for single- and three-phase operation cross over in this region. It must be remembered, however, that at all times the radiation output at the maximum rating is greater for three-phase than for single-phase full-wave operation but especially so at short exposure times where both effects (high current rating and more efficient X-ray production from constant potential) obtain. It is for this reason that three-phase equipment is of prime importance for work involving short exposure times.

Multiple Exposures.—The rating charts and the descriptions of them given so far in this chapter apply to the circumstances when only a single isolated exposure, well separated in time from other exposures, is made. The limitations on the single exposure imposed by the rating charts always apply, but if multiple exposures are made, with only comparatively small time intervals between them, then there are other considerations which may further restrict the exposures which may be made.

It is obvious that it will take a fairly long time for all parts of the X-ray tube to cool down and that if a further exposure is made within this time then the temperature of the various parts of the tube subsequent to this second exposure will be greater than would be the case for a single isolated exposure. There is, in other words, a gradual build-up in temperature as multiple exposures are made, which means that the rating, for each exposure of the series, must fall progressively.

Fortunately, the exposures are rarely made so rapidly that the anode surface temperature is a limiting feature since it is able to dissipate its heat fairly quickly. It is more usual for any restriction to be due to the temperature of the anode structure or of the X-ray tube shield (and contents) as a whole. Although the temperature is the determining factor it is convenient to refer, instead, to the heat capacity of the anode (or tube shield). If a maximum value is assigned to this, it is equivalent to assigning a maximum temperature.

$$\text{Heat capacity} = \text{mass} \times \text{specific heat} \times \text{temperature rise.}$$

Therefore, since mass × specific heat is constant, the temperature rise is proportional to the heat capacity. Furthermore, it is convenient to refer to the heat capacity in terms of the heat units already referred to above. A typical high-power rotating anode unit can have, for example, an anode heat capacity of 110,000 H.U. or a tube shield capacity of 1,250,000 H.U.

Subsequent to an exposure, of course, there is a cooling of the various parts of the X-ray tube. It is again convenient to use heat units and in this case it is the number of heat units remaining in the anode (or tube) after various cooling times which is of interest. *Fig.* 243 shows how the number of stored heat units (viz., temperature) in a typical anode structure falls with time (*note*: in minutes, not in

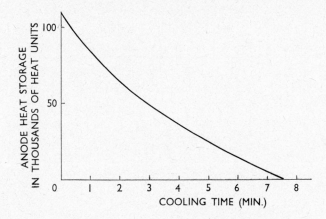

Fig. 243.—Anode cooling characteristic curve.

seconds). It should be noted that the rate of loss of heat is greatest at the higher temperatures, being 30,000 H.U. per min. initially but only 11,000 H.U. per min. after 5 min. This is due to the fact that for all methods of heat loss (conduction, convection, and radiation) the rate of loss of heat depends on the temperature difference, which is, of course, greatest initially.

Now consider the situation, which may arise in some techniques, when it is required to make four exposures each of 90 kV., 500 mA., and 1 sec. in quick succession. The rating chart shows that such exposures are within the normal tube rating for a single exposure. Each exposure represents 45,000 H.U. and if all four are given within say 10 sec., during which time there will be little cooling of the anode, the total heat units given to the anode will be 180,000, which is far beyond its capacity and is therefore not permissible. We can, however, give two of the exposures quickly which will result in a storage of 90,000 H.U. and this is indicated in *Fig.* 244. It is now necessary to wait until there has been a loss of some 25,000 H.U.; that is until the stored heat units have fallen from 90,000 to 65,000. The graph shows that this will take $1\frac{1}{4}$ min., after which a further exposure (of 45,000 H.U.) may be made: the stored heat units rising to the maximum value of 110,000. It is now necessary to wait a further 2 min. during which time the stored heat units will fall from 110,000 to 65,000 units before the fourth exposure can be made.

Other schemes of exposure are possible of course and an alternative method using equal intervals of $1\frac{1}{2}$ min. between the various exposures is illustrated in *Fig.* 241. It is interesting to note that the scheme which brings the anode to the highest safe temperature as quickly as possible leads to a shorter overall time, due, of course, to the greater rate of loss of heat at the higher temperatures.

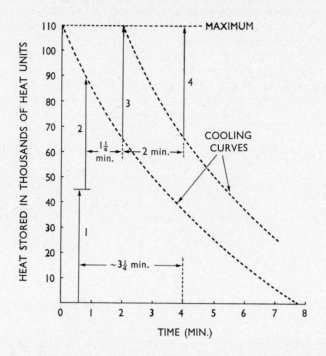

Fig. 244.—The heating, and cooling, of the anode during multiple exposures.

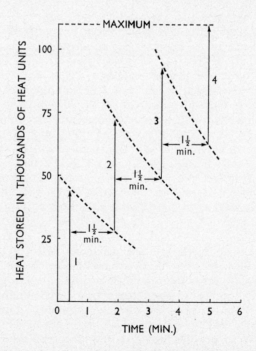

Fig. 245.—The heating, and cooling, of the anode during equally spaced multiple exposures.

Similar considerations apply to the tube shield as a whole and in *Fig.* 246 a typical tube cooling is shown. The times involved are much longer and depend upon whether forced air cooling is used or not. It is only when very long series of exposures are

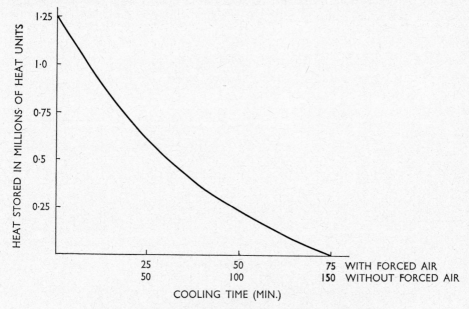

Fig. 246.—Cooling characteristic curve of a typical tube shield.

being made that the heat storage and slow cooling of the tube shield as a whole prove to be a limitation. Calculations similar to the one already done for the anode heat storage can be made to determine the permitted schedule of use.

Continuous Exposure.—The other circumstance in which a gradual build-up of heat in the X-ray tube can occur is during fluoroscopy. *Fig.* 247 shows how the number of heat units stored rises with exposure time. The horizontal line (*a*) is at the level of the maximum anode heat storage capacity whilst the straight line (*b*) indicates the rise which would occur if no cooling were to take place during the exposure. The curve (*c*) shows the actual rise and indicates the large amount of simultaneous cooling which is occurring. It is of interest to note that the curve is becoming asymptotic to the horizontal (*a*) at about $7\frac{1}{2}$ min., which indicates that such a rate of heat input to the target (viz., exposure) may be continued indefinitely as far as the target is concerned. An alternative way of expressing this is to state that at very long times the maximum mA. is independent of exposure time, as was shown earlier in *Figs.* 235 and 236. This is because, for this particular tube, the maximum rate of cooling, which occurs at the maximum permitted temperature, is 30,000 H.U. per min. which is identical to the rate of heat input of 500 H.U. per sec. An equilibrium is thus established, the stored heat being such that the anode is at its maximum temperature and the rate of heat loss by cooling is being balanced by the equal rate of heat input by the exposure. For exposures resulting in a smaller heat input rate the anode will never reach the maximum permitted storage capacity (temperature) as shown by curve (*d*) of *Fig.* 247, whereas for an exposure involving a greater rare of heat input (curve (*e*)) the anode will more quickly reach its maximum temperature after which time the exposure must be reduced to the equilibrium value of 500 H.U. per sec.

The maximum rate of loss of heat is usually quoted by the manufacturer. It is also interesting to note that the maximum rate of loss of heat for the tube shield (which is also usually quoted) is less than that of the anode so that a rate of heat

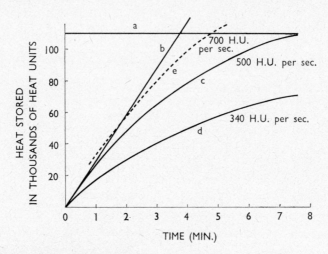

Fig. 247.—The accumulation of heat in the anode during a continuous exposure.

input of 30,000 H.U. per min. can be continued for only a limited time. Eventually after very long exposure times it is the lower rate of loss of heat from the tube shield which will exert the control.

It is very uncommon in practice for such exposures to be made. For example, 500 H.U. per sec. implies an exposure of 100 kV. at 5 mA. which is far above modern screening conditions and which, in any case, should involve intermittent rather than continuous exposure.

Interlocks.—Although all radiographers should be familiar with the principles on which the rating charts and cooling charts are based, they are nowadays considerably helped in their day-to-day work by the provision of various interlocks. These are mechanical (or sometimes electrical) systems which make it impossible to operate the tube if a forbidden combination of kV., mA., sec., or focal spot size is selected. Protection for the single exposure effected in this way is now almost universal on new equipment. Some equipment, but by no means all, is also fitted with circuits which take note of the heat accumulation which, it will be remembered, is of importance when multiple or long exposures are being made.

Optimum Load.—It can be argued that unless the X-ray tube is being used at or just below its permitted rating then it is possible to select, for example, a shorter time and greater tube current combination which will result in a sharper radiograph. In order to facilitate such use, some equipment is fitted with an exposure factor selector system, which indicates the percentage of maximum rating (load) being used or alternately arranges that a tube shall be worked at say 80 per cent of the maximum permitted rating always. In some units it is arranged that the selection of mA.s. automatically provides the maximum mA.–minimum time combination that the tube rating will allow for the particular kV. and focal spot size in use.

Falling Load Operation.—In describing the limitations arising in multiple exposures it was pointed out that a shorter overall time results when the initial input rate is greatest. So it is, and for similar reasons, for the single exposure. If it can be arranged for the current to be high in the initial part of the exposure and then to fall steadily during the exposure it turns out that the same mA.s. can be passed in a shorter overall time than would be the case for a constant current. Some equipment incorporates such a facility which clearly leads to a reduced exposure time and therefore reduced movement blurring.

Although the use of either high percentage loading or falling load operation has its advantage from the point of view of minimum exposure time, the operation of a tube always at its maximum must shorten tube life.

Two exposures at 50 kV. and corresponding to the points A and B on the rating chart shown in *Fig.* 248 give 6 mA.s. and are both within the tube rating in the sense that neither results in an overheated anode. The higher mA. associated with the point A necessitates a higher filament temperature, with which is therefore associated a greater evaporation of tungsten from the filament and consequent shortening of tube life. (It is interesting to note that the rate of evaporation of tungsten from the heated filament varies with the thirty-fourth power of the absolute temperature!) The horizontal dotted line of *Fig.* 248, which is shown on some rating charts, indicates

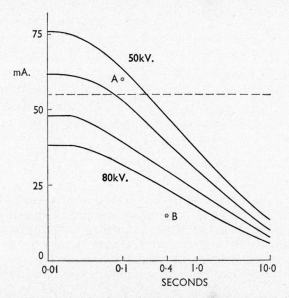

Fig. 248.—Rating chart showing level of tube current that should not be exceeded unnecessarily.

the level of tube current (i.e., filament heating) above which there is excessive evaporation. Exposures involving tube currents higher than this should be made only when there is no alternative and even then the filament should be boosted for the minimum possible time.

The Use of Rating Charts.—The situation is very complex and, clearly, the radiographer cannot be expected to consider all these various features on the occasion of each exposure. Fortunately, all the information required for day-to-day work is contained in the rating charts which, as it will be remembered, are essentially empirically determined by the manufacturer. In conclusion, it is worth while showing how the rating charts for a particular tube may be used in practice. The relevant information is shown in *Fig.* 249, which consists of: (A) the rating chart of the 1·5-mm.-square

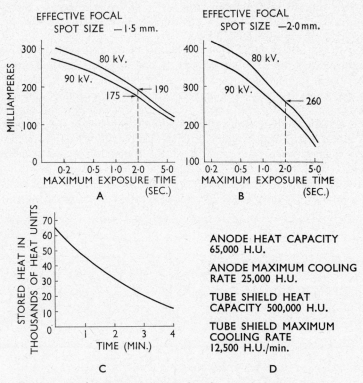

Fig. 249.—Rating charts and other data for a typical X-ray tube.

focal spot, and (B) that for the 2·0-mm.-square focal spot; together with (C) the anode cooling curve, and (D) the values of the anode and tube shield heat storage capacities and maximum cooling rates. On the rating charts ((A) and (B)) the curves for 80 and 90 kV. only are shown since these are the ones to be used; on an actual chart, of course, similar curves for other kV. would also be present.

This chapter has described how there are three items to be considered and these are:

1. The single exposure rating.
2. Any restriction resulting from the anode heat storage capacity and cooling characteristics.
3. Any further restriction resulting from the tube shield heat storage capacity and cooling characteristics.

In the following example each of the aspects is considered in turn.

Example.—A series of three exposures each of 80 kV., 500 mA.s. using an exposure time not greater than 2 sec. and a focal spot of 1·5 mm. square is required. The rating chart (*Fig.* 249 A) shows that at 80 kV. and 2 sec. the maximum current is 190 mA. which is insufficient, a current of 250 mA. being required. The other rating chart for the larger 2-mm.-square focal spot (*Fig.* 249 B) shows that the maximum current is 260 mA. and the required exposure is possible. If the 2-mm. focal spot is acceptable then this revised set of exposure conditions (80 kV., 2 sec., 250 mA., 2·0-mm. focal spot) can be used. An alternative would be to retain the smaller focal spot (1·5 mm.) and to increase the kilovoltage (thus losing a little contrast, which will be presumed to be acceptable). If it is assumed that the effect at the film is approximately proportional to the cube of the kilovoltage (p. 269), a change from 80 kV. to 90 kV. will permit a reduction of the mA.s. from 500 to

$$500 \times \left(\frac{80}{90}\right)^3 = 350 \text{ mA.s.}$$

This is achieved in an exposure time of 2 sec. by using a current of 175 mA. which the rating chart (*Fig.* 249 A) shows is allowed. Hence, although it has not been possible (using this particular tube) to carry out the exposure as originally intended, a slight modification has brought the exposure within the permitted range.

So far only the single, isolated exposure has been considered. It is now necessary to determine whether such an exposure (of 90 kV., 350 mA.s.) may be repeated and if so, how often and how quickly. The number of heat units given to the anode at each exposure is:

$$90 \times 350 = 31,500 \text{ H.U.,}$$

so that three exposures repeated immediately one after the other will deliver a total of:

$$3 \times 31,500 = 94,500 \text{ H.U.}$$

to the anode. The information supplied by the manufacturer (*Fig.* 249 D) shows that this is well in excess of the maximum value (65,000 H.U.). It is, therefore, possible to make only two exposures in quick succession which will result in 63,000 H.U. being given to the anode (point a on *Fig.* 250). It is now necessary to wait until there has been sufficient cooling before the third exposure is made. The anode cooling chart, which is reproduced in *Fig.* 250 and also *Fig.* 249 C, shows that just over $1\frac{1}{2}$ min. (a to b) are needed for the stored heat to fall from 63,000 to 33,500 (i.e., 65,000–31,500). If the third exposure is now made the stored heat will be raised from 33,500 to $33,500 + 31,500 = 65,000$ which is the maximum permitted value. If a further exposure is needed it will again be necessary to wait, this time for about $1\frac{3}{4}$ min. (until the stored heat has again fallen to 33,500 as shown dotted in *Fig.* 250) before the fourth exposure is made. For any subsequent exposures intervals of $1\frac{3}{4}$ min. between each are required. An alternative, but slightly less accurate, way of determining the permitted repetition rate is to equate the mean rate of heat input to the anode and the maximum anode cooling rate. In the example the mean input rate is:

$$31,500 \div 1\frac{3}{4} = 18,000 \text{ H.U./min.,}$$

which is less than the maximum anode cooling rate of 25,000, thus confirming that this schedule is permissible. The difference between the two figures of 18,000 and 25,000 arises because, of course, the maximum rate of cooling obtains only when the stored heat is at its maximum value of 65,000 units and therefore the anode at its hottest. As the anode cools the rate of cooling diminishes. The 18,000 is the mean of the initial value (25,000) and the lower value (13,000) after $1\frac{3}{4}$ min. of cooling. It is because of this complication that the method described first, which used the cooling curve, is preferred.

Although, as far as the anode is concerned, repetition of such exposures can continue at this interval of 1¾ min. indefinitely, it must be remembered that cooling of the anode results in the tube shield and contents as a whole being heated. The tube shield, in this example, has a heat-storage capacity of 500,000 units which represents the accumulated heat of about 16 exposures, which at the rate of an exposure every 1¾ min. will take about 30 min. There will be a little simultaneous cooling of the tube shield during this time, but since this is not large it is usual to ignore it so as to be 'on the safe side'. The tube data sheet (*Fig.* 249 D) records that the maximum cooling rate of the tube shield is 12,500 H.U. per min. which is less than the present input rate of 18,000 H.U./min. It is clear, therefore, that after the

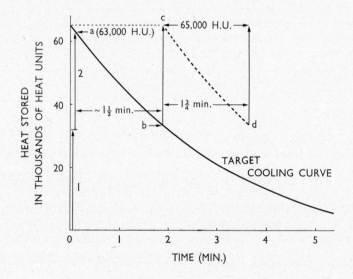

Fig. 250.—Heat storage and multiple exposures.

first sixteen exposures the repetition rate must be reduced to one exposure every 2½ min. which corresponds to an input rate of 12,500 H.U. per min. (31,500 ÷ 2·5 = 12,500). Since the input and cooling rate are now equal, the repetition, at this longer time interval, can be continued indefinitely. The approximate method of equating average input rate to maximum cooling rate is adequate here because of the much greater heat capacity of the tube shield compared with the anode (500,000 compared with 65,000 H.U.), which means considerably less cooling and therefore less change in cooling rate over these time intervals (1¾ min.).

It should be pointed out that it is rare in most day-to-day work to need to consider anything other than the single, isolated exposure rating limitation. The 'natural break' between exposures and patients is usually adequate in even the busiest departments to afford adequate cooling. There are, however, a few circumstances in which the permissible repetition rate must be considered. For example, in serial angiographic work it is sometimes required to make as many as eighteen exposures, each of 75 kV., 100 mA.s., within a space of a few seconds. This corresponds to an anode heat storage of 18 × 75 × 100 = 135,000 H.U. which, although within the capabilities of a modern high-power unit, is well beyond the maximum of many units.

CHAPTER XXV

FLUOROSCOPY

THE use of the fluorescent screen to enable the radiologist to 'see' the X-ray pattern has already been referred to in CHAPTER XIV, and described in more detail in CHAPTER XVII, where it was pointed out that, unless the patient is irradiated by a comparatively intense beam of X-rays, the intensity of the light emitted by the screen is very low and, therefore, the details of the pattern difficult or even impossible to see. This chapter will describe, in somewhat more detail, the effects of these difficulties and indicate how the modern use of image intensifiers and closed-circuit television systems has helped to overcome them. Before doing this, however, it is necessary to give some information about the measurement of visible light brightness and about the way in which the eye operates.

Brightness of Visible Light.—Although the brightness of a surface can be measured by the amount of energy per square centimetre emitted from the surface, it is more usual, for visible light, to use a system of measurement based upon the *standard candle*. The unit used is the *Lambert* (L.) and a surface is said to have a brightness of 1 L. if there is emitted 1 lumen of light per square centimetre. An ordinary 40-W. electric-light bulb is equivalent to about 80 standard candles and a piece of white paper placed about 35 cm. away from it will have a brightness of 50 millilamberts (0·05 L.). This and other examples of the approximate brightness of some typical situations are given in *Table XXVI*. It must also be pointed out that the visual sensation of brightness depends not only on its physical brightness (measured in Lamberts) but also upon the colour of the light.

Table XXVI.—SOME EXAMPLES OF BRIGHTNESS VALUES

Vision Mechanism		Milli-lamberts	Lamberts	Brightness
Cones	Film radiography		16	←——————————Maximum safe brightness
		10,000	10	←——————————Snow in sunlight
		1,000	1	←——————————Clear sky
		100	10^{-1}	
		50 —		←——————————White paper read under 40-W. bulb
		10	10^{-2}	
		1	10^{-3}	
		0·1	10^{-4}	←——————————Moonlight
Rods	Fluoro-scopy	0·01	10^{-5}	←——————————————Thin chest
		0·005		←————Cone threshold
		0·001	10^{-6}	←——————————————A.P. abdomen
		0·0001	10^{-7}	
				←——————————————Lateral abdomen
		0·00001	10^{-8}	
		0·000001	10^{-9}	←————Rod threshold

It can be seen from *Table XXVI* that the eye is capable of working over a very wide range of brightnesses (16 L. down to about 10^{-9} L.: a range of 10^{10}!). It is not surprising therefore that, as already stated on p. 177, the visual sensation is logarithmic.

It is also important to note that the brightness of an object does not depend upon its distance from the eye. Why this is so can be seen by the reference to *Fig.* 251 where the same object is shown, diagrammatically, to be situated at two different distances from the eye. If the object is close, as at A, then a large image is formed on the retina. The amount of light reaching the image is determined by how much light is contained within the cone which extends from the object to the iris of the eye (shown dotted in *Fig.* 251). Since the object is near, this amount of light is large.

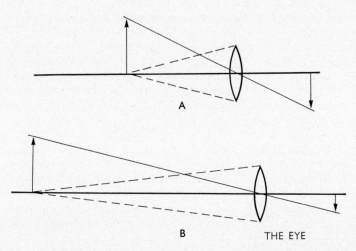

Fig. 251.—Two identical objects, viewed at different distances, appear equally bright.

Conversely when the object is at a greater distance, B, the retinal image is smaller but so is the amount of light entering the eye. The net result is that in both cases the brightness is the same. In the case of a near object a large amount of light is spread over a larger image, whereas in the case of an identical but more distant object an exactly corresponding smaller amount of light is spread over a smaller image.

Rod and Cone Vision.—To cover the very wide range of light intensities there are two distinct mechanisms operating at the retina of the eye.* The retina is the light-sensitive 'screen' in the eye on which the images of the objects being observed are focused by the eye's lens, and is covered by two types of sensitive structures. These, because of their general shape, are called *rods* and *cones*. They are both very tiny and over the surface of the retina there are many thousands of both types. There are rods over the whole area of the retina except for a small region, the macula or fovea centralis, over which there are cones only. In normal vision the pattern created in the observer's brain is determined by the pattern formed on the retina, i.e., by the pattern formed by those cones (or rods) which are illuminated.

The rods are extremely sensitive and, as shown in *Table XXVI*, are capable of detecting a brightness as low as 0·000001 mL., which is called the *threshold* of brightness perception since brightnesses smaller than this do not normally cause any visual

---

* The account given here of the mechanism of vision, although sufficient for present purposes, is necessarily rather superficial. For a more detailed account of the optical, physiological, and psychological aspects of vision the reader is referred to more specialized texts.

sensation. The threshold for cone vision is much higher (viz., 0·005 mL., which, incidentally, is still a very low brightness). The upper limit of cone vision is about 16 L., which is very bright indeed. At brightnesses above this level the retina can be damaged. Because of the way in which they act, which is referred to below, the rods yield very little visual sensation to brightnesses above about 0·02 mL. The situation is therefore that for brightnesses between the lower limit of 0·000001 mL.

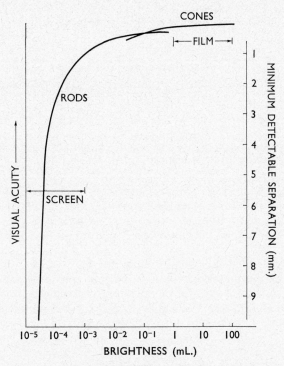

Fig. 252.—Variation, with brightness, of minimum separation at which two objects can just be distinguished.

and about 0·02 mL. the principal method of visual sensation is by means of the rods, whereas above 0·02 mL. it is by means of the cones. It is clear therefore from the data in *Table XXVI* that the pattern on the traditional fluoroscopic screen is seen by rod vision, whereas the reading of a radiograph on a viewing screen utilizes cone vision.

Visual Acuity.—The ability of the eye to distinguish between two objects very close together, that is, to perceive fine detail, is referred to as visual acuity. The acuity of rod vision is very much worse than that for cone vision and furthermore both become worse as the brightness level falls (*Fig.* 252). The difference between the acuity of the rods and cones arises partly from the fact that each cone acts separately and sends its own message to the brain, whereas the rods act in groups (*Fig.* 253), light falling on any one of the rods in a small but finite area will result in the same message being sent to the brain. This means that if the retinal images of two close objects happen to both fall within the same group of rods only one message will be generated and the two objects will not be seen separately.

Acuity is measured in terms of the smallest separation which two objects may have and still be distinguished. For cones the acuity is typically about $\frac{1}{20}$ mm. when the objects are viewed at the normal distance of 20–25 cm. (this corresponds to an angular separation of the objects of less than 1 minute of arc). As is seen from *Fig.* 253, the acuity in rod vision can be very much worse than that for the cones.

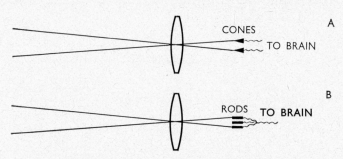

Fig. 253.—A, Two objects are seen separately because their retinal images excite individual cones. B, The same two objects are not resolved at low brightnesses since their retinal images both excite rods in the same group.

When viewing a radiograph (at brightness levels in the region of 10–1000 mL.) the eye is capable, therefore, of appreciating very fine detail and under the best conditions can—unaided—distinguish two objects separated by only one-thousandth of an inch ($= \frac{1}{40}$ mm.). For the fluoroscopic screen, however, where the brightness level is usually in the range 0·0001–0·01 mL., the eye is unable to see such fine detail and detail even as large as several millimetres may not be seen.

Colour Sensitivity and Colour Vision.—The rods and cones also differ in their relative response to light of different colours. It has already been remarked that the eye is not equally sensitive to all colours of light (i.e., equal intensities of light at different colours are observed as different brightnesses). The relative response of the rods and cones is shown in *Fig.* 254. The photopic eye (i.e., one using cone vision) has its maximum sensitivity at about 5600 Å whereas the scotopic eye (i.e., using rod vision) has its maximum sensitivity at 5150 Å.

From the general point of view a most important fact is that in cone vision the different colours of light cause different visual sensations and the observer is said to have colour vision, i.e., he can see the difference between red, orange, green, blue, etc. The rods, on the other hand, do not show this effect and although they have different sensitivities to the different wavelengths they do not produce a different visual sensation and the 'colour' in rod vision is the same for all wavelengths. The rods are said to be completely colour blind. It is for this reason that at low levels of illumination, everything appears to be of the same general grey colour. In other words Cones are responsible for Colour vision whereas the Rods make Romantic the moonlight scene—and all cats are grey after dark!

Contrast Perception.—From the present point of view, however, a more important difference is that the cones are much more capable of detecting differences in brightness than are the rods. It will be remembered that a radiograph placed on a viewing screen shows up its contrast in terms of different degrees of brightness. It so happens that when the brightness is high the cones are able to detect contrast as low as 0·02 (2 per cent), whereas when the brightness is so low that only rods are operative it is difficult for a difference even as great as 0·2 (20 per cent) to be detected. This is, to say the least, unfortunate since the contrasts of interest are often in the region of 2–10 per cent. The ability of both rods and cones to perceive contrast depends upon the brightness of the object and increases as the brightness increases; this is shown in *Fig.* 255.

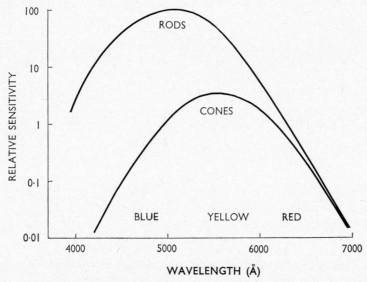

Fig. 254.—Variation in sensitivity of the rods and cones to light of different colours. Note that the scale is arbitrary since the relative sensitivity of the rods to the cones is very much dependent upon the brightness level.

Dark Adaptation.—It is common experience that it is very difficult to see when one moves from a bright environment into a dimly lit one such as often occurs when entering a theatre or a cinema, but that after a short while the eye adapts itself to the lower level of illumination, and visibility improves considerably. This is known as *dark adaptation* and arises from details of the way in which the rods operate. Very briefly, the action of light on the rods involves conversion (as a result of absorption of the light) of a substance known as visual purple which is produced in the eye by a mechanism involving vitamin A. Clearly there can be no sensation of light if there is no visual purple in the rod. This is the case if the light intensity has been high (all the visual purple has been converted). At low levels of light intensity the visual purple can, however, gradually build up and become available for use. There appear to be two mechanisms for the production of visual purple, one of which acts fairly quickly whereas the other is much slower. The result is that the sensitivity of the eye to low levels of illumination (subsequent to being illuminated to high normal brightness) changes with time as shown in *Fig.* 256. There is a fairly quick rise over the first 5–15 min. followed by a slower, subsequent rise: the sensitivity increasing slowly and progressively even after 40 min.

The values quoted earlier for the visual acuity and contrast perception for low-level illumination, poor though they are, apply only to a dark-adapted eye, that is one which has been at the low-light level for something like 20–40 min. Until the eye is dark-adapted the acuity and contrast perception are much lower. Since the rods are relatively insensitive to red light, illumination by such light does not impair the build-up of visual purple and it is possible to acquire and retain dark adaptation by wearing

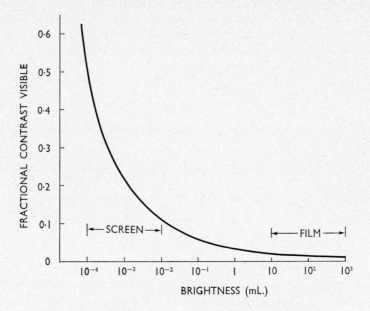

Fig. 255.—Variation, with brightness, of the fractional contrast which can just be detected.

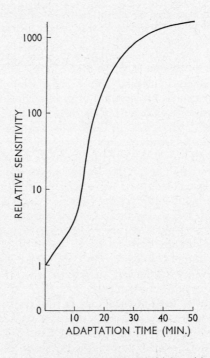

Fig. 256.—Dark adaptation: increase in sensitivity with time spent in
low-intensity illumination.

'red goggles' (i.e., ones which transmit red light only) or by using a red light to illuminate the room. The cones, on the other hand, retain much of their sensitivity in the red end of the spectrum and thus enable the radiologist to 'see' in red light or when wearing goggles. It must be emphasized that exposure of the retina to bright white light even for a fraction of a second will ruin dark adaptation and require a further 15–20 min. to reacquire it.

There is another mechanism which helps the eye to see in dim conditions, namely dilatation of the iris. This enables more light to enter the eye but is, in any case, an immediate, reflex action.

Vision in Practice.—It is clear from the above that the ability to perceive detail and contrast is very much dependent upon the brightness of the object being viewed and that acuity and contrast perception improve as the brightness is increased. The graph of *Fig.* 257 indicates approximately the relationship between the minimum

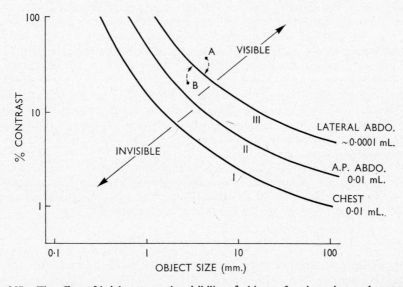

Fig. 257.—The effect of brightness on the visibility of objects of various sizes and contrasts.

contrast and the minimum size of a discernible object at three different levels of brightness. For sizes and contrast above a line (for example, a point such as A in relation to line III) the object is visible: for sizes and contrast below a line (for example, a point such as B for line III) the object is not visible. The three brightness levels indicated are for normal fluoroscopy of the chest (I), the abdomen (II), and a lateral abdomen (III).

It is important to remember that for the level of brightness encountered in radiography, which is about 1 L. (1000 mL.) in the bright regions of the radiograph and about 10 mL. in the dark portions (i.e., a density range of about 2), the contrast perception and acuity can be very high. On the other hand, if the brightness is low then acuity and contrast perception will also be low.

It has already been mentioned in CHAPTER XXI that there is an optimum technique for viewing the radiograph. The same sort of comments apply to viewing at low levels of light intensity. In addition, both general and eye fatigue can set in and the perception of fine detail and small contrasts becomes progressively impaired. Eye fatigue may be associated with failure to build up visual purple and it has even been suggested that vitamin-A deficiency must be guarded against. As regards actual viewing technique it is well known in both astronomy and radiology that faint objects are best seen if they are not looked at! This arises because in the region of the retina known as the macula there are no rods but there is a very high concentration of cones. It is this region of the retina which is used when an object is looked at straight. This has obvious advantages in normal bright vision since acuity will be maximum due to the closeness of the cones. It is equally obvious that such a spot is 'blind' to dim light since there are no rods present. It is found that a faint image is seen more clearly if one looks to the side of it and what is known as peripheral vision is used.

Fluoroscopic Screen Brightness.—The brightness of the fluoroscopic screen is, as already stated, very low and ranges from about 0·05 mL. for a thin chest down to about 0·001 mL. or less for a thick abdomen (*Table XXVI*). It should be noticed that these values are some 10,000 times smaller than the brightnesses at which films are viewed and at these low levels of brightness, at which only the rods are functional, it is very difficult, even for a very experienced, fully dark-adapted radiologist, to see the details of the fluoroscopic pattern because of the limitations of contrast perception and visual acuity described above. There is clearly an advantage to be gained if the screen could be made brighter. Unfortunately, this is not possible for reasons which are obvious when the factors controlling the brightness of the screen are considered. These factors are the intensity of the X-rays incident upon the screen and the efficiency of the screen in absorbing the X-radiation and in emitting visible light as a consequence.

Radiation Dose Rate.—The brightness of the screen is directly proportional to the radiation Exposure rate and clearly an increase in this would therefore produce an increase in brightness. Fairly normal conditions for fluoroscopy are about 60 kV., 3 mA., and a focus–skin distance of about 40 cm. Using the formula given on p. 271 it can be seen that the dose rate on the skin of the patient is:

$$15 \times 60^2 \times 3/40^2 = 100 \text{ mR per sec.}$$

If the accumulated exposure time during a screening session is 4 min., say, then the total skin dose is:

$$100 \times 4 \times 60 = 24{,}000 \text{ mR} = 24 \text{ R,}$$

which is rather a lot of radiation and certainly precludes any possibility of using greater screening currents. In passing, it is worth while noting that the limitation of screen current is one of patient dose and not one of X-ray tube rating. Reference to tube-rating charts indicates that for the usual type of tube employed a current of about 8 mA. could be passed continuously or the tube run at over 50 mA. for up to about 10 min. provided that the anode were rotated and the tube shield fitted with fan cooling. Even with this large increase in tube current and therefore patient dose the increase in brightness would only be by a factor of less than 15, which although it would be helpful is insufficient; an improvement of at least 50 being necessary to bring the brightness into the range of cone vision (0·002–0·1 mL.) and at least 5000 being required to raise the brightness of the fluoroscopic screen to the levels encountered in film viewing (0·002–10 mL.). If it were not for the restrictions of patient dose it is not impossible that X-ray tubes of even higher rating could be constructed even if therapy type continuous forced cooling were thereby needed.

It is fairly obvious therefore that if the patient is not to be subjected to intolerable radiation doses no significant increase in screen brightness is to be obtained by increasing the screening current and therefore the radiation Exposure rate. Rather to the contrary there would appear to be a need to find methods whereby the current and therefore the radiation dose to the patient could be reduced.

A reduction in patient dose rate could be obtained by using a larger focus–skin distance than is normally the case. It is, however, usually necessary to fit the tube beneath the tilting table and the maximum focus–table top (i.e., skin) distance is therefore restricted if the table top is not to be unacceptably high.

The use of a small focus–skin distance means that magnification is high which, although not entirely desirable, is useful in the sense that all the shadows are increased in size and are therefore marginally more visible (*Fig.* 257). The small focal distance tends also to increase geometric and movement blurrings but even so this is not important since their value is still less than that which can be appreciated even by the fully dark-adapted eye, at these low brightness levels.

The use of a high kV. could also lead to a reduction in patient dose for the same screen brightness but this again is not very possible. It will be remembered that the fluorescent screen has a gamma of unity (viz. the brightness is linearly proportional to the X-ray intensity creating it) so that there is no contrast improvement such as that brought about by the film (gamma=4) in radiography. It is therefore important to keep the contrast high by using a low kV.; this is especially true since, as shown by *Fig.* 257, detail perception is very much impaired if the contrast is low, i.e., there is poor contrast perception (*Fig.* 255) at the low brightness levels.

Screen Efficiency.—Zinc cadmium sulphide is the material most commonly used for fluoroscopic screens since:

    i. It is substantially free from after-glow.

    ii. The emitted light is in that part of the spectrum to which the rods are more sensitive (green).

    iii. It has a comparatively high efficiency for converting X-ray energy into visible light especially at the lower kV. used in fluoroscopy.

The screen thickness is rather greater than for intensifying screens in an attempt to increase as much as possible the amount of X-ray absorption in the screen and therefore the brightness. There is a limit to this, however, since if the screen is too thick the light produced in the deeper layers on the screen will be absorbed by the overlying layers and so is not seen. It must be noted that increase of screen thickness will increase the blurring which in any case is rather larger (0·5–1·0 mm.) than that of an intensifying screen, but this is the price which has to be paid in order to gain brightness. It should be appreciated that there is no point in reducing the various blurrings (geometric, movement, or screen) to values which are significantly less than the detail perception of the eye which is worse than $1\frac{1}{2}$ mm. at the low level of brightness. The amount of detail on the fluoroscopic screen is in fact usually rather greater than can be seen by the eye under these conditions since the total blurring is less than the perception of the eye. It is for this reason that the use of a magnifying glass can often increase the amount of visible detail on the screen and why a photograph of the fluorescent screen shows, when viewed at normal room brightnesses, more detail than could be seen on the original screen.

Of the X-ray photons incident upon the fluorescent screen some 15 per cent only are absorbed by the screen and only about 30 per cent of this absorbed energy is converted into visible light. Hence rather less than 5 per cent (30 per cent of 15 per cent = 4·5 per cent) of the incident X-ray energy is converted into light photons. Since the energy of each light photon is very much less than that of the incident X-ray photon there are, in spite of this inefficient conversion of energy, many more light photons leaving the screen than X-ray photons incident upon it (cf. 'Intensifying Screens', p. 192). The inefficiencies do not end here since only a very small fraction of the light produced will leave the screen in the direction of the viewing eye. However, even if it were possible to make the fluoroscopic screen 100 per cent efficient so that all of the incident X-ray energy were absorbed by it and converted into visible light, the improvement in brightness would be by a factor of about 20 only (viz., 5 per cent → 100 per cent) which is again small compared with the desired improvement of more than a thousand times.

Since in radiography the photographic film is placed immediately next to the screen, it absorbs all the light emitted from the screen. The eye, however, is usually at about 20–25 cm. from the fluorescent screen and is only able because of this and of the small diameter of its opening (the iris) to receive and utilize much less than 1 per cent of the light emitted from the screen. In this sense, therefore, the film is much more efficient than the eye. On the other hand, however, the eye is a very sensitive detector of visible light and in spite of its low acceptance of light from the screen it is better than the radiographic film at detecting light. It has been shown that the eye works by integrating light over a period of about 0·2 sec. At the usual screening current of 3 mA. this represents an exposure of $3 \times 0·2 = 0·6$ mA.s. which is far below any possible radiographic exposure. Thus it is not surprising that the radiograph contains much more information in the form of visible contrast and detail since it has required much more X-ray energy to produce the picture.

Role of Fluoroscopy.—In spite of the great technical difficulties of fluoroscopy and of the limited amount of information which can be seen at the low levels of brightness which are obtained, fluoroscopy is a most useful diagnostic method. It has the obvious, trivial, advantage that it is cheap compared with radiography in that it uses no materials such as film and processing chemicals. More important is the fact that it provides an immediate dynamic picture which the radiologist is able, if necessary, to modify by palpation or by the administration of high-density or high-atomic-number contrast materials which, in view of the inherent high contrast which they cause, combat some of the difficulties of fluoroscopy. If adequate detail cannot be seen on the screen then a radiograph can be taken at the instant in time which, the fluoroscope shows, will produce the desired information.

Since fluoroscopy must be carried out in a darkened room, it is uncongenial and inconvenient to both patient and staff. In view of this and its irreplaceable usefulness, it is not surprising that great efforts have been made to overcome its deficiencies of low-contrast discrimination and detail perception. It has already been indicated that no solution is likely to be obtained by increasing the X-ray tube output or by increasing the screen efficiency. A solution has, however, been developed over the past ten to fifteen years in the form of the image amplifier, and now the use of some form of image amplification which makes the fluoroscopic image acceptably bright and within the range of cone vision is becoming almost universal. The use of the traditional, direct vision, fluorescent screen is almost, but not quite, a thing of the past.

THE IMAGE INTENSIFIER

The construction of an electronic image intensifier is shown in a very simplified form in *Fig.* 258. It consists of a fluorescent screen (a) on to which the X-ray pattern is directed as usual. The corresponding pattern of light emitted from this screen is incident upon a second screen (b) which, in practice, is in intimate contact with the fluorescent screen (a). This second screen is composed of a photo-electron emitting material and is called the photocathode. The intensity pattern of the electrons emitted from the photocathode will correspond exactly with the pattern of light incident upon it and therefore to the pattern in the X-ray beam. The electrons are now accelerated across the evacuated envelope by the voltage (about 25 kV.) applied

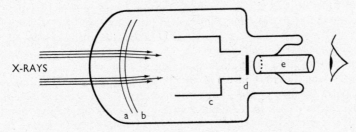

X-RAYS

Fig. 258.—The image intensifier. (a) Fluorescent screen; (b) Photocathode; (c) Electron lens; (d) Output fluorescent screen; (e) Viewing system.

between the cathode and the fluorescent viewing screen (d). The light produced by the absorption of the increased energy electrons in this screen is very much brighter than the light emitted from the initial screen (a) and is in fact sufficiently bright to be seen by cone vision.

The side of the output screen (d) nearest the photocathode is covered by a thin layer of aluminium. This allows the electrons to pass through but stops any light produced in the output screen from passing to the photocathode where it would liberate unwanted electrons. These electrons would eventually produce light, more or less uniformly at the output screen: the whole cycle of events then repeating itself indefinitely. The final effect of this would be a considerable reduction in contrast at the output screen. Clearly this must be avoided.

The pattern, in which the radiologist is interested, is preserved in the electron beam passing from the photocathode (b) to the viewing screen (d) because of the electron lens (c), which, in addition to preserving the pattern, diminishes its size so that the diameter of the original pattern is reduced to about one-fifth, i.e., the diameter of the pattern on the viewing screen (d) is one-fifth that of the pattern on the initial screen (a). Even in the absence of an accelerating voltage across the tube this reduction in size would create an increase in brightness since the same amount of energy is being passed through a smaller area which must therefore appear brighter. If the relative diameters are 1 : 5 then the areas and therefore brightnesses will be in the ratio of 1 : 25 (i.e., 1 : 5^2), thus the reduction to one-fifth size causes a brightness increase of 25 times. The price paid for this increase of brightness is that the image is correspondingly smaller, but this can be compensated by viewing the screen via a magnifying glass (or in practice a specially designed viewing lens system) and so restoring the image to the original full size. This does not automatically reduce the brightness by the factor of 25 since the effect of using a viewing lens is to allow the eye to be placed closer to the screen and, as was shown earlier on p. 342, the brightness of a surface is independent of the viewing distance. An alternative way of looking at this is to say that the system enables a much larger fraction of the light emitted from the original screen to enter the eye. In normal fluoroscopy the radiologist's eye is at some 20 cm. from the screen and thereby gathers only a very small fraction (much less than 1 per cent) of the light emitted from the screen; most of the light is wasted. In the image intensifier almost all of the light emitted from the initial screen (a) is accepted by the photocathode and its energy transmitted via electrons to the output screen (d). The use of the objective enables the eye to be placed much closer to this latter screen and therefore a much greater fraction of the emitted light reaches the eye.

The increase in brightness brought about because of the accelerating voltage can be about 40 times so that, in all, the brightness is increased about one thousandfold. A fluoroscopic image of brightness 0·005 mL. (at which only rod vision is of importance) will, by using an image intensifier, be raised to 5 mL., which, although not equal in brightness to the radiograph on a viewing screen, is well within the range of cone vision, with all its attendant advantages.

Advantages and Disadvantages of the Image Intensifier.—The amplification of brightness made possible by the image intensifier may be utilized in several ways.

Reduction in Patient Dose.—An alternative to having a brightness increase for the same patient X-ray exposure (viz., screening current) would be to reduce the exposure and accept either a reduced or even no increase in brightness. It is now almost universal practice to use a screening current of about 0·5 mA. rather than the traditional value of 3–5 mA. and therefore effect a reduction in patient dose by a factor of between 6 and 10. The brightness increase is then only times 100 which is not usually sufficient to achieve very much in the way of advantage from cone vision (*see Fig.* 252, p. 343); furthermore, viewing in a darkened or semi-darkened room together with some degree, at least, of dark adaptation is still necessary.

More Congenial Working Conditions.—The use of the eye-piece to view the image together with the fact that the image seen is much brighter means that the radiologist need not be fully dark adapted and the room need not be completely dark. This means that the patient is in a much less frightening environment and can see to co-operate. Furthermore, both radiographer and radiologist can see what is happening, can read the case notes, avoid the barium being spilt, etc. In this way the examination is much more congenial, less fatiguing, and, therefore, better for all concerned.

Screen Detail.—Since the screen brightness is greater the perception of detail (i.e., acuity) is much greater and any information on the screen can now be seen. Limitation in detail perception is now the same as in radiography, namely geometric, movement, and screen blurring, all of which were well below acuity at the traditional fluoroscopic brightness levels. In an effort to achieve brightness the traditional fluoroscopic screen had a large unsharpness (*see* p. 202). This is no longer necessary, so the input screen (*Fig.* 258) is one of fine grain whose unsharpness is more like that of an intensifying screen. The output screen (d) must also have a small blurring.

Even the finest output screen will create some blurring and therefore there is a limit to the reduction in size (and increase in brightness) of the image on this screen which may be effected. Excessive reduction will demand a viewing system of high magnification which will, of course, magnify the blur also. By using these 'thinner' screens the brightness is somewhat diminished and a compromise between this and the unsharpness has to be made.

Similarly, especially when television is used (*see below*), the geometric unsharpness can profitably be reduced by using a smaller focal spot size. It will be remembered that a rather small F.S.D. is used in fluoroscopy so that the use of a large focal spot can lead to great geometric unsharpness. It is therefore common practice with many image amplifier systems to use a 0·3-mm. focal spot.

Distortion.—Although no details of the electronic working of image intensifiers are being given here, it is important to realize that the pattern on the output screen

(d) should not have any defects, artefacts, or distortion brought about by the image intensifier tube itself. Just as an optical system has defects which can be corrected by careful design, so does an electron lens system and it must therefore be designed and operated correctly if the final image is to be free from any additional defects.

Field Size.—One of the major defects of the image intensifier is the relatively small size of the area of the patient which can be seen at any one time. In many of the original systems the maximum field of vision was as small as 10–13 cm. in diameter and was regarded as being very restrictive. Efforts to make image intensifiers with large input screens, although successful to a degree, have not proved to be the best solution. Fortunately, a satisfactory solution has been achieved by interposing, as shown in *Fig.* 259, an optical system between the fluorescent screen and the intensifier.

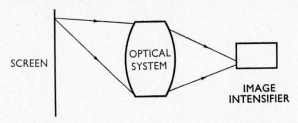

Fig. 259.—Increase in maximum fluorescent screen size by incorporating an optical system.

A fine-grain full-size fluoroscopic screen is used and light emitted from this is focused by means of a lens on to the input screen of the image intensifier, which can now be fairly small. If there is not to be a large loss of light the lens must have a large diameter and if there is to be no distortion, etc., the lens must be free from optical defects.* It is almost impossible, in practice, to devise a system which is efficient from both these points of view and for this reason a system which uses mirror optics together with a special correcting lens is usually employed. One such system is illustrated in *Fig.* 260. An incidental advantage of this system is that the use of mirrors enables the length of the apparatus to be reduced although because of the large diameter needed to collect enough light it is necessarily rather bulky.

Viewing the Image.—The use of an eye-piece to view the output screen ((d), *Fig.* 258) is very inconvenient since it restricts the position of the radiologist; for instance, it can make palpation difficult, if not impossible. It also makes it impossible for more than one person to view the screen at any one time, although ingenious systems of split mirrors have been used to permit vision by two people simultaneously. The solution to this problem which has found most favour is to use a closed-circuit television system to view the output screen of the image intensifier. The type of television camera known as a Vidicon is used, although this is gradually being replaced in many systems by a similar type of camera called the Plumbicon, which has the advantage that there is much less delay between changes in the X-ray pattern occurring and being observed at the television screen. The rather complex details of the many television systems which can be, and have been, used will not be discussed here where only one or two of the important aspects from the user's point of view will be mentioned.

Brightness.—The television camera essentially converts a visible light picture into electrical signals which are then converted back into light at the television screen

---

* For more details of lens systems any textbook on light or optics should be consulted.

(i.e., on the television monitor screen): the camera being connected by a cable direct to the monitor—hence the name 'closed-circuit' television. Once the information about the fluoroscopic pattern is in the form of electrical signals there are many possibilities open. The most important of these is that the brightness of the picture can be as high as desired—almost irrespective of the brightness of the input screen. In other words, further brightness amplification can take place in the television system itself and the monitor screen made as bright as a radiograph on a viewing

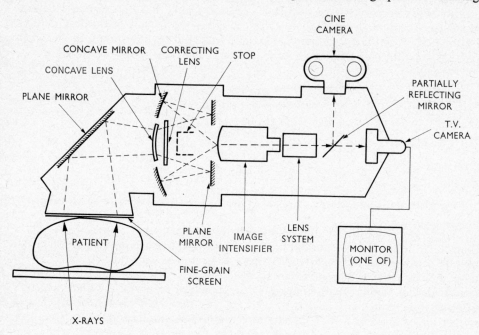

Fig. 260.—Combined image intensifier—television system.

screen. Under such circumstances clearly the deficiencies of the vision associated with low-brightness levels discussed above are of no importance. In one system the image intensifier is, in fact, dispensed with altogether and all the brightness amplification takes place in the television part of the system. For this a rather sensitive and much more costly type of television camera (the Image Orthicon) has to be used. The extra increase in brightness now available makes it unnecessary to work in a much-darkened room (although some reduction in general room lighting is advantageous). In addition, the screening current (mA.) and therefore patient dose can be further reduced. There is a limit, however, to this reduction in patient dose and the amount of intensification which is worth while. As with the intensifying screen (p. 202), if the X-ray Exposure rate is reduced too much then quantum mottle will become apparent and the image quality deteriorate. In addition, if the electronic amplification is too great then defects of the electrical circuits will become of importance and will mar the perception of detail—in the jargon of the electronic engineer, the signal-to-noise ratio will be too low. It turns out that there is little point in increasing the amplification beyond the stage at which the number of light photons affecting the retina is greater than the number of photons present at the stage of the system where the number of photons is a minimum—usually the number of photons being absorbed at the fluorescent screen. In other words, it is not possible to make a fluoroscopic screen image without using X-rays and it would appear that the instrument development has progressed sufficiently far that no further reduction in patient dose is likely. In normal fluoroscopy and even to some extent in radiography it is the defects of the eye which limit the detail perceived: with the image intensifier and television system it is the amount of X-radiation at the fluorescent screen which sets the limit to the detail present in the pattern. It follows, almost without saying, that great care has to be taken with these electronic systems so that distortions and defects are not introduced and the image quality thereby impaired. Although the image quality can be very high when the system is in correct adjustment and is being used correctly, it is very easy to 'twiddle' one or more of the many available knobs and so ruin the picture. Even more insidiously, the image quality can deteriorate slowly, and unnoticed, over longish periods of time due to the electronic system becoming in less than perfect adjustment. It is therefore of great importance to (a) check that the image quality is maintained and (b) that no unnecessary or unknowledgeable knob twiddling occurs. The television system is a complex one which at the present stage of development needs very careful maintenance.

One of the other possibilities of the television system is to change the contrast electronically. This may be to either decrease or increase the contrast, so that, in the latter case, the fluoroscopic image acquired a 'gamma' as in the radiograph. In addition there are many tricks which can be played. For example, the image can be reversed right to left or top to bottom. Furthermore, the television monitor can be made to show the pattern full size or the central portion of the pattern can be magnified and presented on the monitor.

Television Raster.—It is well known that the television picture is made up of a great number of nearly horizontal lines, the brightness of which varies both from line to line and along the length of each line. Therefore, any detail which is smaller than the separation of these lines will not be visible. Using the standard television system of about 400 lines to the picture, the separation of these lines will be little more than $\frac{1}{2}$ mm., if the picture size is 25 cm. which is usual. This is very comparable to the size of the blurrings encountered on the radiograph and is very much better than that encountered in the traditional fluoroscopy. One particular television system uses over 1000 lines to the picture which gives a 'blurring' of less than $\frac{1}{4}$ mm.

General.—It is very difficult to be precise about the relative merits of television fluoroscopy and radiography, but it would appear that under usual operating conditions the radiographic image is substantially better than the fluoroscopic one, principally because of the difficulties of achieving optimal operating conditions for the fluoroscopic system compared with the rather technically more easy radiography. It would appear, however, that when both are being used optimally the radiographic image is only a little better than the fluoroscopic, but what is important is that the latter is much better than the traditional fluoroscopic image. Fluoroscopy and radiography thus remain complementary techniques.

Photofluorography.—Although much good and useful work, particularly in chest examinations, has been and continues to be done by using the simple photofluorographic system in which a full-size fluoroscopic screen is photographed directly by a 35-mm. camera, it must be realized that, here, the radiation dose to the patient is several times greater than for the normal chest radiograph. Alternative systems are now available and, for instance, a single-shot photograph may be taken of the television monitor either full size or on a reduced scale. In neither case is the dose as low or the result as good as the normal radiograph but it can be very comparable, and in many cases more convenient or appropriate.

An alternative scheme, which is incorporated into a specially designed chest unit, utilizes an optical system, similar to that previously described (*Fig.* 260), to direct the light from the initial full-size fluoroscopic screen into the photographic film which is usually 70 or 100 mm. in size.

Other Techniques.—The use of the image intensifier and television system allows several other things to be done. The most simple of these is the use of multiple monitors. Several television monitors may be connected to the camera so that observers in the same or other rooms or even in other buildings can observe the pattern simultaneously. It has even been suggested by a cynic that this is really a disadvantage since eventually the radiologist may prefer to remain at home and watch the screening on the television there! In spite of this, the ability to have several different screens has clear advantages in teaching and consultation.

The making of a cine-radiographic record is also made feasible by the image intensifier. It has always been possible to make a cine-recording by photographing the traditional fluoroscopic screen, but it has not been permissible because of the very high screening current needed and therefore the high patient dose which would be involved. This is no longer the case. Two systems are in use, the first of which directs light from the output screen of the image intensifier, by means of a partially reflecting plane mirror as shown in *Fig.* 260, on the cine-camera. The alternative scheme is to photograph the picture on an additional television monitor screen. In either case normal fluoroscopic screening can continue as the cine-recording is made, but in the latter case care has to be taken that stroboscopic type effects do not occur and the cine-camera has to be driven in exact synchronism with the television picture scan.

It is also possible to make a television recording on magnetic tape (Video recording) and to play back this tape on to a television monitor either immediately or later. This has some advantage over cine-radiography—for example, there is no delay in processing—in some circumstances, although good-quality pictures are difficult to achieve consistently.

A further facility which is not yet fully developed involves the use of a special type of television tube known as an 'image storage tube'. This can operate as a normal television tube but by simply operating a switch, can be made to store the picture existing on the screen at that moment. Returning the switch to its normal position will restore normal operation of the tube. The radiologist is not always interested in the dynamic situation but in using the fluorescent screen rather as an instant, ephemeral radiograph and in examining each part of the screen in turn. Clearly, whilst he is looking at one part of the screen the X-rays being directed on to other parts are being wasted and cause unnecessary dose to the patient. A storage tube enables the full image to be produced by a 'flash' exposure and retained for as long as the radiologist wishes. During this time the patient is receiving no further exposure. Another use could be that, if during a dynamic examination the radiologist sees something which he wishes to look at for a longer time than it is likely to remain there he can do so by storing the image.

As can be imagined, the storage tube is a very complex device and at the present time the coarseness of its screen is a major deficiency. The additional facilities of the storage tube are also available when using Video recording, which, of course, has the further advantage of permanent storage.

In all these various systems the materials used for the input and output fluorescent screens, for the photocathode, and for the television fluorescent screen as well as the type of photographic film used in the cine-camera, must be chosen so as to be compatible with (i.e., emit or be sensitive to) the appropriate wavelengths of light. Although the systems described in this chapter have brought undoubted improvements to the fluoroscopic techniques, they are relatively complicated pieces of electronic equipment. Unless they are adjusted to and maintained in optimum operating conditions the image quality is unlikely to be all that it should be.

In conclusion it must be emphasized that the account given in this chapter of the image intensifier television system is a very superficial one and the exact type of facility available from the various manufacturers is very varied and is being continuously extended further.

CHAPTER XXVI

TOMOGRAPHY

IN normal radiography the character of the pattern on the radiograph formed by the anatomical structures of interest is very often partially or even completely obscured by the shadows cast by overlying or underlying structures. In many cases a distinction can be made by choosing appropriate orientation of the patient, but in others it is necessary to use the technique known as 'body-section radiography' or, more usually, *tomography*. By using the method and apparatus described below the confusing shadows cast by the overlying and underlying structures are blurred out, whilst those of the structures of interest are left sharply defined and therefore visible. To achieve this selective blurring it is necessary to have a controlled, accurate, relative movement of the X-ray tube, film, and patient during the exposure. There are several different types of tomographic movement but the simplest is that due to Twining and is what is known as a *linear* tomographic movement.

THE LINEAR TOMOGRAPH

Fig. 261 indicates, very simply, the movement which takes place. The X-ray tube target is constrained to move along the straight line *TT*, and the film in the opposite direction along a parallel straight line *FF*. The X-ray exposure starts at

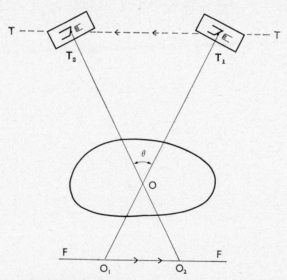

Fig. 261.—The Twining, or linear, tomographic movement.

the instant when the X-ray tube focal spot is at the position such as T_1 and terminates when it is at T_2. The shadow of an object at the point O will therefore be cast, in the plane of the film (*FF*), at O_1 when the target is at T_1 and as the target moves then so will the shadow until finally it reaches O_2 when the target is at T_2. Clearly, therefore,

358

if it can be arranged that, as the target moves in the straight line from T_1 to T_2, the film can also be moved in synchronism a distance equal to O_1 to O_2, the shadow of O will be cast at the same point on the film throughout the whole of the exposure and will not therefore be blurred by the movement. Furthermore, since the film and target move along parallel lines the magnification is constant and the sharpness of the shadow of O will be exactly the same as if a stationary radiograph had been made (except for any extra movement of the patient during the longer exposure required in tomography). The tomographic apparatus is constructed so that this exact relative movement of film and X-ray tube occurs. This may be done by means of a simple attachment to the tube head and Bucky tray which pivots about the point O, or by using a unit specially constructed for tomography. *Fig.* 262 shows a picture of: (*a*) a tomographic attachment, and (*b*) a special tomographic unit.

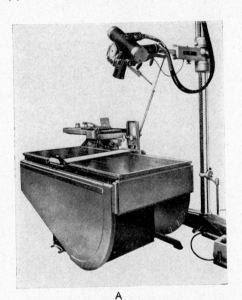 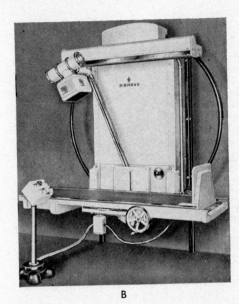

A   B

Fig. 262.—Practical tomographic equipment, showing main features. A, Standard X-ray equipment with tomographic attachment. B, Special tomographic unit.

For structures in the patient lying further from or closer to the film (e.g., X and Y in *Fig.* 263) than O their shadows will move by distances larger or smaller, respectively, than the distance O_1 to O_2, and will therefore move with respect to the moving film and so be blurred. For example, the shadow of X (*Fig.* 263) will move a distance V_x as the target moves from T_1 to T_2 whereas the film will move a distance ($U = O_1O_2$). The shadow of X will therefore be blurred by an amount equal to $V_x - U$. Similarly the shadow of Y will be blurred out by an amount $U - V_y$. These two movements ($V_x - U$ and $U - V_y$) of the shadows, with respect to the film, can be quite large as is indicated by the exaggerated drawing of *Fig.* 263.

By using the fact that triangles T_1OT_2 and O_1OO_2 are similar, it can very easily be shown that if S is the distance moved by the tube target then the distance (U) which the film must move is given by:

$$U = S \times b/a,$$

where a and b are the distances from O to the lines along which the target and film move.

Plane of Cut.—The preservation of the sharpness of the shadow of an object positioned at O, whilst the shadows of deeper and more superficial objects are blurred, applies equally to all objects in the same level. *Fig.* 264 shows two objects O and L at the same level above the film. The tomographic movement (i.e., relative movement of target and film) is such that the shadow of O is sharp (as in *Figs.* 261 and 263). Since O and L are both at the same distance from the film their shadows will move equal distances during the tomographic movement and, therefore, since the shadow of O is stationary on the film, then so will be the shadow of L. This applies to

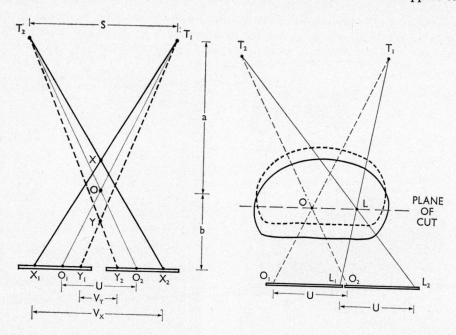

Fig. 263.—Movements of shadows of objects closer to, or further, from the pivot point.

Fig. 264.—The 'plane of cut'. The shadows of objects on the plane move the same amount as the film, and show no tomographic blurring.

all structures on the same level as O and L which is therefore referred to as the 'plane of cut' (sometimes called the 'in-focus plane'). The shadows of all objects in this plane (parallel to the plane of movement of the film) will be free from tomographic blurring, whilst objects not in this plane will have shadows which are blurred to an extent depending on their distance from this plane.

The tomographic apparatus or attachment is designed so that this plane of cut can be placed at any desired level in the patient either by moving the position of the patient (as indicated dotted in *Fig.* 264) or by moving the pivot point (O) of the apparatus.

It should be noticed that in this tomographic movement the focal spot moves along a line parallel to the film movement. During this movement the X-ray tube is itself rotated about the focus as axis in order to keep the beam directed at the film and so achieve uniform exposure rate during the whole of the exposure time. If this is not done the effectiveness of the radiation at the extremes of the swing, and therefore the effective size of the swing, is seriously diminished.

Tomographic Blurring.—The blurring of the unwanted shadows is, of course, nothing more than a particular example of the movement blurring discussed in an earlier chapter. For convenience, however, it is referred to as tomographic blurring. It is important to realize that any lack of synchronism between the corresponding movements of the film and target will cause additional blurring even of the shadows arising from objects in the plane of cut. It is therefore extremely important that the tomographic apparatus be correctly designed, and maintained in accurate adjustment. Failure to achieve this, results not in tomograms but in blurred pictures! Fortunately, however, there is, as always, some room for lack of complete perfection. The other types of blurring (geometric screen and normal movement blurring) are, of course, present simultaneously and following the argument set out on p. 268, it is clear that only when the tomographic blurring is about the same size as the other blurrings will it begin to be noticed. As will be shown below—and as common sense would expect—the amount of tomographic blurring increases as the distance of the objects from the plane of cut increases. There is, therefore, as indicated in *Fig.* 265, a region on either side of the plane of cut which appears to be in focus. In other words, the shadows of any objects between the levels of X and Y (*Fig.* 265) have a tomographic

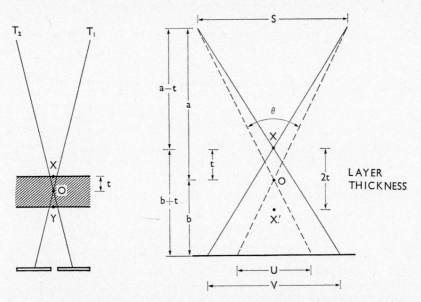

Fig. 265.—The tomographic blurring.

Fig. 266.—The geometric factors controlling the thickness of the layer.

blurring which is insufficiently large to be noticeable in the presence of the usual radiographic blurrings. This region is referred to as the tomographic layer or the 'in-focus layer'. It must be emphasized that in theory, and in practice, there is a continuous increase in the blurring as the distance of the objects from the plane of cut increases and there is nothing sharp about the upper and lower levels of the in-focus layer. Since the eye is only conscious of blurrings above a certain size and tends to ignore blurrings less than this, the idea of an in-focus layer of a definite thickness (2t) is useful and furthermore the size of its thickness can be varied by changing the extent of the tomographic movement.

Factors controlling the Thickness of Cut.—In the diagram of *Fig.* 266 the point *O* lies in the plane of cut and the tomographic movement is assumed to be perfect. A point such as *X*, a distance *t* above the plane, will be blurred by an amount B_m which is assumed to be the maximum tomographic blurring which is just not noticeable. There will be a similar point (*X'*) below *O* and the slice *XX'* will be the tomographic layer. The thickness (2*t*) of this slice can be calculated by reference to *Fig.* 266. The movement of the film (i.e., the movement of the shadow of the object *O*) is given by:

$$U = S.b/a,$$

whereas the movement of the shadow of *X* is given by:

$$V = S(b + t)/(a - t).$$

The movement of this shadow on the film, i.e., the blurring (B_m), is equal to the difference of these two movements, i.e.,

$$B_m = V - U = S.\frac{(a + b)}{(a - t)}.\frac{t}{a}.$$

Now *t* is very much smaller than *a* so that, without significant error,

$$B_m = S.\frac{(a + b)}{a^2}.t$$

or

$$t = B_m.\frac{a}{S} \times \frac{a}{(a+b)}$$

or

$$2t = 2B_m.\frac{a}{S}.\frac{a}{(a + b)}.$$

The angular swing (*θ*) of the X-ray tube about the point *O* is given by:

$$\theta = S/a \text{ in radians.}$$

Inserting this in the previous equation we obtain:

$$2t = 2B_m.\frac{1}{\theta}.\frac{a}{(a + b)}.$$

Hence the thickness of the slice increases as the angle of swing is decreased. This would be expected since smaller movements of the tube will obviously lead to smaller blurrings. The excursion (*S*) of the X-ray tube is the variable which is used in practice to vary the thickness of cut.

Some typical values are:

$\theta = 20°$ or $20/57$ radians; $(a + b) = $ F.F.D. $= 90$ cm.;   and $a = 75$ cm.

Taking 0·7 mm. as a reasonable value for B_m, we have

$$2t = 2 \times \frac{57}{20} \times \frac{75}{90} \times 0.7 = 3\tfrac{1}{3} \text{ mm.}$$

or just over $1\tfrac{1}{2}$ mm. either side of the tomographic plane through *O*.

The thickness of the cut also depends upon the height above the film of the layer being cut. In practice the focus–film distance ($F = a + b$) is constant, as is the angle (*θ*) of swing, so that the thickness of the cut increases as the value of *b* decreases.

In other words, layers cut at a distance from the film are thinner than those cut close to the film. The variation is, however, small and is usually ignored. The magnitude of distance *a* between target and tomographic plane also affects the layer thickness but in practice the control of layer thickness is effected by change of angle of swing only. *Table XXVII* lists some typical layer thicknesses at various angles.

Table XXVII.—Some Approximate Values of Tomography Layer Thickness
obtained with Different Angles (θ) of Movement in Linear Tomography

Angle of Movement (θ)	Layer Thickness
20°	$3\frac{1}{3}$ mm.
10°	$6\frac{2}{3}$ mm.
7°	$9\frac{1}{2}$ mm.
4°	$1\frac{2}{3}$ cm.
2°	$3\frac{2}{3}$ cm.

ALTERNATIVE LINEAR MOVEMENTS

Linear tomography may be performed equally well using the movements due to Grossman, and illustrated in *Fig.* 267 A. In this case the X-ray tube and film move, in synchronism, on arcs of circles centred about the pivot point *O*. The diagram shows three positions of the tube T_1, T_c, and T_2 with the corresponding positions

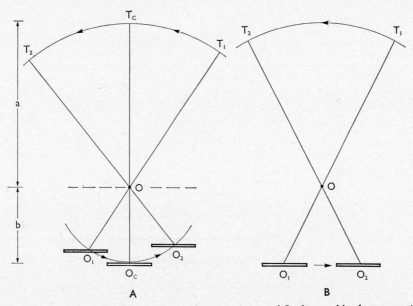

Fig. 267.—A, The Grossman tomographic movement, and B, the combined movement.

of the film O_1, O_c, and O_2, and it will be seen that whilst the film centre follows the arc, the film itself is maintained parallel to the plane of cut (broken line in *Fig.* 267) through *O*. The comments and result of the calculations given previously for the Twining movement apply equally to the Grossman movement. The relative merits of the Twining and Grossman movements depend almost entirely on the success with which they can be engineered, and unwanted blurrings due to uneven and non-synchronous movements avoided. It is usually easier to move the X-ray tube in an arc as in the Grossman system, but easier to move the film horizontally in a plane as in the Twining system. In fact a unit (shown in *Fig.* 267 B) which combines these two movements is produced by at least one manufacturer. Although, theoretically, a simple tomographic cut of uniform thickness is not produced by such a movement, in practice the engineering can be sufficiently successful that the absence of mechanically produced unwanted blurrings more than outweighs these theoretical deficiencies.

Patient Dose.—A typical exposure in tomography is 60 kV., 150 mA., 1·2 sec., and 65 cm. target–skin distance, which results in a dose to the skin of the patient of about 2300 mrad. This is quite a high dose and in addition it is important to realize that in tomographic examinations it is common practice to make several cuts at different levels so that the total dose may be very large by radiographic standards. The total dose to the patient can be considerably reduced by using the multiple cassette, which is illustrated in *Fig.* 268. Instead of using just one film, several films (typically five or six) are contained in a box and spaced at about 1 cm. apart.

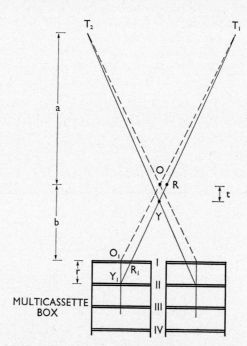

Fig. 268.—Simultaneous multiple 'cuts' are obtained using a multicassette.

It can be seen from *Fig.* 268 that if the plane of cut for the upper film (I) passes, as before, through O there will be an in-focus plane passing through Y which is shadowed on to the second film (II) and similarly other parallel layers for the films (III) *et seq*. The relationship between the distance between the plane of cut (OY) and the film separations ($O_1 Y_1$) is given by:

$$O_1 Y_1 = O Y.(a + b)/a.$$

If, for example, $a = 80$ cm. and $b = 20$ cm. then, in order to make cuts at 1-cm. intervals, it is necessary to space the films by 1·25 cm. The advantage of such a multicassette is, clearly, that several cuts may be made simultaneously during a single X-ray exposure and the patient dose thus reduced substantially.

In order that all the films in the set are of comparable density it is necessary to use a set of intensifying screens of suitably graded speeds. For example, the upper film (l) may be used in conjunction with a single high-definition screen whereas the lower films may use pairs of faster screens.

Circular, Elliptical, and Hypocycloidal Movements.—One of the main objections to linear tomography is that all the blurrings are in straight lines, so that the shadows of extended objects which lie in the direction of the movement, above or below the plane cut, are not particularly well blurred out. This arises because the blurred shadows of various parts of the 'out of plane' objects are superimposed. It can even happen that these blurred shadows build up so as to give the impression of a shadow cast by a real object although no such object is, in fact, present. The possible production of such artefacts must be realized and care taken that they are not misinterpreted.

A second problem is that the extent of the tube travel (S), and therefore angle of swing (θ), cannot be very large. At large angulations both the distance between the target and the film, and the oblique radiation path through the patient are large

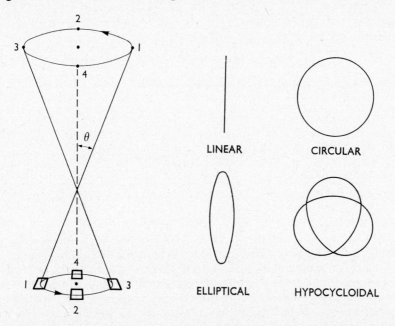

*Fig.*269.—A circular tomographic movement.   *Fig.* 270.—Four types of tomographic movement.

so that the blackening on the film is small, due to the small amount of radiation able to reach it. Hence, even if the angulation is large, most of the exposure of the film takes place during the central part of the swing and therefore the effective angulation is much smaller than is the actual angulation.

More effective blurring out of the shadows of overlying and underlying objects, and therefore decrease in thickness of cut, can be achieved by using movements more complex than the simple linear movement described. Provided that the film is moved, with its plane parallel to the plane of interest in the patient, in synchronized apposition to the movement of the target, then a tomographic cut will always be obtained. The simplest of these more complicated movements is, as indicated in *Fig.* 265, where the film and tube are constrained to move in corresponding circles.

With such a movement the blurrings of the overlying and underlying structures follow circular paths and therefore may not intrude. Clearly any type of simultaneous synchronous movement of tube and film will result in a tomographic cut being made, and the extent of the movement will govern the degree of blurring and therefore the thickness of cut: greater movement leading to thinner cuts. In practice, however, the movements are restricted to: (*a*) linear, (*b*) circular, (*c*) elliptical, and (*d*) hypocycloidal (*Fig.* 270). In each case the extent of the movement can be varied and so control of the thickness of cut effected, with the hypocycloidal giving the greatest possibility of obtaining thin cuts. The shape of the blurring and therefore characteristic artefacts are, of course, different for each type of movement.

Contrast in Tomography.—In the absence of any tomographic artefacts the shadows of the overlying and underlying structures are completely blurred out on the radiograph and the contrasts, from which the radiologist gains the information he needs, are created by the structures within the plane of cut. *Fig.* 271 A, therefore,

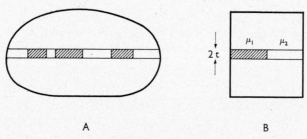

A   B

Fig. 271.—Contrast in tomography.

represents this situation and can be idealized to that shown in *Fig.* 271 B. If $2t$ is the thickness of the tomographic layer then the contrast produced (*see* p. 236) is:

$$C = 0{\cdot}4343\gamma \, (\mu_1 - \mu_2) . 2t.$$

Clearly, if the thickness of the slice is made small by using large tomographic movement the contrast will also be small and, in the limit, not visible. Care must be taken, therefore, that a sufficiently thick layer is used whenever the difference in attenuation of the structures in the layer is not large. On the other hand, if a large difference in an atomic number or density exists then visible contrast can be obtained even if the tomographic layer is very thin. For example, the ossicles in the middle ear are composed of very dense bone surrounded by air: such structures are clearly visible on a tomographic layer which is rather less than 0·2 mm. thick!

It is important to remember that, just as in radiography, there is an interplay between objective contrast and sharpness. In tomography *all* the structures are blurred. In particular even those structures within the layer are blurred more than in normal stationary radiography. This, together with the fact that the contrast can be lowered due to the effectively thin layer creating it, means that the subjective contrast on the tomogram is less than on the radiograph. The character of the pattern is, however, more easily seen because of the removal of the other distracting patterns.

ZONOGRAPHY

Zonography is essentially tomography using larger layer thicknesses of several centimetres rather than the more usual thicknesses of a few millimetres encountered in tomography. It is usually done using a circular movement and an angle of swing of between 1° and 5°. The effect is to produce what looks like a perfectly normal radiograph of the structures of the thick layer but with the confusing shadows of overlying and underlying structures blurred out. Since the movement is small the unsharpness of the structures within the zone is very similar to that in a stationary radiograph. This technique is obviously useful in cases where thick structures or ones not very different in attenuating power from their surroundings need to be seen.

TRANSVERSE AXIAL TOMOGRAPHY

All the tomographic movements mentioned so far are, in practice, limited to producing tomograms of layers parallel to the long axis of the patient. These movements could be used to produce tomograms of layers across the patient by placing the patient vertically between the tube and film movement planes as is shown in *Fig.* 272. This would, however, tend to a very large, unwieldy, almost certainly inaccurate piece of equipment and one which would result in a very large patient dose

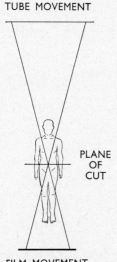

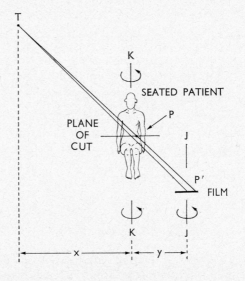

Fig. 272.—A theoretically possible method of transverse axial tomography!

Fig. 273.—A practical method of transverse axial tomography.

—especially to the top of the head! The transverse tomogram is, therefore, produced by using the special type of movement illustrated in *Fig.* 273. The X-ray tube is fixed and points downwards at an angle of 30° to the horizontal. The patient is (usually) seated and can be rotated about a vertical axis *KK* whilst the film is mounted horizontally in the position shown and can be rotated about the axis *JJ*. Both these axes (*JJ* and *KK*) and the X-ray tube focal spot must lie within the same plane.

During the exposure the patient and film are rotated, in exact synchronism, usually for one revolution which takes about 5 sec. As the patient rotates the shadow of the structures at P (*Fig.* 273) which is cast at P' will rotate in a circle centred about the axis JJ as the structure P rotates in a circle about the axis KK. Since the film is also rotating, the shadow of P will remain exactly stationary on the film as will the shadow of all the objects in the same horizontal plane as P. This plane is the tomographic layer.

The shadows and structures above and below this layer will be blurred since they will move with respect to the film. That this is so can be seen by referring to *Fig.* 274, where the shadow cast by an object Q situated above the plane of cut is illustrated. At the start of the exposure object Q is at Q_1 and its shadow is cast on the

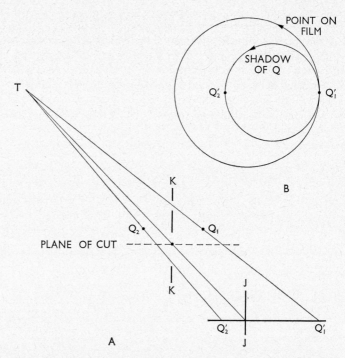

Fig. 274.—The plane of cut and blurring in transverse axial tomography.

film at a point Q'_1. During the exposure the object Q rotates about the line KK and its shadow will therefore trace out a circular path on the film as indicated in *Fig.* 274 B. For example, after half a revolution Q will be at Q_2 and the shadow at Q'_2. The point Q'_1 on the film, at which the initial shadow of Q fell, will also follow a circular path, but, in this case, of larger radius. It can be seen that the movement of the shadow of Q with respect to the film also will be a circle and of diameter equal to the difference in diameter of these two circles.

Layer Thickness in Transverse Axial Tomography.—As in the case of linear tomography the thickness of the layer can be calculated by quite simple geometry (*Fig.* 275). The radius which the shadow of Q traces out at the plane of the film is equal to:

$$r.(a + b)/a,$$

whereas that of the circular path followed by the point of the film on which the shadow of Q initially fell has a radius of:

$$(r + t.\tan \theta) \, (a + b)/a.$$

The blurring (B) is proportional to the difference in the diameters, i.e., to twice the difference in radii and hence:

$$B = 2t.\tan \theta \, (a + b)/a.$$

If B_m is the maximum tolerable blurring then $2t$ is the layer thickness and since $2t$ is small compared with a and b it follows that:

$$(a + b)/a = (a' + b')/a' = (x + y)/x$$

and

$$2t = B_m \cdot \frac{1}{\tan \theta} \cdot \frac{x}{(x + y)}.$$

The normal values for x and y are 150 cm. and 50 cm. respectively, and θ is usually 60°. If B_m is taken as 0·7 mm., the layer thickness is:

$$0 \cdot 7 \cdot \frac{1}{\sqrt{3}} \cdot \frac{150}{200} = 0 \cdot 3 \text{ mm.}$$

Although it is usual to maintain the angle θ constant it can be seen that increase in this angle leads to a decrease in layer thickness.

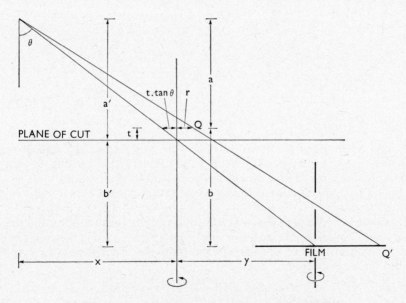

Fig. 275.—Layer thickness in transverse axial tomography.

Difficulties in Transverse Axial Tomography.—The general comments made about the other types of tomography apply equally to transverse axial tomography, in which it is very easy to generate artefacts due to the build up of the shadow and of plane structures. Accurate alinement of the equipment and perfect synchronism

13

of the movements are essential and care must be taken that this is achieved and maintained.

One practical disadvantage is that the patient must remain fixed with respect to the vertical axis of rotation whilst he is rotated and this is difficult to achieve. It is also objected that in many cases a transverse section of a stationary, recumbent patient would be preferable. Such a section can be taken by using the type of apparatus illustrated in *Fig.* 276 in which the patient is stationary, the tube and film rotating in the vertical circular paths shown.

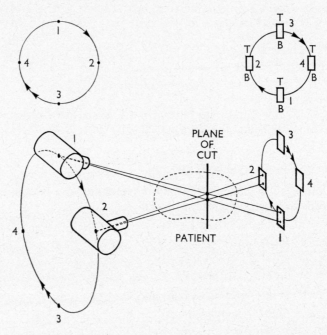

Fig. 276.—Transverse axial tomography for the horizontal patient.

The film is kept parallel to the transverse section of interest and rotated synchronously with the tube rotation. The top (T) and bottom (B) of the film are marked to emphasize that it must remain the same way up during the rotation.

Clearly such apparatus needs to be specially constructed and to date only very few have been made.

Magnification of Tomography.—The large distance between the film and the tomographic layer, especially in transverse axial tomography, means that the pattern on the film is magnified. For example, in the transverse axial tomography apparatus described the magnification is given by:

$$m = (x + y)/x = 200/150 = 1.33,$$

which is much larger than that in normal radiography.

COMPUTER-ASSISTED TOMOGRAPHY

Because of the effects of tissues lying above and below, the visualization even of a structure lying in otherwise uniform surroundings may not be easy in normal radiography. Although there may be a local change of attenuation of several per cent, the consequent effect on film density will be much less because of the attenuation of the over- and underlying material. The types of tomography described above are reasonably successful in overcoming the effect of this 'unwanted' material but the technique is limited by the fundamental difficulty that, as the layer thickness is reduced, the contrast associated with any structure, and therefore its visibility, falls.

However, though the film cannot reveal them, the effect of small (say 2 per cent) differences in attenuation can be revealed by measurements of the X-ray intensity, using a sensitive scintillation detector. It has been realized for a long time that if a number of observations of this kind, using a narrow X-ray beam, could be made in known directions through some part of the body detailed information about the structures present could be obtained; and this without necessary recourse to the use of contrast media.

With the relatively recent availability of sensitive and stable scintillation counters together with small but fast computers and of programs capable of handling the large numbers of calculations involved, the goal is now being achieved. The successful harnessing of these facilities was brought about in the early 1970s by G. N. Hounsfield of E.M.I. His technique, usually known as computer-assisted tomography, was first applied to investigations of the skull and has achieved rapid acceptance and success. Equipment for the examination of other (and larger) parts of the body is now available.

The Equipment and its Use.—*Fig.* 277 is a picture of the scanning equipment for head investigations. It will be seen that it is a little smaller than a conventional X-ray

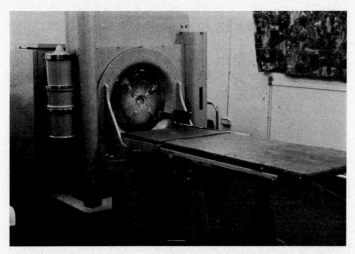

Fig. 277.—The E.M.I. Computer-assisted Tomograph for head studies.

diagnostic set, though this is somewhat offset by the protected area housing the computer and display units as well as the control desk being rather larger than that for the normal diagnostic X-ray controls. In *Fig.* 278 the general principles of its operation are shown.

A narrow X-ray beam is directed through the patient's head and the transmitted intensity measured by a well-collimated scintillation X-ray detector. At the same time the incident intensity is measured, so that the total attenuation along the particular beam path can be computed. This done, the beam and detector (which are rigidly connected) are moved sideways about 1 mm. and the reading and computation carried out again and so on, as shown in *Fig.* 278, until measurements have been taken along 240 lines. This, called scan 1 in *Fig.* 278, takes about 1·5 sec. with the equipment shown.

Then the whole equipment (but not, of course, the head, which must remain stationary) is rotated through a small angle (1° in this equipment) and the whole process is gone through again. This cycle is continued until sets of readings and computations have been taken along 240 lines over 180°. By the time the scanning is

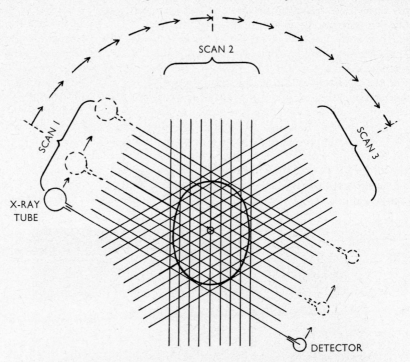

Fig. 278.—The scanning pattern showing linear scans in three different directions.

complete (which takes about 4½ min.) 240 × 180 = 43,200 attenuation values have been calculated and stored, together with details of the directions to which they refer, in the computer. Each value represents the total attenuation along a geometrically well-defined path through the patient's skull, and from the accumulated data can be computed the individual attenuation values of each of the 160 × 160 = 25,600 volume elements (each 1·5 mm.² in cross-section) of the section area examined. Clearly so many calculations can only be carried out by a computer, which, in the practical instrument, completes its work in about half a minute.

The calculated attenuation values are presented on a cathode-ray tube screen in the form shown in *Fig.* 279 A, which is taken from a Polaroid photograph of the image on the screen. A 'print-out' of the actual attentuation values can also be produced, *Fig.* 279 B showing this form of presentation of the same information as shown in *Fig.* 279A. In passing it should be mentioned that, in practice, each scan is double, the attenuation pattern for two adjacent slices of the head (each 13 mm. wide) being obtained simultaneously for, of course, separate display. With this facility the whole head can be dealt with in about five separate scans, taking about half and hour in all.

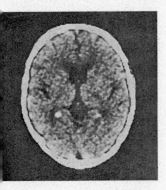
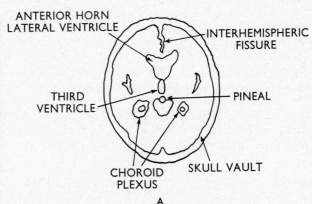

ANTERIOR HORN
LATERAL VENTRICLE
INTERHEMISPHERIC
FISSURE

THIRD
VENTRICLE
PINEAL

CHOROID
PLEXUS
SKULL VAULT

A

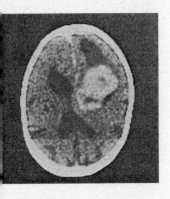
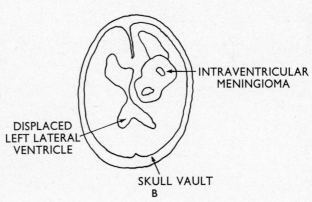

INTRAVENTRICULAR
MENINGIOMA

DISPLACED
LEFT LATERAL
VENTRICLE

SKULL VAULT

B

```
34  22  13  18  17  15  18  14  13  16
36  22  18  18  17  17  18  17  18  17
36  19  20  16  15  16  18  15  13  14
28  18  21  19  18  18  19  13  13  16
25  17  21  15  15  17  15  18  15  14
19  19  17  17  16  19  17  18  14  15
12  14  18  20  16  18  17  14  14  17      C
19  20  24  27  21  14  16  16  16  15
14  24  33  31  29  20  16  16  14  14
15  17  28  29  33  29  25  17  18  15
12  22  31  31  34  32  29  20  18  15
15  25  30  35  39  32  36  27  21  13
14  22  28  32  38  33  35  34  24  13
14  17  22  30  39  36  36  40  32  14
19  18  20  25  27  31  34  35  29  13
16  18  18  22  21  29  28  25  16  20
17  20  18  20  21  15  18  19  16  19
17  15  14  20  18  19  20  21  20  18
18  19  17  12  14  12  20  21  24  17
19  18  18  18  14  14  15  12  11  10
19  17  19  16  14  17  15  12  13  12
19  15  12  15  13  13  13  11  13   7
```

Fig. 279.—Computer-assisted tomographs. A,
A Polaroid picture of a normal scan of the skull
through the level of the posterior part of the third
ventricle. B, A Polaroid picture showing a tumour
enhanced by the aid of an intravenous contrast
medium. C, A typical 'print-out' of part of a
C.A.T. (A and B *by courtesy of Professor Ian
Isherwood, Manchester University and Royal
Infirmary*).

The X-ray Source and the Patient Dose.—In order to be useful, the value of the attenuation needs to be known to an accuracy of better than about 0·4 per cent. This means that a large number of photons must be involved in each measurement otherwise statistical variations (cf. pp. 202, 354, and 414) will introduce excessive uncertainty. Because the time of each measurement is only 5 milliseconds, a high photon flux (X-ray output) must be used and this is provided by using a heavily filtered (to remove low-energy photons which only contributed to the patient dose) beam from a therapy X-ray tube operating at about 120 kV. and 20–30 mA. continuously. Because the method measures attenuation coefficients, which are very dependent on photon energy, a highly stable kilovoltage supply has to be used.

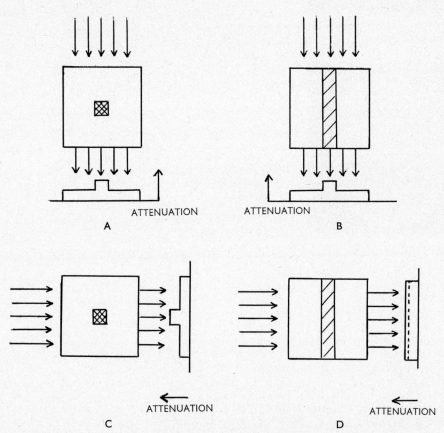

Fig. 280.—The basic principle of computer-assisted tomography. Attenuation measurements taken in two directions enable the two objects in the tank to be distinguished.

In spite of the fact that a high-powered X-ray set is used for a fairly long time on each patient, the radiation dose to the patient is very small, being substantially less, by a factor of 5–10, than for most alternative methods of X-ray investigations of the skull. The reason for this is that although the X-ray intensity is high the beam is small in cross-section, so that any point in the head is irradiated for only a small fraction of the total scan time of $4\frac{1}{2}$ min. Furthermore, the small beam size means that there is little scattered radiation and, hence, that the taking of 'slices' at different levels in the head does not increase the dose, only the volume receiving it.

The Calculations and Display.—The calculations which result in the display pattern are complex in the extreme (25,600 separate attenuations to be deduced from 43,200 facts!), quite beyond the scope of this book, the mathematical competence of its authors and the needs of its readers. Nevertheless, a very simple description of the underlying idea might be of interest and value.

Take the situation shown in *Fig.* 280 A, when a differently attenuating object is placed in a tank of water. If the transmission of a narrow beam of X-rays, directed vertically through the tank and traversed across it, is measured the attenuation pattern

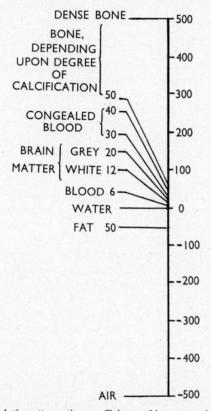

Fig. 281.—Relative attenuation coefficients of important body materials.

shown may be computed. This does not, however, reveal the position or the size of the object nor the attenuation of its material. The same pattern would be produced by a strip of less attenuating material across the tank, as in *Fig.* 280 B.

However, a further series of readings taken with a traversing narrow beam fired horizontally through the tank will distinguish between the two situations—as *Fig.* 280 C and D show—and the position, size, and attenuation of the object determined.

Though obviously enormously more complex, it is along such lines that the computer-assisted tomograph works.

The attenuation values computed and displayed are the *differences* between the mean value for the material at each point and that of water. *Fig.* 281 shows the numerical values of the difference for various body materials at 120 kV. On the scale water is arbitrarily set at zero and the other materials related to this in an arbitrary but linear fashion, bone being about $+500$ and air -500.

Different soft tissues, such as grey and white brain matter, or fat and blood, have values lying within the narrow range -50 to $+30$ or less than 10 per cent of the whole, which is an indication why these tissues cannot be revealed in conventional radiography unless contrast media are used. In computer-assisted tomography they are adequately resolved.

A valuable provision on the practical equipment allows the full range from black to white on the cathode-ray tube display to be used to represent any selected part of the total -500 to $+500$ range. For example, settings may be used by which the limited attenuation difference range from congealed blood to fat occupies the whole presentation range from black to white. These selections and presentation variations are made upon the data stored in the computer which is unaffected by the manipulations, so that any number of different presentations of the information gained from each scan may be tried before the most appropriate is obtained.

Further Developments.—The above is essentially a description of the original E.M.I. head scanner, which seems likely to be the ancestor of a large family of instruments of increasing range and speed. As already stated, it will perform a head scan in $4\frac{1}{2}$–5 min. Already, less than 5 years after the appearance of this original device, scanners are available which will scan the abdomen or thorax in 20 sec. Though the computation of the final result takes much longer than with the head scanner—4–6 min. as against half a minute, because of the much greater number of calculations involved—the fast scan time is a great improvement from the patient's point of view. It is achieved by using a large number of individual X-ray beams, each with its own scintillation detector, for each longitudinal scan and by increasing the angular interval between those scans from 1 to 10 degrees.

In the original scanner the patient's head rested on a cone protruding into a Perspex box filled with water. The object of this arrangement was not only to provide a stable position for the head, but more important, to reduce the range of attenuation differences due to the oval shape of the head. As the scan direction was changed the box (though not the head) moved with it, keeping the path length, through solid or liquid, constant. In this way the calculations were made simpler. In the new generation of scanners it has been found possible to dispense with the water box.

As mentioned earlier, computer-assisted tomography can obtain its results without artificial contrast media being used. There is, however, no reason why its performance should not be enhanced by their use. With these machines, moreover, the media are likely to be physiologically more acceptable than the high-atomic-number liquids or the air used in conventional radiography, often to the patient's considerable discomfort. As with many other facets of the use of this extremely powerful diagnostic acid, the possible use of contrast media is being investigated.

CHAPTER XXVII

ULTRASONICS IN CLINICAL MEDICINE

SOUNDS are produced by vibrating bodies which send out, through the air or any other material, a pattern of higher and lower pressures (compressions and rarefactions) following each other in regular and rapid succession. The pattern is in the form of waves which are usually called sound waves. They are longitudinal waves in so far as the pressure variations are of a 'to and fro' nature along the direction of travel of the waves. This is in contrast to the transverse waves of electromagnetic radiations for which the variations are at right angles to the direction of travel (*see* pp. 7 and 8).

The qualitative effect of these waves upon the ear, in other words the 'pitch' of the sound, depends upon the number of vibrations reaching it per second, that is to say the frequency of the sound—the greater the frequency, the higher, or shriller, the note. Frequencies are now measured in hertz (Hz), one oscillation or vibration per second being 1 hertz. Thus the frequency of middle C on the piano is 256 Hz whilst the note C one octave higher has twice that frequency, namely 512 Hz. (Apologies are offered to the expert musician, who will know that there are, in fact, several 'standard' middle C's!)

Just as the eye can see only a limited range of frequencies of the electromagnetic spectrum (visible light), so the ear can hear only a limited range of sound frequencies. This range is from about 20 Hz to 20,000 Hz (or 20 kHz), though the exact range varies from person to person, older people in general being unable to hear frequencies as high as younger people.

Beyond the audible range there are 'sounds' or varying pressure waves which we cannot hear. Those with frequencies below the audible range are referred to as infrasonic whilst those with frequencies above the audible limit are known as ultrasonic.

Production of Ultrasonic Radiation.—All waves of the 'sound' type are produced in the same way, namely by a rapidly vibrating object. In the case of audible sound, an example is the vibration of the arms of a tuning fork. For ultrasonic radiations the frequency, and hence the rate of vibration of the source, is much higher and the usual source (called a transducer) is a disc-shaped slice of quartz or of a special ceramic, in which the oscillations are produced by the piezo-electric effect.

In this effect the application of an electric field across the material causes that material to expand or to contract depending upon the way in which the field is applied. Thus, as the face of the transducer (e.g., a piece of quartz placed in a suitable fluid) moves forwards and backwards under the influence of an applied alternating electric field, molecules of the surrounding liquid are first pressed together and then drawn apart and a series of waves of higher followed by lower pressure travel through the liquid. The change in thickness of the material is very small, being little more than a few thousandths of a millimetre at most, yet this movement is enough, with suitable frequencies applied to the material, to produce ultrasonic radiations of intensities adequate for clinical work.

Detection of Ultrasonic Radiations.—Just as the application of a voltage across a piece of quartz (or any other material showing the piezo-electric effect) produces a change of shape capable of exerting pressure on the surrounding material, so the squeezing of any 'piezo-electric' material produces a voltage between its faces. Such material, irradiated with ultrasonic radiations, will be subjected to pressure variations which will generate a varying voltage between its faces. The voltage may be amplified and measured and this constitutes the usual method of detecting and measuring ultrasonic radiations. Since it is precisely the opposite of ultra sound generation, we have the great convenience that the same transducer can be used both to generate and to detect ultrasonic radiations (not both at the same time, of course).

The Interaction of Ultrasonic Radiation with Matter.—When ultrasonic radiation passes through matter its intensity decreases with the increasing distance from the emitting transducer (the source). For a simple, plane, non-focused transducer the beam remains parallel for quite a large distance. The actual distance depends on transducer size and ultrasonic frequency but typically it can be about 10 cm. At greater distances the beam spreads out a little so that there is some decrease of intensity with distance for this reason. The main reason for the very rapid reduction of intensity with increasing distance from the source arises from the interaction between the ultrasonic radiation and the atoms and molecules of the material. This results in absorption of sound energy. If, in addition, the material through which the ultrasound is passing is not homogeneous, there will also be some scattering, reflection, refraction and diffraction. As we shall see, the medical use of ultrasound particularly employs reflection by body structures. Absorption and scattering figure mainly as annoying but not disastrous complicating phenomena. Of refraction and diffraction we shall hear no more in this book!

Absorption.—The attenuation of an ultrasonic beam by absorption follows an exponential law, $I = I_0 \, e^{-\mu d}$, where I_0 and I are the initial and reduced intensities respectively, d is the thickness of material traversed and μ is the linear absorption coefficient which depends upon the material concerned and also upon the frequency of the radiation. Over the frequency range likely to be used in clinical work (0·5–10 MHz) the absorption coefficient, in most biological materials (water and bone are exceptions), is approximately directly proportional to the frequency. For water and bone the coefficient is proportional to the square of the frequency. *Table XXVIII* shows values for a number of different types of tissue and a number of points of

Table XXVIII.—Ultrasonic Radiation Absorption Coefficients for Body Tissues

Tissue	Absorption Coefficient μ
Muscle	$0\cdot28f$
Fat	$0\cdot14f$
Blood	$0\cdot04f$
Brain	$0\cdot20f$
Kidney	$0\cdot23f$
Liver	$0\cdot21f$
Bone	$4\cdot6f^2$
Lung	$9\cdot2f$
Water	$0\cdot0005f^2$

f is the frequency in MHz.

importance may be noted. One is the very low absorption in water and another is the high absorption in bone and particularly in lung. For most of the other body tissues the coefficient is approximately the same, averaging about 0·2 per cm. at 1 MHz.

Whilst the relative importance in biological material of the different interaction processes involved is reasonably well known for the various circumstances of interest, the details of the actual mechanisms concerned in the absorption of ultrasound energy are not yet well understood. Fortunately this does not significantly impair our understanding of the important features arising in the medical use of ultrasound. Two effects are, however, of particular importance. Ultrasonic radiation agitates the atoms and molecules of the irradiated material and, therefore, heats it. This is the basis of the calorimetric method of measuring ultrasonic intensities and the effect has clinical uses since quite high temperatures can be achieved with high-power beams. A simple example of these temperatures is given by the fact that a finger placed in a 2-MHz beam, in which the power is 2 watts per cm.^{2}, has to be withdrawn in under a minute because the bone becomes uncomfortably hot even though little or no effect is felt on the skin. This, of course, is because bone is many times more absorbing than the other tissues. In the diagnostic procedures which will be described below, beam intensities of less than a hundredth of that quoted above are used, which means that the heating effect is never noticed.

The second important effect is known as *cavitation*, which is the production and collapsing of bubbles that are mechanically agitated by the radiation. When ultrasonic radiations of adequate intensity pass through a liquid, tiny bubbles are formed and, in the low-pressure regions, they grow to about one-hundredth of a millimetre in diameter. In the next part of the cycle, when the pressure increases, the bubbles are compressed and then collapse. When this collapse occurs, very high, local pressures are generated and there may be many millions of bubbles collapsing at the same time. Cavitation can have a very powerful effect on an irradiated liquid and on biological material in which the changing pressure results in very high forces being exerted on the cell constituents. This phenomenon which occurs most readily at low frequencies is the basis of ultrasonic cleaning baths used industrially to clean metals and also in hospitals for the cleaning of surgical instruments. It may also play a role in the damaging of tissues through which ultrasound passes.

Reflection.—From the point of view of clinical application the reflection of ultrasonic radiations is the most important interaction phenomenon. When ultrasonic waves reach an interface between two different materials, some waves pass on through the second material whilst some are reflected back. The fraction of any beam which is reflected depends on what are called the acoustic impedances (Z_1 and Z_2) of the materials concerned.

Acoustic impedance (Z) is an indication of the resistance to movement of the atoms or molecules which make up a material and values for a number of substances of clinical interest are shown in *Table XXIX*.

Table XXIX.—Values of Acoustic Impedance (Z)

Material	Z (g. per cm.^{2} per sec.)
Muscle	$1 \cdot 70 \times 10^5$
Fat	$1 \cdot 38 \times 10^5$
Bone	$7 \cdot 80 \times 10^5$
Air	$0 \cdot 0004 \times 10^5$

From values such as these the fraction reflected at an interface, which is at right-angles to the direction of the incident beam, can be calculated quite easily from the formula

$$\text{Fraction reflected} = (Z_1 - Z_2)^2/(Z_1 + Z_2)^2.$$

It must be emphasized here that if the incidence is not normal, not only is the reflected fraction reduced but also, since the emitting and receiving transducers are virtually coincident, any reflected ultrasound will not reach the receiver and so will not be detected. The practical importance of this is that in both A and B scanning (*see below*) only structures which are at right-angles to the beam will produce echos. For this reason in B scanning the direction of the beam needs to be suitably oscillated as the transducer is moved round the patient. Some representative examples of the fraction of ultrasound reflected at various interfaces are shown in *Table XXX*,

Table XXX.—Reflection at Tissue Interface

INTERFACE	FRACTION REFLECTED (per cent)
Fat-muscle	~ 1
Muscle-bone	~ 40
Muscle-air	~ 99.9

from which it can be seen that, as might be expected since they are so alike in density and atomic number, little radiation is reflected at the interface between fat and muscle tissue whereas something approaching half of the incident ultrasound comes back from a muscle–bone surface. The almost complete reflection at the boundary between muscle (or any other liquid or solid material for that matter) and air is of particular importance. If a beam of ultrasonic radiation is directed at a patient through the air, hardly any will enter the tissues because of the reflection at the transducer–air interface, so that if ultrasound is to be used for any clinical purpose, such as those described below, there must be good contact between the transducer producing the radiation and the skin. Air must be excluded from between them and this is usually achieved by a layer of oil or gel.

CLINICAL APPLICATIONS OF ULTRASONIC RADIATIONS

Therapeutic.—An intense beam of ultrasonic radiation (say of an intensity of 10 watts per cm.^{2} and frequency of 3 MHz) incident upon the body tissues can change and even destroy them owing to heating, cavitation, or other effects. In the past this has been used successfully in what may be termed ultrasonic diathermy, in which the radiation is focused on to the part to be destroyed. Ménière's disease, a defect of the middle-ear mechanism which results in giddiness and loss of balance, as well as some brain conditions have been treated in this way, though the fact that a 'window' has to be cut through skull bone (because of the greater absorption in and reflection from bone) reduces the attraction of the method.

Ultrasonic radiation of about 0.5 MHz and of intensities of less than about 3 watts per cm.^{2} is used in physiotherapy. The function here is almost certainly restricted to 'internal' heating of the tissues and has comforting, beneficial effects.

Diagnostic.—By far the most important clinical applications of ultrasonic radiations are in the diagnostic field, and these will be considered under two headings. First are the methods using the fact of reflection at tissue interfaces, and second is the method using the fact that waves reflected from a moving reflector are higher or lower in frequency than the incident beam depending upon which way the reflector is moving. The first may be termed 'echo-sounding' or 'sonar' techniques—'sonar' with sound waves being comparable with 'radar' with radio waves—whilst the second is usually called the Doppler method after the man who first explained the general phenomenon.

Pulse-echo Systems

General.—These systems are used to determine the depth of an object or a structure in the body by measuring the time taken for ultrasonic radiation reflected by it to return to the detector.

The general underlying ideas can be illustrated by taking the specific example of the estimation of the depth below the skin of a piece of bone.

A short burst (or pulse) of ultrasound, lasting a few microseconds, is directed towards the bone from a transducer in close contact with the skin, as shown in *Fig.* 282 A. Immediately the pulse has been emitted the transducer is switched to a detecting circuit to be able to register any radiation reflected by the body. When such radiation reaches the transducer it produces a brief piezo-electric voltage pulse which is amplified and usually displayed by the associated electronic circuits. The time between the emission of the initial pulse and the arrival of the echo depends on the depth of the bone and is a measure of that depth. Ultrasonic radiations travel at about 1500 m. per second in muscle tissue, so that if the bone is 1·5 cm. (or $1·5 \times 10^{-2}$ m.) deep, the reflected ultrasound will arrive back $2(1·5 \times 10^{-2}/1·5 \times 10^3$ sec. or 20 μsec. after the emission of the transmitted pulse. The initial figure 2 in the above calculation arises, of course, because the sound has travelled twice the depth of the bone before it gets back to the transducer.

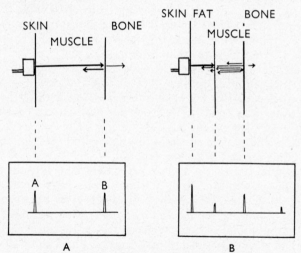

Fig. 282.—Ultrasonic echo sounding or sonar.

The voltage pulse produced by the echo is usually displayed on a cathode-ray tube, the spot of which travels at a constant speed, say from left to right, across the screen and will be deflected upwards by any voltage pulse received. It starts its movement when the original pulse is emitted and a 'spike' (A) indicating the start of the pulse is produced on the display as shown in *Fig*. 282. If the spot moves 1 mm. per μsec. then the voltage pulse due to the echo from the bone will be shown as a second 'spike' (B) 20 mm. from the first. The separation of the spikes thus indicates the depth of the bone, and in practice it is possible to adjust the speed of the spot of the cathode-ray tube so that the 'spike' separation equals the actual depth.

Fig. 282 B illustrates the extension of this sort of system to a slightly more complex situation, namely when the muscle has an overlying layer of fat. In this case the cathode-ray tube screen shows spikes corresponding to reflections at both the fat–muscle and muscle–bone boundaries and it will be noted that the former 'spike' is considerably smaller than the latter. The height of the 'spike' depends on the intensity of radiation reaching the detector and the difference shown here arises because, as already stated, much less (1 per cent) energy is reflected at the fat–muscle boundary than at the muscle–bone interface (about 40 per cent). Notice also the third, quite small, 'spike' to the right of the other two. This is the result of multiple reflections, and 'spikes' of this type could well confuse the interpretation of the type of display by suggesting interfaces where none actually exist—'ghosts'. What happens is that some of the radiation reflected from the bone is reflected back by the muscle–fat interface and some of that reflected radiation is re-reflected by the bone. The third 'spike' shows this multiply reflected radiation and suggests a surface at a depth beyond the muscle–bone surface equal to twice the thickness of the muscle since this is the extra distance travelled. Naturally the third 'spike' is much weaker than the other two. Clearly there could be yet more ghost 'spikes' further out to the right owing to multiple reflections, particularly at the transducer–skin and muscle–fat interfaces. That these are not revealed on the cathode-ray tube trace is owing to a factor not yet taken into account.

Effect of Attenuation.—So far no cognizance has been taken of the attenuation suffered by the incident and reflected radiations as they pass through the tissues. Some radiation will be scattered and some absorbed and, with 2 MHz radiation, for example, the intensity is reduced by a half for every 1·5 cm. or so that it traverses. If we assume, in the example illustrated in *Fig*. 282 B, that the fat layer is 0·75 cm. thick and that the bone surface lies 1·5 cm. below the skin the reflected signal from the fat–muscle interface will be reduced by a half and the echo from the bone by a quarter from the values expected when attenuation is ignored. The multiply reflected signal, in this case, would be reduced by a further factor of a half (to one-eighth of the value ignoring attenuation) because of the extra 2×0.75 cm. it travelled. Any signals resulting from more reflections (which are already basically weak because only a fraction is reflected at any surface) would be reduced even more by attenuation. This is useful in fading out potentially confusing multiple reflection echoes.

However, this attenuation is far from an unmixed blessing because, as shown above, it affects the genuine as well as the 'ghost' signals and is increasingly severe on reflections from deeper structures. For example, the intensity of the signal reflected from an interface 9 cm. deep would be reduced by a factor of 2^{12} for the 2 MHz radiation quoted above since the total distance travelled (18 cm.) is equal to twelve times the 'half-value layer' of 1·5 cm. In other words the signal, on this simple picture, would be reduced to at least one four-thousandth of the value it would have had without attenuation. In practice the situation would probably be worse and a reduction by a factor of 10^4 quite likely.

Thus, echoes from two similar interfaces at different depths in the body will differ by large factors so that, unless some corrective measures are taken, the distant reflections will pass unnoticed. The remedy is to increase the amplification ('gain') of the received signals progressively with time from the moment of the emission of the initial pulse. At the beginning the 'gain' is small and reaches its full value by the time the cathode-ray tube spot has reached the end of its path. In this way quickly returned echoes are less amplified than those returning later, which, coming from deeper structures and therefore being more attenuated, need greater amplification. Ideally the size of the 'spike' from similar interfaces should be the same regardless of their depth.

Operating Frequency.—A reduction in the effects of attenuation could be achieved by reducing the frequency of the ultrasound being used since, as shown above, absorption increases with increasing frequency. Such a solution, however, introduces other difficulties, and in particular it affects the *resolution* attainable by the method. The range resolution (i.e., the ability to distinguish separate structures in the direction of the ultrasonic beam) decreases as the frequency is reduced. For example, when using 10 MHz radiation, objects can be distinguished when they are only a fraction of a millimetre apart, whereas with 1 MHz radiation objects 3 mm. apart can just be detected as separate. As so often in clinical work, a compromise has to be made. For investigations of the brain, for example, 2 MHz radiation may be used, whereas for studies of the eye (when the dimensions are small) 15 MHz may be employed.

A-scanning.—The echo-sounding or sonar use of ultrasonic radiations takes several practical forms and the above is almost a complete description of the first and simplest technique used—what is now called A-scanning. The only practical detail that has to be added to the general picture given above is that the echo-sounding radiation pulse is repeated about 500 times per second, a *pulse repetition frequency* high enough to give a steady and readily visible trace on the display screen and yet not so rapid that the transducer has to be switched over to send out another pulse before it has finished receiving echo-pulses from the last. Although direct measurements are often made on the cathode-ray tube screen, a permanent record is usually made photographically using a Polaroid film camera, the record being completed almost immediately.

Provided the position and direction of the ultrasonic beam, relative to the body, are known, the depth of any identifiable structure can be obtained. For example, A-scans are particularly valuable for the determination of the position of the midline of the brain, in the case of accident or disease; the measurements of the internal dimensions of the eye, especially when the lens has become opaque; and for accurate measurements of the foetal head size.

B-scanning.—A-scans provide quantitative but limited information. The display itself does not indicate the part of the body being investigated nor the direction in the patient to which the trace applies. B-scans are designed to build up a cross-sectional picture of the various structures in a chosen plane through the patient. They thus contain much more information than A-scans and the equipment is more complex and expensive.

The echo-sounding principles of B-scanning are the same as for A-scanning (and B-scan equipment can be used for A-scans), but there are two important practical differences. In the first place, the echo is not displayed as a 'spike' on the cathode-ray tube but as a dot, provided the strength of the echo is above a preselected value. When there is a weak (or no) echo the base line is suppressed. Secondly, the direction of movement of the spot across the screen—and therefore the line along which the echo dots are formed—is in a direction related to the direction of the ultrasonic beam through the body whilst the start of the display trace corresponds with the position of the transducer. This is achieved by an ingenious and complex linkage between the transducer head and the electronic controls to which further reference will be made later.

A simple example of the relationship between the transducer beam direction and the cathode ray tube display is shown in *Fig.* 283 A, in which the transducer is shown in two positions, A and B, firing the ultrasonic beam as indicated. For transducer position *A* the display tube spot moves along the line *AA* and dots are produced on the screen at A_s (for the emission pulse and skin position since the transducer is in close contact with the skin) and A_x for the position of the reflecting structure X. For position B the display spot moves along BB producing its echo spots at B_s and B_y for the skin and structure Y. It will be noted that B_s is closer to the intersection of AA and BB than is A_s taking cognizance of the fact that the transducer is closer to the centre of the body when at B than it is when at A.

In practice the transducer is moved steadily over the surface of the body in the plane being investigated and, as indicated diagrammatically in *Fig.* 283 B, the large

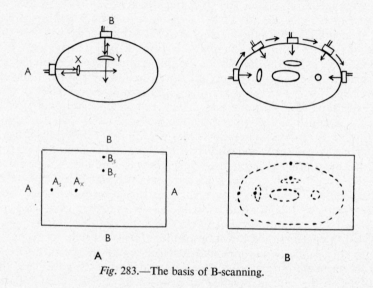

Fig. 283.—The basis of B-scanning.

numbers of dots resulting from the various transducer positions build up, on the cathode-ray tube screen, outlines of the echo-producing surfaces. The cathode-ray tube screen used is a special type known as a storage screen, on which the image persists. A permanent record of the screen patterns may be made on Polaroid film. Some examples of pictures obtained in this way are shown in *Fig.* 284 and illustrate the very considerable amount of information that can be obtained by B-scanning.

Equipment.—A typical piece of apparatus for B-scanning is shown in *Fig.* 285. The console carries all the electronic circuits needed for the production and detection of the ultrasonic radiation and the cathode-ray tube for the display. At one end of the scanning arm, which permits free movement of the transducer in one plane, is the small transducer. The frame above the patient contains the mechanical-electrical equipment which 'tells' the circuits responsible for the display exactly where the transducer is relative to some fixed point and the direction in which the beam is being pointed. This ensures that the sweep of the cathode-ray tube spot is in the correct direction across the screen and that it starts at the correct point, otherwise the displayed cross-section will be distorted. Although it looks simple the scanning arm is quite a master-piece of ingenuity and precision, for whilst being capable of free and complex movement, the linkages are such that a spot on the screen can be reproduced to within about 1 mm.

As was commented on page 383 with reference to A-scans, the resolution of structures in the direction of the beam can be quite high also in B-scanning. However, the resolution of objects separated in a direction normal to that of the ultrasonic beam is much less high. This arises owing to the finite width of the beam, which is often 1–2 cm. in diameter. Increase in lateral resolution may be obtained (at a preselected depth) by using a suitably focused transducer and in other ways too complex for description here. In general practice the low lateral resolution is usually acceptable.

Grey Scale.—The B-scan described above is black and white in the sense that either the dot appears on the screen if the echo strength is higher than a preselected value or it does not appear if the echo strength is less than this value. Since the structures in the

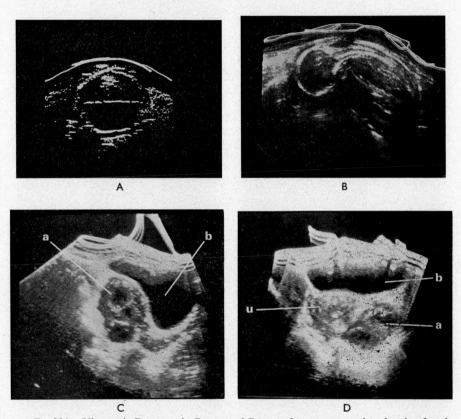

Fig. 284.—Ultrasonic B-scans. A, Compound B-scan of transverse section showing foetal skull and midline. Photographed from a storage oscilloscope (*by courtesy of Dr. Higginbotham, Withington Hospital, Manchester*); B, Grey scale longitudinal view of abdomen showing foetal head, spine, and heart (*by courtesy of Mr. D. Jenkins, Lancaster School of Radiography*); C, Grey scale longitudinal scan showing large pelvic abscess (a) and the bladder (b). Three areas of liquefaction within the abscess are shown as different levels of greyness; D, Grey scale transverse scan through the above abscess (a) showing that it lies alongside but not within the uterus (u). (C and D *by courtesy of Dr. Hylton B. Meire, Northwick Park Hospital.*)

section being scanned produce different echo strengths depending on their nature—or, more accurately, depending on the relative nature of the two materials on either side of the echo-producing interface (i.e., the acoustic impedance)—it is not surprising that there is an interest in using the echo strength information to help identify the nature of the structures, and also to observe other structures whose echoes are too weak to be seen in conventional B-scanning. The technique adopted is the so-called grey scale.

This is done by arranging for the brightness of the dot to be controlled by the strength of the echo. Unfortunately this cannot be done directly on the storage tube normally used in B-scanning, and one solution of this difficulty is to use a non-storage tube. The picture is then obtained by setting up a camera in front of the screen and opening the shutter at the start of the scan. A very real disadvantage of this method of working is that it is not possible to view the scan picture during the scanning unless a second

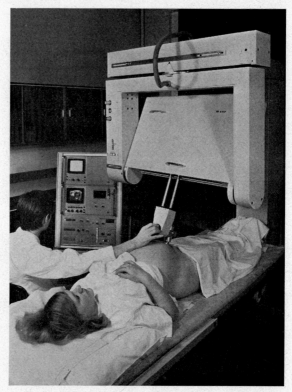

Fig. 285.—Ultrasonic compound B-scope being used for obstetrical examination.

display 'scope is available. Even with such a second display a great deal of skill (and luck!) is needed to acquire a good picture. A serious problem is that the same structure may be scanned more than once and so the brightness of the associated point on the picture will give a false representation.

A more satisfactory method is to use the so-called scan converter. This is a device which stores the pattern of dots and their intensities on a semi-conductor matrix memory. The associated electronic circuits are such that information about the echo strength associated with the structure at each point in the cross-section is acquired only once and so the difficulty referred to above is avoided. The pattern of intensities stored is displayed continuously during the scanning on a normal television screen. With this system it is therefore possible to continue and adjust the scanning until a satisfactory picture is obtained. A permanent record may be obtained by photographing the TV screen.

The scan converter grey scale system offers a considerable improvement over previous displays not only in the quality of the picture but the relative ease with which it can be made. For these reasons the scanning of organs such as liver and kidneys is becoming increasingly popular and useful.

Time-position Scanning.—A-scanning is used to observe and measure the size of stationary structures. A slightly modified system—called time-position scanning—can be used to observe the movement of identifiable structures, e.g., the mitral valve of the heart. How this is done can be described by reference to *Fig.* 286. A stationary

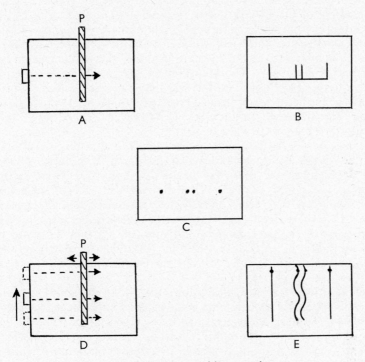

Fig. 286.—Time-position scanning.

structure (*P*) contained in a rectangular tank of water (*Fig.* 286 A), if examined by an A-scan, will produce the display shown in *Fig.* 286 B. The electronic circuit system is modified so that this *A*-display appears as shown in *Fig.* 286 C, i.e., rather like one single line of a B-scan.

The circuit is further modified so that over a period of about 4 sec. the line along which the displayed dots lie is moved vertically up the face of the display screen. If now the previously stationary object is vibrated to and fro as indicated (*Fig.* 286 D), the associated display will be as shown in *Fig.* 286 E. The stationary entry and exit walls of the tank will show as two straight vertical lines whilst the echoes from the moving surfaces of the oscillating object show the pattern of movement. The pattern on the display screen is in fact a graph of position (horizontal) against time (vertical). Arrangements are usually made to present the displayed pattern on a sheet of paper for permanent record.

Although specially designed equipment is often used for time-position scanning it is worth noting that most B-scan equipment can be operated as a time-position scanner: the display being presented on the storage 'scope.

As indicated above, one typical and important use of this technique is the examination of the detailed pattern of movement of the various components of the heart, particularly the valves.

'Doppler Shift' Systems

Everyone will be familiar with the change of note of a police car siren as it passes by: the note is shriller as the vehicle approaches than when it recedes. This is a fairly common example of the Doppler 'shift' (named after the Austrian physicist who predicted this type of phenomenon for visible light over 130 years ago). What happens is that as the sound source approaches, each successive wave is given out a little closer to the hearer and therefore reaches his ear rather more quickly than would be the case had the source been stationary. Thus the waves are much more bunched together—they have a higher frequency. In the same way when the source is receding each succeeding wave has a little further to travel than its predecessor and so arrives a little later than had the source been at rest. In this case fewer waves per second reach the ear—the sound frequency is reduced.

This change, or shift, of frequency applies equally to ultrasonic radiations and can be used to detect the movement, rather than the depth, of surfaces. In the case of ultrasonic Doppler systems the change of the frequency of radiation reflected by a moving surface or object is the basis of the measurement. This is achieved by comparing the frequency of the original and reflected radiations and generating (electronically) a new signal whose frequency is equal to the difference between the original and reflected frequencies, i.e., the Doppler shift. Since the frequency difference, produced by rates of movement in the body, is small, the generated frequency is in the audible range and in most clinical equipment using the Doppler shift the output is a loudspeaker.

The technique is particularly suitable for investigating rhythmic events like heartbeats and blood-pulses. It is becoming quite widely used in pregnancy for detecting and measuring foetal heart movements and in more general medicine for blood-flow studies in arteries and veins. The ability to establish quickly and, particularly, without any surgical or other equipment the presence or absence of flow in particular vessels is very valuable. Methods for measuring the rate of blood-flow have also been developed, but because the reflection of radiation is from large numbers of blood corpuscles travelling with a range of velocities the interpretation of signals and the obtaining of accurate quantitative measurements is very difficult. However, the method is full of promise.

POSSIBLE HAZARDS OF THE DIAGNOSTIC USE OF ULTRASOUND

Although X-rays are powerful agents in medical diagnosis some hazards may be consequent upon their use. As pointed out on p. 84 and discussed at greater length in CHAPTER XLIII, ionizing radiations produce biological effects so that their use may lead to damage to the patient and may, through genetic effects, damage future generations. One consequence of these hazards is that X-ray examinations during pregnancy are seldom undertaken and pelvic radiography of women of child-bearing age is usually restricted as described in CHAPTER XLV.

Though some of the hazards were recognized early, the possible genetic consequences of radiography were only generally realized relatively recently. Consequently any new diagnostic agent is scrutinized with particular care since the absence of short-term effects is no guarantee that there will not be any long-term damage. That ultrasonic radiations can produce biological effects has already been mentioned.

Therefore, until the contrary is proved, it must be assumed that there is some risk even with the small amounts of ultrasonic energy involved in diagnostic procedures.

A large range of animal experiments has demonstrated that effects can be produced by ultrasonic radiation in many body tissues but has failed to show any harmful effects at the intensity levels used in any of the diagnostic procedures described. All current evidence suggests that present methods of ultrasonic radiation diagnosis have a wide margin of safety. There is still a lack of information about long-term consequences and all concerned with the use of ultrasonic radiations must be constantly alert for hitherto unsuspected effects. That said, however, it seems fairly safe to conclude that ultrasonic radiations will continue to offer, especially in obstetrics and gynaecology, far safer methods of investigation than X-rays.

CHAPTER XXVIII

RADIOACTIVE ISOTOPES IN CLINICAL MEDICINE

As CHAPTER IV has already indicated, radioactive isotopes of practically every element can now be produced 'artificially', that is to say by neutron or proton bombardment, or from the 'fission fragments' of the uranium fission process. With the widespread development of atomic (or, more correctly, nuclear) energy resources, abundant supplies of these isotopes are readily available in a wide variety of chemical forms. They are used in medicine in four different ways:

1. As gamma-ray beam sources.
2. As alternatives for radium or radon in plesiotherapy.
3. For internal administration for therapeutic purposes.
4. For 'tracer' studies for diagnostic or research purposes.

The first two of these uses, which exploit the materials solely as sources of radiation will be discussed in CHAPTERS XXXVIII and XL. The third and fourth uses exploit both the radioactive (radiation emitting) and the isotopic (same chemical properties) features of the materials. If a substance is known to play some part in a process in the body, it may be possible to introduce a radioactive version of that substance (often spoken of as a 'labelled' material) into the system where it will behave exactly like its

Table XXXI.—SOME RADIOACTIVE ISOTOPES IN CLINICAL USE

RADIOACTIVE ISOTOPES	SYMBOL	HALF-LIFE	RADIATION EMITTED	PRINCIPAL γ-RAY ENERGIES IN MeV.
Hydrogen 3	$^{3}_{1}H$	12·3 yr.	β^-	None
Fluorine 18	$^{18}_{9}F$	1·9 hr.	β^+	0·505
Sodium 24	$^{24}_{11}Na$	15 hr.	$\beta^-\gamma$	1·37 and 2·75
Phosphorus 32	$^{32}_{15}P$	14·3 dy.	β^-	None
Chromium 51	$^{51}_{24}Cr$	27·8 dy.	$\gamma^\star$	0·323
Iron 55	$^{55}_{26}Fe$	2·7 yr.	$\gamma^\star$	0·006
Iron 59	$^{59}_{26}Fe$	45 dy.	$\beta^-\gamma$	Mainly 1·10 and 1·29
Cobalt 57	$^{57}_{27}Co$	270 dy.	$\gamma^\star$	Mainly 0·122 and 0·136
Cobalt 58	$^{58}_{27}Co$	71 dy.	$\beta^+\gamma^\star$	0·51 and 0·81
Cobalt 60	$^{60}_{27}Co$	5·26 yr.	$\beta^-\gamma$	1·17 and 1·33
Selenium 75	$^{75}_{34}Se$	121 dy.	$\gamma^\star$	Mainly 0·14 and 0·27
Strontium 85	$^{85}_{38}Sr$	65 dy.	$\gamma^\star$	0·513
Strontium 87m	$^{87m}_{38}Sr$	2·8 hr.	$\gamma\dagger$	0·388
Technetium 99m	$^{99m}_{43}Tc$	6 hr.	$\gamma\dagger$	0·140
Indium 113m	$^{113m}_{49}In$	1·7 hr.	$\gamma\dagger$	0·390
Iodine 125	$^{125}_{53}I$	60 dy.	$\gamma^\star$	0·035 and 0·027
Iodine 131	$^{131}_{53}I$	8 dy.	$\beta^-\gamma$	Mainly 0·36
Iodine 132	$^{132}_{53}I$	2·3 hr.	$\beta^-\gamma$	0·38 to 1·39
Xenon 133	$^{133}_{54}Xe$	5·3 dy.	$\beta^-\gamma$	0·081 and 0·16
Mercury 197	$^{197}_{80}Hg$	65 hr.	$\gamma^\star$	0·069 and 0·077
Gold 198	$^{198}_{79}Au$	2·7 dy.	$\beta^-\gamma$	Mainly 0·412

$\star$ These materials exhibit K-electron capture and hence characteristic X-rays.

$\dagger$ These isomers exhibit internal conversion and emit high-energy electrons and characteristic X-rays.

non-radioactive counterpart. This may be done either to deliver a therapeutic dose of radiation to particular tissues or, for diagnostic purposes, to enable the interaction of the material with the body to be followed with the aid of emitted radiations—often called 'tracer studies'. The properties of some of the radioactive materials found useful for these purposes are given in *Table XXXI*.

In the main, radioactive isotopes have been a great disappointment as internal therapeutic agents, though it must be confessed that some of this stemmed from the initially exaggerated expectations of their value. Theoretically, the ability to incorporate a radioative element into almost any chemical substance opens up the attractive possibility of getting selective absorption of radioactive material into at least some malignant growths. If this could be achieved, much greater radiation doses would be delivered to the tumour than to the normal tissues and the tumour would, therefore, have 'committed suicide'. Unfortunately, such dramatic events are very rare and the prospect of discovering new ones does not seem great. It must be realized that very high relative concentrations in the tumour are needed—say thirty times more than the general concentration in the rest of the body. This is because of the extreme sensitivity of the body to whole-body irradiation, and especially to irradiation of the blood-forming organs. Even if a particular part of the body selectively absorbs some administered isotope, an amount of that material will be circulating through, and irradiating, the rest of the body. It is this dose that normally sets a limit to the use of selectively absorbed radioactive materials and, as a result, there are now only a few regular uses of internal radioactive isotope therapy.

In contrast, the use of radioactive isotopes in clinical diagnosis is great in range and importance, so much so that some regard it as a specialty in its own right (often known by the somewhat misleading title of 'nuclear medicine'). Here only its more important general principles can be described and some examples of their application given.

RADIOACTIVE ISOTOPES IN CLINICAL DIAGNOSIS

Radioactive isotopes are particularly valuable tools because they enter into any chemical reaction or metabolic process in exactly the same way as would their stable isotopes and, furthermore, because they reveal their presence by the radiation they emit. It is thus possible to 'label' with radioactive materials a substance which will behave in the body and enter into metabolic processes in exactly the same way as would the same material without its radioactivity. Such 'labelled' substances are often called 'radiopharmaceuticals' and they may be followed by a suitable radiation detector (usually a scintillation counter) appropriately positioned near the patient for *in vivo* measurements or by measurement, by counters, in the laboratory, of the radioactivity of samples of tissues, body fluids, or excreta taken from the patient (*in vitro* studies).

The Selection of Radioactive Isotopes.—A great advantage of the use of radioactive isotopes in 'tracer studies' is the extreme sensitivity of the method. For the type of investigations or tests that will be described the amount of radioactive material used weighs about one ten thousand millionth of a gramme (10^{-10} g.) or probably a thousand times less than could be detected by any other test. This means that studies can be carried out without any chance of the test method affecting the system being investigated.

However, although the amounts of radioactive isotopes used will be small, it must be remembered that they may be widely distributed throughout the body for some time after their administration and will, thus, give rise to widespread, even if low-level, irradiation. Since it is always desirable to avoid unnecessary irradiation, careful thought has to be given to the kind, as well as the amount, of radioactive material used in any investigation.

The paramount aim is to obtain the desired information with as much certainty and as little irradiation of the patient as possible. To achieve this the following are the desirable (though not always entirely attainable) features of the 'tracer material'.

1. *The Tracer Substance.*—This should, as far as possible, be identical in its chemical and biological properties to the stable substance being investigated, so that following the former inevitably means that the latter is also being followed. Such a tracer substance is achieved when one of the elements making up the substance being investigated is represented by one of its radioactive isotopes. For example, in studies concerning vitamin B^{12} (cyanocobalamin) the stable cobalt atom is replaced by an atom of one of the radio-isotopes of cobalt.

In some cases exact substitution is not practicable, as, for example, where radioactive strontium is used in studies of calcium metabolism. When results obtained in this type of case are being interpreted care must be taken to allow for any differences in chemical behaviour introduced by the change of element.

2. *The 'Label'.*—The 'labelling' isotope should remain attached to the 'labelled' tracer substance throughout the investigation. Failure to satisfy this requirement could mean that quite a different system from that intended was being studied. At the very least it increases the difficulty of result interpretation.

3. *Isotope Half-life.*—Any radioactive material used in an investigation will, as already stated, be irradiating much if not all of the patient. To keep the dose as low as possible it is necessary for the radioactive material to be present for as short a time as possible. This means that the half-life should be as short as is compatible with the investigation being carried out. Too long a half-life means a larger dose than is desirable; too short a half-life means that, towards the end of the test, the activity may be too low for accurate assessment or that, with the activity changing so much over a measurement period, accuracy is difficult to attain. Whilst hard-and-fast rules cannot be laid down, a rule-of-thumb could be that the half-life should be of the order of the period over which measurements have to be taken.

In this connection it should be noted that the amount of radioactive material in any biological system decreases with time, not only because of radioactive decay but also because of removal of the material by metabolic and excretory processes. Thus to the fraction (λ_R) removed per second by radioactive decay (cf. p. 29) must be added a comparable fraction (λ_B) removed biologically. The total fraction lost per second is, therefore, given by

$$\lambda_E = \lambda_R + \lambda_B,$$

where λ_E is the *effective* decay constant for the two effects.

λ_R is, of course, an absolute constant for any particular radioactive isotope (*see* pp. 27 and 28,) whereas λ_B is not. Its value depends on the material in which it is incorporated and the biological system involved as well as on the current metabolic state of the patient under investigation. (A patient starved of iodine is likely to retain any administered iodine longer than would a patient with a normal iodine complement, for example.) Nevertheless, average values can be established which are an acceptable guide for this purpose.

Since

$$\lambda = \frac{0 \cdot 693}{T}$$

where T is the half-life (see p. 30), it follows that

$$\frac{0 \cdot 693}{T_{\mathrm{E}}} = \frac{0 \cdot 693}{T_{\mathrm{R}}} + \frac{0 \cdot 693}{T_{\mathrm{B}}},$$

where T_{E}, T_{R}, and T_{B} are, respectively, the effective, the radioactive, and the biological half-lives of the radioactive material in the biological system concerned.

Hence

$$\frac{1}{T_{\mathrm{E}}} = \frac{1}{T_{\mathrm{R}}} + \frac{1}{T_{\mathrm{B}}}$$

or

$$T_{\mathrm{E}} = \frac{T_{\mathrm{R}} \times T_{\mathrm{B}}}{T_{\mathrm{R}} + T_{\mathrm{B}}}.$$

Since the effective half-life is always shorter than either of the other values it is the effective value which should be considered when choosing an isotope for a particular role. A good example will be seen on p. 400 in the account of the Schilling test for pernicious anaemia.

4. *Radiation Energy.*—In most of the common diagnostic tests using radioactive isotopes detection is via gamma rays because of their considerable penetrating power. For *in vivo* tests gamma rays are essential and, from the point of view of their penetrating through body tissues to reach the detector, the higher their energy the better. However, the efficiency with which they are detected by the scintillation counter is greater at lower energies, as is the protective efficiency of the shielding placed round the detector to exclude, as much as possible, radiation coming from any direction other than that of immediate interest. Therefore, a compromise has to be reached between these opposing effects and, if possible, mono-energetic gamma rays in the energy range 100–500 keV. are used.

5. *Other Radiations.*—Any beta rays accompanying the gamma rays contribute radiation dose to the patient but, because of their very limited range (e.g., *see* pp. 26 and 27), little or nothing to the measurements. Therefore, it is desirable that the beta-ray emission should be as small, or of as low energy, as possible. The ideal would be to use a pure gamma-ray emitter, and this can be achieved by using isotopes which exhibit K-electron capture or by using radio-isomers, those radioactive nuclei which, as described on p. 24, only emit gamma rays. In practice, however, radio-isomers are not purely gamma-ray sources owing to the phenomenon of 'internal conversion'. In this a nuclear gamma-ray interacts, photo-electrically, with one of the orbital electrons of its atom (usually in the K shell). This results in the emission of a fast electron (a photo-electron) whose energy equals the gamma-ray energy less the electron binding energy, together with X-rays characteristic of the material concerned. These internal conversion electrons, as far as their effects are concerned, are indistinguishable from beta rays, which are, of course, fast electrons (*see* p. 22), but they only occur for a small fraction of gamma-ray emissions rather than in 100 per cent of emissions in the normal beta–gamma-ray decay process.

An additional advantage of isomers for much tracer work is their short half-lives, though these create considerable supply problems unless a local source is available. For example, technetium 99m (half-life 6 hours), which is widely used in diagnostic procedures, would decay to only 6 per cent of the activity dispatch if in transit for only 24 hours, whilst in the case of indium-113m (half-life 1·7 hours) only about one sixty-five thousandth would remain. Fortunately relatively simple local sources for isomers and other short-lived radioactive isotopes are available and full advantage can be taken of their desirable properties.

'**Generators' for Short-lived Isotopes.**—A number of short-lived radioactive isotopes of value in clinical work are produced by the decay of a parent radioactive material of longer half-life. For example, iodine 132, which has a half-life of 2·3 hours, is the 'daughter' product of tellurium 132 which has a half-life of 78 hours. Similarly technetium 99m (6 hours), indium 113m (1·7 hours) and strontium 87m (2·8 hours) are, respectively, decay products of molybdenum 99 (67 hours), tin 113 (118 days) and yttrium 87 (80 hours). In each case the 'daughter' is chemically different from the 'parent' and can be separated from it chemically. This is the basis of the 'generators' (or 'cows' as they are often called) which can, in a hospital department, provide supplies of short-lived isotopes over several days.

Fig. 287 A shows the principle of the 'generator' used for obtaining ^{132}I from tellurium 132. A glass funnel contains a cylindrical column of sodium tellurite 132 absorbed on to alumina, with nylon mesh above and below it to keep the column in place.

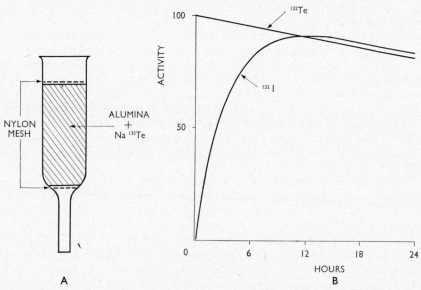

Fig. 287.—A, A ^{132}Te 'column' for the production of ^{132}I. B, The decay of ^{132}Te and the rise and decay of the accumulated ^{132}I.

The ^{132}I, produced by the decay of ^{132}Te, accumulates in the column until removed by pouring over the column a very dilute solution of ammonia to which a little 'hypo' has been added. This addition is necessary to ensure that the iodine is in the form of an iodide rather than iodate which is not readily absorbed by the thyroid gland, for investigations of which the ^{132}I is normally used. Such a washing (or elution) with 20 ml. of solution removes about 60 per cent of the accumulated ^{132}I and the process can be repeated after the iodine has had time to re-establish equilibrium with its 'parent'. This, as *Fig.* 287 shows, takes about 12 hours. In practice the column (or 'cow') is eluted (or 'milked') daily over about a week, after which time it is too weak to satisfy most clinical demands, the activity of the tellurium being down to about one-quarter of its original value.

Technetium 99m can be obtained by eluting, with saline, a generator of similar design containing molybdenum 99 absorbed on to a resin rather than on to alumina. The reasons for the different column materials are complex. Basically, however, the material chosen must retain the parent but not the daughter radioactive material so that, ideally, elution removes all the latter but none of the former. In practice, as already indicated for [132]I, complete removal is not achieved.

An important difference in design between the generators for iodine 132 and for technetium 99m (or indeed any other isotope used in injected material) is that the generator for the latter is completely enclosed so that the strictest sterility can be attained and the eluted material be kept free from pyrogens and other dangerous organisms.

Elution Technique.—For any standard radioactive isotope test, sources of the same strength are required on each occasion so that the elution technique used with any 'generator' must be able to provide such sources, in spite of the fact that the amount of daughter radioactive substance present decreases continuously as the parent substance decays. For example, the amount of [132]Te present (and therefore the amount of [132]I) after 3 days will be roughly half that present initially. (The half-life of [132]Te is 78 hours.) The normal procedure (which may be repeated as frequently as daily) is to use the same volume of eluting fluid at each elution, that volume being enough to remove a high proportion of the daughter product present. The resulting solution— at least over about a week—will be more concentrated than is required for normal use so that dilution is necessary. Samples of the required strength can therefore be achieved each time by reducing the dilution in step with the reduction in the amount of material present.

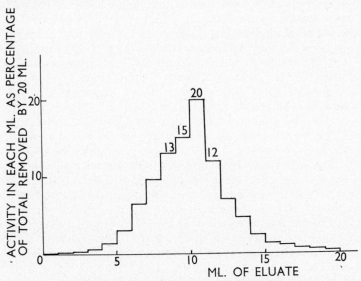

Fig. 288.—The elution of a ^{99m}Tc generator.

An example may make the procedure clear. Assume that solutions containing 0·1 mCi per ml. are required, and that initially the elution produces a solution containing 1·0 mCi per ml. If 9 ml. are added to each millilitre of this solution, the required concentration is achieved. Some time later, due to source decay, the elution material contains 0·5 mCi per ml. Then the addition of 4 ml. of diluting fluid will produce the required strength. When the elution only produces 0·25 mCi per ml. an additional 1·5 ml. has to be used, and so on. In each case the final solution contains 0·1 mCi per ml.

When particularly concentrated samples are needed, as, for example, for the labelling of some chemicals, advantage can be taken of the special pattern of the release of the radioactive material from the generator into different volumes of eluting fluid. If, for example, 20 ml. of fluid are poured through the column a considerable percentage of the available radioactive material will be removed, but if this volume is collected as twenty separate samples of 1 ml. each it will be found, as *Fig.* 288 shows, that very little is removed in the first few millilitres whilst succeeding millilitres each remove progressively more until the eleventh removes most. Thereafter successive equal volumes produce weaker sources as the amount remaining in the generator becomes less and less. If, for example, 1 ml. of maximum concentration is required, 10 ml. should be passed through the column, collected but not used. The next 1 ml. added will remove 20 per cent of the total possible yield and will thus be four times as concentrated as the solution obtained by using 20 ml. (i.e., 20 per cent in 1 ml. against 100 per cent in 20 ml.). If a larger volume is required, discarding (to a properly safe store) the first 8 ml. used and collecting the next 4 will give a total of 60 per cent of the maximum yield in these, i.e., 15 per cent in 1 ml.

TYPES OF DIAGNOSTIC TEST

The tests which can be carried out with radioactive isotopes can be loosely divided into three groups, namely metabolic and other physiological studies, the measurement of body composition or body 'spaces', and organ and tumour localization and visualization. A few illustrative examples of each type will be given.

Metabolic and other Physiological Studies.—In these the total amount of material that an organ takes up, and the rate at which it takes it up or excretes it, may be measured, and departures from the normal used as indications of the possible existence of malfunction.

Thyroid Function Tests.—The main role of the thyroid gland is the taking of inorganic iodine from the blood for the production of hormones which are mainly involved in growth and growth control. Iodine administered to the patient is, after circulating in the blood, selectively absorbed by the thyroid and relatively little is stored in other parts of the body. The fraction of any administered iodine which is absorbed by the gland, and the speed at which this takes place, depend on its state of health or disease. Radioactive iodine is used to study the uptake pattern, and *Fig.* 289 shows the sort of differences which occur between underactive, normal, and overactive glands. One feature of the overactive condition that is worthy of note is that its high initial uptake of iodine may be followed by a rapid loss so that, after a day or so, the uptake appears similar to that in the normal gland. This is one of the reasons why uptake measurements are usually taken within a few hours of the administration of the radioactive material.

A known activity of radioactive iodine, usually in a very dilute solution of sodium iodide, is given orally to the patient and, at some precise time later, the amount of radioactive material in the thyroid gland is measured. The time interval varies between centres but is usually between 2 and 4 hours: the description below assumes a '2-hour uptake test'.

Fig. 290 shows one measuring arrangement. The patient lies down and the scintillation counter is positioned over the neck, with its crystal at some fixed distance (about

25 cm.) from the thyroid. A substantial lead collimator surrounds the crystal to exclude, as far as possible, any radiation except that coming from a region of 12–15 cm. diameter at the level of the patient's neck. This collimator is necessary because a substantial fraction of the administered radioactive iodine will be distributed through the rest of the body, and thus must not be included in the measurement. The effect of any soft scattered radiation can be reduced by placing a filter of 1–2 mm. of lead in front of the crystal. Better still, the smaller 'pulses' produced by the scattered radiation can be eliminated from the measurement of a suitable setting of the 'discriminator' (*see* p. 121).

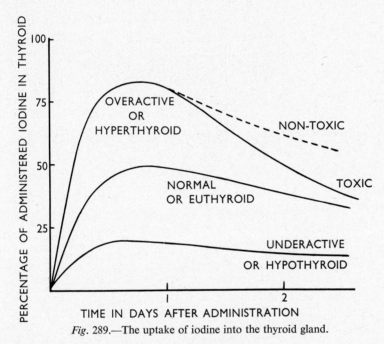

Fig. 289.—The uptake of iodine into the thyroid gland.

Measurements: Measurements are then taken of the thyroid activity, which is, say, A counts per minute. This value will be mainly due to iodine in the thyroid (which is what we want to measure), but there will also be a contribution from iodine surrounding the gland and from the inevitable 'background' which was discussed in CHAPTER XI. Repeating the measurement with the thyroid covered with a piece of lead about $\frac{1}{2}$ in. thick (as shown in *Fig.* 290) gives an indication of the unwanted contribution—say A_B counts per minute. The iodine in the thyroid may thus be said to give $(A-A_B)$ counts per minute.

To calibrate the counter and to determine the fractional uptake of the thyroid the above measurements are repeated with, instead of the patient, a radioactive iodine source of known strength inside a standard neck phantom. This phantom consists of a cylinder of paraffin wax, or similar material, 10–12 cm. in diameter, and 15–20 cm. long, and in it the radioactive source is placed at a position corresponding to that of the thyroid gland in the neck, i.e., with its centre at about 2 cm. deep. When the iodine was administered to the patient a source of equal strength was kept and this is used as the calibration source, thus automatically allowing in the comparison for any physical decay that has occurred. If readings made with the phantom, both with and without the screening block of lead, were respectively S and S_B counts per minute then the percentage uptake by the thyroid gland must be

$$\frac{A - A_B}{S - S_B} \times 100.$$

Technical factors: So far nothing has been said about the isotope to be used or how much of it should be used.

For any short-term test, such as the 2-hour uptake test, iodine 132 with its 2·3 hour half-life is preferred to iodine 131 (8 days) because of the considerable reduction in

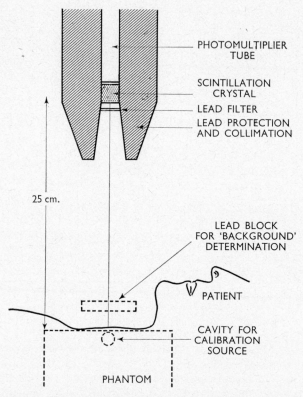

Fig. 290.—Measuring the radioactive iodine in the thyroid gland. The position of the lead block inserted for the determination of the 'background' contribution is shown dotted, as is the position of the calibration phantom and source.

dosage resulting from its use. The dose to the gland (1–2 rad per microcurie of iodine 131) is reduced by a factor of about a hundred whilst the whole-body dose is reduced more than tenfold. The amount of radioactive material needed for the test depends on the sensitivity of the measuring equipment: with a scintillation counter not more than about 10 μCi of iodine 132 will be called for.

When the work load is too small to justify having a local 'generator' for iodine 132, or where for some other reason one cannot be made available, iodine 131 can be obtained, from the Radiochemical Centre at Amersham, England, for example, in capsule form, at a variety of levels of activity ranging from about 8 to 100 μCi. Having a much longer half-life than iodine 132, they can be kept and still have usable activities ɔver much longer periods. This activity, at any time, is easily estimated since they are ɔolour coded to indicate their activity at some known time and since decay tables are eadily available.

Diagnostic value: A simple test such as this, in which the patient drinks a small volume of sodium iodide solution, and the activity of the thyroid is measured, does ıot, of itself, provide complete answers to a diagnostic problem. As with all simple ests the answer given must be considered in relation to other clinical evidence. No ɔhysical test yet devised replaces the trained observation and judgement of the experienced clinician: it brings extra evidence to aid him in reaching a decision.

Such is the variability of human beings that there will always be a range of response :o any test. Not all normal thyroid glands take up the same amount of iodine, nor will all overactive glands have the same increased uptake. The best that can be hoped s that ranges of values in which the various conditions might lie may be established. For example in the '2-hour uptake test' and a particular technique:—

Uptake of more than 25 per cent of administered iodine	Overactive thyroid
Uptake between 20 and 25 per cent of administered iodine	Borderline
Uptake between 5 and 20 per cent of administered iodine	Normal

This test, by itself, does not distinguish between hyperthyroidism and the relatively rare non-toxic goitre. The distinction has to be made on clinical grounds or by additional tests. Neither is it particularly useful for hypothyroidism (under active thyroid gland) where the initial uptake may be at a reasonably normal rate but this is not maintained so that the total uptake is low. Where this condition is suspected a test measurement after 24 hours (a '24-hour uptake test') is more likely to be useful. For such a test the longer half-life ^{131}I rather than ^{132}I needs to be used in order that the observed count rate after 24 hours would be large enough for accurate measurement. (In 24 hours the physical decay of ^{131}I would be about 8 per cent leaving 92 per cent of the initial material present. With ^{132}I a mere 0·1 per cent would remain.)

These last figures, however, indicate another advantage of ^{132}I over ^{131}I in many cases. Its short half-life allows a repeat test to be carried out quite soon after the ınitial test since, for example, 2 days after the test a millionth of the ^{132}I remains— assuming no biological removal—compared with over 80 per cent for ^{131}I.

Renal Function.—The chemical substance ortho-iodohippurate (Hippuran) is exclusively and quickly removed from the blood by the kidneys and excreted by them. The pattern of this removal and excretion can be used to study renal function. For this work Hippuran 'labelled' with ^{131}I is rapidly injected into the patient's bloodstream and its accumulation in, and its clearance from, the kidneys is observed by placing a scintillation counter over each kidney. As in *Fig.* 290, the counters are shielded and only receive radiation from a limited region—they each 'see' only one kidney. The electrical output from each counter is fed into a pen-recorder voltmeter so that an ink trace records, for each kidney, the variation, with time, of the radioactivity of each kidney. Examples for the sort of records obtained are shown in *Fig.* 291.

Both traces on the left are normal, both kidneys behaving very similarly and showing a fairly rapid build-up of activity in the kidney as the Hippuran is removed from the blood, followed by a rather slower excretion. In the centre record there is indication of acute obstruction of the right kidney (the build-up is fairly normal but there is no evacuation) with a normal left kidney. Finally the right-hand traces show a normal right kidney whilst the left is non-functioning.

Not all traces are as straightforward as these especially chosen examples, but there is no doubt that this method is a valuable complement to radiography in the evaluation of kidney disease. Although its indications are more qualitative than quantitative it is very useful for comparative studies such as the revealing of unilateral disease, and for serial studies either of the progress of the disease or the results of remedial procedures.

Vitamin B₁₂ and Pernicious Anaemia.—Vitamin B_{12} is essential for the normal development of red blood-cells. If, for some reason, it is not absorbed by the body

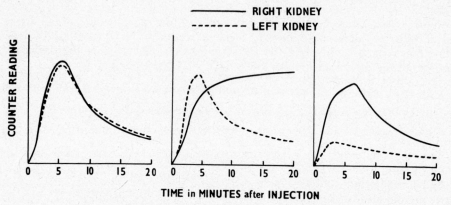

Fig. 291.—The uptake into and excretion from the kidney of Hippuran.

an anaemia results. Under the influence of a normal chemical constituent of the body, known as the 'intrinsic factor' secreted by the stomach, the vitamin is absorbed by the terminal ileum and stored in the liver. Failure of the stomach to secrete the factor results in pernicious anaemia, and this can be diagnosed by the aid of a relatively simple radioactive isotope test, the Schilling test.

As already mentioned, the molecule of vitamin B_{12} contains an atom of cobalt and therefore, can be 'labelled' using radioactive cobalt. A small amount of this 'labelled' material is given orally to the patient, and a little later, a very much larger dose of non-radioactive vitamin is given intramuscularly. This latter dose is large enough to satisfy the demand for vitamin B_{12} by the plasma and other tissues needing it. Therefore, any radioactive vitamin B_{12} absorbed through the gut is not needed and will be excreted in the urine, the radioactivity of which is an indication of the ability of the gut to absorb the vitamin. All the patient's urine is collected for 24 hours and its radioactivity measured, usually by placing the Winchester, in which the litre or so of urine is contained, inside a large 'well-type' counter or on top of a large, flat crystal detector. Small amounts of radioactivity are involved (about 0·25–0·5 μCi) and, therefore, high sensitivity of detection is needed. In normal patients between 10 and 30 per cent of the labelled material administered orally will be found in the collected urine, whilst a total of less than 5 per cent indicates defective absorption but not necessarily pernicious anaemia. There may be some other defect of the stomach mucosa or terminal ileum.

To eliminate that possibility the test is repeated after a period of a week to 10 days (during which time the radioactive material present will have been considerably reduced, partly by radioactive decay but mostly by biological elimination). At this second test, the patient is also given a dose of 'intrinsic factor'. If normal excretion is now observed, pernicious anaemia is confirmed: if it is not, there is some other cause of the malabsorption.

So far nothing has been mentioned about which of the radioactive isotopes of cobalt is used. Three are available and the selection of cobalt 57 is a good example of the application of the principles for the choice of isotope which have already been given above. Cobalt 60 emits 1·2 MeV. gamma rays and has a half-life of 5·3 years; cobalt 58 gives 0·8 MeV. gamma rays and its half-life is 71 days, whilst cobalt 57 is a source of 0·13 MeV. radiation with a half-life of 270 days. Of the three the choice is clearly between the last two, the very acceptable 0·13 MeV. gamma rays of cobalt 57 being offset by the long half-life, whilst, with cobalt 58, the more acceptable half-life goes with a rather too high gamma-ray energy. The ultimate choice of cobalt 57 stems from the effect of the rapid *biological* removal of vitamin B_{12} from the body. The biological half-life is about 6 days with the result that the effective half-life is practically the same whichever isotope is used. Assuming that the biological half-life is 6 days, then the effective half-lives for cobalt 60, 58, and 57 are, respectively, 5·98, 5·53, and 5·87 days.

Red-cell Survival Time.—Radioactive isotopes can also be used to measure the survival time of a patient's red blood-cells. The technique is simple, though the interpretation of the results calls for caution. A small sample of the patient's blood is incubated at 37° C. for about half an hour with about 100 μCi of ^{51}Cr (in the form of sodium chromate). During this process the ^{51}Cr attaches itself to the red blood-cells. The blood, having been carefully washed to remove any unattached chromate, and therefore unattached radioactivity, is reinjected and a further sample of blood taken from the patient 24 hours later and daily thereafter for 3 or 4 weeks. When the activity of the other samples is compared with the activity of that taken at 24 hours it is found to fall steadily due partly to the natural decay of the radioactive material, which can be allowed for, and partly through the removal of the aged red cells from the blood-stream. However, there is another factor which makes more difficult the deduction of the life span from these observations. Some of the chromium gets detached, or 'eluted', from the red cells and since this chromium is not in the blood samples the number of red cells seems less, and therefore the survival time shorter, than is in fact the case. The average normal survival time of the red cell is about 120 days though this type of experiment would yield an answer of about 50 days.

Because of this problem it is usual to measure the length of time for the amount of ^{51}Cr in the circulation to fall to half its original value, and to use variations from the normal range as indicators of blood disease. In the normal person this 'half-life' usually lies between 28 and 35 days: anything significantly shorter suggests that an abnormal process of red-cell destruction is at work.

Melanoma Detection.—All rapidly growing tissues need phosphorus and therefore it was felt that malignant tumours, whose main distinction is uncontrolled growth, might be revealed by their greater uptake of any administered ^{32}P. It has been claimed that breast tumours do this, and that they could be detected by the greater amount of radiation over the tumour than over the corresponding area on the other breast when the patient had had an injection of ^{32}P. Unfortunately many breast tumours are at such a depth in the mammary tissue that none of the beta rays from them can reach the surface. The test is thus of very limited value and is not generally used.

Melanomas (the malignant versions of the pigmented mole), on the other hand, are generally superficial and any difference in phosphorus uptake will not be masked by overlying tissues. For the test the patient is given an intravenous injection of about

14

50–400 µCi of ³²P in the form of sodium phosphate solution. One hour later the 'uptake' in the suspected lesion is compared with that in normal tissue at the corresponding site on the other side of the body. If the suspect area shows an uptake of more than 1·8 times that in normal tissue the presence of a malignant melanoma is indicated, though an inflammatory condition is not ruled out. Like all simple tests it is not infallible; like all other laboratory or physical tests it must be considered in conjunction with the clinical observations which it complements but for which it is no substitute.

Body 'Space' or Volume Determination.—This type of investigation employs a 'dilution' technique in which a known amount, A, of radioactive material is mixed into a system whose volume, V, is to be measured. After mixing a sample volume, v, is taken and its radioactivity measured and found to be a. Since the activity per unit volume must be the same in both the whole volume and the sample it follows that

$$\frac{A}{V} = \frac{a}{v} \quad \text{or} \quad V = \frac{Av}{a}.$$

Of these quantities A, v, and a can be measured directly and hence V can be found.

Measurements of the radioactivity in this sort of work are usually carried out in a 'well-type' scintillation counter, the general design of which is shown in *Fig.* 292. A hole is cut into the scintillator crystal into which a small test-tube containing the sample may be inserted. Because the sample is almost completely surrounded by the

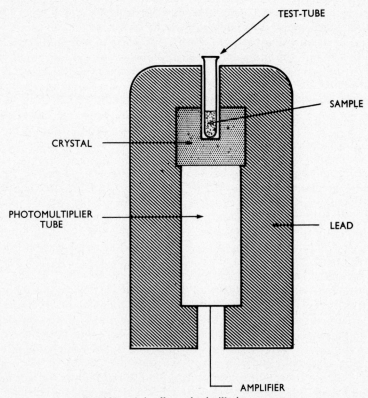

Fig. 292.—A 'well-type' scintillation counter.

crystal, radiation emitted in practically every direction must pass through it and hence high-detection efficiency is obtained. Radiation from outside sources is greatly reduced by surrounding the crystal and photomultiplier tube by several inches of lead, as shown.

Total Blood-volume.—The normal haematological measurements of haemoglobin concentration, of packed-cell volume, and of the red-cell count may not reflect the whole-blood condition: a knowledge of the total blood-volume may also be needed for, among other instances, patients suffering from burns or following major surgery, when shock or cardiac failure may complicate recovery.

To determine the blood-volume one method uses blood that has been labelled with ^{51}Cr in the way described for red-cell survival studies. About 10 ml. of blood labelled with a measured activity of ^{51}Cr (about 20 μCi) are reinjected into their donor and allowed to mix into the main blood. Although peripheral mixing is very rapid, equilibrium throughout the vascular space is rather slower so that 10 min. are usually allowed before a known volume of blood is removed, its activity measured, and the blood-volume calculated by the above formula.

Red-cell and Plasma Volumes.—To find the red-cell volume or the plasma volume it is necessary to know the haematocrit, that is the fraction of the volume of whole blood that is occupied by red cells. If V_T and V_R are, respectively, the total and red-cell volumes the haematocrit (H) is given by

$$H = V_R/V_T.$$

The value of the haematocrit is determined by centifuging a volume of blood so that all the red blood-cells are packed together in a solid column at one end of the centrifuge tube. By comparing the length of this column with the total column length a measure of H can be found. If H and the total blood-volume V_T are known, V_R can be calculated and also the plasma volume (V_p) since

$$V_T = V_R + V_p.$$

Unfortunately the simple haematocrit measurement described above is subject to two errors which may have to be taken into account. In the first place, a proportion of the plasma is trapped in the red-cell column, the exact amount depending upon the speed and length of time of the centrifugation. A reasonable correction for this phenomen is to reduce the value of H, as calculated above, by 3 per cent. The other source of error is physiological in basis. The blood flowing in the minute blood-vessels has a lower haematocrit than that of blood in the larger vessels, to the extent that the mean value of the haematocrit for all the blood in the body is about 10 per cent lower than that for arterial or venous blood.

Because of these uncertainties direct measurement of plasma volume is often undertaken or the red-cell and plasma volumes (and hence the body haematocrit) are determined simultaneously by a double-isotope technique.

Plasma Volume.—By using human serum albumin labelled with ^{125}I the plasma volume may be determined directly. About 5–10 μCi of the radio-iodinated serum albumin (RISA) are injected intravenously into the patient and an equal sample kept as a standard. Mixing takes about 10 min. after which a sample of blood is taken and centrifuged to separate the red cells from the plasma, the activity of a known volume of which is measured in a 'well-type' counter (*Fig.* 292). If this activity is compared with the activity of the standard RISA sample the dilution suffered by the injected material can be measured and hence the plasma volume calculated. Since the normal plasma volume is of the order of 3 litres, the activity of the plasma will be about one three-thousandth of the activity of an equal volume to the standard. It is therefore convenient, and usual, to dilute the standard to about the same strength by the addition of a known amount of water. Both samples can now be measured on the same range on the instrument and the accuracy of measurement improved.

An example may make the method clearer. Assume that a small volume of RISA was injected into a patient and an equal volume kept as a standard. After mixing, about 10 ml. of blood were taken from the patient and after centrifugation 4·0 ml. of plasma were counted in a well counter, giving 2880 counts per min. The standard was diluted by the addition of 3000 ml. of water and 4·0 ml. of this mixture also counted. It gave 2640 counts per min. Both these count rates include, of course, the inevitable 'background' count (*see* p. 122) which in this case was 120 counts per min., and must be allowed for.

$$\text{Plasma activity} = 2880 - 120 = 2760 \text{ counts per min.}$$

$$\text{Activity of diluted standard} = 2640 - 120 = 2520 \text{ counts per min.}$$

It will be remembered that before being mixed in the body or diluted with water the two samples were equally active. Their activity is now distributed throughout the volumes with which they were mixed, and the counts per unit volume multiplied by the total volume must be the same for each sample. If the plasma volume in the body into which the one sample was mixed is V_p and the volume of water into which the standard sample was mixed is V_s (in this case 3000 ml.) then

$$\text{Volume} \times \text{counts per ml.} = V_p \times 2760/4 = 2520 \times 3000/4$$

or

$$V_p = 2739 \text{ ml.} = \text{plasma volume.}$$

Red-cell and Plasma Volumes—a Double-isotope Technique.—This type of measurement is possible because the scintillation counter can discriminate between radiations of different energy. The red blood-cells are labelled, as before, with chromium 51, which emits 0·33 MeV. gamma rays, whilst the iodine 125 used to label the albumin for the plasma determination emits 0·035 MeV. photons.

A mixture of the two labelled preparations having been injected into the patient, and time allowed for thorough mixing with the blood, a sample of blood is taken as in the previously described separate estimations of whole-blood and plasma volumes. Its activity is then measured in a 'well-type' scintillation counter with the operating conditions set first to detect one gamma-ray energy and then the other. Thus each of the radioactive isotopes is estimated separately and the whole blood and plasma volumes can be determined directly. Knowing these two, the red-cell volume and the whole-body haematocrit can be deduced.

There is one complication in the counter measurements which has to be taken into account. Whilst the counter will not detect the 0·035 MeV. radiation from the iodine 125 when set for the chromium 51 (0·33 MeV.) radiation, when it is set for the iodine radiation it will also measure some radiation from the chromium 51. This is scattered radiation (what is called the 'Compton tail') that inevitably arises when radiation passes through any material, and some of it will be in the energy range the counteris, set to measure.

Allowance can be made for this extra radiation by measuring a standard solution. of labelled red blood-cells only, under counter conditions for chromium 51 and then iodine 125 radiation.

Organ Visualization.—Radiography relies on the different opacity to X-rays of the different parts of the body, and when this does not naturally exist it can be created by the use of artificial contrast media such as have been described in earlier chapters.

This technique does not, however, allow the detail of organs like the thyroid gland or the liver to be revealed radiographically. It is fortunate, therefore, that radiography can be complemented by the use of radioactive pharmaceuticals. Using artificial contrast radiology the information gleaned stems largely from the displacement or distortion of normal structure. With radioactive isotope techniques it is possible, because of different amounts of radioactive material taken up, to determine the size, shape, and position of an organ or space-occupying lesion in relation to its surroundings, or to reveal the distribution within the organ of some substance, which might be related to its normal or abnormal function.

Scanning.—The radioactive isotope tests so far described have been concerned with the total amount of a particular material in some part of the body or in a sample. In scanning, interest is centred on the detailed distribution of the material within the system of interest. To obtain this information a scintillation counter, which is heavily shielded except for a small hole (or in practice a series of specially directed small holes, which will be described later) which 'sees' only a small part of the patient at one time, is moved slowly backwards and forwards in straight lines over the region being studied. Each successive sweep across the area is displaced from its neighbours by a small distance along the body, and in this way the whole area is 'scanned'. *Fig.* 293 shows a typical commercially available automatic scanning machine used in this

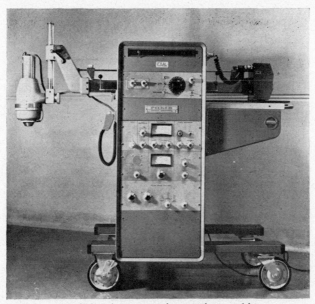

Fig. 293.—An automatic scanning machine.

sort of investigation. On the left of the control console is the scanning 'head' which contains the collimator, the scintillator, and the photomultiplier tube, whilst on the right is the recording apparatus which produces the visual representation of the readings. The whole equipment is fairly mobile on its wheels and can be positioned over any part of a patient lying on a suitable couch or stretcher trolley.

Collimation and Detail.—The narrow-hole collimator is used because it is desired to detect, and indicate, variations in radioactive isotope concentration from place to place, and this cannot be done satisfactorily with other than small holes, as *Fig*. 294 shows. This diagram shows a scintillation counter centred over the thyroid gland and having, in turn, a wide, a narrow, and a very narrow collimator hole. It is assumed that the gland contains a uniform distribution of radioactive iodine except for the three zones, A, B, and C. In A the concentration is three times that in the bulk of the gland, whilst in B the concentration is five times above the general level. Zone C contains no radioactive material and it is also assumed that there is none in the tissues around the gland. To investigate the isotope distribution each counter is

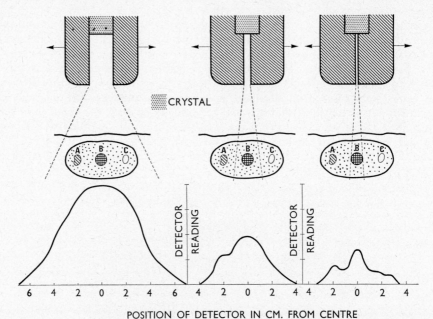

POSITION OF DETECTOR IN CM. FROM CENTRE

Fig. 294.—The effect of collimator size on the detail revealed by a scintillation counter (i.e., its resolving power). A large-aperture collimator (left) has considerable sensitivity but does not reveal detail. The medium-sized collimator, in the centre, gives a smaller reading and some detail. Good resolution, revealing both high concentration zones and hinting at the absence of activity in C, is shown by the right-hand counter with the very narrow aperture. The readings, however, are considerably reduced. Relative isotope concentrations: Gland in general, 1; Zone A, 3; Zone B, 5; Zone C, 0; outside the gland, 0.

traversed across the gland as indicated by the arrows, and the variation in its reading is given in graphical form below. A quite different 'profile' (as the graph is often called) is obtained in each case.

It will be seen that when the large collimator is used, radiation from the whole of the gland can reach the detecting crystal, which can be moved at least 1 cm. on either side of the central position before any of the gland lies outside the zone from which the crystal can receive radiation. The counter response is insensitive to position and only gives a crude indication of the isotope distribution. There is hardly any suggestion of the three special zones.

The narrow collimator, shown in the centre, only 'sees' part of the gland from any position. In the position indicated it 'sees' the whole of zone B but A and C are outside its sensitive region, whereas if it is moved 1 cm. to the left it will receive radiation from part of A and part of B. Its readings give some indication of the presence of A and B but do not really show that C is present.

Finally, with the very narrow collimator, quite a small part of the gland is measured from each position. If, for example, the apparatus is moved 1 cm. from its central position, it can 'see' none of the special zones and its reading indicates the activity of the general bulk of the gland. The 'profile' produced by this collimator is much closer to that which might be expected from the known distribution of radioactive isotope. The 'hot spots' A and B show clearly and at approximately the right intensities, whilst there is a small indication of the presence of C, though this is not very definite.

From these results some important generalizations may be made. If information about variation is needed the collimator must be small, but if so, then the apparatus sensitivity will be small. The large collimator gave a large reading, but was unable to separate out the special zones (it was unable to 'resolve' them), and it indicated that radioactivity was spread over a much wider zone than we know to be the case. In contrast the very narrow collimator 'resolved' the 'high spots' and suggested the presence of the low spot, whilst indicating a gland size not far from the truth. Against this, of course, its response is very small.

Collimation for 'Scanning'.—Because 'scanning' is used to investigate isotope distributions, it calls for a fine collimator and hence will be a much less sensitive process than, for example, an uptake study. A further reduction of sensitivity arises from the fact that the detector is moving, so that each place is measured only for a very limited time. Therefore it is usual to have to use more radioactive material for 'scanning' than for measurements with a static counter, and also to have the detection much closer to the patient. There is, however, a further aid to sensitivity which is of considerable importance, and that is the so-called 'focusing collimator'. Good resolution—the ability to reveal detail—calls for narrow collimation, but this does not mean that only one hole has to be used. Greater sensitivity, without loss of resolving power, can be achieved by using a number of holes pointing at one spot, as shown diagrammatically in *Fig.* 295. In such a focusing collimator a number of tapered holes all point towards the point A which is usually at about 10 cm. from the crystal. A typical collimator used with a 3-in. sodium iodide crystal has about 30 holes, each of about 4 mm. diameter at its lower end.

It must not be imagined, however, that this type of collimator receives radiation from only one point or level in the patient. Just as in a radiograph the pattern of the film is the result of different attenuation at all levels in the part irradiated, so the radiation received by the detector crystal through any collimator hole comes from all depths in the zone 'seen', as *Fig.* 296 A shows. The counter responds to the total radioactivity in the 'seen' zone and gives no indication of the level at which it occurs. In this respect too the focusing collimator has an advantage over the single-hole collimator, as *Fig.* 296 B shows. Collimator hole 1 'sees' radioactivity anywhere in zone ABHG whilst hole 2 'sees' CDEF and the counter response depends on the total activity in all this volume. However, the activity in the overlapping (hatched) region is, as it were, 'seen' twice and, therefore, its effect upon the counter is doubled. With three holes the effect of the zone 'seen' by each hole would have three times the effect of any zone 'seen' by one hole, and so as the number of holes is increased the effect of the zone common to all holes is more and more enhanced compared with the effect of the rest of the region. In this way a relatively small zone around the 'focus' point (hatched in *Fig.* 296 C) contributes most to the output of the counting system, so that if the counter is 'scanned' across the patient the activity between the dotted lines in *Fig.* 296 C will be emphasized in any output pattern (e.g., graphs like those in *Fig.* 294 or dot pictures as discussed below). To some extent, at least, the output from a 'focusing' collimator represents the distribution of radioactivity in the patient in a layer on either side of the focus point. By raising or lowering the counting head relative to the patient information about different layers can be obtained if desired. The contribution from the rest of the body must not, however, be forgotten. On either side of the zone where all the holes overlap there will be regions 'seen' by several though not all the holes and these, especially when closer to the counter, will produce

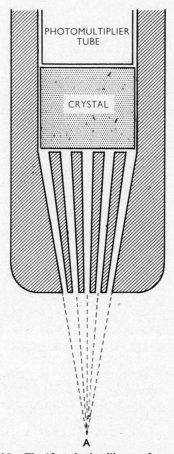

Fig. 295.—The 'focusing' collimator for scanning.

a marked effect. The effect of the main zone will therefore be overlaid with effects from other parts to the detriment of contrast and of the sharpness of delineation of any structure being studied.

Presenting the Answer.—Each time a photon interacts with the crystal, a flash of light (a scintillation) is generated and this is converted, as already described, into an electrical pulse by the photomultiplier tube. How can these pulses be handled so that the distribution of radioactivity is revealed?

The simplest method is indicated in *Fig.* 294. As the counter is moved, either by hand or mechanically, across the area being studied, the meter indicating the pulse rate is read at suitable intervals and a graph like those at the foot of the diagram is plotted (or the output can be fed into a pen-recorder and the graph obtained automatically). There will be one such set of readings, or graph, for each traverse by the counter, and from them an iso-count chart (made up of a series of lines joining points of equal count rates) can be produced in much the same way as an iso-dose chart is obtained for an X-ray treatment. (*See*, for example, CHAPTER XXXII.)

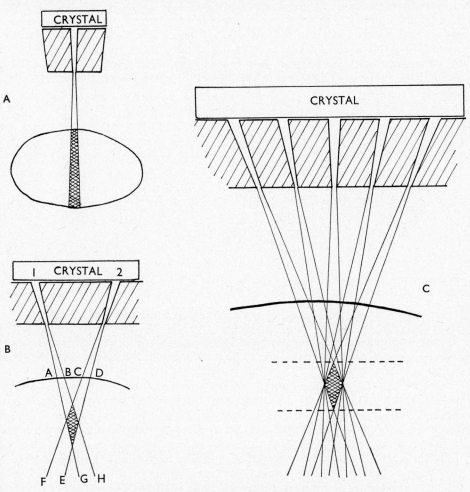

Fig. 296.—The principle of the mode of action of the focusing collimator.

Such a method is simple but slow, and most modern scanning equipment uses mechanical display systems, as well as a mechanical drive for the scintillation counter. A popular method is to have a printer which makes a mark on a piece of paper every time a predetermined number of scintillations (say 8) has been recorded from the detector. The printer moves along with the counter and where there is concentrated radioactivity the marks on the paper will be close together, whereas when there is little isotope the paper will receive few marks. An ingenious extension of this is to make the colour of the marks different for different count rates. Thus the marks are not only closer together for high count rates—and therefore high activity—but their colour will be different from that used for the sparser points at low count rates. Whether this system, which is undoubtedly impressive, actually conveys more information or conveys information more readily to the trained observer is not certain. *Fig.* 297 shows a typical iso-count diagram and the dot-presentation for the same scan of a thyroid gland.

A complete scan of, for example, a liver may take up to 40 min. during which time the distribution of and amount of radioactive isotope in the organ should not change appreciably otherwise the picture may give a completely false impression. The need for this relative constancy has to be taken into account in the selection of the pharmaceutical to be used—it must not be metabolized or removed too quickly —and of the radioactive substance used to 'label' it, which must not have too short a half-life.

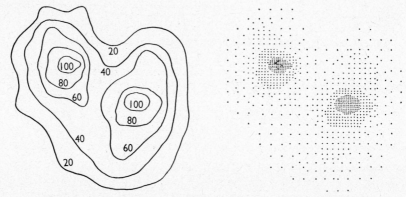

Fig. 297.—An iso-count diagram and a dot diagram for the same thyroid gland.

Thyroid Scanning.—Thyroid 'scans' are the easiest of all to perform not only because of the high selective uptake of radioactive material, but also because the gland is close to the skin. ^{131}I or ^{99m}Tc is usually used.

Brain 'Scanning'.—Under normal circumstances what is known as the 'blood–brain barrier' prevents many materials from entering the brain from the blood-supply. When disease is present the barrier may be disrupted and because of this it may be possible for some materials to 'seep' through the affected area into the brain. If these materials are 'labelled' with radioactive atoms the presence and extent of the 'breakthrough', and possibly of the disease, may be detectable. Brain 'scanning' is now widely used for tumour diagnosis and localization, and it is claimed to give valuable information concerning the existence and position of brain lesions in about 80 per cent of cases.

Until recently the most commonly used radioactive isotope for brain 'scanning' was mercury 197 (half-life 67 hours), labelling the drug neohydrin. Now technetium 99m in the form of sodium pertechnetate is preferred because of its much shorter but adequately long (6 hours) half-life.

Liver 'Scanning'.—One of the normal functions of the liver is to remove particles from the blood and either to break them down or metabolize them prior to excreting them. This function can be used to introduce radioactive material into the liver to aid the diagnosis of suspected malfunction or disease or to reveal the liver outline, which cannot be obtained radiographically because no X-ray artificial contrast material can easily be deposited in the liver. Gold-198 colloid was originally used but the dye Rose

Bengal (which the liver will remove from the blood) labelled with ^{131}I was generally preferred until recently when a more suitable material became available. The difficulty with Rose Bengal is that its metabolism in the liver proceeds fairly rapidly so that by 20–30 min. after its injection into the patient, and while the scan is still proceeding, excretion is already taking place. A misleading picture may therefore be presented. The difficulty is overcome by using a sulphur colloid labelled with ^{99m}Tc. The colloid particle size is more suitable for remaining in the liver and stays there longer than would the Rose Bengal, whilst the ^{99m}Tc is superior to ^{131}I in so far as it has a shorter half-life and practically no beta rays accompanying its gamma-ray emission.

In addition to revealing the liver outline, 'scanning' can provide information which is valuable in the diagnosis of hepatitis, of cirrhosis of the liver, and also of abscesses or tumour metastases which appear as blanks (because they are inactive as far as liver function is concerned and therefore take up no radioactive material) in the 'scan' picture.

The Gamma Camera.—The value of the 'scanner' described above is limited by the time that it takes to perform its task. In the 30–40-min. taken for the 'scanning'

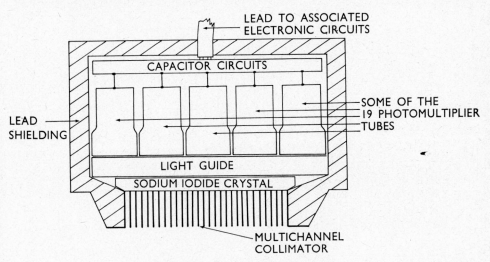

Fig. 298.—The Anger gamma camera.

head to 'observe' all the region to be examined, the pattern of the radioactivity may change—as, for example, with Rose Bengal in the liver. As already stated, a misleading picture of a distribution may be given unless the material chosen has a fairly lengthy stay in the part being examined. The 'scanner' cannot be used in dynamic studies—it cannot be used to follow the progress of an isotope in or out of any organ or its movement inside that organ. The gamma camera avoids this difficulty by recording the activity in all parts of the organ at the same time. It is, therefore, particularly useful for studying dynamic situations as well as producing much more quickly (though unfortunately at much greater expense) the information given by the moving scanner.

The principle of the gamma camera (or Anger camera as it is often called after its developer) is shown in *Fig.* 298. A sodium iodine crystal, about 30 cm. in diameter and 1 cm. thick, is used as the detector and any scintillations in it are detected by a number of photomultiplier tubes arranged in a hexagonal pattern over a Perspex 'light guide' plate about 4 cm. thick placed directly over the crystal surface. In the originally available cameras 19 tubes were used. Now 37 are commonly used and some equipment uses 61. Between the crystal and the radiation source is a collimator plate of about 3 cm. thick lead pierced by a very large number of parallel holes each about 3 mm. in diameter. As with any other scintillation counter the whole is light-tight and the crystal, light guide, and photo-multiplier tubes are surrounded by a lead shield to reduce the 'background' radiation as much as possible.

How the Gamma Camera works.—A complete description of how the gamma camera produces its ultimate picture would not only be very lengthy but also very complex. It would be beyond the scope of this book and the needs of its readers for whom, however, the admittedly much simplified description given below may be useful.

The role of the collimator is to ensure, as far as possible, that the pattern of scintillations in the crystal corresponds to the isotope distribution within the tissue being examined, and, as in most practical exercises, a compromise has to be reached. *Fig.* 299 illustrates one aspect of the problem. Imagine a disk of radioactive material

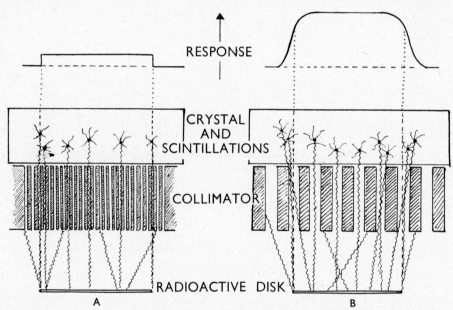

Fig. 299.—Anger camera collimation. Fine holes (A) give a sharp image of small brightness. Coarse holes (B) give a brighter image which is less sharp.

underneath the gamma camera which, in one case (A), has a very fine-holed collimator whilst in the other (B) it has a collimator with larger holes. For complete correspondence between the scintillation pattern and the radioactive object all the scintillation must take place within the dotted lines in the crystal. This is achieved with the very fine holes since only radiation arising immediately below the holes can pass through them. Any oblique rays are stopped by the collimator. The scintillation pattern across the crystal is depicted by the graph above the diagram, and it will be seen to fall off sharply to zero at the edge of the area of correspondence. Thus the ideal correspondence is achieved but at the price of very little radiation reaching the crystal —the system is in fact too insensitive. More radiation must be allowed to reach the crystal, and this is done by using the larger diameter holes. As a result some oblique rays can pass through to reach the crystal and to produce scintillations outside the zone of correspondence. In this way the scintillations are spread over a rather wide zone and, as the right-hand graph shows, a blurred edge replaces the sharp edge of the previous pattern, but at the gain of increased sensitivity. In practice 3-mm. holes represent a satisfactory compromise between the competing demands of sensitivity and image sharpness.

When a scintillation counter occurs in the crystal, light from it is received by every photomultiplier tube, the amount received by each, as *Fig.* 300 shows, being dependent

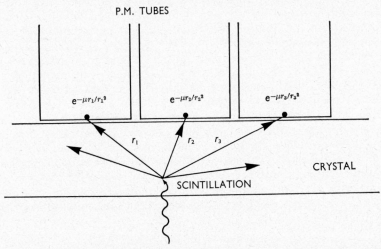

Fig. 300.—The amount of light reaching each photomultiplier tube depends on the position of the scintillation relative to it.

upon the position of the event relative to the tube. Because of the operation of the inverse square law and of attenuation in the crystal most light is received by the two or three tubes nearest the event, the amount received by more distant tubes being relatively negligible. The voltage pulses resulting from the light received by the various tubes are fed into complex and elaborate electronic circuits which work out (from their relative magnitudes) the position at which each scintillation occurred, and also cause a dot of light to appear at the corresponding point of the output screen on which the picture is displayed. This screen is of the storage type, which means that the light persists for a long time and the picture is built up as the individual scintillations occur at different parts of the crystal. These events follow one another very quickly but it must be remembered that they are quite separate events arising from complete random individual radioactive decays. Because the 'dead time' of the crystal-photomultiplier tube system is very small (*see* p. 121) the very large majority of the events are separately and correctly recorded. When, after a few minutes' exposure the picture can be regarded as complete, it is photographed to form a permanent record for study purposes.

Picture Quality.—It has been seen that the reading obtained with a Geiger-Müller counter or a scintillation counter cannot be taken directly as an indication of the activity of a source: corrections have to be applied for the inevitable 'background' radiation and also for radiation from other parts of the body leaking through the surrounding protection. By the same token gamma camera and scinti-scanner pictures must not be taken at their face value. They, too, will receive a contribution (which may vary in time) from 'background' and 'leakage' radiation, for which direct allowance cannot be made as readily as in simple counting techniques. Then there are defects in the picture, which stem from the fact that the collimator design is a compromise which leads, as already discussed, to structures appearing blurred or two separate objects appearing as one (they are not 'resolved'). Finally, there are random effects due to what is technically known as 'noise' in the detecting system, which may add to the picture details not present in the original.

There are two separate facets to this particular problem: one is due to the electronic equipment and the other to the radioactive material. In any electronic equipment there are always tiny spurious effects which are unimportant except when the effects being measured are also tiny. Then the spurious effects may enhance the current or voltage being measured and make it, temporarily, appear to be greater than, in fact, it is. One example of this 'noise' is provided by the photomultiplier tube, the photocathode of which may spontaneously emit an electron which produces the same effect as would an electron produced by a light photon. This 'dark current', which is variable, will make any light intensities being measured appear greater than they are and vary more than they do. Radioactivity, as pointed out in CHAPTER III and on p. 123, is a random process so that the amount of radiation given out by a source in successive equal short intervals of time will not be constant, the importance of the fluctuations being much greater with a small source than with a larger one. For example, on p. 122 the results are given of a series of 1-min. observations and the range, for an average value of 100, is from 88 to 112. With a weaker source the series could well go

$$10, \ 9, \ 12, \ 13, \ 8, \ 11, \ 7, \ 8, \ 11, \ 10$$

showing a variation of ± 30 per cent. To keep the dose to the patient as small as possible the amounts of radioactive material used are kept as small as possible with the result that the random (statistical) variations in output are more important than with large activities. Thus the picture of a uniformly radioactive area may have variations across it and suggest a pattern in the original which does not exist. Unless the user is aware of these possibilities and that the significance of small change must not be regarded too highly, false conclusions may be drawn. The experienced observer learns to take these possibilities into account and he can now be helped by the output of 'scanner' or gamma camera being subjected to complex scrutiny by a computer. For instance, the computer can test whether the difference between two different areas on the picture can be taken to indicate a real difference in the original or whether it could be due to the naturally occurring 'noise'. In this sort of way the information content and usefulness of the final picture are considerably enhanced.

The Scanner and the Gamma Camera—a Comparison.—Until recently most departments with radio-isotope visualization facilities were equipped with scanners, partly because they were less expensive than gamma cameras and partly because they had important practical advantages over them. Although the scanner is unsuitable for dynamic studies it had the advantage of greater resolving power and of being able to reveal a larger area of the body. Much of this has now changed.

With any device which produces images (pictures) an important question is 'What is its resolving power?' By this we mean, in simple language, how close can two similar objects be and still be shown to be separate? The smaller this distance the greater the resolving power, or resolution, of the system and the finer the detail it can reveal. Until recently the resolution of the scanner was superior to that of the gamma camera, mainly because of the relatively small number of photomultiplier tubes used in the latter. Now cameras are available with 37 tubes (as against 19 in the early models), and with a resolving power slightly superior to the scanner. With the 61-tube models, now being developed, marked superiority will be attained. At the present time the scanner can resolve (show as separate) objects 8–10 mm. apart whilst for the gamma camera the figures are 5–6 mm.

The area that the gamma camera revealed at any time was roughly equal to the area of its detection crystal, namely about 30 cm. in diameter. Now, however, a scanner facility has been added whereby as the camera is moved over any area of the body the instantaneous picture is continuously stored in the associated computer 'memory' until the end of the scanning movement. Then the whole area covered is displayed. In its stationary mode the camera can still be used for dynamic studies.

Thus, apart from the cost, in which the scanner still has an advantage, the gamma camera is now generally the superior instrument and most users would opt for it. In passing, it must be pointed out that the resolving powers of both the radioactive-isotope scanner and the gamma camera are considerably inferior to those obtainable using X-rays (e.g., see p. 208). However, the comparison is not particularly apposite since the scanner and camera reveal patterns that cannot be revealed by conventional radiography. Relatively crude though they are, these radioactive-isotope visualization techniques are valuable diagnostic aids. What would be the effect on their use if the even more expensive computer-assisted tomography became widely available is a subject of interesting speculation.

Whole-body Counters.—So far the tests and equipment that have been described have been concerned with the radioactivity of small samples of material or relatively limited zones of the body. Sometimes, however, it may be desirable to be able to determine the total amount of radioactive material already in, or taken up by, a patient, and for this purpose special *whole-body counters* have been developed.

The precise design of this type of equipment depends on the type of study being undertaken and on the kind and amounts of material that are expected to be present, but one essential feature of any design is that, as far as possible, the total response is independent of the distribution of the radioactive material within the body. To achieve this large detectors are placed round the body so that practically all the emitted photons are detected, or alternatively one or two small detectors are placed at positions which are chosen so that the photons they receive are a representative fraction of the total emission. In one version of the latter technique the patient lies as nearly as possible in an arc of a circle, at the centre of which the detector is placed. This is shown diagrammatically in *Fig.* 301 A, whilst *Fig.* 301 B shows an alternative approach in which the patient sits on a reclining chair with his legs at right-angles to his thighs which are at right-angles to his trunk. The detector in this case is vertically over the intersection of the back and seat of the chair at about 35 cm. from the middle of the legs and trunk.

In both these cases the detector is shielded except for the face towards the patient since, as usual, it is desirable to reduce the 'background' effects as much as possible. 'Background' radiation is of particular importance in studies with the whole-body counter which may have to measure very small amounts of radioactivity, the gamma-ray emission from which may be very little greater than, or could even be less than, the intensity of cosmic rays and the inevitable radioactive contamination of all surrounding materials, including the air. In such circumstances the 'background' is reduced by the use of special shielding.

For clinical work the 'shadow shield' technique is the most popular. In this, as *Fig.* 301 C shows, quite massive shielding is arranged around the detector and even under the patient to cast a 'shadow' as far as 'background' radiation is concerned over the area 'viewed' by the detector. No *direct* background radiation can reach the detector without passing through the shield, and a fiftyfold reduction in 'background' can be achieved in this relatively simple way. It should be noted that in this

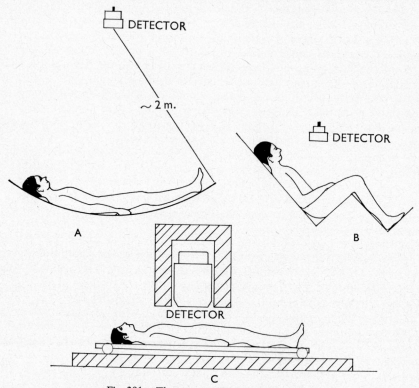

Fig. 301.—Three types of whole-body counter.

type of counter whole-body measurements are achieved by moving the patient slowly from one side to the other under the detector.

When very low level activities have to be measured, more extensive and expensive shielding is called for and in such a case the whole-body counter is placed inside a small room shielded on all sides with about 15 cm. of steel. Because modern steel may be slightly contaminated with radioactive material used in 'tracer' tests during its production, old steel is preferred. Steel plates from some old battleships have found peaceful and useful 'retirement' in this way.

Whole-body counters were originally to measure the amount of radium in people who had been working with that material, and they have since been extensively used to determine the amounts of a variety of radioactive materials, any of which may have been ingested by workers. In such cases not only can the levels of radioactivity be measured but the progress of the effects of any remedial action followed. In like manner the whole-body counter can be used, in metabolic studies, to measure how much of a deliberately given radioactive isotope is retained in the body, or how quickly it is excreted. Such an approach obviates the necessity of collecting and measuring faeces and urine, which is not only unpleasant but may not be accurate if the collection is not complete. An alternative to the Schilling test, already described for the estimation of vitamin-B_{12} absorption and the diagnosis of pernicious anaemia, has been developed, whilst the counter is also used for the measurement of the absorption of iron and of the absorption and excretion of chromium-51 in gastro-intestinal or menstrual blood-losses in some anaemic patients. The loss is both intermittent and variable in amount which makes direct measurement very difficult. Using iron 59, however, and the whole-body counter a simple method has been evolved which allows the loss over periods up to about 3 months to be measured.

Much work has also been done on the potassium content of the body, using the whole-body counter to measure the naturally occurring radioactive isotope, potassium 40, which constitutes about 0·01 per cent of normal potassium. In this case there is no need to administer anything to the patient—a material of considerable importance already present can be studied by its own radioactivity (^{40}K emits beta particles and 1·46-MeV. gamma rays). Much valuable information about the body's potassium in sickness and in health has emerged from these studies, and there is no doubt that in these, and other directions, the whole-body counter is of steadily increasing clinical importance.

Calibration and Standardization.—If reliable and comparable results are to be obtained standard source strengths must be used and equipment performance must be as constant as possible, otherwise a particular response—picture or count—will not have the same meaning on different occasions. Methods of source calibration and equipment standardization have, therefore, to be available: their nature will depend upon the volume of work being undertaken and its variety.

In a department doing a large number and wide range of tests and investigations an ionization chamber will probably be available for source calibrations. This will probably be quite large—a cylinder about 30 cm. in diameter and 40 cm. long with a co-axial hole into which the source to be measured is placed—to compensate for the inherently lower sensitivity of the ionization chamber compared with the Geiger-Müller or scintillation counter. In spite of this lower sensitivity (which, however, is adequate for calibration purposes), the ionization chamber is preferred for this purpose because it is not only much more reliable but also because its response is far more independent of radiation energy, which makes it more suitable for measuring a wide range of isotopes.

The price of the so-desirable high sensitivity of the Geiger-Müller and scintillation counters is that they do not have constant stability over long periods, so that they have to be subjected to frequent checks and adjustment if satisfactory reproducibility of results is to be achieved. The simplest check is to use a standard test source of some long-life radioactive material—for example, radium or caesium 137. This is placed in a fixed position relative to the apparatus and the controls adjusted, if necessary, to give a standard reading. It must be remembered, however, that any single source only checks the performance for the energy of radiation which it emits and not at quite different energies. For this purpose it is usual to obtain a number of standard sources of different isotopes covering a wide range of energies and to use these for periodic absolute checks. Such sources are obtainable from the Radiochemical Centre at Amersham in Great Britain or from the National Bureau of Standards. Unfortunately they are usually of short-life isotopes and are only available from time to time so that it may be necessary to supplement them with tests carried out with locally prepared isotope sources.

Table XXXII.—SOME FURTHER CLINICAL USES OF RADIOACTIVE ISOTOPES

STUDY	ISOTOPE AND ACTIVITY USED	LABELLED MATERIAL AND TECHNIQUE	COMMENT
Organ scanning Brain	Indium 113m, 7–10 mCi	Chelated substance injected intravenously. Scan 1–5 hr. later	More difficult to prepare than ^{99m}Tc but longer half-life generator. High-energy gamma rays are disadvantage
Kidneys	Mercury 197, 150 μCi	Chloromerodin. Scan after 1 hr.	Same agent but in larger doses (700 μCi) can be used in brain scanning
Lungs	Technetium 99m, 1 mCi	Macroaggregated serum albumin. Scan at once	Lengthy preparation
	Iodine 131, 150–300 μCi	Macroaggregated RISA. Scan at once	Eight-day half-life. Suitable sources can be purchased
	Indium 113m, 1 mCi	Indium hydroxide. Scan at once	More easily prepared. Long half-life generator but gamma-ray energy rather high
Spleen	Chromium 51, 300 μCi	Heat-damaged erythrocytes. Scan after several hours	Long preparation time
	Mercury 197	Erythrocytes damaged by BMPH. Scan several hours later	Shorter preparation time but expensive material
Bone	Strontium 85, 100 μCi	Strontium chloride	Long physical half-life leading to higher radiation dose
	Strontium 87m, about 1 mCi	Strontium chloride	From yttrium generator. Lower dose—short half-life
	Fluorine 18, about 1 mCi	Sodium fluoride	Rapid elimination. Very short half-life. Can only be used clinically if site of production close at hand
Pancreas	Selenium 75, 200 μCi	Selenomethionine. Scan $\frac{1}{2}$ hr. later	Liver image must be subtracted from scan picture to enable pancreas to be seen. Liver alone by using labelled colloid
Placenta	Chromium 51, about 50 μCi	Erythrocytes	Placenta is in the region of highest count rate
	Technetium 99m, 0·5–1·0 mCi	Albumin	
Clearance and blood-flow studies Cerebral blood-flow	Xenon 133, about 1 mCi	Xenon dissolved in saline solution	A number of counters positioned over each hemisphere can give information about regional blood-flow
Liver function	Iodine 131, 50 μCi	Rose Bengal	Activity changes over liver and precordial region recorded
Cardiac output	Iodine 131, 30 μCi	Serum albumin	Counter placed over precordial region
Metabolism and body-space determinations Fat absorption	Iodine 131, 25–50 μCi	Triolium administered orally	Percentage of dose excreted in faeces measured over several days. Not always reliable
Gastro-intestinal blood-loss	Chromium 51, 30–40 μCi	Erythrocytes administered intravenously	Activity in faecal samples can be used to estimate gastro-intestinal blood-loss
Iron metabolism	Iron 59, 3–10 μCi	Ferric citrate administered intravenously	Rate of disappearance from plasma gives an index of erythropoieseis
Exchangeable body-sodium	Sodium 24, 20–100 μCi	Sodium chloride intravenously or orally	Like red-cell and plasma-volume measurements, method depends on dilution principles
Total body water	Tritium ($^3_1$H), 200–500 μCi	Tritiated water	

A small department will generally use only a limited range of isotopes, but will not usually have the expensive apparatus or a range of standard sources. Other arrangements for source calibration and equipment standardization have to be made.

In the case of long-life materials it is usual, and satisfactory, to rely on the stated strengths of radiopharmaceuticals offered by suppliers like the Radiochemical Centre. For example, capsules of strength suitable for direct administration to the patient can be purchased, whilst other sources can be prepared by diluting the known activity of a phial and taking appropriate fractions of the diluted material to obtain a source of the required strength.

Short-lived isotopes present a more difficult problem because they have to be prepared locally, but a satisfactory solution can be found which combines source measurement and instrument standardization. A long-life standard should be available as a basic performance check and the final adjustment of the instrument carried out with the amount of isotope to be used in a particular test. Approximately the right amount of isotope may be eluted from a generator, the strength and elution characteristics of which will be known. Assume, by way of example, that the amount to be used is in a syringe ready for injection. The syringe may then be placed in a fixed position relative to the detector and the reading brought to a standard value by control adjustment. Since answer (count or picture) depends on both the instrument sensitivity and source strength this method of testing adjusts the one appropriately for the other. Should the source be rather weaker than desired the sensitivity has to be increased, whilst a stronger source will call for a rather lower sensitivity. This method, it should be noted, is acceptable because, and provided, there is confidence that the amount of isotope prepared is near to that desired.

General.—These then are examples of typical tests and procedures which exploit radioactive isotopes for clinical diagnostic purposes. The descriptions given are designed to emphasize the principles involved in each test and must not be regarded as recipes for the carrying out of the tests or the interpretation of the results. The former can be obtained from specialized texts on the subject, such as *Principles of Nuclear Medicine*, edited by Wagner and published by Saunders (1968) or *Radioisotopes in Medical Diagnosis*, by Belcher and Vetter published by Butterworth (1971), whilst the latter comes from such textbooks and from clinical experience. Finally it must be stressed that the examples given are but a fraction of those in common use, the number and sophistication of which increase all the time. A few more examples are given in outline, in *Table* XXXII.

INTERNAL THERAPEUTIC USES OF RADIOACTIVE ISOTOPES

When radioactive isotopes first became available in quantities sufficient for treatment purposes, a whole range of treatments and a variety of isotopes were tried. Of these only three remain of sufficient importance or interest to be worthy of mention, namely:

1. Radioactive iodine in thyroid disease.
2. Radioactive phosphorus in blood diseases.
3. Radioactive gold in colloid form.

Radioactive Iodine.—Because the thyroid gland selectively absorbs iodine and little is stored elsewhere in the body, it is possible to achieve a sufficiently high concentration of radioactive iodine in the gland to deliver a useful dose to it, without excessive irradiation elsewhere. (Details of the dosimetry of internally administered isotopes will be given later in this chapter.)

Unfortunately, thyroid cancer tissue usually takes up less iodine than normal thyroid tissue so that it is not possible to achieve a higher concentration, and hence a higher dose, in the malignant tissue than in the normal. This does not entirely preclude the use of radioactive iodine in thyroid cancer—it is very valuable, for example, for treating metastases after the removal of the cancerous thyroid gland —but its use is very limited. On the other hand, it can be valuable for dealing with overactive thyroid glands (hyperthyroidism). Here a relatively small amount (about 3–6 mCi) of radioactive iodine (^{131}I), given in the form of a simple drink of a dilute solution of sodium iodide, will reduce the thyroid activity because the radiation destroys some of the thyroid gland. This simple treatment has been widely used.

Radioactive Phosphorus.—In contrast to iodine, which is almost entirely taken up by the thyroid, phosphorus is widely distributed throughout the body and so will be any radioactive phosphorus (^{32}P) given to the body. This material may, therefore, be used where it is desired to give a 'whole-body' treatment. Because of the sensitivity of the blood-forming tissues (mainly the bone-marrow) to ionizing radiation, useful treatment can be given to them in this way without excessive damage to other, more radiation-resistant tissues. Radioactive phosphorus has been mainly used in the treatment of certain types of leukaemia, and of polycythaemia rubra vera.

Radioactive Gold.—Whereas both iodine and phosphorus play important parts in the working of the body, gold is not normally used in the body (except for 'filling' faulty teeth!) and its use in internal radiotherapy followed lines quite different from those described above. Radioactive gold (^{198}Au) is introduced into body cavities, in colloidal form, to irradiate the tissues lining those cavities. Whereas a solution would pass through the lining tissues, the larger-sized particles which make up the colloid cannot do so, and therefore the radioactivity is not disseminated beyond the cavity. Colloidal gold 198 was most used in the pleural or the peritoneal cavities for the treatment of malignant effusions in those places, but now it has almost entirely been superseded by cytotoxic drugs.

THE DOSEMETRY OF INTERNAL RADIOACTIVE ISOTOPES

For radiotherapy it is essential, and even for the diagnostic use of radioactive isotopes it is important, to be able to estimate the radiation dose which will be delivered by any radioactive isotope introduced into the body. The dose clearly depends on the type and energy of the radiation emitted by the isotope being used, the concentration of that isotope in the tissue concerned or other tissues and the length of time for which the isotope remains in the tissues, i.e., on its effective half-life. A complication is the very different attenuation and absorption patterns of the two types of radiation (beta rays and gamma rays) that may be involved, whilst the problem is made even more difficult because the distribution of the isotope in any particular type of tissue may not be uniform and is often not known accurately. In general, therefore, calculated values of absorbed doses are no more than estimates, though valuable nevertheless.

Because of their marked differences beta-ray and gamma-ray dosage calculations will be considered separately.

Beta-ray Dosage.—Beta rays travel only a few millimetres in tissue so that their dosage is almost entirely confined to the tissues containing the radioactive material. Any neighbouring tissues will be practically unaffected. The absorbed dose in rads (100 ergs per gramme) is therefore easily calculable (assuming uniform distribution of isotope) from a knowledge of the total energy emitted by the radioactive material, i.e., the energy emitted per beta ray emitted times the number of nuclei that decay. On this basis the beta ray absorbed dose (R_β) is given by

$$R_\beta = 73 \cdot 8 \bar{E}_\beta \times T_E \text{ rads per microcurie per gramme,}$$

where $\bar{E}_\beta$ is the average energy in MeV. of the beta particles and T_E is the effective half-life in days of the isotope in the situation under consideration.

It should be noted that both for beta rays and for gamma rays, as described below, the absorbed dose depends upon the isotope concentration, which implies a knowledge of both the isotope activity and the mass of tissue involved. Both, and especially the latter, may be difficult to determine accurately, which introduces a further uncertainty into the final estimate.

Examples: (1) What beta-particle dose, in rads, would be received by a thyroid gland estimated to weigh 35 grammes, and containing 1·75 millicuries of ^{131}I? The effective half-life of the isotope can be taken as 5 days and its average beta-particle energy ($\bar{E}_\beta$) is 0·187 MeV.

$$\text{Isotope concentration} = \frac{1750}{35} = 50 \, \mu\text{Ci per gramme.}$$

$$\therefore R = 73 \cdot 8 \times 0 \cdot 187 \times 5 \times 50$$

$$= 3450 \text{ rad.}$$

This is a relatively small dose compared with some given in radioactive iodine therapy of the thyroid gland.

(2) A patient weighing 65 kilograms is given 13 millicuries of ^{32}P. Assuming that this is uniformly distributed throughout the body, what dose will be delivered by the complete decay of the radioactive isotope? The average beta-particle energy is 0·69 MeV. and the effective half-life is 12 days.

$$\text{Isotope concentration} = \frac{13,000}{65,000} = 0 \cdot 2 \, \mu\text{Ci per gramme.}$$

(N.B.: 1 mCi = 1000 μCi and 1 kg. = 1000 g.)

$$\therefore \text{Absorbed dose} = 73 \cdot 8 \times 0 \cdot 69 \times 12 \times 0 \cdot 2$$

$$= 121 \text{ rad.}$$

Although this dose is numerically much smaller than that calculated for the thyroid gland in the first example it must be remembered that this would be given to every gramme of the body, and is a large whole-body dose.

Gamma-ray Dosage.—For a volume of tissue throughout which a beta-particle emitter is uniformly distributed, the absorbed dose calculated as above will be received uniformly by all that tissue with the exception of a thin shell around the volume, where the dose falls rapidly from its full value to one-half of that value at the surface. The thickness of the shell is the range of the beta particles—a few millimetres at most. Beyond the surface there is falling beta-ray dose through another layer of tissue, equal in thickness to the particle range, and beyond this, nothing. The short range of the beta particles leads to confined, uniform, and relatively easily calculable dosage.

With gamma rays the situation is quite different because of their very considerable penetrating power. A volume of tissue containing a gamma-ray emitter will receive a dose of radiation which is highest at the centre, falls off steadily towards the surface, and whose magnitude depends not only on the concentration of the isotope and its gamma emission rate, but also, in a complicated way, on the energy of the radiation and the size and shape of the tissue concerned. Furthermore, there will be a considerable contribution of radiation dose to tissues well away from those containing an isotope. The development of the formula for the calculation of the absorbed dose requires the use of quite complicated mathematics, but the answer is that the gamma-ray absorbed dose (R_γ) is given by:

$$R_\gamma = 33 \cdot 1 \times 10^{-3} \Gamma \times T_E \times G \text{ rads per microcurie per gramme,}$$

where Γ is the gamma-ray emission rate (roentgens per hour at 1 cm. per millicurie) T_E is the effective half-life in days and G is a geometrical factor which takes into account the size and shape of the tissues involved and the position at which the dose is being estimated. For example, the value of G at the centre of a sphere of diameter D cm. is $2\pi D$, whilst the average value, $\bar{G}$, for spheres of up to 20 cm. diameter is given by $\bar{G} = 1 \cdot 5 \pi D$.

These factors tend to over-estimate the absorbed dose which would be received in the human body because radiation attenuation is ignored in their derivation. If it is taken into account the average dose is reduced by about 30 per cent. Furthermore, of course, most parts of the body, and certainly the whole body, approximate more closely to cylinders than to spheres. Since, as the elongation increases a greater proportion of gamma rays escape, doses in cylinders are less than in spheres of the same volume. For a cylinder whose height is five times its diameter the mean dose would be a half of the dose in a sphere of the same volume.

Radiation from a gamma-ray emitting isotope penetrates far beyond the tissue in which the isotope is deposited, so that quite distant tissues will be irradiated even though they contain no radioactive material. The absorbed dose (R) to reach distant tissues can be estimated by the formula

$$R = \Gamma \times T_E \times M e^{-\mu d}/d^2 \text{ rads,}$$

where M is the total activity, in millicuries, in the active tissue, μ is the attenuation coefficient for the gamma radiation in body tissue, and d is the mean distance from the radioactive material to the tissue or organ at which the dose is being calculated. A reasonable value of μ is $0 \cdot 03$ cm.$^{-1}$, which means that the radiation dose rate is halved for each 23 cm. of tissue penetrated.

Radioactive Isotope Concentration.—For the calculation of the dose with either of the formulae it is necessary to have a knowledge of the concentration of radioactive isotope in the tissue in question, and this is not easy to obtain accurately. In the case of the thyroid gland uptake, for example, it is possible to calibrate a counter by using a dummy neck with a known amount of radioactive iodine in the dummy thyroid, and thus be able to make a fairly accurate estimate of the *total amount* of radioactive iodine in the patient's thyroid. However, the *concentration* depends also on the size of the thyroid, the accurate estimation of which can be very difficult, so that any statement of isotope concentration can only be of limited accuracy.

When the radioactive material is widely distributed through the body, the average concentration is found by dividing the amount administered by the known body-weight. This assumes equal uptake in all parts of the body which, again, is seldom true. Care must therefore be exercised in the importance given to dose values calculated on this basis, since some tissues may receive much higher values due to selective absorption therein.

As already stated the dosemetry of internally distributed isotopes is not very accurate, nevertheless it gives valuable guidance.

Dosage: Summary and Example.—
Beta-particle dose: $R_\beta = 73 \cdot 8\ \bar{E}_\beta T_E$ rad per microcurie per gramme,
Gamma-ray dose: $R_\gamma = 33 \cdot 1 \times 10^{-3}\ \Gamma T_E G$ rad per microcurie per gramme,
where $\bar{E}_\beta$ is the average beta-particle energy in MeV.; T_E is the effective half-life in days, Γ is the gamma-ray emission rate, and G is a geometric factor.

Example: A patient, who weighs 64 kg. and whose thyroid gland is estimated to weigh 34 grammes, is given 16 mCi of ^{131}I for the treatment of cancer of the thyroid. It is estimated that 51 per cent of the administered iodine is taken up by the thyroid, and that the effective half-life is 5·5 days. What will be the total absorbed dose delivered to the thyroid for the complete decay of the isotope? For ^{131}I the value of Γ is 2·3 R per hour and of $\bar{E}_\beta$ is 0·187 MeV.

Assuming that the thyroid gland is spherical, its diameter would be approximately 4 cm. and therefore the value of $\bar{G}$ will be $1 \cdot 5\pi D = 6\pi = 18 \cdot 9$.

$$\text{Isotope concentration in the thyroid gland} = \frac{16 \times 1000}{34} \times \frac{51}{100}$$

$$= 240\ \mu\text{Ci per gramme.}$$

$\therefore R_\beta = 73 \cdot 8 \times 0 \cdot 187 \times 5 \cdot 5 \times 240 \qquad = 18{,}217\ \text{rad}$

and $\quad R_\gamma = 33 \cdot 1 \times 10^{-3} \times 2 \cdot 3 \times 18 \cdot 9 \times 5 \cdot 5 \times 240 \quad = 1{,}890\ \text{rad}$

Giving a total absorbed dose of $\qquad\qquad\qquad\qquad 20{,}107\ \text{rad}$

It will be noted that the gamma-ray contribution to the thyroid dose is relatively small, and, in fact, it is often ignored.

SECTION III. RADIOTHERAPY

CHAPTER XXIX

THE PHYSICAL PRINCIPLES OF RADIOTHERAPY

The Concise Oxford Dictionary defines 'radiotherapy' as the 'treatment of disease with X-rays or other forms of radiation'. Nowadays the disease concerned is mainly, but not exclusively, cancer, the basis of the value of radiotherapy in the treatment of that disease being the fact that ionizing radiation (always damaging to living tissue) produces more damage in malignant than in non-malignant tissues. A dose of radiation sufficient to kill cancer cells will produce considerable, but not irreparable, damage to normal tissue, so that the latter recovers whereas the malignant tissue does not.

Excessive irradiation, however, leads to the destruction of the normal tissues (radiation necrosis) as well as the cancer, whilst inadequate dosage fails to kill the cancer cells, so that after a time they recover from such damage as they have sustained, regain their vitality, and start to multiply again (tumour recurrence).

This is, of course, a simplified and, inevitably, incomplete description of very complex processes, but it will serve to indicate why it is necessary to have a good understanding of the ways in which radiations interact with matter. It also stresses the importance of dosemetry, especially since the margins between inadequate and adequate dosage, and between adequate and excessive dosage, are relatively small.

Safe and efficient treatments can only be carried out when at least approximate optimum dosage levels have been established, and these can only be known after considerable clinical observation of the effects of known doses of radiation. Not only accurate, but also constant dosemetry is essential to good radiotherapy. Furthermore, because of the undesirable consequences of under- or overdosage, the general aim of radiotherapy is to deliver as uniform a dose of radiation as possible to all parts of the tumour-bearing zone. Outside this zone, as low a dose as possible is aimed at. The steps that have to be taken, and the apparatus needed to achieve these aims, will be the subject of subsequent chapters.

Radiation dose magnitude is not, of course, the only parameter that influences the biological effects of radiation. The time over which the treatment is spread has an important bearing; the shorter the time, the greater will be the effect of any given dose. Another important factor is the pattern of ionization produced by the radiation. The spacing of ionization along the track of ionizing radiations differs with the type and energy of the radiation—there is much more ionization per unit length, or energy deposited per unit length by alpha rays than by electrons, and rather more by 200-kV. X-rays than by those generated in the megavoltage range. These differences are usually expressed as the 'relative biological efficiency' (or effectiveness) of two radiations. Thus 4-MV. X-rays have a relative biological effectiveness (R.B.E.) compared with 250-kV. X-rays of about 0·90 by which we mean that:

$$\frac{\text{Absorbed dose of 250-kV. X-rays for a given effect}}{\text{Absorbed dose of 4-MV. X-rays for the same effect}} = \text{R.B.E.}_{\text{4 MV -250 kV.}} = 0\cdot9.$$

Expressed in another way, this means that for the same effect the absorbed dose of

424

4-MV. rays has to be 10 per cent greater than that of 250-kV. radiation. The differences between other radiations may be very much greater.

It must be stressed, however, that differences in R.B.E. do not necessarily indicate differences in ability to cure cancer—4-MV. radiation is certainly not 10 per cent less efficient than 250-kV. for that important work. In this respect it is the therapeutic ratio that is important, that is, the ratio of the damage sustained by the tumour compared with the damage to normal tissue. Any increase in this ratio would be extremely valuable but, as yet, it does not seem that change of physical factors has any effect upon it, though such changes may be advantageous from other points of view.

A full discussion of these aspects of radiotherapy are beyond the scope of this book, in which most attention is being given to X- and gamma rays. In their use, as in the use of any other therapeutic agency, it is the radiotherapist's responsibility to decide what absorbed dose should be delivered, and what sort of treatment pattern should be used. The treatment is planned with the aid of the physicist, or using material provided by the physicist, who is responsible for dosage accuracy. Responsibility for carrying out the treatment plan rests with the radiographer (or radiotherapy technician). However, this precise division of responsibilities, whilst useful in some ways, must not be allowed to obscure the fact that radiotherapy is very much a collaborative exercise in which the three disciplines of the radiotherapist, physicist, and radiographer must be welded together in the closest possible teamwork. Each must appreciate the others' problems—the physicist must learn something of anatomy and physiology; the radiologist and radiographer must know something of the physical basis of their subject. To help in this latter is the object of this book.

Though the aim is the same in each case—the delivery of a known and uniform dose of radiation to a zone believed to encompass the tumour, and as little radiation as possible elsewhere—radiotherapy can conveniently be divided into three sections, each with quite different approaches, and each calling for quite different physical information.

1. Teletherapy.—'Tele' is the Greek word for 'far', so that 'teletherapy' is the general term applied to treatments when the external source of radiation is many centimetres from the part being treated. Beams of X- and gamma rays, high-energy electrons, and neutrons have all been used in this way. Using X- or gamma rays, it is the most widely used of the three therapeutic methods, and the one which will receive most attention in this book. Dependent upon the depth of the tumour in the body, it calls for beams of various penetrating power, and for the various tumour shapes and sizes, beams of different shapes and sizes which are produced by suitable beam collimation by 'applicators' or by variable diaphragms. Details of these will be given in CHAPTER XXXV, which will also describe beam-direction devices, with the aid of which accurate aiming of beams is ensured.

Penetrating power, for X-rays, depends mainly upon the generating voltage and filtration being used, and upon the distance from source to surface (the source–surface distance, or S.S.D.). In cancer therapy, three quite distinct sets of treatment conditions can be recognized:

'Superficial' therapy	60 to 140 kV.	5 to 15 cm. F.S.D.	1–3-mm. Al filter
'Deep' or kilovoltage therapy	200 to 300 kV.	50 cm. F.S.D.	1–2-mm. Cu or ½-mm. Sn filter
Megavoltage therapy	2 to 10 MV.	70 to 100 cm. F.S.D.	—

Mention may also be made of 'Grenz' ray therapy, used for very superficial dermatological conditions, and employing 10–30-kV. radiation. This is not suitable for cancer therapy because the radiation has too little penetration, even for the most superficial malignancy.

Dosage information for teletherapy is usually presented in two sets of data. The first of these deals with the amount of radiation being delivered per minute—that is the *output* of each radiation beam, whilst the second set of data concerns the penetration of the radiation into the tissues, and presents the **percentage depth dose** values, either in tables or as **isodose charts.**

Uniform dosage throughout the zone being treated can often be achieved by using several beams aimed consecutively, from different directions, towards the same point. Such efforts may, however, be thwarted by body inhomogeneities like lungs, cavities, and bones, by body curvatures, or by the desirability, or necessity, of using a small number (often two) of fields. Special **compensators** or **wedge filters** enable many of these difficulties to be overcome, whilst *correction factors* are available to enable the effects of body details to be allowed for, if necessary.

2. Plesiotherapy.—'Plesios' is the Greek word for 'near', and this prefix is usually applied to indicate those forms of radiotherapy where the radiation source is close to the tissues being treated. Strictly speaking, plesiotherapy can include X-ray treatments in which the S.S.D. is only a few centimetres, but it is usually reserved for treatments where small beta- or gamma-ray sources are placed within a centimetre or two of the body surface, or gamma-ray sources are actually implanted into the tissues. Most attention will be given to gamma-ray plesiotherapy.

Originally it was carried out exclusively with radium or radon in suitable tubes or needles. Now, however, a number of other gamma-ray sources are available, for example cobalt 60, caesium 137, iridium 192, and gold 198. For the short distances between the sources and the tissues being treated, it is usually assumed that radiation attenuation is negligible, and that doses can be calculated by means of the inverse-square law and the known gamma-ray dose rate of the isotope. Dosage uniformity is achieved by arranging the sources according to predetermined patterns, such as those prescribed by the Manchester Dosage System.

3. Internal Therapy.—This form of treatment is entirely by means of radioactive isotopes which, in some form or another, are incorporated into body tissues. The radiations involved are beta particles, gamma rays, or both. As already discussed in CHAPTER XXVIII, radioactive isotopes have not fulfilled the early (and probably over-optimistic) hopes that were placed in them, but a few, either because they are selectively absorbed in specific organs, or because they are widely distributed throughout the body, are used as internal irradiators. Their dosemetry is, often, rather difficult because their distribution is not uniform. However, reasonable average values can be calculated, and the method can be said to be a useful, if limited, means of treatment.

CHAPTER XXX

TELETHERAPY DOSAGE DATA: GENERAL CONSIDERATIONS

IN teletherapy, as in any other form of radiotherapy, it is necessary to know the *absorbed dose* of radiation at points within the patient, and since direct measurement of absorbed dose is fraught with great difficulties (*see* CHAPTER XII) it is usual to determine *Exposure* and to convert to absorbed dose using the expression

$$\text{Absorbed dose} = \text{Exposure} \times f,$$

where f is a factor (already described in CHAPTER XII) which converts Exposure (in roentgens) into absorbed dose (in rads) in a particular tissue; f, it will be recalled, depends upon the radiation quality and upon the type of material being irradiated. Values of this factor will be given later, in CHAPTER XXXIII.

The Exposure at any point depends upon many physical factors and especially, of course, upon the time for which irradiation is continued. It is convenient, therefore, to discuss Exposure rate rather than total Exposure, and so eliminate one of the variable factors.

$$\text{Absorbed dose} = \text{Exposure rate} \times \text{irradiation time} \times f.$$

Since the Exposure rate at a point in its turn depends upon such factors as the depth of that point, the size and shape of the beam, possibly the method of beam collimation, as well as upon the tube operating factors (mA., kV., filter, and S.S.D.), it has been found to be convenient to arrive at the dose at any point in two stages. First, the *output* of the apparatus at some standard *reference point* is determined for each set of operating conditions in use. Exposure rates at other points are then established relative to the output values. Hence, as a generalization it can be said that:

$$\text{Absorbed dose at any point} = E \times R \times f \times t,$$

where: E is the Exposure rate at the reference point for the operating conditions in question, i.e., it is the *output*;

R is the Exposure rate at the point of interest expressed relative to E;

f is the roentgens to rads conversion factor appropriate to the operating conditions; and

t is the irradiation time.

Though different workers have favoured different reference points, and different methods of output determination, as will be described in CHAPTER XXXII, the most commonly used now is the surface of the irradiated material for kilovoltage radiations, and the point of maximum absorbed dose for megavoltage beams. In such cases R is expressed as a percentage of the Exposure rate (*output*) at the reference point and is called the *percentage depth dose*. Its value at the reference point is, of course, 100.

Since Exposure rate (or output) and percentage depth doses depend differently on the same factors, or sometimes upon different factors, it is convenient to consider them separately, and this will be done in later chapters. Furthermore, it is convenient, both historically as well as physically, to give separate consideration to radiations generated by kilovoltages and those generated by megavoltages. The division line is inevitably indistinct, and the choice, here, of 1 MV. is quite arbitrary though, as should be apparent later, not at all unreasonable.

427

Although the object of these considerations is to establish the absorbed dose at some point in a patient, for fairly obvious reasons it is impracticable to make the required measurements either on, or inside, patients. Therefore some material has to be found which attenuates the beam and absorbs radiation energy as closely as possible to the way in which the human body attenuates and absorbs. Such material then can be used as a 'phantom' in which measurements can be made.

Because of the complexity of the body, with its different tissues such as muscle, bone, fat, and blood, and its cavities, like the mouth, the lungs, or the nasal sinuses, it is impossible to find a single material which will simulate them all. Attention, therefore, has been focused upon finding a substance which behaves, to X-rays, like the most important body tissue—muscle. In passing, it may be noted that tumours are generally composed of soft tissue and mostly grow in soft tissue.

Phantom Materials.—To have closely similar attenuating and absorbing properties, two materials must have very similar atomic numbers, densities, and electron densities. For muscle tissue the values of these quantities are, respectively, 7·42, 1·0, and $3·36 \times 10^{23}$ electrons per gramme and the common material with the closest resemblance to these values is water ($Z = 7·42$, $\rho = 1·0$, and electron density $= 3·34 \times 10^{23}$ electrons per gramme). Because of these values, coupled with its almost universal availability, constant composition, and low cost, water has been generally regarded as the most acceptable material for standard radiation dosemetric measurements.

However, water is not without its disadvantages. Being a liquid it can only be used in a suitable container, the walls of which may interfere with the measurements. Happily, the advent of plastics like perspex (also known as lucite or plexiglas), which has an atomic number, etc., not unlike those of water, has decreased the magnitude of this problem. In addition, because water is slightly conducting, care must be taken to sheathe ionization chambers lest moisture ruin their vital high insulation. Again, such protection, unless carefully designed, may interfere with the general 'tissue equivalence' of the phantom system. Sheaths of perspex, nylon, or similar plastics are generally acceptable.

Nevertheless, for many purposes a phantom of solid material is more convenient, and many different materials have been tried. These have included 'unit-density' waxes, mostly made of paraffin wax with additives like beeswax or resin; proprietary hardboards of the Masonite 'Pressdwood' type and the more recent plastic 'Mix D', developed at the Mount Vernon Hospital, near London. In general, it is not difficult to satisfy one of the three requirements (density, atomic number, or electron density) but a completely satisfactory material has proved very difficult to concoct. By far the most successful of the materials listed is 'Mix D' which is commercially available in sheets each about 1 cm. thick and 40×40 cm. in area. It can readily be machined into any shape to make special measuring phantoms, as well as being more convenient than water for the conventional cubic phantom. It is also much more expensive!

Almost equally 'water equivalent' (and therefore soft-tissue equivalent) are 'Lincolnshire Bolus', so named because it was developed at the Radiotherapy Centre of that county, and 'Spiers Mixture', suggested by Professor F. W. Spiers of Leeds. The former is made up in the form of tiny spheres of about ¼-mm. diameter (very like the familiar cake decoration 'hundreds and thousands') and consists of 87 per cent sugar and 13 per cent magnesium carbonate, whilst Spiers Mixture is a powder mixture of 60 per cent rice flour and 40 per cent sodium bicarbonate. Both materials, though they could be used in phantoms, are more widely employed in radiotherapy as 'bolus', i.e., packing material to correct for body-contour variations, as will be discussed more fully in a later chapter.

It might be commented, at this stage, that the use of the word 'phantom' here does not indicate that the device has any ghostly or spiritual properties, as anyone having to carry a normal-sized 'phantom' will soon realize. The name is simply a convenient piece of technical jargon, indicating that the material is being used in place of the body, or, more strictly, of its soft tissue. Typical water and 'Mix D' 'phantoms' are shown in *Fig*. 302. The walls of the water 'phantom' are of perspex, and the thin waterproof perspex sheath for holding the ionization chamber can be clearly seen protruding through one side of the 'phantom'. It will be noted that the 'Mix D'

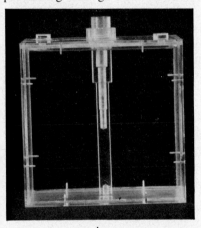 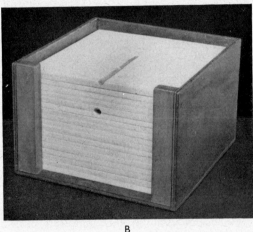

A   B

Fig. 302.—A, Water and B, 'Mix D' 'phantoms' for X-ray measurements.

'phantom' is made up of sheets of that material placed on top of one another. One of the sheets contains a specially drilled hole into which an ionization chamber fits snugly for measurements at various depths, which are obtained simply by placing more or less sheets of material above or in front of (depending upon the direction of the beam) the hole-carrying block. The groove for surface measurements can also be seen in *Fig*. 302. When lying in the groove the chamber centre is at the level of the surface of the 'Mix D' sheet, and the chamber is said to be in the 'half-sunk' position.

In *Clinical Dosemetry*, a report published by the International Commission on Radiological Units, it is recommended that for standard measurements a 'phantom' should be 'at least 30 × 30 cm. in cross-sectional area and at least 15 cm., preferably 20 cm., deep'.

The Patient is not a Phantom!—Unlike 'phantoms' such as those shown in *Fig*. 302, a patient is neither cubic nor homogeneous in composition. Dosage data obtained from measurements in a 'phantom', therefore, can only be approximations to the doses being received at corresponding points in a patient. The approximation is often surprisingly good but, for the most accurate work, allowance may have to be made for the curvature of the patient's surface, or for the fact that the beam may have to pass through bone (more attenuating than soft tissue) or through lungs or air-filled cavities (less attenuating) on its way to the point of interest. Or, again, the part being treated may be much smaller than the 'phantom' in which measurements were made. A later chapter (CHAPTER XXXIII) will describe the magnitude and application of some of these corrections.

CHAPTER XXXI

TELETHERAPY DOSAGE DATA FOR CLINICAL USE

1. KILOVOLTAGE RADIATIONS

Up to 1946 the great majority of teletherapy was carried out with X-ray beams generated by voltages up to 250 kV., and it is only in the last decade or so that the great swing to higher radiation energies—to 'megavoltage radiations'—has taken place. There is, however, still a considerable place in radiotherapy for the lower-energy radiations and it is not out of place, even today, to consider them in some detail, especially as many points of principle apply as much to them as to the higher-energy rays.

'OUTPUT' VALUES

In the early days of radiotherapy it was difficult, even when numerous fields from different directions were used, to deliver adequate absorbed doses to a deep-seated tumour without, at the same time, delivering a high dose on the surface at each field. This was because the maximum generating voltages available were little more than 200 kV.—often less—so that the penetrating power of the radiation was relatively low. Surface doses were often the limiting factors of a treatment and therefore an accurate knowledge of them was most important. For this reason the centre of the field on the surface became universally accepted as the standard reference point for 'output' statements, and though it is now known that this convention has some serious disadvantages (which will be discussed later) it is too well established to be likely to be superseded. For radiations generated at up to 1 MV. then, the reference point for dosage statements is at the surface at the centre of each field.

Surface Output.—The Exposure rate (R) at any point in an irradiated material is made up of two components—primary radiation (P) coming directly from the tube, and scattered radiation (S) from the irradiated material. In the case of the surface output it is useful to consider the two components separately.

Primary Radiation.—The Exposure rate of primary radiation depends on how much radiation is being generated at the target of the X-ray tube; on how much and what material the radiation has to pass through to reach the surface; and on how far the surface is from the target.

Recalling CHAPTER V it can be said that:

$$P \propto I.E^2.Z,$$

where, in practical terms, I is the tube current in milliamperes, E is the applied kilovoltage, and Z the target atomic number.

In addition, there is the effect of the 'wave form' of the applied voltage and this effect cannot be stated so succinctly. However, as also outlined in CHAPTER V, a constant potential supply gives an output greater than that for either full or half-wave rectification.

The effect of the 'filtration' through which the beam has to pass (and this includes the inevitable X-ray tube wall material, as well as any material deliberately inserted for filtration purposes) has been discussed in CHAPTER XIII, on the basis of which discussions it can be said that the greater the thickness of the material and the greater its atomic number, the smaller the amount of radiation that is transmitted. In other words, the primary surface output decreases with increase of filter thickness or atomic number.

The Exposure rate will also depend upon the distance (*d*) from the focal spot to the reference point on the surface, because of the operation of the inverse square law. In practical terms, the primary Exposure rate is inversely proportional to the square of the S.S.D.*

Finally, it must be remembered that the primary contribution is *independent* of beam size or shape. It is the same for all fields.

Scattered Radiation.—It will be clear that the Exposure rate of the scattered radiation will always be directly proportional to the Exposure rate of the primary radiation, no matter what else it depends on. And to this extent the Exposure rate

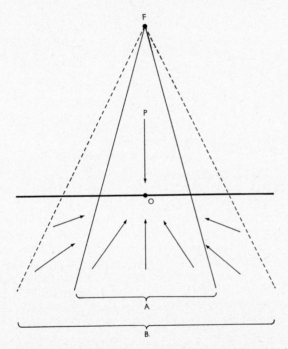

Fig. 303.—The dependence of backscatter on beam size. The scattered radiation reaching O from the larger field (B) includes that from field A.

depends upon all the factors mentioned above. It is therefore convenient to consider the percentage scatter, i.e., the Exposure rate of the scattered radiation expressed as a percentage of the primary Exposure rate which is producing the scatter—and the factors upon which it depends. For a point on the surface this is often called the

---

* The distance from the focal spot to the surface of phantom or patient has been known, for many years, as the focus–skin (or surface) distance or F.S.D. Recently, however, the International Commission on Radiological Units suggested that source–skin (or surface) distance, or S.S.D., is to be preferred, since it may be applied to gamma-ray as well as to X-ray sources. This suggestion has been accepted in this book.

percentage backscatter and its magnitude depends chiefly upon the size and shape of the X-ray field, and upon the radiation quality.

Beam Dimensions.—As a simple generalization it can be said that the larger the beam the greater the percentage backscatter. This is because the greater the volume irradiated the greater the amount of scattered radiation generated, as indicated in *Fig.* 303. Percentage backscatter does not, of course, vary in direct proportion to the beam size, simply because scattered radiation generated in the outer parts of an irradiated zone suffers more attenuation in reaching the reference point than does that generated nearer the centre. The general effect of this is shown in *Fig.* 304, the line on which shows the variation of percentage backscatter (for circular and square beams) with beam area.

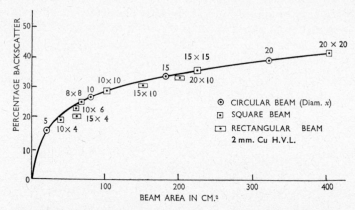

Fig. 304.—The variation of percentage backscatter with beam area. Note that rectangular beams have smaller values than circles or squares of the same area.

Notice that the percentage backscatter does not increase indefinitely but reaches what might be called a 'saturation' value, when a further increase in beam size produces practically no increase in the scattered radiation reaching the centre. When this state is reached, any scattered radiation generated at the periphery is practically completely absorbed by the intervening material before it reaches the centre.

Another notable feature shown in *Fig.* 304 is the effect of beam shape upon percentage backscatter. The values for circular and square beams, of the same area, are practically identical—the values for circles and squares lie on the same curve—

Table XXXIII.—DEPENDENCE OF PERCENTAGE BACKSCATTER ON FIELD SHAPE

Radiation 1·0 mm. Cu H.V.L.

FIELD AREA	36 cm.²				100 cm.²			
Dimensions	6×6	9×4	12×3	18×2	10×10	12·5×8	20×5	25×4
Percentage backscatter	25·2	23·8	21·7	18·0	35·7	35·0	30·8	27·8

but for rectangular beams, and especially those of marked elongation, the scatter are values always smaller than for squares and circles of the same area. *Table XXXIII* shows this trend for different beam shapes of two beam areas.

The reason for this lower scatter contribution in the more elongated rectangles can be explained with the aid of *Fig.* 305, and stems from the same effect as causes the backscatter curve for large beams to 'saturate', i.e., the attenuation of scattered

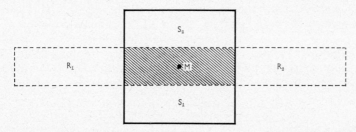

Fig. 305.—Why square fields have more scatter than rectangular fields of the same area.

radiation before it reaches the point of measurement. In *Fig.* 305 the square and the dotted rectangle are equal in area (the one being 12 × 12, say, and the other 36 × 4). The shaded area is common to both areas and its scattered radiation contribution will be the same to M, whether it is part of a square or of a rectangular beam. On the other hand, the areas S_1 and S_2 will contribute more than the equal areas R_1 and R_2 because they are generally closer to M.

Radiation Quality.—*Fig.* 306 shows how the percentage backscatter, for one size of beam, varies with the quality (as measured by the half-value layer) of the beam, and

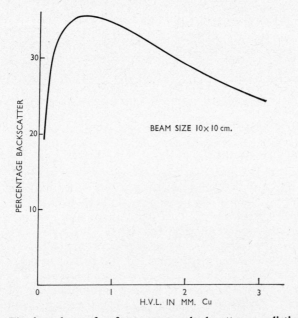

Fig. 306.—The dependence of surface percentage backscatter on radiation quality.

reveals a situation which is partly what would be expected and yet is partly very surprising. It will be recalled, from CHAPTER VI, that the likelihood of radiation being scattered (normally expressed as the scatter attenuation coefficient σ) decreases as the

15

energy of the radiation increases. The steady fall in the percentage backscatter at the higher-quality end of the graph is therefore to be expected, and as will be especially seen later in the case of megavoltage radiation, this reduction of the relative amount of scattered radiation is one of the major advantages of using high-quality beams. What is unexpected, and what—at first sight—would seem to be at variance with theoretical predictions, is the marked falling off of scattered radiation at the lower qualities.

There is, however, no contradiction between theory and observation: it is simply that the amount of scattering suffered by the primary radiation is not the only factor involved. As in the cases of the backscatter for large beams, and for rectangular

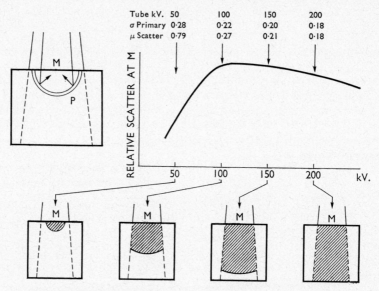

Fig. 307.—An explanation of the shape of the scatter–radiation quality curve.

beams, the ability of any scattered radiation to reach the point of measurement must be taken into account. (A similar situation has been discussed in CHAPTER XX where the amount of scattered radiation emerging from a patient undergoing diagnostic radiography is described.)

Consider, by the way of example, the irradiation of a cube of material, and the scattered radiation reaching a point M on its surface. This scattered radiation can be considered as being made up of contributions from a series of concentric hemispherical layers like the shell P shown in Fig. 307.

How much scattered radiation such a layer will contribute to M obviously depends on the amount of scattered radiation generated in it (that is to say, it depends on σ), and also upon how much of that scattered radiation reaches M (that is to say, it depends on μ, the total attenuation coefficient appropriate to the energy of the scattered radiation). Taking a very simple picture of the process (which in fact is very complex) the contribution of the shell P to the point M will depend on $\sigma e^{-\mu d}$, and by integrating (or adding up) this sort of term for each of the layers such as P into which the irradiated zone can be divided, a curve such as is included in Fig. 307 is obtained. Its general shape resembles the experimental curve in Fig. 306, closer agreement could hardly be expected from such a simplified approach.

Explaining the phenomenon in words rather than symbols, it can be said that the greater amount of scattering of the lower-energy radiations is more than offset by its much lower penetrating power, and this is demonstrated in an alternative way by the small diagrams at the foot of *Fig.* 307. In these the shaded areas are those contributing the bulk of the scattered radiation which reaches *M*. Any scattered radiation generated outside these zones suffers more than a 99 per cent reduction by attenuation, and therefore makes a negligible contribution to the total. The magnitude of this total obviously depends on the contributing volume as well as upon how much radiation is scattered per unit volume. Therefore, although 50-kV. radiation suffers at least 50 per cent more scattering than that produced at 200 kV., the very small contributing volume at the lower energy compared with the contributing volume at the higher energy outweighs the higher scatter production. However, when the whole irradiated volume can contribute scatter to *M*, then the percentage backscatter depends almost entirely upon the amount of scatter produced (σ) and so decreases steadily with increasing energy. Observation and theory are not in conflict: they are in complete accord when all the factors are taken into account.

Source–Surface Distance (*S.S.D.*).—Percentage backscatter mainly depends upon the factors which have just been discussed, but there are some other factors which might have some influence, and the most obvious of these is the distance from the source to the surface. However, it turns out that except possibly for very short values, percentage backscatter on the surface is independent of S.S.D.

'Applicators' and Diaphragm Systems.—Although they do not necessarily affect the *back* scatter, beam-defining devices such as diaphragms and '*applicators*' (details

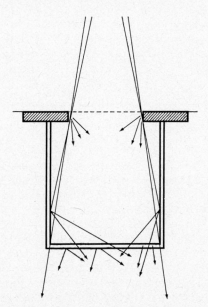

Fig. 308.—Scatter generated by a beam collimation 'applicator'. Wherever radiation is incident some scatter radiation is produced and added to the beam.

of which will be discussed later) may add scattered radiation to the beam, and thus be a contributory factor in the variation of tube output with operating conditions. As *Fig.* 308 attempts to demonstrate, radiation may be scattered from the edge of any diaphragm, from the sides of any collimator, and from the closed end of such a device. Just how the magnitude of this scattered radiation contribution varies with beam size and shape can hardly be predicted theoretically and can only be determined by measurement. With a well-designed system the contribution will be small, but it will vary from one type of equipment to another when different collimation systems are used. For this reason, among others, output measurements on one piece of equipment can seldom be applied to another. It is also a reason why the surface is not perhaps the ideal place for making output calibration measurements, a point which will be discussed further in CHAPTER XXXII.

Position in the Beam.—Output statements and percentage backscatter values generally refer to the Exposure rate at a standard reference point which, for kilovoltage beams, as already stated, is at the centre of the beam at the surface. However, the Exposure at other points on the surface is of importance and *Fig.* 309 gives an example

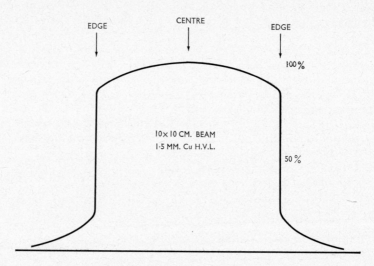

Fig. 309.—Variation of Exposure rate across a beam. Note the scattered radiation outside the beam edge.

of its variation across a beam. The reason for the falling-off of the scattered radiation towards the beam edge is that this edge is generally further away from much of the beam than is the centre, and therefore scattered radiation reaching the edge has generally suffered more attenuation.

Just how important this falling-off of scattered radiation is depends on the beam size, being much greater for large beams than for small ones. Nor is this the only falling-off that occurs: the primary Exposure rate is smaller at the edge than at the centre of the field because of the effect of the inverse square law. The edge is further from the source than is the centre, and once again the magnitude of the effect depends on the beam size, being greater for larger fields, as *Table XXXIV* shows. For the bigger beams the drop must not be forgotten in clinical work.

One other factor must be mentioned here. Those so far mentioned operate equally on either side of the central ray because they are geometric. Whilst in the plane at right-angles to the electron stream, the X-ray emission is symmetrical on either side of the central axis, in the plane of the stream, as pointed out in CHAPTER V, more radiation emerges from the target side of the central axis of the beam than from the filament side. This effect is counteracted to some extent by different attenuation in the target, so that the precise result is not easy to predict. Details will be discussed later in this chapter but the effect must not be overlooked here.

Table XXXIV.—VARIATION OF SURFACE DOSE AT EDGE OF FIELD, WITH FIELD DIAMETER

1·5 mm. Cu H.V.L.

Field diameter in cm.	5	6	7	8	10	12	15	20
Edge dose as percentage of central dose	95	94	93	92	90·5	86·5	85·5	81·0

Another important effect shown in *Fig.* 309 is the considerable amount of scattered radiation beyond the geometric edges of the beam, that is to say, in the region not receiving any primary radiation. This can be very important in the clinical use of radiation: organs and tissues outside the geometric beam may well be exposed to amounts of radiation that are not negligible.

SUMMARY OF OUTPUT

The total Exposure at the usually accepted point for 'output' statement, i.e., the centre of the beam on the surface, is made up of two distinct components, primary radiation and scattered radiation. Although the latter depends on the former the factors on which they depend can be enumerated separately as below. The factors above the broken line can usually be controlled and varied at will by the operator of the equipment: those below the line are fixed for any one set of equipment. Where the variation obeys a simple law, this is indicated in the brackets.

Primary Exposure Rate depends on:
1. Tube current   ($\propto$ mA.)
2. Tube kilovoltage ($\propto$ kV.^{2})
3. S.S.D.   [$\propto (1/\text{S.S.D.})^2$]
4. Any added filter

Percentage Backscatter depends on:
1. Size of beam
2. Shape of beam
3. Quality of radiation

_____

5. Tube-wall thickness and material
6. Target material   ($\propto Z$)
7. Voltage wave form

4. Design and detail of collimation

DEPTH DOSE DATA

The output of an X-ray tube is thus the Exposure rate at the centre of the field at the surface (for kilovoltage radiations) and this has to be determined for all conditions likely to be used in treatment. How this is done will be described later. What is then required for the computation of the absorbed dose at any other points in a phantom is the appropriate data concerning the penetration of the beam into the irradiated material—that is to say, the appropriate *percentage depth dose* data.

The percentage depth dose at any point is, strictly, the ratio (expressed as a percentage) of the absorbed dose (or absorbed dose rate) at that point to the absorbed dose (or rate) at the dosage reference point, i.e.,

$$\text{Percentage depth dose} = \frac{\text{Absorbed dose rate at the point}}{\text{Absorbed dose rate at surface}} \times 100.$$

The absorbed dose rate at any point is the Exposure rate there multiplied by the appropriate Exposure to absorbed dose conversion factor (roentgens to rads). Now this factor changes very slowly with radiation quality and the same value can be used for the surface and for points inside the phantom, so that we can say that:

$$\text{Percentage depth dose} = \frac{\text{Exposure rate at the point}}{\text{Output}} \times 100$$

without introducing more than a very small inaccuracy.

Tabulated values of percentage depth doses for points along the central ray of the X-ray beam (central axis percentage depth doses) are usually provided for each beam size and shape in use. Values for points off this axis are obtained from *isodose curves*.

In the discussion of the factors upon which percentage depth dose depends, attention will be fixed first upon values for points on the central axis of the beam. More general points will be considered later, though, fortunately, there is very little extra to be said.

FACTORS INFLUENCING PERCENTAGE DEPTH DOSE VALUES

Depth.—The most important parameter affecting the percentage depth dose (*D*) at a point is the depth of that point below the surface. In general, for any particular beam, the greater the depth the smaller the value of *D*, a fact to be expected from the

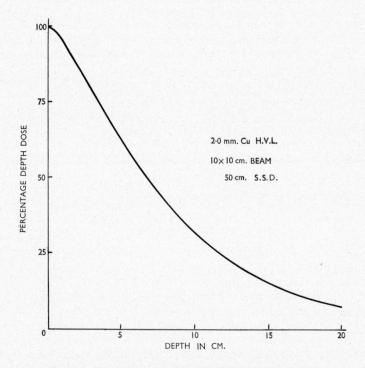

Fig. 310.—Variation of percentage depth dose with depth.

operation of the inverse square law and from the increasing attenuation that must be suffered by the beam, the greater the thickness of material through which it has to pass. A typical central axis percentage depth dose curve, showing the way in which *D* changes with depth, is given in *Fig.* 310.

Beam Dimensions.—As in the case of the output at the reference point, so with values of D, at any depth, there is a steady, though not linear, increase as the beam area increases. And again for any particular area the values of D are smaller for rectangular than for square or circular beams. This is illustrated in *Fig.* 311.

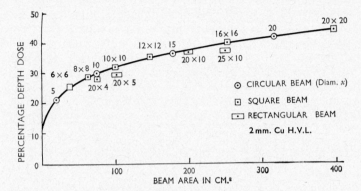

Fig. 311.—The dependence of percentage depth dose on beam area. Note again the relatively lower values for rectangular beams.

The reason for the changes is exactly the same for percentage depth dose values as for output values, i.e., the effect of scattered radiation. Not only at the surface, but everywhere within the irradiated zone, the Exposure is made up of

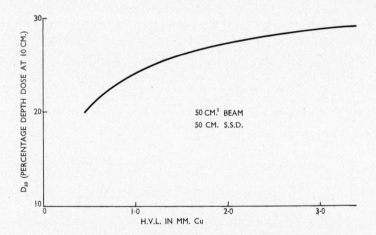

Fig. 312.—How percentage depth dose varies with radiation quality.

contributions from primary and from scattered radiation, the former being independent of beam area, whereas the latter increases with beam size.

Radiation 'Quality'.—'Quality' in radiology indicates the penetrating power of radiation, and, as is to be expected, percentage depth dose values increase with increasing half-value layer. The magnitude of the increase is not, however, as great as might be expected partly because of the influence of scattered radiation, which contributes a considerable fraction of the total radiation at a depth, and which does not alter much with quality changes. Furthermore, it must be remembered that part of the fall of percentage depth dose with depth is due to the inverse square law, and change in quality has no effect on this factor.

Because of the influence of scattered radiation the change in D values with quality is more pronounced for small (where there is less scatter) than for large beams. Even so, as shown in *Fig.* 312, a threefold increase in half-value layer only increases D_{10} (i.e., the percentage depth dose value at 10 cm. deep) by about 20 per cent even for the relatively small (50 cm.^{2}) beam chosen.

This, of course, has an important practical consequence. It is, in general, not very efficient to attempt to increase percentage depth dose values by increasing filtration. As has been pointed out in CHAPTER XIII, there are limits to half-value layers that can be obtained by filtration changes, so that quite large filtration changes (and the consequent considerable reductions in tube output) produce remarkably little increase

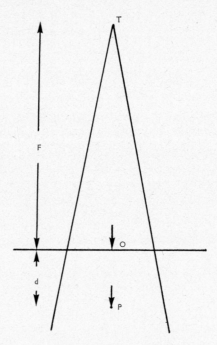

Fig. 313.—S.S.D. and depth.

in percentage depth dose values. If greater percentage depth dose values are needed, higher radiation energies (and therefore usually new equipment) are called for. Even so, however, only considerable changes produce worth-while increases and it was to achieve these that much of radiotherapy turned from radiations generated in the 200–300-kV. range to those in the megavoltage range, of which more anon.

S.S.D.—The general effect of change of source–surface distance upon percentage depth dose values is easily stated: percentage depth doses increase when the S.S.D. is increased. Why this should be so is perhaps not so easily seen, though a simplified example might help to make the reason clearer.

Consider the situation represented in *Fig.* 313, where a beam of radiation at an S.S.D. of F cm. falls upon a phantom, and where the percentage depth dose (D_p) at a point d cm. deep is to be studied. For the sake of simplicity only the primary radiation will be considered. The Exposure rate at P (E_p) will be controlled by the inverse-square law and also by the exponential attenuation law, and can be found from the equation:

$$E_p = \frac{k}{(F+d)^2} e^{-\mu d},$$

where μ is the linear attenuation coefficient for the phantom material for the radiation used.

Similarly the Exposure rate (E_O) at the reference point O is given by:

$$E_O = \frac{k}{F^2},$$

from which it follows that:

The percentage depth dose $D_p = \dfrac{E_p}{E_O} \times 100 = \dfrac{F^2}{(F+d)^2} e^{-\mu d}.$

For any given depth, then, the greater the value of F the greater the fraction $F^2/(F+d)^2$ and hence the greater the percentage depth dose. For a simple example, take d as 10 cm. in each case, and compare the percentage depth dose at that depth for $F = 40$ cm. and 50 cm. In the former dose the value of $F^2/(D+d)^2$ is $40^2/(40+10)^2$

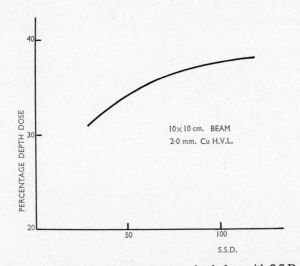

Fig. 314.—The variation of percentage depth dose with S.S.D.

or 0·64, whilst in the latter case ($F = 50$) the fraction is $50^2/(50+10)^2$ or nearly 0·7. Since $e^{-\mu d}$ will be the same in each case, it would appear that an increase of 10 cm. in S.S.D. increases the percentage depth dose by almost 10 per cent.

In practice the increase would be considerably less, for the same reason that has already been mentioned in connexion with changes of percentage depth dose values with quality. The primary radiation is only part, and often a relatively small part, of the total exposure at any point: scattered radiation makes up a considerable fraction and, in general, is not greatly influenced by S.S.D. changes. So the increase will be smaller than calculations involving primary radiation only would indicate, but nevertheless the changes are far from negligible, as the values given in *Fig.* 314 show.

Effect of S.S.D. Change on Output.—From what has been said it might appear that the simplest way to achieve adequate percentage depth dose values for any radiotherapy situation would be to increase the S.S.D. appropriately. Such a procedure would give increased values (though not to an unlimited extent, since the attenuation factor always plays a part) but any such gain is, in any case, at the expense of even greater decreases in surface output, which is inversely proportional to the square of the S.S.D. Thus treatments might become impractically long if too great S.S.D. values were used. For example, doubling the S.S.D. from 40 to 80 cm. produces about a 12 per cent increase in the 10-cm. deep percentage depth dose of a moderately sized beam with 2·0-mm. Cu H.V.L. radiation. At the same time the output falls by a factor of 4. In practice the chosen S.S.D. is a compromise giving reasonable depth dose values and output: for apparatus working in the 200- to 300-kV. range the most widely used value is 50 cm.

Position in the Beam.—As at the surface, so at any depth the Exposure rate falls off to either side of the central ray for reasons that should be clear from *Fig.* 315 A. The primary radiation contribution to P_1, for example, will be smaller than that to

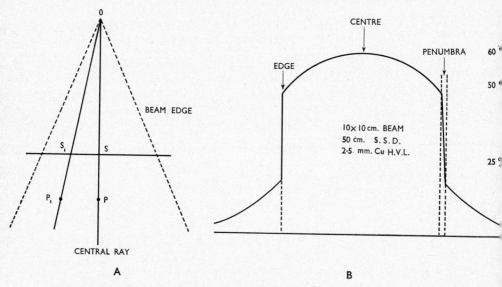

Fig. 315.—A, Why, and B, how, Exposure rate varies across the beam at any depth. Note the difference between the left- and right-hand sides of section B illustrating the effect of focal spot size.

P not only because OP_1 is greater than OP but also because S_1P_1 is greater than SP. Both inverse square law and attenuation combine to make the primary Exposure rate at P_1 less than that at P.

The scattered radiation contribution at P_1 will also be less than at P for the reason already given to explain the reduction in surface scatter towards the beam edge, i.e., the fact that P_1 is generally further than P from the regions contributing scatter, which therefore suffers more attenuation in getting to P_1 than to P.

As a net result of these effects the percentage depth dose across the beam at any depth varies as shown in *Fig*. 315 B—greatest at the central axis and falling off progressively towards the beam edge. Attention must be drawn to the region outside the confines of the geometric beam, for although no primary radiation can reach it, it is not completely unirradiated since it receives a contribution of scattered radiation, which falls off as the distance from the edge increases. Notice should also be taken of the difference between the two sides of *Fig*. 315 B. On the left-hand side is the situation which would exist if the focal spot were, in fact, a point source (instead of an area of a few square millimetres) and the defining system perfect. The beam has a sharp edge, there being a sharp break in Exposure rate when the edge is reached: to the right there are primary and scattered contributions, to the left, scattered radiation only. In practice, of course, these ideal conditions do not hold, for the focal spot has some area and the defining system is never perfect, so that the beam has no sharp edge but is surrounded by a zone of penumbra, as indicated on the right-hand side of *Fig*. 315 B. In this region the Exposure rate break is less abrupt since there is some primary contribution in the penumbra zone (diminishing, in this case, from left to right) which tempers the suddenness of the change.

The extent of the penumbra, which can be seen again in *Fig*. 316, depends mainly on the focal spot, or source size, and the position of the defining diaphragms relative to the skin. Though this matter will be discussed in greater detail later, in CHAPTER XXXV, which deals with beam diaphragms in general, it can be stated that the larger the source size or the further the beam-defining system is from the surface the greater will be the penumbral zone.

ISODOSE CURVES

To find the absorbed dose at any point in an irradiated phantom or patient, central axis percentage depth dose data are inadequate since many points of interest lie off that axis. Information about percentage depth dose values for such off-axis points (as well as for points on the central axis) is, therefore, presented by means of *isodose charts*, a typical example of which is shown in *Fig*. 316. These charts are essentially contour maps of the dosage distribution in, and around, the beam, since the *isodose curves*, which make up the charts, link up points of equal percentage depth dose. Percentage depth dose values at points lying between the lines are generally found by interpolation—that is to say, by the exercise of judgement. For example, in *Fig*. 316, the point *P* lies between the 40 per cent and 50 per cent isodose curves, and since it is rather closer to the latter than to the former line, may be judged to have a percentage depth dose of 46 per cent.,

On isodose charts such as that shown, the falling-off of dose towards the beam edge can readily be seen, as can the small, but not negligible, and quite wide-ranging scattered radiation beyond the geometric confines of the beam.

Primary and Scattered Radiation.—Although our main concern is with the percentage depth dose values at a point, it is of some value to consider the primary and secondary radiation contributions to the dose there, and especially their relative quantities. For example, it is instructive to note that the amount of scattered radiation, for any beam, increases with depth over the first few centimetres and then, as would be expected in view of the general falling-off of the beam, the amount of scattered radiation falls off too. This is shown in *Fig*. 317 A, whilst *Fig*. 317 B illustrates what is possibly a more important aspect of the same phenomenon. In the latter diagram is shown the fraction of the total contribution which is provided by scattered radiation, and it will be seen that this latter contribution becomes increasingly important with depth, making up practically three-quarters of the total radiation at 10 cm. deep, for example.

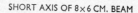

SHORT AXIS OF 8×6 CM. BEAM

50 CM. S.S.D.   2·5 MM. Cu H.V.L.

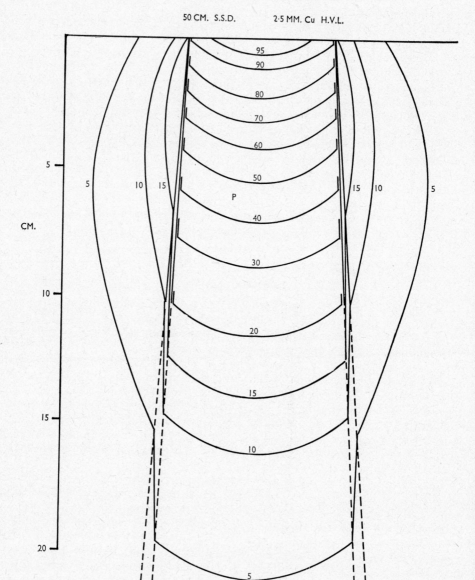

Fig. 316.—A typical isodose chart for a kilovoltage beam. Note the penumbral region (between the dotted lines) on each side of the beam.

For higher-energy beams the importance of scattered radiation becomes progressively less, as *Fig.* 318 shows. Nevertheless, in the kilovoltage range which is mainly illustrated in this diagram, scattered radiation still constitutes a considerable

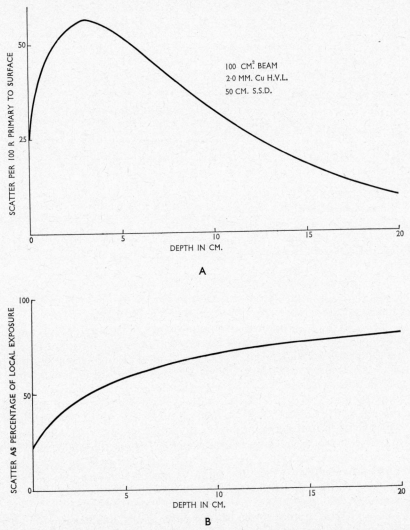

Fig. 317.—The variation of the amount of scattered radiation with depth in a phantom. A, The amount of scatter per 100 R of primary radiation delivered to the surface; B, The scatter as a fraction of the total dose at each depth.

part of the total dose at depths of interest in treatment. For example, it still makes up 50 per cent of the total at 10 cm. deep for radiation generated at 500 kV. (6·3 mm. Cu H.V.L.). It is only for radiations in the megavoltage range that scattered radiation becomes the minor partner in the total dose at a point.

Thus, for any beam, the radiation quality inside the phantom or patient is less than that of the primary beam. This is because of the added scattered radiation, the energies of the photons of which are always lower (longer wavelength) than those of the original primary photons because the scattering arises from the Compton process. This quality difference may be quite marked for low-energy beams but becomes progressively less important as the primary beam energy is increased, simply because

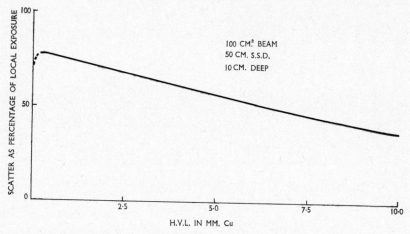

Fig. 318.—The reduced importance of scattered radiation with the high-energy radiations.

there will be progressively less scattered radiation in the beam. As will be seen in the next section of this chapter, the influence of scattered radiation in megavoltage beams is very small indeed.

The 'Heel Effect'.—An implicit assumption that has been made so far is that the beam is symmetrical about the central ray or, put in another way, that the left-hand side of an isodose chart is identical with the right-hand side. So far also, nothing has been said, for kilovoltage radiations, about any factor limiting the size of beam from any tube. In both these questions the so-called 'heel effect' is involved.

In the discussion, in CHAPTER V, of the spatial distribution of the radiation coming from an X-ray target it was pointed out that the natural tendency for rather more radiation to be produced in 'forward' directions, even at kilovoltages, was compensated by greater attenuation in the target by rays such as OC which are more intense than, for example, OA (*see Fig.* 319 which recalls *Fig.* 31, p. 56). By appropriate choice of the target angle (θ) effective output symmetry on either side of the central ray (OB) can be achieved, at least for fields of reasonable diameter. For working voltages between 200 and 300 kV. an angle of 30° is normally used.

There is, of course, a limit to the field size over which compensation takes place. The difference in radiation intensity in the various directions is not great and the changing thickness quite soon produces more attenuation than is needed to cope with the distribution differences. For example, the attenuation in OZ much more than compensates for the rather greater intensity in that direction. Therefore the output falls off quite quickly for the outer parts of larger fields and in practice the largest field usually used is a diameter which is half as big as the S.S.D. The angle between the extreme rays in this case is about 28°.

However, although the distribution may be satisfactory when the tube is new, an asymmetrical distribution may develop as it is used, if local 'pitting' or roughening of the face occurs. *Fig.* 319 B shows, in exaggerated fashion, the principle of what happens. Radiation generated at the point O_1 travels through thicknesses of target material which are quite different from those corresponding to the same directions in *Fig.* 319, i.e., when the tube was new. A good distribution is thereby upset and also there may well be some loss of output due to the increased attenuation in the target, and in any evaporated tungsten deposited on the X-ray window.

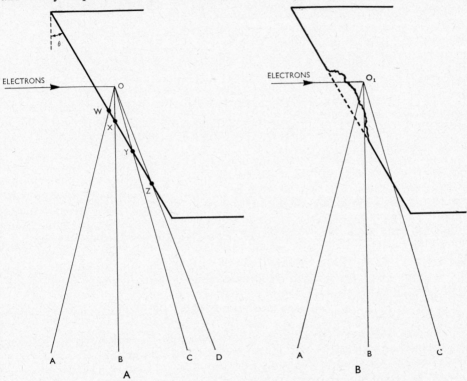

Fig. 319.—The 'heel effect' at an X-ray target. **A**, With a new target. **B**, With a target where 'pitting' has occurred. The dotted line shows the original target face.

Routine checks of radiation distribution should be taken periodically 'in air' to ensure that satisfactory conditions are maintained or to detect any changes. Any falling-off in output should prompt a distribution check since it may result from 'pitting' which may upset the distribution.

2. MEGAVOLTAGE RADIATIONS

The division of the consideration of the dosage data for teletherapy into two distinct sections—those for beams generated at below 1 MV. and those for beams generated above that level—may at first seem artificial. In fact, it is not only convenient, and with a good historical basis, but it also has a very sound physical basis.

Up to 1939, with very few exceptions, X-ray teletherapy was carried out with radiation generated at 250 kV. or less. A few pioneer machines working at about 1 MV. had been developed to take advantage of the greater penetrating power that radiation generated at such energies could be expected to possess, but it was not until after 1945 that technical advances enabled the even more advantageous still higher voltages to be attained. Nowadays 'megavoltage' machines are almost as common as those working round 250 kV., the most popular being linear accelerators working at 4 to 8 MV. and large sources of radioactive cobalt (^{60}Co) which give beams of almost mono-energetic radiation which, as far as penetrating power is concerned, is equivalent to that produced by an X-ray tube operating at 3 MV. A few machines work in the 10–20-MV. range and a number at 30 to 35 MV. By a quirk of history rather than by a conscious scientific development, it has happened that very little use has been made of radiation generated between 300 kV. and 1 MV., which means that it is possible to divide the field into the 'kilovoltage' and 'megavoltage' categories without introducing any important boundary difficulties or misunderstandings.

Megavoltage Radiations.—The main advantage of megavoltage radiations over those generated at kilovoltages is, from what has been said up to now, their greater penetrating power. Another advantage, closely linked with the first, is the much smaller scattering suffered by the higher-energy radiations and the fact that such scatter as occurs is predominantly in a 'forward' direction. There is also a major difference in the scale and pattern of the ionization produced by the electrons set in motion by the photons.

Ionization.—The effects of X-radiation are produced by the ionizations and excitations produced in turn by the electrons liberated when photons interact with matter. Reiterating what has already been written in CHAPTER VIII, these primary electrons possess considerable energy and in their passage through matter produce hundreds of ionizations and excitations in atoms near to which they pass before being brought to rest. As a result of these processes, chemical or biological changes may ensue. 'Kilovoltage' radiations liberate electrons which travel only a fraction of a millimetre in tissue, water, or tissue-like material, and so it is fair to say that the original transfer of energy from beam to material, and the ultimate effect of that energy on the material, take place essentially at the same point. Another way of stating the same fact is to say that the Exposure at a point is a direct measure of the absorbed dose at that point.

In contrast, electrons liberated by 1-MV. radiations can travel about 1 mm. in water whilst those ejected by 4-MV. and 20-MV. X-rays traverse up to 2 and 8 cm. before being brought to rest. Since electrons, like all other charged particles, produce most of their ionization towards the final end of their track (the Bragg effect already outlined in CHAPTER III), it will be clear that the effects of these high-energy rays may well be produced at some distance from the point at which the energy was initially extracted from the photons of the beam. In other words, the absorbed dose at any point may arise from Exposure at a point some little distance away.

Then there is the difference in spatial distribution between the ionization produced by kilovoltage and megavoltage radiations. Round about 250 kV. the primary electrons are emitted roughly equally in all directions, whereas with megavoltage rays the primary electrons go predominantly in a 'forward' direction, that is to say, in the direction of the X-ray beam.

How these differences of ionization pattern as well as the different penetration and scattering characteristics affect the distribution of radiation within a patient can now be considered.

The Central Axis Depth Dose Values.—Perhaps the most striking difference between megavoltage and kilovoltage radiation beams is in the pattern of their respective absorbed dose variation with depth. *Fig.* 320 shows how the absorbed dose varies along the central axis of a 10 × 10 cm. field of 4-MV. radiation and it will immediately be seen to be very different from the variation of 250-kV. radiation with depth, which is indicated by the dotted line. The greater penetrating power of the

higher-energy radiation is revealed by the slower fall of the depth dose values below
1 cm., but the striking difference is the extremely small absorbed dose at the surface
for the megavoltage beam and its rise over the first centimetre. Kilovoltage radiations show no such 'build-up'.

The 'Build-up'.—There are several effects contributing to the 'build-up'
phenomenon, but the most important are the pattern and distribution of ionization
produced by megavoltage radiations, the general features of which have been discussed

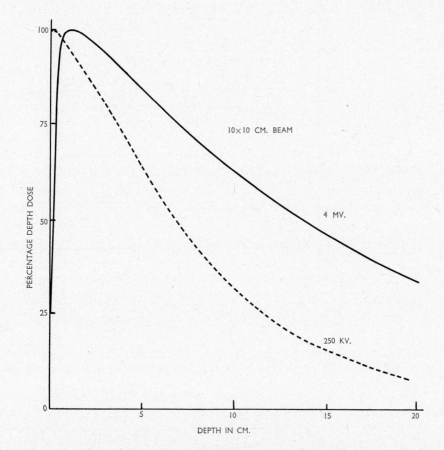

Fig. 320.—The variation of central percentage depth dose values with depth for a
4-MV. X-ray beam. Note the 'build-up' of dose in the first centimetre. The dotted curve is
for 250-kV. radiation for comparison purposes.

above. A greatly simplified, but not unrealistic, picture of what happens is shown in
Fig. 321, in which a beam of photons is depicted as irradiating a block of material,
and interacting at various depths. At each interaction between the photons and the
material it is assumed that the electron is ejected in a 'forward' direction, and that it
travels in a straight line to the end of its range. In passing through the material each
electron produces ionization, and to make allowance for the Bragg ionization effect
it will be assumed that 6 per cent of the total ionization occurs in the first millimetre,
with 9, 25, and 60 per cent respectively in the next three millimetres, the total range

being 4 mm. These percentage values are the figures entered along the 'tracks' in the diagram.

Consider now what happens. Some photons from the beam interact with surface atoms and their electrons penetrate to 4 mm. deep (as with photon A). Other photons can be imagined as penetrating to 1 mm. deep before interaction (as photon B) and

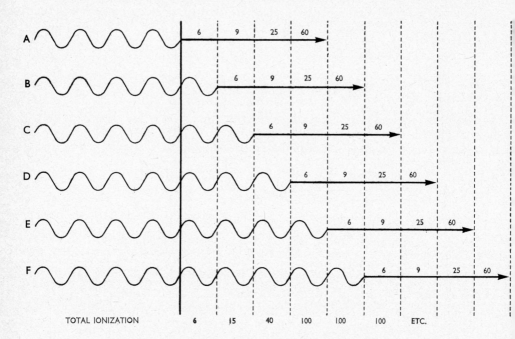

Fig. 321.—A simplified explanation of the 'build-up' phenomenon.

their electrons will get as far as 5 mm. (i.e., 4 + 1 mm.) deep. Yet others will interact at 3, 4, 5, and so on millimetres deep, with electrons penetrating 4 mm. beyond their point of generation in each case.

The total ionization at any place will obviously be the sum of all the effects shown, and numbers representing this pattern are given at the foot of *Fig.* 321. They clearly show a 'build-up' to a maximum, which in the case of this simple picture is the same for all depths greater than the fourth millimetre. In practice the ionization decreases beyond the peak of the 'build-up' because of the effects of the inverse square law and of photon attenuation, both of which have been ignored in this simplified picture.

Though photons do not interact simply at 1-mm. intervals, but throughout the depth of the material, and though the primary electrons do not only travel forward and certainly do not travel in straight lines, the 'build-up' of ionization does occur in this sort of way. It comes about because the electrons ejected by megavoltage photons have a not inconsiderable range, that they travel predominantly 'forward', and there is an increase of ionization along their tracks towards the end of their range. However, this build-up would not occur, or at least it would not be so marked, were it not for the very small amount of radiation scattered back by the phantom at megavoltage qualities. Any scattered radiation travelling generally in the opposite direction from that of the main beam would eject its electrons towards the surface and thus counterbalance the 'build-up' effect described. Such a process does occur with megavoltage radiations, but because its magnitude is small the effect is not

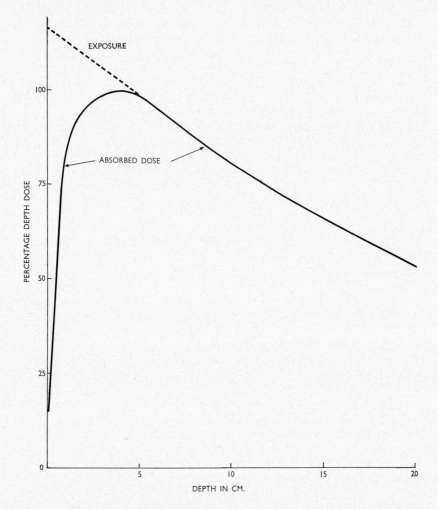

Fig. 322.—The central percentage depth dose curve for 20-MV. radiation. The dotted curve indicates the variation of Exposure with depth in the first few centimetres. Beyond the peak of the absorbed dose curve, the Exposure and absorbed dose curves are essentially the same.

great and marked 'build-up' of dose below the surface is a feature of megavoltage beams.

Exposure and Absorbed Dose.—It should be noted that in discussing the 'build-up' it has been the ionization in the material (which is directly related to absorbed dose) and not the ionization of air in an ionization chamber (which is related to the Exposure) that has been involved. Exposure, which is a function of the beam, has its maximum at the surface and falls steadily with depth through the joint influence of the inverse square law and beam attenuation (*Fig.* 322). Beyond the peak of the 'build-up', however, Exposure and absorbed dose vary in almost exactly the same way. At these depths Exposure measurements (in roentgens) can be directly converted into absorbed doses (in rads) as for lower voltage radiations. In the 'build-up' region absorbed doses can only be found by means of measurements made in special ionization chambers with thin walls.

Dosage Reference Point.—Because of the 'build-up' effect the standard reference point is not taken on the phantom surface but at the depth of the maximum of the depth dose curve on the central axis. *Fig.* 322 shows the percentage depth dose curve for a 20-MV. X-ray beam and it will be seen that the maximum dose occurs at about 4 cm. deep, since electrons generated by these X-rays are able to penetrate to this depth. Hence, for a 20-MV. X-ray beam the dosage reference point—the 100 per cent of the curve—is at about 4 cm. deep. In this diagram the variation of Exposure with depth has been included to emphasize its difference from the absorbed dose in the 'build-up' region, and its close similarity beyond the peak.

With these explanations of how the main features of megavoltage dose distributions arise, consideration may be given to their variation with different factors.

OUTPUT

The operating factors of megavoltage X-ray tubes are generally much less easily variable than the corresponding factors at kilovoltage levels. Nevertheless, if they can be varied, it would be found that the Exposure rate at the standard reference point would be proportional to the square of the applied voltage, to the number of electrons hitting the target (i.e., to the tube current—usually micro-amps in this type of machine), and to the atomic number of the material of the target. In other words, the simple law—first stated in CHAPTER V and repeated earlier in this chapter—that:

$$P \propto I . E^2 . Z$$

holds just as much for megavoltage as for kilovoltage radiations. So too does the inverse square law, so that output here is also inversely proportional to the square of the S.S.D.

The effect of filtration in this energy range is rather different and more complex than with kilovoltage beams. As for lower-energy radiations, the placing of material in the beam reduces the Exposure rate but the filtration effect (i.e., the removal of unwanted lower-energy radiations) is generally negligible in the case of radiations generated at between 2 and 10 MV., whilst for higher generating energies added material tends to remove high-energy photons rather than those with lower energies.

It must be remembered that because megavoltage X-rays are mainly produced in a 'forward' direction relative to the electron (or cathode) stream in the X-ray tube, a 'transmission' type target is always used in these high-energy tubes. This means that many of the photons have to pass through quite a thick layer of high atomic number before emerging from the tube and so suffer a considerable degree of 'inherent' filtration, which removes the bulk of the low-energy end of the spectrum. The 'unfiltered' beam is thus already quite heavily filtered when it leaves the tube!

The effect of using a lead filter (such as is used with up to about 2-MV. X-ray beams) on beams of higher energy has already been described in CHAPTER XIII, but may conveniently be recalled here with the aid of *Fig.* 323, which shows the variation of the mass attenuation coefficients of lead and water with changing photon energy. Round about 2 to 8 MeV. the coefficient in lead changes little so that lead has no selective effects in this energy range. Above 10 MV., on the other hand, lead removes high-energy photons more readily than those of lower energy, which is undesirable since the higher-energy photons continue to be more penetrating in water up to at least 50 MeV. 'Filtration', as usually understood with kilovoltage beams, has no place in megavoltage work.

As with kilovoltage radiations, the radiation reaching the dosage reference point consists of both primary and scattered radiation contributions. However, for mega-voltage beams, the amount of scattered radiation is small. For example, for a

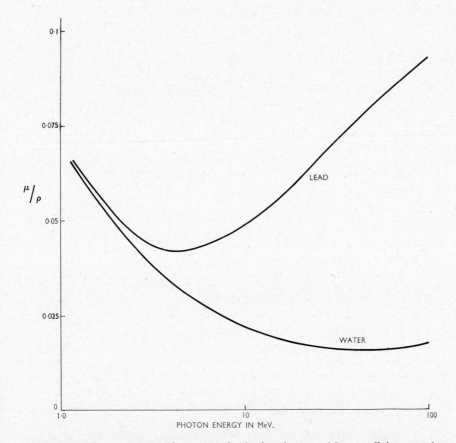

Fig. 323.—The mass attenuation curves for lead and water. Mass coefficients are here plotted to enable both curves to be displayed close together and therefore easily compared. The linear coefficient, which is needed for assessing actual filtration effects, is found simply by multiplying the mass coefficient by the density of the material.

400-cm.^{2} field at 4 MV. the percentage backscatter is about 10 per cent, whereas at 1·5 mm. Cu H.V.L. the value is 45 per cent. This has two important practical consequences. The first is that in the megavoltage range output is almost independent of field shape, whilst the second is that output varies very much less with field size than it does in the kilovoltage range. There is, for example, a 25 per cent output increase between a 4 × 4 cm. field and a 20 × 20 cm. field at 1·5 mm. Cu H.V.L. At 4 MV. the change is only 8 per cent, whilst at 20 MV. there is no variation at all.

PERCENTAGE DEPTH DOSE VALUES

As has already been mentioned earlier in this chapter, megavoltage X-rays are more penetrating, and suffer less scattering, than their kilovoltage counterparts and these facts have an important bearing on the percentage depth dose values and other features of megavoltage beams. However, the factors which influenced kilovoltage beams have similar, though often less marked, effects on megavoltage beams, as will be seen below.

1. Generating Voltage.—As before, the percentage depth dose at any depth increases as the voltage increases, as shown in *Fig.* 324.

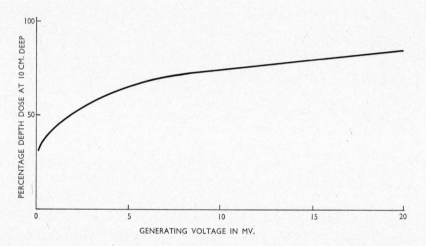

Fig. 324.—The increase of the percentage depth dose at 10 cm. deep with increasing generating megavoltage.

2. S.S.D.—An increase in source–skin distance produces greater percentage depth doses just as with kilovoltage radiation, but the change is greater here. This is because there is less scattered radiation in the megavoltage beams. As was pointed out earlier, the amount of scattered radiation at any depth alters little with S.S.D. changes, which therefore mainly affect the primary beam. The smaller the scatter, therefore, the greater the influence of S.S.D. on percentage depth doses.

In this connexion it should be pointed out that because of the much greater output of megavoltage (remember that the amount of radiation produced is proportional to the square of the applied voltage) it is possible and usual to use much greater S.S.D. values than can be used with kilovoltage radiation. For example, the usual S.S.D. with kilovoltage beams is 50 cm.; with 4-MV. apparatus 100 cm. is normally employed. This greater S.S.D. augments the greater penetrating power of the megavoltage rays and enhances their depth dose superiority over kilovoltage beams.

3. Beam Size and Shape.—As previously with kilovoltage radiations, the larger the beam size the larger the percentage depth dose value at any depth. But, as in the case of the output at the standard reference point, the much smaller amount of scattered radiation produced from megavoltage beams means a much smaller variation in percentage depth doses with beam size and also practically no variation with beam shape.

By way of example, it may be recalled that for 1·5-mm. Cu H.V.L. radiation the percentage depth dose value at 10 cm. deep increases 100 per cent between a 4 × 4 cm. and a 20 × 20 cm. beam (the actual values are 20·3 and 41·2 respectively). At 4 MV., on the other hand, the corresponding beam size increase raises the percentage depth dose value by only 16 per cent (from 57·2 to 66·2). With 20-MV. radiation the same beam size increase produces no such change.

4. Depth.—This is, of course, the main factor influencing percentage depth dose values and the variation of central percentage depth dose values has already been illustrated in *Figs.* 320 and 322. Apart from the 'build-up' region, which does not occur at lower energies, the chief feature of the megavoltage curve is its much slower rate of decrease with depth, compared with what happens for kilovoltage beams. This is, of course, a direct consequence of the greater penetrating power of the radiation and is the main advantage of the high-energy beams.

5. Position in the Beam.—For kilovoltage radiation it was found that, at any particular depth, the amount of radiation was greatest at the centre of the beam and fell off towards the edges (*see*, for example, *Fig.* 315 B, p. 442). This effect was ascribed to a reduction of scattered radiation towards the beam edge and to a reduced primary dose contribution due to the effects of the inverse square law and increased attenuation (*see Fig.* 315 A, p. 442). Provided the target angle is correctly chosen or

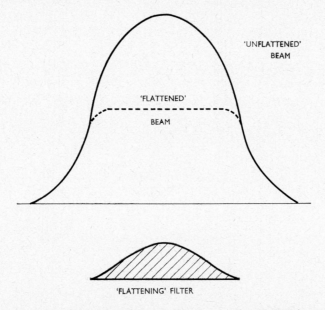

Fig. 325.—The variation of Exposure rate across the beam of a 20-MV. betatron, and the effect of introducing a 'flattening' filter (general shape shown) into the beam.

other measures taken to allow for the 'heel effect', it is reasonable to assume (as discussed in CHAPTER V) that the same intensity of primary radiation is emitted in all directions (i.e., that radiation is emitted 'isotropically' from the target).

Such an assumption cannot be made for megavoltage radiation, for radiation is emitted mainly in a 'forward' direction and its intensity falls off quite quickly on either side of the central ray. The rate of fall-off is often indicated by the distance from the central ray at which the Exposure rate is 50 per cent of the central value.

At 100 cm. S.S.D. this distance is about 25 cm. for 4-MV. radiation, whilst at 20 MV. it is only 7 cm. By way of comparison it should be noted that with a 250-kV. beam the Exposure rate would have fallen by 2 per cent in 7 cm. and only by 20 per cent in 25 cm.

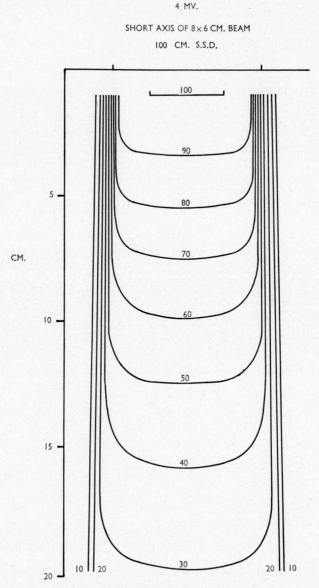

4 MV.

SHORT AXIS OF 8×6 CM. BEAM

100 CM. S.S.D.

Fig. 326.—A 4-MV. X-ray beam isodose chart.

Thus, though there is very little scattered radiation associated with megavoltage beams, they fall off relatively quickly away from the central axis, as shown in *Fig.* 325, and in this state is completely unsuitable for radiotherapy. Therefore, it is essential to introduce, into a megavoltage X-ray beam, a 'beam-flattening' filter or, more properly, compensator to eliminate the rapid variation of primary Exposure rate across the beam. Such a compensator will be thickest in the middle and taper away to nothing towards the beam edge. A diagram of a common shape, and an indication of its effect on the primary beam, are shown in *Fig.* 325.

With the aid of such compensators the Exposure variation across megavoltage fields is much smaller than the variation in the case of kilovoltage beams.

6. Isodose Charts.—*Fig.* 326 shows an isodose chart for 4-MV. radiation and whilst it follows the same pattern as those for kilovoltage radiations, of which *Fig.* 316, p. 444, is a typical example, comparison with that diagram reveals a number of important differences. Perhaps the most striking of these are the much smaller amount of scattered radiation outside the geometric limits of the beam, and the smaller changes in percentage depth dose across the beam at any depth. These 'flatter' isodose curves are mainly the result of the 'beam flattening' compensator already referred to, though its efficiency at considerable depths is due to the reduced scatter for the high-energy radiation. The much greater percentage depth doses at corresponding depths will also be noted.

CHAPTER XXXII

OUTPUT MEASUREMENTS AND THE USE OF ISODOSE CHARTS

ATTENTION must now be turned to the provision of the basic dosage data which are required for clinical work; to the consideration of how this information is to be used; and to deciding what other information may be needed or what other measurements may be required on an X-ray set or teletherapy unit being used for radiotherapy. It will be assumed that the 'quality' of the beam is known, either from half-value layer measurements such as have been described in CHAPTER XIII or, in the case of a gamma-ray 'beam' unit, from a knowledge of the radiation emitted.

For each beam being used, two separate sets of information are called for:

a. The 'output' of the machine, at the selected standard reference point, and

b. The dose distribution throughout the irradiated material—this is provided by central percentage depth dose tables and isodose charts which give the doses at any point relative to that at the reference point. As has been outlined in foregoing chapters, percentage depth dose values depend upon field size and shape, on radiation 'quality', and on the S.S.D. They are but little affected by the detailed design of the beam-producing equipment, so that information obtained with one X-ray tube can, quite reasonably, be applied to another working under similar conditions (provided certain precautions, to be mentioned later in this chapter, are taken). It is, therefore, quite practicable—and often to be recommended—to use data measured by others, of which there is a considerable selection, published in the radiological literature. In 1963 the International Atomic Energy Agency in Vienna took over the service of data distribution pioneered since 1944 by the Hospital Physicists' Association and can provide a very wide selection of isodose charts. Direct measurement, in a water or wax phantom, of radiation exposures at a large number of points so that an isodose chart may be produced is seldom necessary except for some very novel equipment or special beam shape. It will therefore be assumed that percentage depth dose data are available; tube output values have to be obtained.

'OUTPUT' MEASUREMENTS

By contrast with depth dose data, it cannot be said that two X-ray machines even of the same type, working under apparently identical conditions, will give identical output values. Because of its dependence, to some extent, on small details of tube construction—for example, the X-ray tube wall-thickness may differ from one tube to another—'output' has to be measured separately for each piece of equipment and, of course, frequently remeasured to ensure constancy of working conditions.

Two main methods have been used for this, and they are illustrated in *Fig*. 327. They are usually called the 'Output with Backscatter' and the 'Output in Air' methods.

Output with Backscatter.—This is the method that has found most favour in Britain, the measuring ionization chamber being placed with its centre at the reference point on the surface of (for kilovoltage radiations) or inside (for megavoltage radiations) a phantom. *Fig*. 327 A shows the so-called 'half-sunk' method used for kilovoltage radiations.

458

The method measures both the primary radiation coming from the tube and the backscattered radiation from the phantom, and hence gives directly the 'output' which is needed for clinical purposes. Two important points must, however, be made. The first is that with this approach a separate measurement has to be made for each field size and shape in use, since both these factors influence the scattered radiation component of the beam. The second is that, when the field is defined by an applicator, the measured value has to be corrected for the fact that when the measurement is

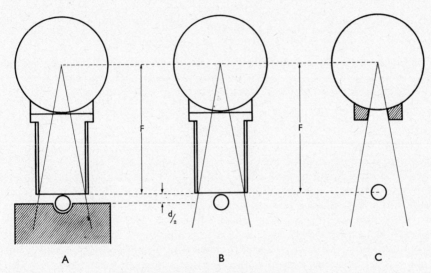

Fig. 327.—Output measurements. A, With backscatter; B, In air—with applicator. C, In air—with adjustable diaphragms.

being made the applicator end cannot be brought in direct contact with the surface (as it would be in treatment) but stands back by half the diameter ($d/2$) of the measuring system. Consequently the true output is rather greater than that measured, the latter having to be corrected by multiplication by a factor based on the inverse square law. If, as indicated in *Fig.* 327 A, F is the S.S.D., the factor is:

$$\left(F + \frac{d}{2}\right)^2 \Big/ F^2.$$

Since F is usually of the order of 50 cm. and d is about 1 cm., the correction factor is only about 2 per cent—nevertheless it should not be forgotten.

Where the beam is defined by movable or fixed diaphragms, such as is illustrated in *Fig.* 327 C, no such correction is needed since the chamber can then be placed at the correct distance from the machine.

Output 'in Air'.—The alternative method, generally favoured in the United States, and which is illustrated in *Fig.* 327 B, measures the primary radiation (P) only, since no phantom is present during the measurement. To this measured output must then be added an appropriate scatter contribution, values of which—as percentage backscatter—are given in many publications. If D represents the total output and s is the percentage backscatter (i.e., the amount of scatter per 100 units of primary radiation) then:

$$D = P\{1 + (s/100)\}.$$

In some publications the scatter component is given as a 'backscatter factor' (f), by which the primary contribution is *multiplied* to give the required total. Thus:

$$D = P.f.$$

Comparing the two equations it will be seen that:

$$f = \{1 + (s/100)\}$$

or

$$\text{Backscatter factor} = 1 + (\% \text{ Backscatter}/100).$$

The position may be made clearer by a simple example. If the percentage backscatter for a particular set of working conditions (quality, S.S.D., field size) is 15 per cent then the backscatter factor will be:

$$1 + (15/100) = 1\cdot15.$$

If the 'in air' output (i.e., the primary radiation Exposure rate) is measured as 60 R per min. the output 'with backscatter', which is the output appropriate to the treatment of a patient, will be $60\{1 + (15/100)\}$ or $60 \times 1\cdot15$, i.e., 69 R per min.

'In air' output measurements are not easily applicable to megavoltage radiations though the approach can be used. For kilovoltage beams it has the advantage (theoretically, at least) that only one measurement has to be made for any set of working conditions (quality, mA., and S.S.D.), since the primary contribution is regarded as being independent of field size and shape, which factors only influence the scattered radiation. However, this advantage is more apparent than real since, in fact, the 'in air' measurement—if carried out for a number of field sizes—shows an irregular, though small, variation, due to scattered radiation from the field-defining system. Therefore, for accurate work the 'in air' measurement has to be carried out for each field.

Where closed ended applicators are used, 'in air' measurements like those 'with backscatter' have to be corrected for the inverse square law effect, since the chamber centre is a small distance away from the applicator end.

An Alternative Approach to Output Calibration.—Although many tables of percentage depth dose values have been published for kilovoltage radiations, their most striking feature is their lack of agreement! This poses to the would-be user the question: 'Which set is correct and which must be rejected?' Enigmatically the answer is: 'All—and none.' The discordance between the different sets is more apparent than real and can almost certainly be eliminated by a change from the normal approach.

It will be recalled that kilovoltage percentage depth dose tables are all based on the surface dose as 100 per cent. Yet surface doses are probably the most difficult of all to measure and are much more affected by minor features of tube and collimator design than are doses deeper in the material. Nevertheless, all published data have been based on this shaky foundation: no wonder there is discordance, the extent of which can be gauged from *Fig.* 328 A. This diagram shows three recently published curves for the same field size, S.S.D., and radiation quality, and it will be noted that there are considerable differences between the three sets of values. The only place of agreement is in fact at the surface and this is only because this is 100 per cent for each curve.

Fig. 328 B shows the same data presented rather differently. Instead of having all the surface values the same, the values have been 'normalized' at 5 cm. deep—that is to say, they have been presented as if the basic measurement were made at that depth and all other measurements are quoted with reference to it. Immediately it will be obvious that the three sets of apparently discordant data are in excellent agreement, *except close to and at the surface.* And lest it be thought that the smallness of the diagram cloaks differences, the actual percentage differences at several depths are

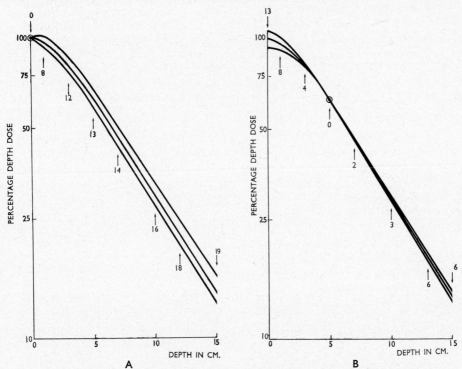

Fig. 328.—Percentage depth dose data presentation. Three different sets of data for the same radiation conditions (1·0 mm. Cu H.V.L., 50 cm. S.S.D., and 100 cm.² field) presented. A, Conventionally, i.e., 'normalized' to 100 per cent at the surface. B, 'Normalized' to the same value at 5 cm. deep. The numbers near the arrows indicate the percentage differences between the upper and lower values at the indicated depths, e.g., at 12 cm. deep in A, the upper curve shows 25 per cent and the lower 20·5 per cent, i.e., 18 per cent less.

shown on each diagram, emphasizing the great improvement achieved. The three sets of data agree at clinically important depths and are only discordant near the surface.

Since, in good radiotherapy, surface doses seldom have to be known with as great an accuracy as is desired for depth doses, the above facts have led to the proposal (backed by the International Commission on Radiological Units) of a new calibration technique which, whilst eliminating many of the difficulties, leaves established methods of output statement and depth dose calculation undisturbed.

The method can be summarized as follows:

1. For each beam size and shape measure the output at 5 cm. deep in a suitable phantom.

2. Any modern percentage depth dose tables, appropriate to the radiation conditions employed, can be used for depth dose calculation purposes.

3. From the known percentage depth dose value for 5 cm. deep, and the measured output value for the beam in question, the surface output 'with full backscatter' can be calculated for that beam. Thus the radiologist is provided with the same type of basic data as previously and his calculations of the dose at any depth can proceed along established lines.

An example may be helpful both to demonstrate the shortcomings of the traditional methods and to show the advantages of the method now being advocated, as well as illustrating how it is used.

Assume that, for the conditions being used in a particular department, there are two sets of published data (A and B) which seem equally appropriate. A choice has to be made between them. The discordance between them is obvious: the correct choice is not. By way of illustration it will be assumed that it is required to find the Exposure rate at 10 cm. deep. Using the two methods of calibration in general use and also the proposed new method, the following steps would be taken:

Measured Data.—

Exposure rate with 'full backscatter'	(D_B)	70 R per min.
'in air'	(D_A)	54 R per min.
at 5 cm. deep	(D_5)	44·5 R per min.

Tabulated Data.—

	Data A	Data B
Backscatter factor (f)	1·293	1·286
Percentage depth dose at 5 cm. deep	63·3	68·7
at 10 cm. deep	32·4	35·5

Note: (a) Exposure rate with backscatter = Exposure rate in air × backscatter factor.
   (b) Exposure rate at any depth = D_B × %DD/100.
   (c) Exposure rate with backscatter also = D_5 × 100/%DD for 5 cm. deep.

Calculations.—

1. *Using 'in-air' output value*

	Data A	Data B
Calculated Exposure rate with backscatter	54 × 1·293	54 × 1·286
	= 69·8	= 69·5
Hence Exposure rate at 10 cm. deep	= 69·8 × 32·4/100	= 69·5 × 35·3/100
	= 22·6 R per min.	= 24·7 R per min.

2. *Using full backscatter output value*

Exposure rate at 10 cm. deep	= 70 × 32·4/100	= 70 × 35·5/100
	= 22·7 R per min.	= 24·9 R per min.

3. *Using '5 cm. deep' output value*

Calculated Exposure rate with backscatter	= 44·5 × 100/63·3	= 44·5 × 100/68·7
	= 70·3 R	= 64·8 R
Hence Exposure rate at 10 cm. deep	= 70·3 × 32·4	= 64·8 × 35·5
	= 22·8 R per min.	= 23·0 R per min.

Thus although ostensibly for the same radiation conditions, the two sets of data give values for the Exposure rate at 10 cm. deep which differ by about 8 per cent (22·6 or 22·7 compared with 24·7 or 24·9), whichever of the conventional methods of output calibration is used. On the other hand, with the new method, the difference is only 1 per cent. Thus it is immaterial which set of data is used, both give the same answer for the Exposure rate at a point in the region in which the tumour is likely to lie. The fact that two sets of data give the same answer does not necessarily prove that that answer is true. However, that assumption can be made quite justifiably when *Fig.* 328 B is also taken into account, since that shows that all data lead to the same depth dose values, provided the appropriate reference point is used.

Data A were obtained by careful measurements on the type of apparatus on which the quoted measurements were made, and this is why each method of determining the output gives almost the same answer. The fact that data A obtained under quite different circumstances give the same answer when the proposed calibration method is used, underlines its correctness and value.

It will be noted that the surface output values obtained from the two sets of data are not in agreement, but the important point is that *whichever of these is used*, with its appropriate depth dose data, *the correct answers for the tumour depths are obtained*. Skin doses may be in some doubt, and this is not important in good radiotherapy: tumour doses will be accurately known, and that is important.

TREATMENT DOSAGE CALCULATION

As can be seen from many diagrams in this book, the absorbed dose of radiation (except in the megavoltage 'build-up' region) decreases with depth in the phantom or patient. In order to build up an adequate dose at a tumour deep inside the body, without at the same time producing excessive doses in more superficial tissues, it is necessary to use a number of beams directed towards the tumour from a number of different directions. Usually the central rays of beams lie in one plane, which greatly simplifies the computation of the dosage distribution arising from this sort of treatment.

The Production of the Combined Isodose Pattern.—To find the dose pattern produced by a multifield treatment it is necessary to have isodose charts for the beams being used and a full-sized outline of the cross-section of the patient at the level of the

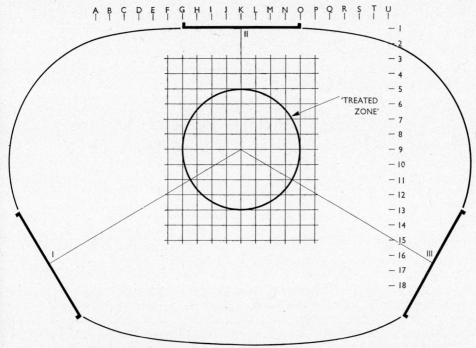

Fig. 329.—Body outline drawn for isodose chart production. Part of the grid of lines of the graph paper is shown, together with the field and central ray positions. The outline of the 'target volume' is also given.

treatment. To illustrate one—and probably the best—method of computing this sort of dose distribution, the case of a cancer of the bladder to be treated by three 4-MV. X-ray beams will be considered in detail.

The body outline, obtained by means of a flexible rule, a plaster-of-Paris moulding, or more sophisticated methods, is drawn out on a sheet of graph paper and the position of the three fields marked on, as well as the outline of the zone to be treated (often known as the 'target volume'). Graph paper is used because the corners of its larger (1 cm.) squares form a regular and useful pattern of points at which dosage may be assessed. *Fig.* 329 shows a typical outline and the positions and central rays of the three fields as well as some of the lines of the graph paper. Not all are shown to avoid excessive complexity. It is convenient, but in no way essential, if the point of intersection of the three central rays falls at one of the corners of the grid. For ease

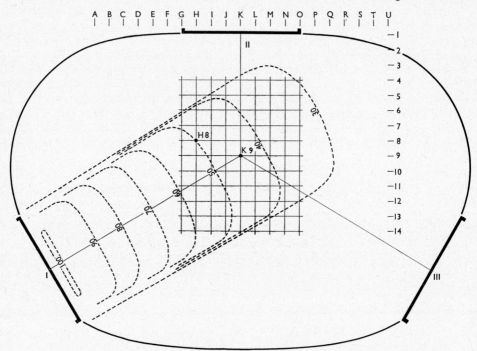

Fig. 330.—Body outline diagram—as in *Fig.* 329—showing field isodose chart in position for the reading of contributions to the grid points.

of identification the vertical lines are lettered and the horizontal lines numbered as shown. Thus the point K 1 is the centre of the anterior field, on the skin, whilst K 9 is the point of intersection of the three central rays—in this case, as usually, the tumour centre. On this diagram the radiotherapist also usually indicates the area which he wishes to raise to high and uniform dose—the 'target volume'. The appropriate isodose chart is then laid upon each field position in turn and the dose contributions to the corner of each square of the grid read off. *Fig.* 330 shows the isodose chart for an 8 × 10 cm. field, in position for the left posterior oblique field, and from this diagram it can be seen that the contribution at K 9 is 44 per cent, whilst at H 8 it is 50 per cent. The values of all such contributions should then be entered into a table such as *Table XXXV*, in the compilation of which it is advantageous to enter individual contributions for each point in the same order each time. This has been done in *Table XXXV* and, as the top left-hand square indicates, the left-hand figure in the top row is the contribution from the left posterior oblique field (I), the centre number shows what comes from the anterior field (II), whilst the right-hand number shows what the right posterior oblique field (III) contributes. The single number below shows the total contribution at each point—on the assumption that equal doses (in this case 100 rad) are delivered to the reference point of each field.

Table XXXV.—PART OF TABLE RESULTING FROM READING CONTRIBUTIONS OF EACH FIELD AT THE GRID POINTS. EACH FIELD DELIVERS 100 TO ITS REFERENCE POINT

	F (AND P)	G (AND O)	H (AND N)	I (AND M)	J (AND L)	K
3	I II III Total	2 60 28 90	3 94 29 126	5 96 30 131	7 96 25 128	10 96 10 116
4	3 5 28 36	2 70 29 101	5 92 31 128	5 93 32 130	20 93 34 147	36 93 36 165
5	5 6 29 40	5 70 31 106	12 87 33 132	31 88 34 153	39 88 36 163	38 88 38 164
6	10 6 30 46	30 70 32 132	44 81 34 159	42 83 36 161	41 83 38 162	40 83 40 163
7	49 7 32 88	49 65 33 147	47 77 35 159	45 78 38 161	43 78 40 161	42 78 42 162
8	54 8 32 94	52 62 34 148	50 72 36 158	47 73 39 159	45 74 41 160	43 74 43 160
9	57 9 33 99	54 60 35 149	52 68 37 157	49 69 40 158	47 70 42 159	44 70 44 158
10	60 10 33 103	57 59 36 152	54 63 38 155	51 64 41 156	48 65 43 156	46 65 46 157
11	62 10 31 103	59 55 35 149	56 59 39 154	53 60 42 155	50 61 43 154	47 61 47 155
12	65 10 10 85	61 52 30 143	58 55 38 151	54 56 42 152	51 57 44 152	48 57 48 153
13	67 10 5 82	63 50 5 118	59 52 20 131	55 53 40 148	51 53 45 149	48 53 48 149
14	69 10 2 81	64 47 2 113	60 49 5 114	55 50 5 110	51 50 20 121	45 50 45 140
15	70 9 2 81	64 44 2 110	59 45 2 107	50 46 5 101	20 47 6 73	8 47 8 63

Inspection of such a completed table (and it should be remembered that the table presented is only a part of what would be used in an actual treatment charting) gives an immediate impression of the main features of the dosage pattern. Even from the limited area illustrated, the build-up of dose in the region of the tumour, and the falling-off of dose elsewhere, which is the aim of multifield treatments, can be seen. A second point which also emerges is that there is a falling-off of dose from the front to the back of the zone which it is desired to treat. For example, the dose at K 4 (= 165) is about 15 per cent above that at K 14 (= 140). Whilst this is not excessive it would be better if they were equal, and this can be achieved quite easily.

16

So far, in this example, it has been assumed that equal doses are being delivered by each field. This is not essential, and it is by having different doses from some, or all, of the fields that a more uniform dose pattern can be achieved in this example, as well as in general. A number of methods have been used to find what these different doses should be, one of the simplest being through the 'balancing' of the dose at two points on either side of the point of central axis intersection.

Consider, for example, the points K 6 and K 12, and assume that it is desired that the resulting dose distribution shall be symmetrical on either side of the central axis of the anterior field (i.e., about the line K). When equal dose contributions are made on each field (100 at the reference point of each) then the doses at our two points are:

	At K 6	At K 12	Change in Contribution
From anterior field	83	57	83−57 = 26, falling, from front to back
From two posterior fields	80	96	96−80 = 16, falling, from back to front
	163	153	

For the dose at K 6 to be the same as at K 12, the fall-off of the contribution of the anterior field must be matched by the opposing fall-off of the contribution from the other two fields along the same direction. That is to say, if the posterior fields give 16 less to K 6 than to K 12, the anterior field should give 16 more; equal doses on each field give a difference of 26. The balance sought can be achieved by reducing the dose delivered by the anterior field by a factor of 16/26, that is from 100 to 61·5. All the contribution from this field must therefore be reduced by the factor, and thus our two points receive:

	At K 6		At K 12	
From anterior field	$83 \times 16/26 =$	51	$57 \times 16/26 =$	35
From two posterior fields		80		96
		131		131

The doses at the two chosen points are thus 'balanced' and, as Table XXXVI shows, a corresponding reduction in all the contributions from the anterior field yields a much more uniform dosage pattern.

The Practical Approach.—Normally it is not necessary to do all the work outlined above—done here to make the method clear—and to compile Table XXXV. In practice, the contributions at K 6 and K 12 (or similar points) would be determined as above, and the 'balancing' calculation carried out to determine the relative contribution from the anterior field. Only when this was done would the doses over the whole area be determined and Table XXXVI produced.

An Alternative Method.—The 'balancing' method is particularly useful where, as here, there is some symmetry and two of the fields can be assumed, from the outset, to deliver equal doses. This is not always so, and an alternative method of attaining the desired uniform dose pattern is to require each field to deliver the same dose to K 9, the point of central ray intersection. In the above example the anterior field delivers 70 and each posterior field 44, when they all give the same doses to their reference points. For them to deliver equal contributions to K 9, the anterior field contribution must be reduced by 44/70 or from 100 to 63—which is in good agreement with the 'balancing 'method.

The Dosage Calculation.—The decision concerning the magnitude of the dose to be delivered and the time over which it is to be spread rests with the radiotherapist, and such decisions do not concern us here. It will be assumed that the dose is to be 6000 rad, to be delivered in 15 treatment sessions spread over 3 weeks.

Table XXXVI.—As for *Table XXXV*, except that the Anterior Field only delivers 61·5 for every 100 from the Oblique Fields. The Contributions from Field II, listed in *Table XXXV*, have all been reduced by a Factor of 0·615

	F (AND P)			G (AND O)			H (AND N)			I (AND M)			J (AND L)			K		
3	I	II	III	2	37	28	3	58	29	5	59	30	7	59	25	10	59	10
		Total			67			90			94			91			79	
4	3	3	28	2	43	29	5	57	31	5	57	32	20	57	34	36	57	36
		34			74			93			94			111			129	
5	5	4	29	5	43	31	12	54	33	31	54	34	39	54	36	38	54	38
		38			79			99			119			129			130	
6	10	4	30	30	43	32	44	50	34	42	51	36	41	51	38	40	51	40
		44			105			128			129			130			131	
7	49	5	32	49	40	33	47	47	35	45	48	38	43	48	40	42	48	42
		86			122			129			131			131			132	
8	54	5	32	52	38	34	50	44	36	47	45	39	45	46	41	43	46	43
		91			124			130			131			132			132	
9	57	6	33	54	37	35	52	42	37	49	42	40	47	43	42	44	43	44
		96			126			131			131			132			131	
10	60	6	33	57	36	36	54	39	38	51	39	41	48	40	43	46	40	46
		99			129			131			131			131			132	
11	62	6	31	59	34	35	56	36	39	53	37	42	50	38	43	47	38	47
		99			128			131			132			131			132	
12	65	6	10	61	32	30	58	34	38	54	35	42	51	35	44	48	35	48
		81			123			130			131			130			131	
13	67	6	5	63	31	5	59	32	20	55	33	40	51	33	45	48	33	48
		78			99			111			128			129			129	
14	69	6	2	64	29	2	60	30	5	55	31	5	51	31	20	45	33	45
		77			95			95			91			102			123	
15	70	6	2	64	27	2	59	28	3	50	28	5	20	39	6	8	29	8
		78			93			90			83			55			45	

But what, precisely, is meant by this statement? Is 6000 rad the dose at some particular point, and if so, which point? Or is it the maximum dose, or the minimum dose, or the average—or what is it? All these interpretations have been placed upon the dosage statement at different times or in different departments, and it is partly because of this that different centres disagree about dosage levels to achieve the same ends—say the cure of some particular type of cancer. In truth they disagree, in part —at least—because their doses mean different things.

Recently it has been suggested, and the suggestion has received considerable support, that the quoted dose should be the *modal* dose over the high dose zone. This may sound rather mathematical, but in fact is quite straightforward since the *mode* or *modal* number of any group is that which occurs most frequently. In practice it may be found by noting the number of times a particular number occurs, or more often, a brief inspection will reveal the answer. For example, it will quickly be apparent that a reasonable choice for the representative number for the high dose zone in *Table XXXVI* (bounded by the heavier line) is 130 or 131, and in fact the latter occurs more frequently. Having decided this, we proceed as follows:

The representative figure of 131 is equivalent to 6000 rad, and to achieve this each oblique field gave 100 to its reference point, with an anterior field contribution of 61·5.

Therefore   131 represents 6000 rad
so that   100 represents 4580 rad
and   61·5 represents 2820 rad.

In other words, a modal dose of 6000 rad over the tumour area can be achieved if each oblique field delivers 4580 rad to its reference point (this is often called its 'given dose') whilst the anterior field has a given dose of 2820 rad. What daily dose would be given on each field will depend on local treatment policy, e.g., whether each field is treated every day, or whether, for instance, one field only is treated per day.

PRESENTATION OF THE DOSAGE PATTERN—
THE COMPLETE ISODOSE CHART

Although a table of the type of *Table XXXVI* contains all the necessary information, its impact upon any user is small and its interpretation somewhat difficult. Much more effective is the presentation of the same data in diagrammatic form, as the

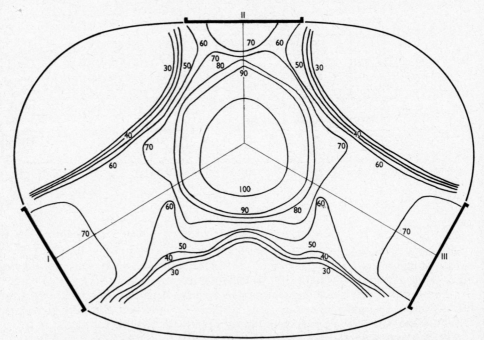

Fig. 331.—The isodose chart of the complete treatment when the dose delivered by the anterior field (II) is 0·615 of the dose delivered by each posterior oblique field (I and III) to the respective reference points.

isodose chart of the combined dose distribution. This is made up of lines joining up points receiving 10, 20, 30, etc., up to 100 or even 110 or 120 per cent of the stated tumour dose. The drawing of these lines involves some interpolation, but this is not difficult when doses are known at points which form a regular pattern, such as that used above.

For example, if 131 represents 6000 rad, then 80 per cent of this stated dose is represented by $131 \times 80/100 = 105$ (to the nearest round number). Now from *Table XXXVI* it will be seen that the total is 105 at G 6, which is obviously a point on the 80 per cent isodose curve. Also, since the value is 111 at H 13 and 95 at H 14, it is not unreasonable to infer that somewhere between these two points there is another at which the value would be 105. This point would be expected to be rather closer to H 13 (111) than H 14 (95), and the 80 per cent line passes through it. *Fig.* 331 shows a more complete dose distribution pattern so produced.

Charts of this sort, however, may not be particularly easy to interpret since each line has the same visual effect and there are many of them. Recently, therefore, colours have been used to place more emphasis on dosage 'areas' rather than on lines. Such a system immediately indicates the vital features of a treatment, revealing the extent of the zone adequately treated; the width of zones receiving marginally effective doses; the presence of any particularly high or low dose areas, and so on. Any number of colours can be used but great variety only confuses, and the following scheme, shown in *Table XXXVII*, has been found, in practice, to be effective and informative with relatively few colours.

Table XXXVII.—Colour Zones for Isodose Chart Presentation

Zone (Per cent)	Colour	Isodose Curves bounding Zone (Per cent)
120	Purple	125–115
110	Bright orange	115–105
100	Blue	105– 95
90	Dark green	95– 85
75	Light green	85– 65
50	Pale yellow	65– 35

Coloured areas are used in *Fig.* 332 to present the dosage pattern of our example in terms of zones rather than the lines of *Fig.* 331.

The Use of Computers for Treatment Plan Production.—So far, in this chapter, only 'hand' methods for the production of radiation distribution plans have been described. In these methods a suitably trained person places beam isodose charts on body outline diagram, reads off contributions at specified points, modifies these as necessary, and finally, from the added values, compiles a complete isodose chart. Such a method is time- and labour-consuming and, as a general rule, has been used only to produce charts in the plane of the central rays of the beams, because charts for other planes are usually much more difficult to obtain.

Over the past few years, however, there has been growing enthusiasm for the use of computing machines (usually digital computers) in this work, since they work quickly, can save much labour, and, usually, are not as subject to errors as a human being might be. In addition, a computer may well be able to do many things of which 'hand' methods are simply not capable.

The information previously presented as an isodose chart for a particular radiation beam is usually supplied to the computer as a mathematical formula which, more or less, represents the basic information. Therein lies a strength, and a weakness, of the use of computers. From the formula the dose distribution anywhere in the beam— not merely in the plane of the usual isodose chart—can easily be computed. Similarly, distributions in any plane—not merely the plane of the central rays as earlier in this chapter—can be investigated. In this way the amount of information available to the radiotherapist about his proposed treatment is much greater than heretofore, and it is conceivable that hitherto unsuspected shortcomings might be revealed, whose correction could improve the treatment.

On the other hand, the formula is usually empirical (chosen to fit the data as closely as possible) and may not be completely accurate. Simplifying assumptions may have

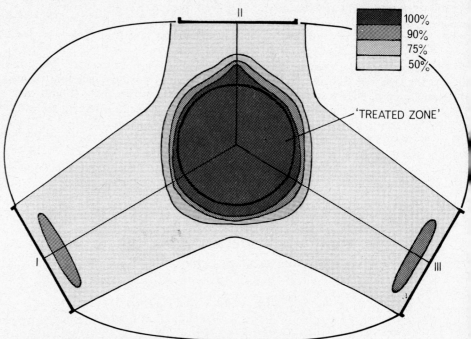

Fig. 332.—The complete isodose chart in terms of zones. The outline of the 'target volume' is also given to show that the whole of the zone required to be treated, and very little more, is raised to the desired level or within 5 per cent of it.

to be made and approximations introduced. The resulting computed dose distribution will be affected by these, and its accuracy may well be less than that attained by 'hand' methods. Furthermore, the inaccuracies will be hidden, and hence more dangerous.

Up to the present computer programmes have been of greatest value in rotation therapy treatments (see CHAPTER XXXVII), for which dose distribution calculations are particularly time-consuming and laborious. It is also possible to calculate fixed field treatment distributions and to allow for beam obliquity and surface irregularities, but so far the problem of allowance for body-tissue inhomogeneities has not been adequately solved. There is no doubt, however, that this difficulty will be resolved in the near future, for, as CHAPTER XXXIII will describe, it is now possible to make this sort of allowance in 'hand' methods.

There is little doubt that the computer has an important role to play in radiotherapy, as it has in so many human activities. It is likely to be especially useful in investigating wide ranges of approaches to various situations and trying out arrangements not previously used because evaluation of their dose distributions was too difficult to be attempted by 'hand' methods.

The provision of more accurate dosage information and treatment plans is of the greatest value to radiotherapy, provided that the treatment they represent can be applied with equal accuracy to the patient. If this cannot be done their production is a waste of time and effort. To put any 'paper' treatment scheme into accurate effect calls for care, thought, and specialized apparatus such as will be described in CHAPTER XXXV. It is imperative that advances that may come from the use of the computer are matched by increased attention to these more mundane but vital parts of the whole treatment sequence.

CHAPTER XXXIII

PATIENT DOSAGE

THE dosage data discussed in the last chapter all refer to what happens when a 30-cm. sided cube of water is irradiated. A patient is neither cubic nor composed entirely of water (nor of any other homogeneous material) nor, in general, can he or she provide dimensions 30 cm. long in each of three directions at right-angles to one another. As a result, any dosage computations or distributions based on the standard data may differ appreciably from the values that apply to an actual treatment. For accuracy, allowance must be made for:

a. Patient size and shape, and

b. Patient inhomogeneities.

Effect of Patient Size.—Since the part of the patient being treated is usually smaller than the standard measuring phantom there may be less scattered radiation and hence doses may be *smaller* than those deduced from the standard data. In general it will

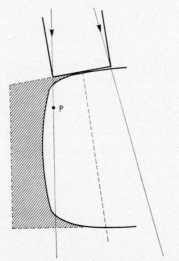

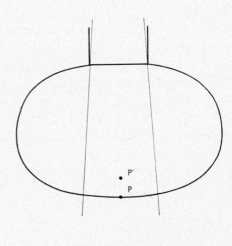

Fig. 333.—A beam close to the surface of a patient. The shaded portion indicates added 'bolus' material.

Fig. 334.—The exit dose problem.

be points close to surfaces that will be most affected, whilst megavoltage radiation with its much smaller scatter component is much less affected by the size of the part than is kilovoltage radiation.

    a. Entrance Surface.—So long as the part being treated is more than 10 cm. thick, or, if less, is 'backed' by some material like a mattress or table-top, the data provided by the standard tables are correct.

    b. Points near the Beam Edge.—Where, as illustrated in *Fig.* 333, the edge of a beam runs close to a body surface, local doses, such as at point P, will be less than suggested by the isodose curves due to lack of lateral scattering material. In the case of kilovoltage radiations the reduction in dose may be as much as 12 per cent, whereas with megavoltage radiations at most it will not exceed 5 per cent. Should either of these reductions be regarded as clinically important, full dosage can be restored by packing 'bolus' around the open surface, as indicated by the shaded area in the diagram.

c. *Points near the Exit Surface.*—The dose at points like P and P′ in *Fig.* 334 would also be smaller than would be estimated from isodose charts, because of the reduced amount of material beyond them, compared with that in a measuring phantom. *Table XXXVIII* shows the order of the dose reductions, giving factors by which the value from standard data should be multiplied to allow for the lack of 'backscatter'. Note that the factor is smaller, the smaller the amount of material beyond the point considered. Thus, for example, the exit dose (i.e., at P) for a 100-cm.^{2} field is 28 per cent less than the value indicated on the isodose curve, whereas for a point (P′) 4 cm. inside the surface the reduction is only 7 per cent. Should the patient be lying on a mattress or other support these differences are virtually eliminated. In general these reductions are clinically advantageous, rather than the reverse, since points near an exit surface are seldom being treated and the lower dose is desirable.

Table XXXVIII.—FACTORS BY WHICH PERCENTAGE DEPTH DOSE VALUES SHOULD BE MULTIPLIED TO ALLOW FOR LACK OF UNDERLYING TISSUE

a. H.V.L. 1·5-mm. to 2·5-mm. Cu.

THICKNESS OF UNDERLYING TISSUE PP[1]	FIELD AREA (sq. cm.)			
	25	100	200	400
0 cm. (P)	0·81	0·72	0·68	0·66
2 cm.	0·93	0·87	0·84	0·82
4 cm.	0·97	0·93	0·91	0·89
6 cm.	0·99	0·97	0·96	0·95

b. ^{60}Co and 4-MV. radiations.

Factor never less than 0·96 even for exit surface.

Effect of Patient Shape.—Isodose curves and central axes depth dose data are usually obtained with beams directed at right-angles to the plane surface of a phantom, whereas during treatment the beam is often directed on to a surface of a curved and complex form. In addition, the central ray may be inclined at an appreciable angle to the general slope of the surface, as depicted in *Fig.* 335. To such a situation normal isodose curves and depth dose data obviously cannot be directly applied, and two courses are open for dealing with it. Either the 'missing' material must be restored to the beam or corrections applied to allow for its absence.

'*Bolus*'.—The simplest method of dealing with the problem is to fill the gap between applicator end and skin with 'bolus', that is to say, with some material whose attenuating and scattering properties are closely similar to those of soft tissue. Most suitable for this purpose is 'Lincolnshire Bolus', already described in CHAPTER XXX. These tiny spheres, usually contained in small linen bags, 'mould' easily into the various shapes needed and restore the treated volume to the regular shape used in the measurement of the isodose curves. These can therefore be applied without further correction to the calculation of doses. *Fig.* 336 shows the 'bolus' in position and the isodose curves superimposed. If treatment is being carried out with the aid of a 'shell'

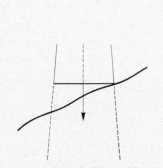

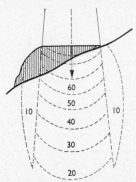

Fig. 335.—A beam incident obliquely on to a irregular surface.

Fig. 336.—Obliquity correction by 'bolus' (shown shaded) enables normal isodose charts to be used without correction.

of plaster bandage, or plaster, a shaped and permanent block of wax may be used instead of the 'Lincolnshire Bolus'.

Tissue 'Compensators'.—Using 'bolus', as described, is the method of first choice for kilovoltage radiations. For megavoltage radiations, where, it will be remembered, the high-dose zone only starts a few millimetres or more below the surface, the use of 'bolus' would bring high dosage on to the skin, which is often—though by no means

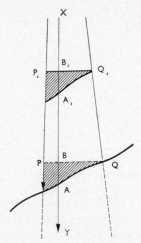

Fig. 337.—The principle of the tissue 'compensator'.

always—undesirable. The alternative is to use a tissue 'compensator' as illustrated in *Fig.* 337. In its simplest form such a 'compensator' would be of tissue-equivalent material, such as 'Mix D' or other wax, shaped so as to be a replica of the missing material, but taken back in the beam some distance away from the surface. Thus, though the width of the 'compensator' P_1Q_1 is smaller than the width PQ of the beam t the surface, the thickness A_1B_1 equals the thickness AB of the missing material long the ray XY. In this way the dose at Y will be the same as would have been there ad the surface been plane, but by having the 'compensator' at least 15 cm. from the cin, the dose still 'builds up' below the surface and skin doses are still low.

In making 'compensators' of this type it is not essential to use tissue-equivalent aaterial, but merely to ensure that along any ray there is added attenuation equal to hat which would have been provided by the 'missing' tissue.

This method is only readily applicable to megavoltage radiations for which the mount of scattered radiation is small. For kilovoltage radiation the lack of material aeans more radiation reaching the tissue because some attenuation is missing, but

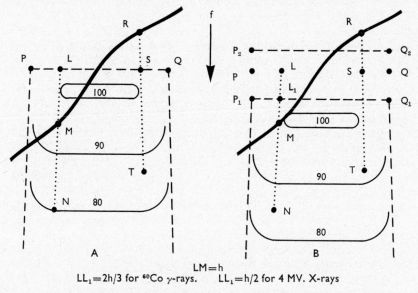

$LM = h$

$LL_1 = 2h/3$ for ^{60}Co γ-rays. $LL_1 = h/2$ for 4 MV. X-rays

Fig. 338.—Allowance for beam obliquity by the 'isodose chart shift' method.

his is partially offset by the fact that the 'missing' material would have added cattered radiation to the other tissues. To use the simple 'compensator' described bove, under these circumstances, would have restored the missing attenuation but ot provided the ameliorating scatter. It would have 'over-corrected' the situation.

Isodose Curve Corrections.—There are occasions when the dose distribution roduced by an oblique beam may be more suitable to the treatment required than the istribution produced with the aid of 'bolus' or a tissue 'compensator'. In such ircumstances some method is needed by which correct doses can be obtained easily om standard data. The most easily applied, illustrated in *Fig.* 338, is the so-called sodose chart shift' method and may be applied with considerable accuracy for beams f megavoltage radiation. It is less accurate for kilovoltage qualities because of the reater importance of scattered radiation.

PQ shows the width of the beam at the normal S.S.D. (f). If the treated surface ere flat it would be against this level that the isodose chart would be placed for osage assessment purposes. *Fig.* 338 A shows it so placed, the percentage depth ose at the point N being indicated as 80 per cent. This reading, however, is rroneous because the primary radiation reaching N has suffered less attenuation

than the chart suggests because the material LM is absent. Point N, in fact, receive
more radiation than is indicated.

To an acceptable degree of accuracy the dose at any point can be found simpl
by shifting the isodose chart to a new position P_1Q_1 as shown in *Fig.* 338 B and readin
off the dose directly. Thus at N the percentage depth dose is 84 per cent. All tha
has to be decided is how much the chart should be moved. For 4-MV. radiation th
move is equal to half the thickness of the missing material, whereas for cobalt-6
beam units a move equal to two-thirds of the thickness is needed. For the point 1
for which the primary beam has to travel through the extra thickness RS, the cha
would be moved upwards from PQ to P_2Q_2.

It will be realized that this is a purely empiric method, balancing the effects (
changed source–skin distances and extra or reduced attenuation. It does not wor
in the 'build-up' region.

Effect of Body Inhomogeneities.—Water is used as the phantom material fc
standard dosage measurements since its density, average atomic number, and electro
density are almost identical with those of muscle tissue and blood, and close to thos
of fat. Such measurements can, therefore, be used to estimate doses in those tissue
without any correction. Other tissues, however, do not resemble water so closely an
for these water phantom data need some correction. The important examples of thes
differing tissues are bone, and air-filled cavities, particularly lung.

It will be recalled, from CHAPTER VI, that the attenuation suffered by radiatio
depends on the thickness, the density, and the atomic number of the material throug
which it passes. Lung tissue is very similar to any other soft tissue of the body (i.e
the atomic number is the same), but the presence of large quantities of air in the
means that the density of healthy lungs is much lower than the value (approximate
1·0) of most soft tissue. The precise value is a matter of some debate, but if it
taken as 0·3 the error will not be great.

In contrast, bone is not only denser than soft tissue—its density varies betwee
about 1·8 for compact bone and about 1·2 for spongy bone—but its average atom
number, at about 13, is almost twice as great. Thus, whereas the attenuation in a give
thickness of lung is less than that in the same thickness of muscle, a piece of bone (
equal thickness would produce much greater attenuation. The precise effects a
somewhat complex and deserve some detailed consideration. In fact they must t
divided into two parts: the first of these concerns the influence that a layer of lung (
bone will have upon the radiation reaching tissues beyond them, whilst the secon
which will be discussed rather later in the chapter, concerns the actual radiatio
energy absorbed in these tissues which may, or may not, be the same as would t
absorbed in soft tissue.

Lung.—As has been indicated, a beam of radiation passing through healthy lun
will suffer less attenuation than would the same beam passing through an equ
thickness of muscle tissue. This means that tissues beyond lungs will receive a great
amount of radiation than that indicated by the standard percentage depth dose tabl
or isodose curves. Unfortunately, the situation is complex and it is difficult to gi
anything better than general indications of the magnitude of the effect. The low
density leads to increased transmission of radiation but this, to some extent, is offs
by the fact that the lower density material scatters less radiation (this is part of t
reason for the increased transmission!). Therefore tissues beyond the lung will recei
less scattered radiation than they would from unit density material, so that the amou
of radiation reaching them will not be increased by as much as might be expected
first sight.

Fig. 339 shows what happens when the 5 cm. of muscle between 5 and 10 cm. deep are replaced by 5 cm. of lung and allowance is made for the increased transmission only. *Fig*. 340 shows the rather lower values obtained when the reduction in scatter is also allowed for. Only at some distance from the lung surface does the dose reach the full value that might be expected from consideration of attenuation alone.

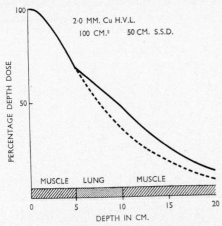

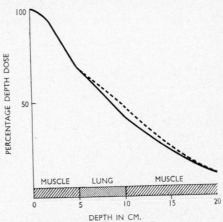

Fig. 339.—Central percentage depth dose values for a beam passing through a body section containing lung. Tissue thicknesses and positions indicated. Solid curve shows values obtained by allowance for attenuation only. Dotted curve shows water phantom values.

Fig. 340.—The modifying influence of scattered radiation. Solid curve shows actual values. Dotted curve shows values obtained by allowance for attenuation only in the solid line of *Fig*. 339.

Only at some distance from the lung surface does the dose reach the full value that might be expected from consideration of attenuation alone, as *Fig*. 340 indicates.

For the tissues close to the lung surface (which are often those in which the dose is most important) it is only possible to give approximate values for the correction factors which have to be applied to allow for the effect of the lungs. However, it will be clear that the factor will be smaller in the case of megavoltage radiation than for kilovoltage beams because of the greater penetration of the former through all materials. Furthermore, the compensating effect of scattered radiation will be smaller for the higher energies, since for these there is a smaller scattering coefficient. *Table XXXIX* gives some examples of the increases in dose beyond healthy lung that might be expected with beams of different energies. Where the lung contains fluid or solid tumour no increase is to be expected, since then it behaves as ordinary soft tissue.

Table XXXIX.—INCREASES IN DOSE TO TISSUES IMMEDIATELY BEYOND LUNG

300-kV. X-rays	+ 8 per cent per cm. of healthy lung
^{60}Co γ-rays ($\approx$ 3 MV. X-rays)	+ 4 per cent per cm. of healthy lung
4-MV. X-rays	+ 3 per cent per cm. of healthy lung
20-MV. X-rays	+ 2 per cent per cm. of healthy lung

Bone 'Shielding'.—As has already been said, the attenuation of a beam of radiation passing through a layer of bone is greater than that suffered when it passes through an equal thickness of soft tissue, because of the great atomic number and density of the bone. Tissues beyond bone will, therefore, receive a smaller exposure than would be indicated by standard dosage data, as *Fig*. 341 shows. Unfortunately, because of the complexity of the attenuation and scattering phenomena in an actual irradiation, especially when only part of a beam passes through bone, correction for the effects of bone on tissues beyond can only be approximate. Nevertheless, it is better to apply some factor than none at all, and *Fig.* 342 shows some appropriate values at different radiation energies. In this graph is given the percentage reduction brought about when 1 cm. of bone replaces 1 cm. of muscle tissue, and it will be noticed that the shielding effect diminishes quite rapidly as the radiation energy

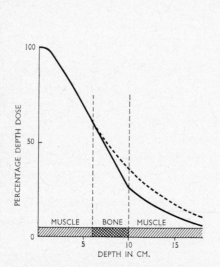

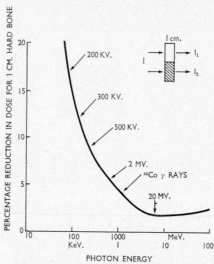

Fig. 341.—Central percentage depth dose values for a beam passing through a body section including a layer of bone. Dotted curve shows water phantom values.

Fig. 342.—The shielding effect of 1 cm. of bone for various photon energies. The values for different practical beams are indicated by the arrows.

increases into the megavoltage range. This is, of course, due to the greatly decreased effect of photo-electric absorption at higher energies. For radiations generated at between 500 kV. and 4 MV. practically all the attenuation is due to the Compton process and therefore the shielding effect in bone is entirely due to its greater density. For radiations generated at more than a few megavolts the shielding effect increases again because of increasing pair production—a process which it will be recalled is greater in materials of higher atomic number.

In so far as 'shielding' is a disadvantage in radiotherapy, in that it tends to reduce the amount of radiation reaching the deeper tissues, it will be clear, from *Fig.* 342, that megavoltage radiations are therapeutically superior to those generated at kilo-voltages, and that those generated in the range 2 to 10 MV. are best from this point of view. For bone thicknesses that occur in the body, the shielding effect for radiations generated between 2 and 10 MV. is very small, and it is one of the therapeutic advantages of these radiations that the dosage pattern indicated by their isodose curves is practically unaffected by the presence of bone.

THE CONVERSION OF EXPOSURE TO ABSORBED DOSE— ROENTGENS TO RADS

The final objective of all our dosemetric endeavours and data compilation is to find the absorbed dose at any point in the irradiated material. How can this be done from the output data (Exposure rates in roentgens per minute) and depth dose data (which are ratios of Exposure)? In principle the answer is quite simple and has been discussed at length in CHAPTER XII; the absorbed dose rate at any point is given by:

Absorbed dose rate (rad per min.) = Output (R per min.) × %DD value × f,

where f is the factor converting roentgens into rads in the substance irradiated and for the radiation energy being used. Some typical values of f have been given in *Table XI*, p. 132.

In practice, however, there is a difficulty. The values quoted in *Table XI*, for example, refer to homogeneous beams (monochromatic) of the stated energy, whereas the radiation at any point in an irradiated phantom, or patient, is a mixture of primary and scattered radiation, the constitution of which changes with depth and field size. The selection of the appropriate value for f may, therefore, present difficulties.

Fortunately, however, as *Fig.* 75 (p. 132) also shows, the factor changes slowly with radiation quality. It is, therefore, possible to choose, for a particular radiation quality, a single factor which will, to an accuracy of a percent or so, apply to any point in the irradiated material no matter what field size is used. *Table XL* shows the effective radiation energy at a number of depths for a small, a medium, and a large field for 1·5- and 2·5-mm. Cu H.V.L. primary radiation. The marked decrease in effective energy with increasing depth and field size is very obvious. In the lower part of the table the corresponding roentgen-to-rad factors are given, and it will be seen that their range is much smaller than that of the energies. Using a single factor for all field sizes and depths for each quality (0·944 for 1·5-mm. H.V.L. and 0·956 for the harder beam) greatly simplifies the estimation of rad doses in any treatment and only introduces errors of 1 or 2 per cent. However, it should be noted that the values selected are significantly less than the factors that would apply to the primary radiation in each case.

Table XL.—THE QUALITY OF RADIATION IN A UNIFORM PATIENT AND THE CORRESPONDING ROENTGEN-TO-RAD FACTOR

	H.V.L.		1·5-mm. Cu			2·5-mm. Cu		
PRIMARY BEAM	Effective Energy (keV.)		97			122		
	Factor		0·955			0·966		
		Depth (cm.)	*Field Diameter (cm.)*			*Field Diameter (cm.)*		
			5	10	15	5	10	15
BEAM IN PHANTOM	Effective energy (keV.)	0	92	86	79	118	111	107
		2	89	84	78	113	105	100
		5	87	80	76	109	98	93
		10	84	77	70	104	91	86
		15	82	73	66	100	87	79
	Factor	0	0·952	0·948	0·945	0·965	0·962	0·960
		2	0·950	0·947	0·944	0·963	0·959	0·957
		5	0·949	0·944	0·940	0·961	0·956	0·954
		10	0·947	0·941	0·935	0·959	0·951	0·948
		15	0·945	0·938	0·930	0·956	0·949	0·943
	Average factor		0·944			0·956		

Values of the roentgen-to-rad conversion factor (f) for some typical radiation qualities used in radiotherapy (and in the calculation of which the effect of scattered radiation in treatment conditions has been allowed for) are given in *Table XLI*. These values, of course, apply to soft tissues—they are not valid for the calculation of the absorbed dose in bone, which is a very complex subject, already discussed in CHAPTER XII and touched upon again later in this chapter.

Table XLI.—ROENTGEN-TO-RAD CONVERSION FACTORS FOR TREATMENT PURPOSES

Primary Radiation Quality	Roentgen-rad Factor (f) for Soft Tissues
1·0-mm. Al H.V.L.	0·930
2·0-mm. Al H.V.L.	0·935
1·0-mm. Cu H.V.L.	0·940
1·5-mm. Cu H.V.L.	0·944
2·0-mm. Cu H.V.L.	0·950
2·5-mm. Cu H.V.L.	0·956
^{60}Co γ-rays	0·965
4-MV. X-rays	0·965

ABSORBED DOSE IN OTHER TISSUES

Lung.—The actual tissue of the lungs is very similar, in for example atomic number, to any other soft tissue of the body; it is only their density as a whole which is different. Therefore, the absorbed dose in the lung tissue can be found simply by multiplying the local Exposure by the same roentgen-to-rad factor as would be applied to normal muscle tissue. It is a general rule that for any material the absorbed dose in rads (i.e., essentially in ergs per gramme) is independent of its density.

Bone.—In contrast to the simplicity of the absorbed dose situation in lung tissue, bone presents a most complicated problem. This has already been discussed at length in CHAPTER XII, and it will suffice here to recall the main features of the

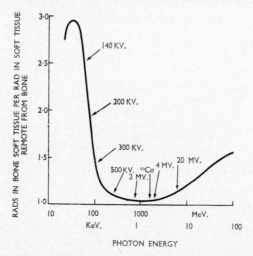

Fig. 343.—Rads in bone with various radiation energies.

problem. Therapeutically, the important absorbed dose is that in the living soft-tissue elements in the bone: the absorbed dose in the inorganic matrix material is, by comparison, unimportant. For reasons outlined in CHAPTER XII, the absorbed dose in this soft tissue, or in any soft tissue attached to bone surfaces, is greater than that received by soft tissues remote from bone. The factor by which the dose is greater depends upon the quality of the radiation being greater for low-energy radiation than it is for high-energy photons. For example, with radiation of 1·0-mm. Cu H.V.L. the average dose to the soft tissues in bone (what we will call the 'bone dose') is about twice that received by ordinary soft tissue, whereas at 2·5-mm. Cu H.V.L., the factor has fallen to 1·4.

With megavoltage radiations between 1 and 10 MV., pair production is still relatively unimportant in bone, practically all absorption being due to the Compton effect. Thus, since this is practically the same for all materials any excess dose to the bone soft-tissue elements is associated with the greater density of bone, which results in the 'bone dose' being only a little greater than that in ordinary muscle tissue, as *Fig.* 343 shows. Since excess dose to any tissues is clinically undesirable, the near equality between the 'bone dose' and normal soft-tissue dosage is one of the major advantages of megavoltage radiations generated between 1 and 10 MV. Above these values increasing pair production builds up the 'bone dose' again, so that for radiations generated at about 25 MV. the situation is as bad as it was at about 250 kV.

MEGAVOLTAGE VERSUS KILOVOLTAGE BEAMS IN RADIOTHERAPY

At various places in the preceding pages hints have been given of the therapeutic superiority of the higher-energy radiations. It is desirable to summarize these now and to consider whether or not there is any optimum generating voltage for X-ray therapy. The main advantages of megavoltage radiations and the consequences that flow from these advantages are:

1. Much improved percentage depth doses. *Fig.* 344 shows how the value of the percentage depth dose at 10 cm. deep steadily increases with generating voltage. This improvement means that fewer beams are needed to treat deep-seated tumours which, in turn, means that treatments are simpler and there is a valuable reduction in the amount of healthy tissue that has to be irradiated.

2. Because of the 'build-up' phenomenon, the surface dose is low, whilst the maximum dose occurs at a depth which increases with radiation energy increase, as illustrated by *Fig.* 345. This low surface dose (25 per cent or less of the peak dose) means that, with megavoltage radiation, there is practically no skin reaction. (This is often called the 'skin sparing effect'.) In one way this might be considered a slight disadvantage in so far as skin reactions have provided for some radiotherapists a guide to treatment progress. The considerable variation of reaction from one person to another greatly reduced the value of this guide, so that its absence is a very small price to pay for the major advantage of sparing the patient the considerable discomfort which usually accompanied the marked skin reaction to lower-energy treatments. However, if the lesion being treated comes near the skin, it is essential to cover that skin with a sufficient thickness of material to ensure that full dosage is delivered to the skin.

3. Smaller amount of scattered radiation. Not only does this aid the 'build-up' but it also means that there is a considerable reduction in the dose outside the main beam, thus reducing the unavoidable damage that the therapeutic use of a beam inevitably entails. The general debilitating effect of the irradiation is thus decreased, and important structures lying close to, but outside the treatment beams, suffer less damage than with

kilovoltage beams. The smaller scatter also makes the design and use of
'wedge' filters or 'compensators' much more simple, as will be indicated
later.

4.   Smaller shielding of tissues by bone and smaller extra dosage to the soft-
tissue elements growing in bone, as already discussed, and illustrated in
Figs. 342 and 343.

Clinical experience over more than a decade has shown that these advantages are
very real and, though kilovoltage radiation still has an important part to play in

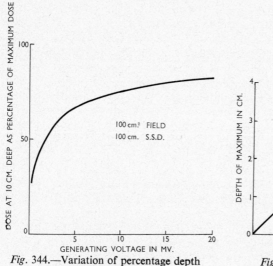

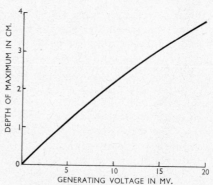

Fig. 344.—Variation of percentage depth
dose with beam energy.

Fig. 345.—The increase of the depth of
the maximum dose as the radiation energy
is increased.

radiotherapy, megavoltage radiations will, more and more, become the main agents.
Nevertheless, it must be confessed that the established advantages are physical and
technical—as yet there is no spectacular evidence of any great clinical advantage.

THE OPTIMUM ENERGY

Since percentage depth dose values, at say 10 cm. deep, increase steadily with
increasing radiation energy, at least up to 40 or 50 MV., and since increasing energy
also gives progressively less scattered radiation, smaller surface doses, and ever
deeper peaks of the depth dose curve, it might be concluded that the higher the radiation energy the better. Such a conclusion, however, is not justified, for there are other
factors which must also be considered, and which indicate that in some respects the
higher energies are definitely disadvantageous.

Two of these features have already been discussed and are illustrated in *Figs*. 342
and 343. For generating voltages above about 20 MV. there are increases in both
the shielding effect of bone and the excess dose in the living elements of bone, and
therefore, for very high energies, the disadvantages of kilovoltage radiation (in this
respect) are simply reintroduced. Another point to be remembered is that, although
higher energies mean lower skin doses on the side through which the beam enters the
patient, they also mean higher doses on the exit side (because of higher percentage
depth doses). There is obviously no advantage in reducing skin doses on one side

erely to transfer the possible skin reaction effects on the other. Assuming that the
atient is 20 cm. thick, entrance and exit doses are equal for 5-MV. radiation. For
energies greater than this the skin on the exit side will develop the greater reaction,
ad from this point of view, therefore, there is nothing to be gained by greater
enerating voltages.

This latter effect is of relatively minor importance. Of much greater importance
the natural narrowness of the beam for very high energy radiations. Reference has
een made to this earlier, and a typical variation of exposure across a megavoltage
eam is shown in *Fig*. 325, p. 455. This diagram also indicates the usually adopted
ure' for this situation—the 'beam flattening' filter or 'compensator'. With this, the
atural concentration of photons around the direction of the electron stream and the
latively rapid falling off to either side are 'corrected' by the filter being thickest in
e middle and thinning out towards the edge. Output is lost but a considerable
egree of uniformity of exposure across the beam is attained. The output loss usually
ts a limit to the size of beam that can be used. Normally a central output of reduc-
on of 50 per cent is acceptable. Under these conditions the maximum practical beam
ze at 20 MV., and 100 cm. S.S.D., is of 15 cm.-diameter. At 50 MV. a mere 6-cm.
eam at 100 cm. S.S.D. is all that can be used. Up to 10 MV. no such difficulties are
acountered.

Finally, there is the question of the cost and size of the apparatus and the cost and
ulk of the protective barriers that have to go with it. All these increase rapidly with
enerating voltage, and whilst increased cost should (ideally, at least!) be no con-
deration if the product is better for the job, increased size is a positive disadvantage
ecause, beyond a certain point, at least, it makes accurate treatment more difficult
attain and, therefore, less likely to be attained.

Taking all factors into account it can be fairly claimed that the optimum generating
oltage *for X-ray therapy* lies between 3 and 8 MV., and that if a single value had to be
ated, it would not be far from 5 MV. Whether higher voltage generators yielding
enetrating electron beams have a special place in radiotherapy will be discussed in
HAPTER XLII.

INTEGRAL DOSE

The damage produced by radiation depends upon the amount of radiation energy
aat has been absorbed by the material concerned. Cell damage depends on how
uch radiation energy has been absorbed by the cell, the damage sustained by the
amour depends on its absorbed dose. Though the destruction of the cells in the
calized tumour is of main interest in radiotherapy, it must not be forgotten that
diation energy is absorbed, and damage caused in many other places in the body,
esides the tumour region. This absorption of albeit small amounts of radiation
nergy by large volumes of tissue produces undesirable (though sometimes inevitable)
rstematic effects upon the patient and it is desirable to keep it as low as possible.
he total energy absorbed by the body, or by some specified part of it, is usually
alled the integral absorbed dose, and it is measured in gramme-rads (or mega-
ramme-rads since large numbers are often involved). 1 gramme-rad is 100 erg since
rad is 100 erg per gramme.

In concept the unit is quite simple: if a block of tissue weighing 100 grammes is
niformly irradiated to an absorbed dose of 50 rad, the integral absorbed dose is
00 × 50 = 5000 gramme-rad. In practice the determination is much more difficult
ecause uniform irradiation, except for relatively small parts of the irradiated volume,
seldom achieved. What should be done is to assess what volume of material receives

each dose, multiply these two figures (volume and dose) together, and then add up all
the values for the whole body. An example of how this is done is shown in *Fig.* 346,
which shows the isodose curves of a 10 × 8 cm. X-ray beam (2·5-mm. Cu H.V.L.).

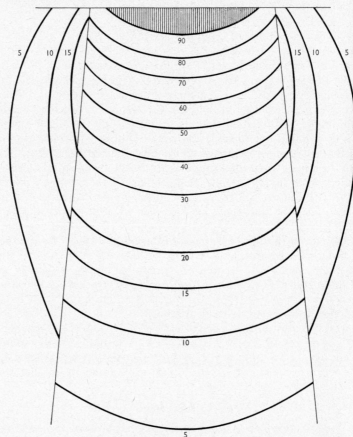

Fig. 346.—Volume in 10 × 8 cm. X-ray beam which may be considered to receive an average
of 95 rad per 100 rad at the skin.

If such a beam delivers 100 rad at its reference point, then the mass of tissue between
the 90 per cent isodose curve and the surface (shown hatched in the diagram) can be
regarded as receiving an average of 95 rad. Similarly, the material between the 90
and 80 per cent lines gets 85 rad on average, whilst that between 80 per cent and 70 per
cent gets 75 rad, and so on. To compute the integral absorbed dose for such a beam
it is simply necessary to know the mass of material between each zone: unfortunately
this is far from easy, especially for rectangular fields.

An approximate formula for calculating integral absorbed dose (Σ) has been
devised by Mayneord, and is:

$$\Sigma = 1\cdot 44 D_0 A d_{\frac{1}{2}}\left(1+\frac{2\cdot 88 d_{\frac{1}{2}}}{f}\right),$$

where D_0 is the delivered dose, A is the field area, and $d_{\frac{1}{2}}$ is the depth of its 50 per cent
isodose curve. f is the S.S.D., and the expression inside the brackets takes account of
the spread of the beam.

An example may make clear the use of this formula. Assume that a dose of 350 rad is delivered to the surface of an 8×8 cm. field, by radiation whose half-value layer is 2·0-mm. Cu, and at an S.S.D. of 50 cm. The value of $d_{\frac{1}{2}}$ for this beam, S.S.D., and radiation quality is 6·8 (50 per cent isodose curve at 6·8 cm. deep),

$$\therefore \ \Sigma = 1.44 \times 350 \times 64 \times 6.8 \ \left(1 + \frac{2.88 \times 6.8}{50}\right)$$

$$= 219,331 \ (1 + 0.392)$$

$$= 300,000 \text{ gramme-rad or } 0.3 \text{ mega-gramme-rad.}$$

The multiplication does not lead to exactly 300,000 gramme-rad, as has been written, but to quote the correct answer of something a little over 305,000 would be to suggest an accuracy that is unwarranted. This approximate formula in general accounts for something like half the total energy that the beam delivers to the body, some of which, of course, escapes in the transmitted beam or in the scattered radiation leaving the body. It can be regarded as providing a lower limit to the integral absorbed dose.

An alternative approach to the problem is to calculate how much energy enters the body when the beam delivers, say, 1 rad at the reference point. If it is assumed that all this energy is absorbed in the body then we have an upper limit to the integral absorbed dose. The assumption is not unreasonable with radiations generated at about 200 kV., but is progressively less satisfactory for higher energies, for which, however, some correction can be applied.

It must be recalled that the rad measures the energy abstracted from the beam: the total energy in the beam can readily be calculated from this fact, if the appropriate absorption coefficient is known, since the energy absorbed per gramme is essentially the product of the mass absorption coefficient and the energy in the beam. *Table XLII*

Table XLII.—ENERGY FLUX PER RAD FOR A RANGE OF RADIATION BEAMS

Generating Voltage or Radioisotope	H.V.L.	Mass Absorption Coefficient	Energy Flux
200 kV.	1·5 mm. Cu	0·0250	40·0 gramme-rad
250 kV.	2·0 mm. Cu	0·0256	39·1 gramme-rad
250 kV.	2·5 mm. Cu	0·0262	38·2 gramme-rad
300 kV.	3·0 mm. Cu	0·0270	37·0 gramme-rad
500 kV.	6·0 mm. Cu	0·0306	32·7 gramme-rad
^{137}Cs		0·0327	30·6 gramme-rad
2 MV.	About 12 mm. Cu	0·0323	31·0 gramme-rad
^{60}Co		0·0301	33·2 gramme-rad
4 MV.	About 16 mm. Cu	0·0292	34·2 gramme-rad

gives values of the mass absorption coefficient for water for a number of therapeutically popular beams, and also the energy flux (that is to say, the energy passing through 1 cm.² of beam area) for a rad at the reference point. One striking, and quite useful, feature of this table is the relatively small variation in the absorption coefficient, and hence the energy flux, over a wide range of radiation energy; 35 gramme-rad per sq. cm. of beam area for 1 rad delivered to the reference point is a useful generalization for the energy delivered to the body for most beams used in radiotherapy.

This, of course, does not mean that these are the values of the integral absorbed dose per sq. cm. per rad because some radiation is transmitted and some 'escapes' as scattered radiation. However, they are reasonable approximations for radiations round about 200 kV. but become progressively less so at higher energies. Fortunately, correction for transmitted energy, at least, is easy and *Fig.* 347 shows how it can be done. In that diagram the isodose chart for a 10 × 10 cm. beam of 4-MV. radiation is laid over an outline of a cross-section of the trunk, and it will be seen that the unit percentage depth dose (at the lower surface) is about 34 per cent. Thus for every rad

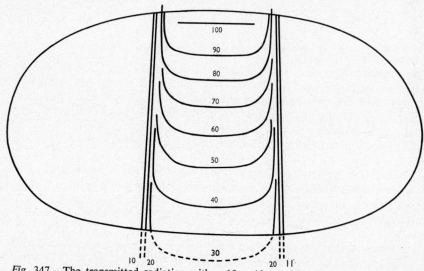

Fig. 347.—The transmitted radiation with a 10 × 10 cm. beam of 4-MV. X-rays. The dotted isodose lines represent radiation passing through the patient and therefore contributing nothing to the integral dose.

delivered to the reference point energy equivalent to 0·34 rad leaves the body as transmitted radiation, and allowance can be made for this, as the example below shows.

Assume an absorbed dose of 200 rad to be delivered by the 10 × 10 cm. field. The radiation is generated at 4 MV., for which energy *Table XLII* gives a value of 34·2 gramme-rad per rad as the energy flux per sq. cm. of beam air. The unit percentage depth dose (D_x) is 34, for an S.S.D. of 100 cm.

Estimated integral absorbed dose = Absorbed dose at ref. point × flux × area of
$$\text{beam} \times (100-D_x)/100$$

$$= 200 \times 34{\cdot}2 \times 100 \times (100-34)/100$$

$$= 450{,}000 \text{ gramme rad or } 0{\cdot}45 \text{ mega-gramme-rad.}$$

It is of interest to compare this result with that which would be obtained with the Mayneord formula. This gives, since $d_{\frac{1}{2}} = 13{\cdot}5$ cm.,

$$\Sigma = 1{\cdot}44 \times 200 \times 100 \times 13{\cdot}5 \left(1 + \frac{2{\cdot}88 \times 13{\cdot}5}{100}\right)$$

$$= 0{\cdot}54 \text{ mega-gramme-rad.}$$

This agreement is very satisfactory, and much better than would be obtained by comparing the formula answer and the incident flux answer for the lower-energy radiation used in the earlier example. For the conditions for which the formula gave an answer of 0·3 mega-gramme-rad the incident flux calculation gives 0·79 mega-gramme-rad (allowing for 10 per cent transmission). This large discrepancy arises partly because the formula, as already stated, gives the integral absorbed dose only to the 10 per cent isodose curve and so ignores a considerable mass of tissue which, though receiving low dosage, makes a quite large contribution to the total effect. For megavoltage radiation there is much less scattered radiation and the discrepancy is less. The second reason for the difference arises similarly—the flux calculation overestimates the effect because it makes no allowance for escaping scattered radiation, an effect larger at the lower energy than the high.

On balance, the most accurate estimate of integral absorbed dose is probably obtained by taking the average of the values obtained from the formula and from the energy flux calculation.

Clinical Significance.—The value of a knowledge of integral absorbed dose is limited, and in general it gives a scientific basis to long-established clinical rules, such as that which recognizes that large volumes of the body cannot be irradiated to as high doses as can smaller volumes. Except in the case of large-volume irradiation, integral absorbed dose is seldom a limiting factor in radiotherapy. However, in so far as it is an indication of unwanted (though possibly inevitable) damage to the patient, integral absorbed dose is a useful guide when treatments are being compared. When two different approaches, for example, yield the same tumour dose, the method giving the smaller integral absorbed dose is to be preferred.

No distinction is made between integral absorbed dose and the tissues in which the energy is absorbed and this may well be one of the reasons why clinical effects (such as blood changes) so often do not correlate closely with integral absorbed dose values. Energy absorbed in the kidney, or in bone-marrow, is likely to have quite different effects from those of the same amount of energy in fat or in the big toe!

CHAPTER XXXIV

BEAM MODIFICATION

ALTHOUGH, in the majority of instances, the collimated beam emerging from an X-ray tube can be directly applied to the patient, there are circumstances where it is desirable to modify the spatial distribution of radiation within the patient by the insertion of material into the beam. Such deliberate changes can conveniently be considered under four separate headings, though they have many features in common, and they are:

a. Alterations to the shape of the beam to reduce or, as far as possible, eliminate the radiation dose at some special parts of the zone at which the beam is directed. This may be called 'shielding'.
b. Alterations to the natural beam because its spatial distribution renders it unsuitable for radiotherapy. This is usually called 'beam flattening'.
c. Alterations to enable normal distribution data to be applied to all, or part, of the treated zone when the beam enters the body obliquely and/or it passes through different types of tissue. These involve the use of tissue 'compensators'.
d. Alterations to produce special spatial distributions for particular types of treatment. The most common of these modifications call for 'wedge filters'.

Some of these modifications have been dealt with at various places in previous chapters: even at the expense of some repetition it is advisable to deal with them all again here.

The General Problem.—The radiation reaching any point in a scattering medium is made up of a mixture of primary and scattered photons, a fact which influences the effect of any material introduced into the beam to modify it. For example, the radiation reaching the point Q, in *Fig.* 348 A, is made up of primary photons (P) travelling along OAQ and scattered photons from all directions. When material is put across the beam, as in *Fig.* 348 B, the primary contribution to Q is reduced by an amount which depends on the thickness (BC) of the material that has to be traversed by the photons passing through Q. The effect on the scattered radiation will be complex: that from the right of AQ will be reduced more than that from the left, since the primary contributions to the right are more reduced (because of the thicker filter) than those on the left. The result of introducing any modifying filter, therefore, depends very much on the relative amounts of primary and scattered radiation and is, generally, not easily predictable.

A specific example may help to make this clear. Imagine, as shown in *Fig.* 349, that a thick strip of lead is inserted across a beam to shield some tissues from the incident radiation (as is often done when it is desired to shield the uterine cervix, already adequately irradiated by intra-cavitary radium sources, when parametrial tissues are being irradiated with external beams). This strip (F) can be sufficiently thick so that practically no primary radiation passes through it. Nevertheless, the point T will not go unirradiated because of scattered radiation from the irradiated zones on either side. If the aim were to give to T complete protection from radiation,

488

this would not be achieved because of the scattered radiation. The effect on the radiation reaching T due to the introduction of the beam modifier (F) is less than the effect produced on the primary beam by attenuation in F, because of the 'blurring' effect of the scattered radiation. This is found, to a lesser or greater extent, in all attempts at beam modification.

Shielding.—The example just discussed, and illustrated in *Fig.* 349, is of course a case of shielding, and it will be realized, from what has been said, that complete

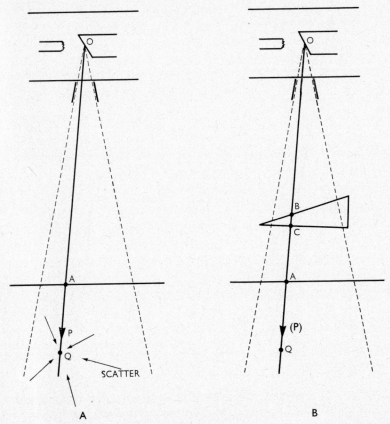

Fig. 348.—A, The radiation reaching any point in a scattering medium. B, The introduction of a modifying filter.

protection can never be afforded in this way to any part of an irradiated body. Worth-while reductions in the dose to previously irradiated, or specially sensitive, or important tissues can, nevertheless, be achieved, and more easily with high-energy radiations than with those of lower energy, simply because the amount of scattered radiation associated with the former is so much less. This is well illustrated in *Fig.* 350, which shows the effect of introducing the same block of lead into a 250-kV. and a 4-MV. X-ray beam. Although the block must attenuate the lower-energy primary beam much more than the higher-energy primary beam, there is considerably more radiation in the 'shadow' with the 250-kV. radiation. The shielding aim is more nearly achieved with megavoltage rays than with those of lower energy. A similar state of affairs will be found with all the other modifications that are to be discussed—

they are all more easily achieved with megavoltage radiations where scattered radiation is so much less important.

Another point worthy of mention is also illustrated in *Fig.* 350, and refers to the dose of radiation at any point such as W (*Fig.* 349) in the fully irradiated zone. The presence of the shielding block (F) will, to some extent, reduce the dose at W, since by shielding some material from radiation it cuts out scattered radiation which would otherwise have originated in this material and contributed to the total dose at W.

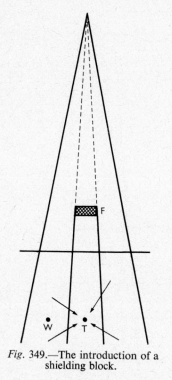

Fig. 349.—The introduction of a shielding block.

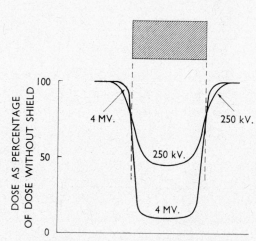

Fig. 350.—The effect of a shielding block on a beam of kilovoltage and a beam of megavoltage radiation.

Fig. 350 shows that the effect, though not great, is also not negligible near to the 'shadow' for kilovoltage radiations, whereas there is practically no effect with megavoltage radiations.

Beam 'Flattening'.—*Fig.* 351 shows the variation of Exposure rate across two beams, one generated at 250 kV. and the other at 20 MV. In both cases the rate at the centre is greater than the rate out towards the beam edge. The reasons for this have already been given in CHAPTER XXXI. As the reader may wish to be reminded, these reasons are partly that there is more scattered radiation in the centre (important at the lower energies), partly because the beam edge is always further from the focal spot than is the centre (the inverse square law effect holds at all energies), and partly because there may be a greater Exposure rate along the central axis than to either side due to the natural spatial distribution of radiation (especially at high energies).

Since the aim of radiotherapy is to produce radiation distributions which are as uniform as possible, this variation is undesirable. The variation across the lower energy beam is not too great to be acceptable, though there are instances where this may not be so, as will be outlined later. The 20-MV. beam shown in *Fig.* 351 B is quite unsuitable and has to be modified. This is done by a 'beam-flattening' filter ('attenu-ator' would be a better term) which reduces the central Exposure rate relative to that near the edge of the beam, to give, as nearly as possible, a constant rate across the

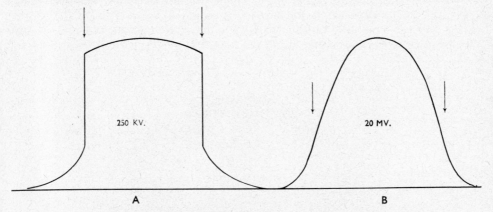

Fig. 351.—Variation of Exposure rate at about 10 cm. deep for A, 250-kV. and B, 20-MV. radiation. The arrows indicate the geometric beam width.

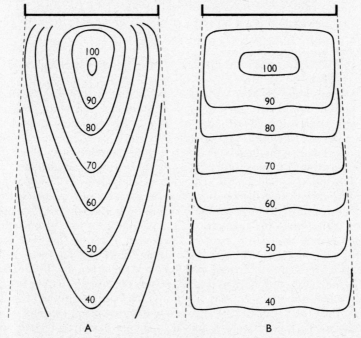

Fig. 352.—Isodose curves for 20-MV. X-ray beams. A, Without, and B, With a 'beam-flattening' filter.

beam. The 'flat' isodose curves resulting from such modifications are shown—in comparison with those of the natural beam—in *Fig.* 352.

To achieve this result the filter must be thickest at the centre and taper off to nothing towards the edge, as can be seen in *Fig.* 353. Copper or aluminium is usually used for these devices. The precise material is unimportant for there is no question of 'hardening' the beam—in fact, 'hardening' of the beam, with its consequent increase of penetrating power, is to be avoided since this would make 'flattening' more difficult. Because 'hardening' is avoided the introduction of beam-flattening filters alters the distribution of radiation in the beam but it does not alter the central axis percentage depth dose values. Much more important than the material for any filter is its accurate positioning in the beam and the maintenance of this position.

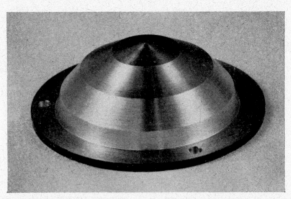

Fig. 353.—A beam-flattening filter for a 20-MV. betatron. The material is copper.

Misplacement will only exaggerate the unsatisfactory situation being corrected and therefore the correctness of the placing of any beam flattening filter should be frequently checked.

The 'flattening' of a 20-MV. beam is a fairly extreme example, but its principle is the same as that found necessary in most megavoltage machines of lower energy. Most modern megavoltage machines now have a beam-flattening filter fitted as a routine item, and this means that special care must be exercised in using for one machine isodose charts obtained on another. Unless their flattening filters are designed to produce the same flattening, other data will not be strictly applicable.

Kilovoltage Beams.—The lateral falling-off in kilovoltage beams does not prevent satisfactorily uniform dose distributions from being obtained in the central plane of multi-field, co-planar treatment, as *Fig.* 354 A shows. But what of the dose on either side of that plane; how, for example, does it vary along a line through O, at right-angles to the plane? *Fig.* 354 B provides the answer, showing that the dose does fall off on either side of the central plane, the doses shown in *Fig.* 354 A being greater than the corresponding doses on any parallel plane on either side of the centre. Such falling-off is inevitable with normal beams and it is customary to limit its influence by using fields whose dimensions in the direction at right-angles to the central plane are rather larger than the size of the high dose zone required might suggest. For example, if the volume to be treated were spherical, a square field might seem appropriate, whereas, in fact, a rectangular field with its long side at right-angles to the central plane should be used to carry the fall-off of dose which occurs towards the beam edge out beyond the edge of the required treatment zone. (*See*, for example, *Fig.* 354 B.)

This solution has the clinical disadvantage, however, that it is achieved at the expense of the irradiation of larger volumes of normal healthy tissue than are strictly necessary for the treatment of the tumour. It was in an attempt to avoid this unnecessary irradiation that beam-flattening filters, now almost exclusively used for megavoltage

eams, were first devised for kilovoltage beams. They partially succeeded: they
roduced 'flat' isodose curves over a range of depths of about 5 or 6 cm., as *Fig.* 355
1ows, but not over the wide depth range for which megavoltage beam-flattening filters
ork. For depths much greater than that for which the flattening was devised the
;odose lines become curved again, whilst more superficially there are considerable

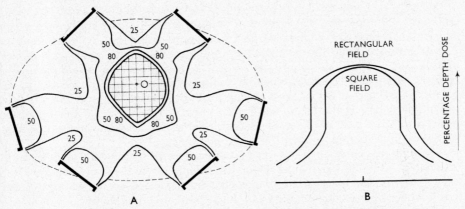

Fig. 354.—A, The combined isodose curves for a multi-field treatment with 250-kV. beams.
B, Variation of Exposure rate across square and rectangular beams.

hot spots' of radiation near the beam edges and the surface. The reason for this
lefect is the much greater change of scattered radiation associated with the kilovoltage beams at the different depths.

A specific example may help to demonstrate the extent to which this additional
scattered radiation complicates the situation with kilovoltage beams and why

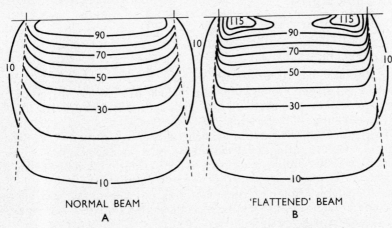

Fig. 355.—Isodose charts for normal and 'beam-flattened' 250-kV. beams.

modification is so much easier and more successful with megavoltage beams. Consider
the Exposure rates at 5 cm. deep on the central axis and at the edge of the long axis
of a 20 × 7·5 cm. rectangular field for both 250-kV. and 4-MV. radiation. The rates,
in roentgens per minute, are as follows:

	250 kV.		4 MV.	
	Centre	*Edge*	*Centre*	*Edge*
Total Exposure rate	88	70	85	76
Primary Exposure rate	35	33	77	70
Scattered Exposure rate	53	37	8	6
Centre–edge variation	About 26 per cent		About 12 per cent	

Not only is there more scattering in the 250-kV. beam, but it also causes a greater cross-field variation and hence presents a more difficult 'flattening' problem. T equalize the centre and edge rates the former must be reduced by 26 per cent an 12 per cent respectively for the kilovoltage and megavoltage radiations, and this ca only be done *by altering the primary radiation.* Because scattered radiation come from all parts of the irradiated material, the scattered radiation contribution at an point is not related in any simple way with the local primary Exposure rate. In orde to bring about the desired 'flattening', for example, the kilovoltage primary contribu tion has to be reduced by about 40 per cent, whereas for the megavoltage radiation change of 13 per cent in primary Exposure rate suffices.

The primary contribution has to be overcompensated to allow for the effect of th scattered radiation at a particular depth. At a depth where the scatter is proportion ately less (i.e., nearer the surface) the modification is excessive—the central Exposur rate is reduced more than necessary and 'high spots' are produced towards the edge a shown by the following superficial Exposure rates—at the surface for 250 kV., at 1 cm deep for 4 MV.:

	250 kV.		4 MV.	
	Centre	*Edge*	*Centre*	*Edge*
1. *Unmodified rates*				
Total Exposure rate	132	114	100	92
Primary Exposure rate	100	94	97	90
Scattered Exposure rate	32	20	3	2
2. *After modification*				
Primary reduced by	40 per cent	0	13 per cent	0
Primary Exposure rate	60	94	86	90
Scattered Exposure rate	28	19	3	2
Total Exposure rate	88	113	89	92

Some allowance has been made for the fact that the scattered radiation will be reduced by the 'flattening' procedure, and the final effect at these superficial levels is that the Exposure rate is some 28 per cent higher towards the edge than at the centre for 250-kV. radiation. For the 4-MV. beam the 'hot spot' is a mere 3 per cent high.

The reverse of these effects occurs at depths greater than those for which 'flattening' is attempted. At these there is relatively more scatter and therefore the compensation applied to the primary beam is inadequate and non-flat isodose curves result, the dose being higher in the middle again—as with non-modified curves.

These undesirable features of 'beam-flattening' of a kilovoltage beam are shown in *Fig.* 355, and are the reasons why 'beam flattening' nowadays is almost exclusively reserved for megavoltage beams.

The 'Heel' Effect.—Although, for the reasons just given, 'beam-flattening' filters are not generally used in kilovoltage therapy, they may be necessary where the 'heel' effect, discussed in CHAPTER XXXI, introduces an asymmetry into the beam. If such correction is needed frequent checks are necessary to confirm that it continues to perform its allotted function. As already pointed out, use of a tube results in a roughening of the target face and, to some extent at least, 'pitting' which may alter the initial distribution markedly. Hence a filter designed for one set of circumstances may have to be modified as time goes on, to keep pace with target changes.

'**Compensators**'.—Another type of beam modification which is almost entirely concerned with megavoltage beams is 'compensation' for absent tissues so that normal depth dose data and isodose charts may be used for situations to which they could not normally be applied. Standard isodose charts are usually obtained from measurements made in cubic phantoms into which the beam enters normally—i.e., at right-angles to the surface. They cannot be directly applied, therefore, where the beam enters the patient obliquely or through a curved surface, and it is to this sort of situation that the type of compensation being discussed is applied. Some reference to this has already been made in CHAPTER XXXIII.

A general example of this type of situation is shown in *Fig.* 356 A, where a beam is shown entering obliquely through a curved surface. The line AB indicates the position of the end of an applicator which might be used for defining the beam or is at the standard S.S.D. where no applicator is used. It will be clear, immediately, that more radiation will reach P and Q respectively than would be indicated by any isodose chart since to reach those points the beam has suffered less attenuation than it would in the plane-faced cubic-measuring phantom.

To allow for the 'missing' material and to enable standard data to be used, the simplest expedient is to replace the material missing from the beam by filling the space with wax or other 'bolus' material, as is shown in *Fig.* 356 B, and labelled I. Such a solution is not generally acceptable, however, with megavoltage beams. It will be recalled that with such beams the absorbed dose 'builds up' below the open surface of any irradiated material, the actual surface receiving materially less dose than tissues immediately below it. If the skin is the surface through which the beam enters the patient, it receives quite small doses with megavoltage beams and this 'skin-sparing' effect can be one of the advantages of megavoltage, over kilovoltage, beams. Placing any material on the skin will place that skin nearer to the peak of the 'build-up' curve and so, possibly unnecessarily, throw away an advantage.* Moving the material 10 or 15 cm. away from the skin (into the position labelled II) would, however, mean that it did not affect the 'build-up'. The only question, then, is whether it would produce the desired effect.

The amount of primary radiation reaching P will be the same whether the added material is in position I or position II, provided that A'C' equals AC. Similarly, the dose at Q is unchanged by the move if D'E' equals DE. And so for all points in the irradiated zone, provided that the thickness of the compensating material remains the same in position II as in position I, *but its lateral dimensions must be shrunk in proportion to the amount that it is moved towards* O, because of beam divergence. For example, if AB is at 100 cm. from O and A'B' is at 85 cm., then if AB is 6 cm., A'B' should be:

$$6 \times (85/100) = 5 \cdot 1 \text{ cm.}$$

Under such conditions, compensation of the *primary radiation* for the missing material is achieved equally well whether the material is at I or II. However, there is also the question of the scattered radiation to be considered. The amount of scattered radiation contributed from the block in position II will be much less than would reach points such as P or Q from it in position I. Thus, strictly speaking, there will be a

---

* To bring the skin into the high dose zone is not universally undesirable, of course. Where the lesion to be treated is close to the skin, it is often necessary that the skin should receive the full tumour dose. In such a case, with megavoltage treatments, 'build-up' material ('bolus') is deliberately placed on the skin to secure the desired end.

reduction in the radiation reaching P and Q when the compensating block is transferred from position I to position II.

For kilovoltage radiation the contribution of scattered radiation can be quite considerable and therefore true compensation can only be achieved by using block I.

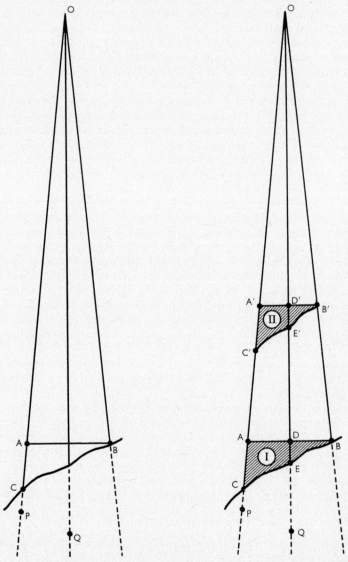

Fig. 356.—The need for, and principle of, the tissue compensator.

With megavoltage radiation the scatter contribution is so small that block II gives acceptable compensation for all points—except those close to the surface. Close to the surface, of course, there will be the usual 'build-up' of dose with megavoltage radiations. Elsewhere the isodose curves will be those indicated by the standard isodose charts.

Compensators in Practice.—In the kilovoltage range, compensation such as that provided by block I in *Fig*. 356 is achieved by the use of unit density wax, or 'Lincolnshire Bolus', or other similar material, in bags. Such materials are obviously unsuitable for megavoltage compensation because of the difficulty of maintaining the required thickness whilst 'shrinking' the lateral dimensions to suit the position for the compensator.

Nor, of course, is it essential to maintain the same thickness of compensator. What, in fact, is needed is that the attenuation in A'C' or D'E' should be the same as

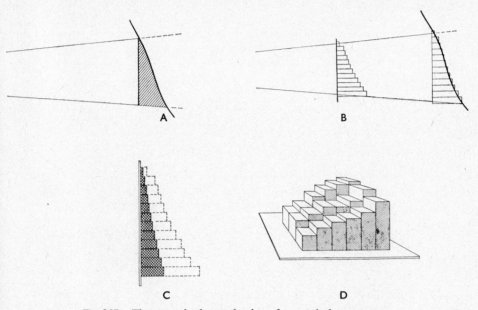

Fig. 357.—The stages in the production of a practical compensator.

the attenuation in AC or DE; a smaller thickness of a more attenuating material would be equally acceptable. Hence aluminium or even brass is usually used in these devices.

The practical design of a compensator will be more readily understood if considered, with the aid of *Fig*. 357, in three separate stages. First, the material indicated by the shading in *Fig*. 357 A can be replaced by a series of square-section 'sticks' (*Fig*. 357 B). The replacement is not exact, having a castellated instead of a smooth outline, but the differences are negligible in their effect. In practice, if used in this position, each 'stick' would have an end-section 15 mm. square. However, since the actual compensator is placed at, say, 80 cm. instead of 100 from the source, as shown in *Fig*. 357 B, the necessary 'shrinkage' would be achieved with 'sticks' which are 12 mm. square (12 mm. $= \frac{80}{100} \times 15$). This completes the second stage. The third involves the replacement of the unit density material, which by implication, at least, has been discussed so far, with some more practicable material—say aluminium. Instead, therefore, of the 'sticks' in the compensator being of the same length as those close to the skin, they are of such shorter lengths as would provide the same attenuation (*Fig*. 357 C).

Having produced the correct lengths they must be carefully and correctly assembled and positioned in the beam. To this end they are screwed or glued on to a base-plate which fits into an accurately reproducible position on the X-ray tube or gamma-ray beam unit. Although this description has been confined to compensation in one plane, that of the paper, compensation must apply in all planes, and a completed compensator will appear something like that shown diagrammatically in *Fig.* 357 D.

'Wedge' Filters.—There are often situations in radiotherapy when it is desirable to treat from one side of the patient only, though it is necessary to use more than one beam. A typical example could be a lesion of the middle ear, for which treatment by two beams angled as shown in *Fig.* 358 might be contemplated. Unfortunately, this approach gives a very inhomogeneous dose pattern over the zone common

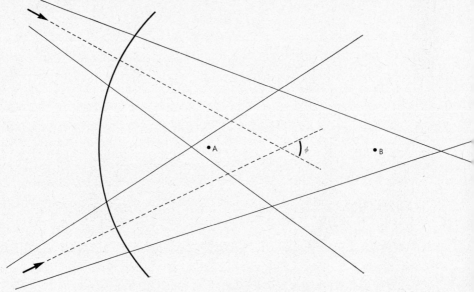

Fig. 358.—The need for a 'wedge' filter.

to both fields, the dose falling steadily from left to right. The reason for this inhomogeneity can clearly be seen by considering just two points, A and B. The former is not only closer to both radiation sources than is B, but also radiation reaching A will have traversed less tissue, and hence suffered less attenuation than that reaching B. Hence the dose at A is greater than that at B.

What is needed is some form of beam modification that will reduce the dose contributions to A relative to those to B, with proportional reductions for points in between. And this can be done by using what are usually called 'wedge' filters, which turn through an angle θ (the value of which depends upon the design of the filter) isodose curves which normally cut the central axis at right-angles.

It can be shown that if the isodose curves for two intersecting fields lie parallel to one another (usually they intersect) then a considerable proportion of the zone common to both fields will be uniformly irradiated. The dose distribution patterns produced by normal (often called 'plain') beams and those incorporating 'wedge' filters are shown in *Fig.* 359. The treatment is that already indicated in *Fig.* 358 and the left-hand drawings refer to plain beams. *Fig.* 359 A shows how the plain isodose curves intersect, whilst the sketch below it shows the falling dose pattern already discussed. For the right-hand sketches 'wedge' fields are used and *Fig.*

359 B indicates that the modifying filters have been chosen so that the isodose curves from the two fields run parallel to one another, thus producing uniform irradiation over a considerable part of the zone of overlap, as the lower part shows.

The purpose of this type of beam-modifying attenuation is to change the cross-field radiation distribution from the normal, which is symmetrical about the central

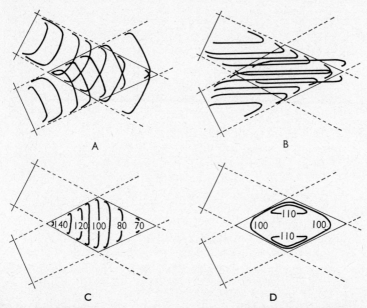

Fig. 359.—Isodose charts for a pair of fields: A, Using normal beams, and B, Beams modified by 'wedge' filters. Upper diagrams show basic curves. Lower diagrams show final distribution.

axis, has been illustrated previously, and is shown again in *Fig.* 360, into one where the dose progressively falls from one side of the beam to the other, as *Fig.* 360 also shows. To achieve this the attenuator (or filter as it is more usually called) is thicker at one end and tapers to nothing at the other: in other words, it is wedge-shaped, and hence the name usually applied to it.

Whilst 'wedge' filters have been successfully applied to both kilovoltage and megavoltage beams (they were first devised by Drs. Ellis and Miller of Sheffield, for kilovoltage beams), their chief value, and almost exclusive modern use, is with mega-voltage radiations. Just as with 'beam-flattening' filters, the considerable amount of scattered radiation associated with a kilovoltage beam in a patient makes modification difficult. For example, the angle through which the beam is turned changes with depth (gradually getting smaller) and there is generally a rather large 'hot spot'—high dose zone—near the surface. With megavoltage beams neither of these effects is large enough to be important. Furthermore, the design of filters to produce curves at any particular angle is not difficult, since whatever changes are made in the primary beam (and these can be calculated if the attenuation coefficient and relevant thickness of the 'wedge' filter are known) are almost exactly reproduced in the total doses.

The material used for 'wedge' filters is relatively unimportant especially in the megavoltage range since there is no question of 'hardening' of the beam and, weight for weight, almost all materials attenuate to the same extent. Local convenience and the availability of material will often be the deciding factors rather than any physical properties. Aluminium, copper, brass, or lead are most used, the denser materials having the advantage over the less dense if space is at a premium, since they give thinner filters than does aluminium.

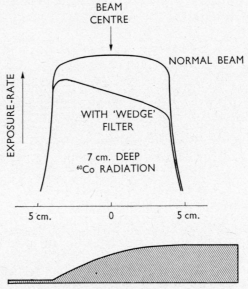

Fig. 360.—The variation of Exposure rate across a beam without and with a 'wedge' filter with a sketch of the 'profile' of the filter.

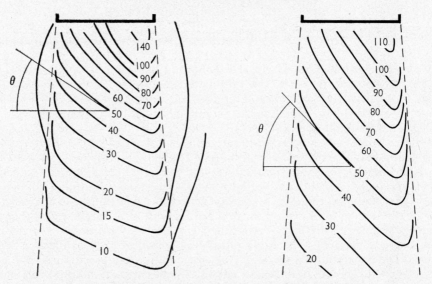

Fig. 361.—Isodose charts for a 250-kV. and a 4-MV. X-ray beam.

In *Fig.* 361 typical 'wedge' filter isodose charts for kilovoltage and megavoltage beams are given, and the 'wedge isodose angle' or 'wedge angle' (θ) is indicated. This angle has been described by the International Commission on Radiological Units as 'the complement of the angle which the isodose curve for 50 per cent makes with the central ray', but equally well, and perhaps more understandably, it can be described as the angle through which the 50 per cent isodose curve has been turned from its position in a normal beam. It will be noted that a particular curve is specified: this is necessary with kilovoltage beams because the angle of isodose curve slope varies with depth. As has been said, this variation is much smaller with megavoltage beams. (*See Fig*. 361.)

An important question that now has to be answered concerns the values of θ which are needed in clinical practice. Geometric considerations show that the value of θ depends on the angle ϕ—*see Fig*. 358—between the central rays of the two intersecting fields. This angle is usually called the 'hinge angle' and its relationship to θ to satisfy the condition required for uniform dosage, i.e., parallel isodose curves, is:

$$\theta = 90 - \phi/2.$$

Thus if the fields are at right-angles to one another ($\phi = 90°$) the wedge angle should be 45° and, to take an extreme case, if $\phi = 180°$ (that is to say the fields are opposite one another—a 'parallel opposed pair') $\theta = 0$, which means that normal isodose curves are needed.

Theoretically, the formula requires a different value of θ, i.e., a different isodose chart and hence a different filter, for every value of ϕ that is used. Fortunately, however, to produce a high dose zone which is clinically acceptable (over which there is a variation of no more than ± 5 per cent, say) it is not necessary for the isodose curves to be strictly parallel. With any 'wedge' filter there is a small range of 'hinge angle' values for which satisfactorily uniform distributions are obtained. Furthermore, the range of values of ϕ normally employed is somewhat limited and it is found that three 'wedge' filters (giving values of θ of about 35, 45, and 55°) will cope with the large majority of practical situations.

Theoretically, too, there should, for each value of θ, be a different 'wedge' filter for each field size, but again the small amount of scattered radiation associated with megavoltage beams simplifies the problem for that energy range (the only range to which wedge filters are seriously applied, now) and it is possible to use the same filter for a range of field sizes. There is, in fact, a small steady reduction of θ with increasing field size, but this offers no real disadvantage—in the first place it is only a few degrees over the range of fields used, and furthermore the isodose charts for each field size will indicate the angle θ for that field, so that treatment planning is on an accurate basis.

Firstly for this reason, but even more for a reason best explained with the aid of *Fig*. 362, it is not usual to use one filter for a very wide range of fields. The 'wedge' filter XYZ produces isodose curves with the same 'wedge angle' for both the large and small fields shown (and, of course, for other sizes as well). However, for the smaller field only the portion ABC is producing any 'wedge' effect. The extra material ACDE simply attenuates equally all parts of the beam and so merely reduces the output for that field size. Using the same filter for too great a range of field sizes, therefore, merely reduces unnecessarily the output efficiency of the smaller fields. Usually one filter is used for fields up to about 10 cm. long, and another for the larger fields.

The importance of exact positioning of 'beam-flattening' filters has already been stressed: with 'wedge' filters the need is just as great but the problem is, in general, more difficult because it is more complicated. For any radiation source there is usually only one 'beam-flattening' filter and that is fixed to the apparatus. On the other hand, a number of 'wedge' filters are usually available with each machine, and many treatments will be carried out with none of them in the beam. Therefore provision has to be made not only for exact positioning, but also to ensure that the filter is in the right way round, and also that the correct filter is used. Much thought has been given to the prevention of the serious consequences which could flow from any of the errors

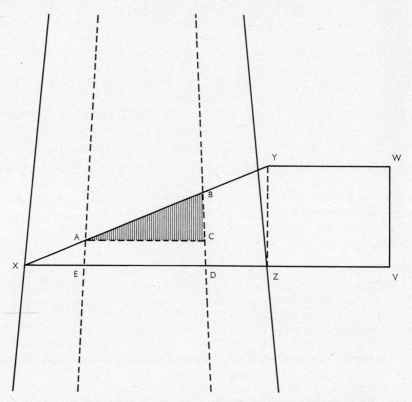

Fig. 362.—The 'inefficiency' of using one 'wedge' filter for all beam sizes.

inferred in the above and a number of ingenious systems have been described in the radiological literature. In this book it must suffice to stress that in this as in all other aspects of the use of radiations on patients, the 'price of safety is eternal vigilance'.

CHAPTER XXXV

COLLIMATORS AND 'BEAM-DIRECTION' DEVICES

WHEN isodose curves and isodose patterns have been discussed and described in earlier chapters it has been assumed that radiation beams, confined to the desired size and shape, were available. So far, however, no indication has been given as to how this desired effect can be achieved.

Even though the size of the *useful* beam may be restricted by the 'heel effect' with kilovoltage radiations and by the tendency of megavoltage photons to be emitted in the direction of the electron stream, some radiation is given out in every direction, and even the useful beam is far greater than is needed for most treatments.* Because radiation damages all tissues, it is obviously desirable to keep the irradiation of normal tissues as small as possible, and one way of doing this is to use beams which are just big enough to irradiate the desired zone, and no bigger. Methods have, therefore, to be found of producing beams of the shapes and sizes called for by the radiotherapist —in other words, the radiation must be *collimated*. In practice this is usually achieved in two stages, which might be described as Master, or Fixed, and Treatment, or Movable, Collimation. The general aim—never completely achieved, of course—is to have uniform irradiation over the whole area of the beam, and none outside the beam. Usually there is a falling-off of Exposure rate towards the beam edge, as already discussed, and a 'leak' of radiation of about 0·5 per cent of the beam intensity through the collimating materials.

THE MASTER, OR FIXED, COLLIMATION

Fig. 363 illustrates three aspects of the problem with which this part of the collimation system has to deal. Because of the 'heel effect' it is not usually possible, for X-ray tubes operating at kilovoltages, to produce satisfactory beam symmetry about the central axis for beams with a total angle of more than 30°—that is of about 15° on either side of the central ray. Nevertheless, as *Fig*. 363 A indicates, radiation is emitted in other directions and it is necessary to prevent any of this from reaching the patient, to whom it would serve no useful purpose and only do harm.

To remove this radiation the tube is surrounded, except for a thin 'window', with sufficient lead for the purpose: there are many ways in which this is done, one of which is shown in *Fig*. 363 A. There the X-ray tube is mounted in a metal box (which also serves to contain the insulating, and possibly cooling, oil associated with the running of the tube—*see* CHAPTER XXXVIII), which is lined with lead except for a small area through which the useful beam emerges. An alternative that has been used is to construct the main body of the tube of lead glass, which is highly attenuating, and only allow radiation to escape through a thin 'window' of the much less attenuating soda glass.

In the megavoltage range the maximum beam size usually accepted is one for which the primary exposure rate at the edge is 50 per cent of that at the centre. With 4-MV. radiation, for example, the beam falls off to 50 per cent of its central value at about

---

* Radio-isotope teletherapy units are even worse, since radioactive materials emit their radiations isotropically (equally in all directions).

10°—in other words, the beam angle is about 20°. Again, however, as shown in *Fig.* 363 B, radiation is emitted in other directions and this also has to be prevented from reaching the patient, and this again is achieved by shrouding the source with a sufficient—which in this case is several inches—thickness of lead, through a hole in which the useful beam emerges.

With the so-called telecurie radioactive isotope sources which provide beams of high-energy gamma rays, and for most purposes can be considered as X-ray machines,

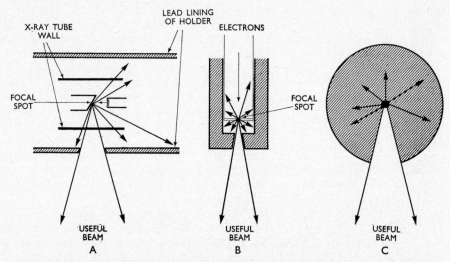

Fig. 363.—Master, or fixed, collimation. A, Kilovoltage tube (with 'reflection' target). B, Megavoltage tube (with 'transmission' target). C, Radioactive isotope telecurie unit. In each case only radiation emitted over a relatively small angle is used; the rest is cut off by the collimation.

the problem is rather different. Since radiation is emitted equally in all directions, there is no limitation upon the beam size such as is imposed by the 'heel' effect on kilovoltage beams and, by the natural forward emission, on megavoltage beams. However, there is a limit set by the need to keep the movable collimation to a reasonable size, and in practice the beam has an angle of about 20°. The fixed collimation in this case is provided (in principle at least) by having the source at the centre of a sphere of lead (*see Fig.* 363 C) from which a cone running to the centre has been removed for the emergence of the largest beam that the apparatus can give.

Table XLIII.—MAXIMUM BEAM SIZES (WHICH ARE EASIER TO VISUALIZE) FOR THE DIFFERENT BEAM ANGLES

Source	Maximum Angle used	Maximum Field Size
250-kV. X-rays	30°	27-cm. diam. circle at 50 cm. S.S.D.
^{60}Co γ-rays	20°	26-cm. diam. circle at 75 cm. S.S.D.
4-MV. X-rays	20°	35-cm. diam. circle at 100 cm. S.S.D.*

* Usually, for other reasons, the maximum field size is restricted to about 26 cm. diameter.

The master, or fixed, collimator then protects the bulk of the patient from radiation and dictates the maximum beam size that the source can give. This is greater than is needed for the majority of treatments—it is usually circular and of diameter between 20 and 30 cm., as *Table XLIII* shows. Therefore some means have to be provided for obtaining the various shapes and sizes of beam required for radiotherapy. This is done by means of the Treatment, or Movable, Collimation, of which there are two main forms.

TREATMENT, OR MOVABLE, COLLIMATION

The Applicator.—A typical design of treatment 'applicator' or 'cone' is shown as a photograph and as a diagram in *Fig.* 364. As will be seen from that illustration, it has a metal plate which positions it in guides over the X-ray 'window' of the tube for which it is used. Immediately under this plate is a sheet of lead several millimetres thick (the precise thickness depending upon the energy of X-rays with which the

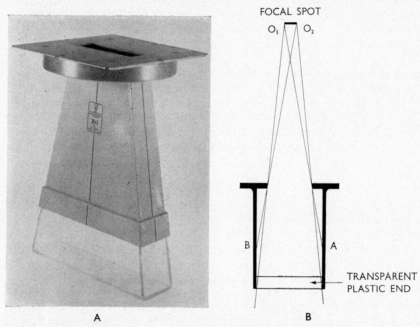

A   B

Fig. 364.—A typical treatment applicator for radiation generated at about 250 kV.

applicator is to be used) with a hole of appropriate size and shape cut into it. This layer of lead provides the major collimation, cutting out more than 99 per cent of the radiation incident upon it. Also attached to the top plate is a wooden or steel 'box' whose lower end is usually closed with a thin transparent plastic cap. When wood is used in this part it is provided with a lead lining, often with a thin layer of copper and aluminium on the inside to remove characteristic radiation that may be emitted from the lead when absorbing incident X-ray energy. Because the top layer of lead provides the main collimation and also because any rays striking the side do so at an oblique angle, the thickness of lead or of steel required in it is quite small, and most modern applicators now have walls of steel of about 1·5 mm. thick.

The steel, or lead-lined wooden, box serves three purposes, the first of which is demonstrated in *Fig.* 364. As has been emphasized, the main collimation is performed by the thick lead plate, but because the source of radiation is never a point source, the beam passing through the hole in that plate will always have some penumbra. When the hole in the lead is correctly cut and positioned, this penumbral radiation (rays O_1A and O_2B in the diagram, for example) strikes the applicator sides and is effectively removed. The box, therefore, serves a very useful purpose in reducing the penumbra which inevitably occurs.

Applicators also play an important role in the achievement of accurate treatment dosage. Not only do they indicate immediately the size and shape of the beam being used, and its position on the skin, but they also give a useful indication of its direction. More important, however, they position the patient at the desired distance from the tube and show whether or not this distance has been maintained.

Positioning is made easier if guide marks on the skin, for example, can be seen during the 'setting-up' process, and for this reason it has become common practice that the last few centimetres of the applicator should be made of some transparent material, usually plastic, as the diagrams indicate. This plastic material also closes the applicator end and thus enables the applicator to serve yet another purpose. This is to provide what is usually called 'compression', though in fact it is quite often the pushing aside of tissues rather than actually compressing them. It is always advantageous to bring the applicator end, and hence the X-ray focus, as close as possible to the tumour, thus increasing the percentage depth dose to the tumour. This can be achieved in parts of the body where no bony structures intervene, by pressing the applicator end into the tissues. Some mobile tissues are pushed aside by this, others are somewhat compressed (but not sufficiently to push the tumour deeper too, which would vitiate the whole procedure), thus reducing the skin to tumour distance as desired. A further advantage of 'compression' is that it helps to immobilize the patient during treatment—an important factor in accurate radiotherapy.

In superficial therapy—using X-rays generated at up to 150 kV.—compression is, of course, quite unnecessary since only superficial lesions are being treated and therefore open-ended applicators are usually used.

It will be clear that there must be a separate applicator for each beam size and shape that is used, which means that some 20 or 30 are usually called for. If some beam shape other than that provided by the available applicators is required, it can be achieved by cutting an appropriately sized and shaped hole in a sheet of lead, usually 2 mm. thick at 250 kV., and placing this between the end of an applicator, giving a rather larger field, and the skin. This, however, should be regarded as an expedient and should not be used as a reason for not having an adequate range of beam sizes: neither should the fairly high cost of the applicators—about £30 each.

This cost should, however, be one reason—though not the most important—for treating applicators with care. The more important reason, of course, is that mishandling can easily damage them, resulting in their being distorted and so giving different field shapes, or, if the box is bent in any way, giving a misleading impression of the direction of the beam.

Movable Diaphragms.—Applicators for use with 250-kV. (or thereabouts) radiations weigh some 9 or 10 lb., and therefore—though not light—the labour involved in lifting them on and off the tubes as different beam sizes are called for is not unduly great.

The situation is quite different with megavoltage beams, where the thickness of lead required for satisfactory collimation is measured in centimetres rather than millimetres. Any applicator of the type just described would therefore be far too heavy to be lifted on and off the tube, let alone carried about. The various field sizes needed are therefore provided by movable diaphragms, rather than by a series of separate applicators.

Typical movable diaphragms are those used on the 4-MV. linear accelerator, their main features being illustrated in *Fig.* 365. This diagram, of course, only shows one pair of 'jaws', the other pair moving in the direction at right-angles to the plane of the

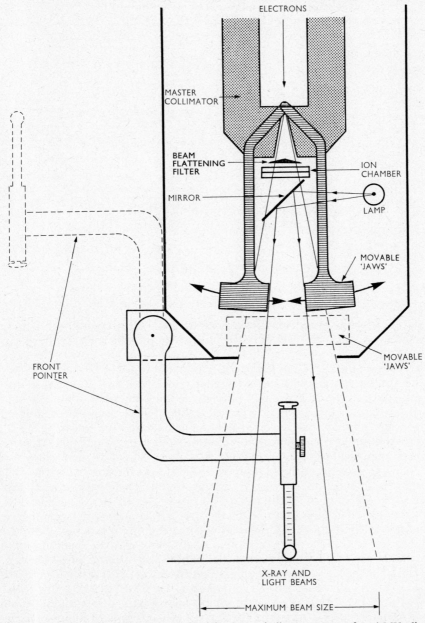

Fig. 365.—Adjustable diaphragms and light beam indicator system for 4-MV. linear accelerator. The 'front pointer' is also shown in its operative and (dotted) retracted positions.

paper, and being immediately above or below (in the case illustrated) the other pair. Such an arrangement can, of course, only yield rectangular or square fields. Where circular fields are called for (and their use is becoming rarer in modern radiotherapy) they are usually provided by trapping, between the movable jaws, a square-sectioned block of lead in which the appropriate conical hole has been drilled.

The jaws are usually blocks of lead which by a suitable mechanical linkage can be made to move in and out at the turn of a handle (each pair is, of course, adjustable separately). It is also arranged so that the jaws move in such a way that their inner

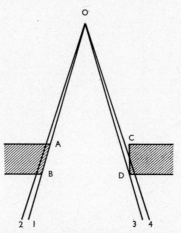

Fig. 366.—Diaphragm face design.

faces always lie on lines radiating from the focal spot. The reason for this, and the advantage it provides, are demonstrated in *Fig.* 366, in which the left-hand jaw is shown with its face AB along a radial line, whereas the right-hand jaw has its face CD parallel to the central ray. If the desired beam is that bounded by OB and OD it will be clear that the 'cut-off' provided by the left-hand jaw will be much sharper than that by the right-hand jaw. Ray 2 has to pass through the whole thickness of the collimation, whereas ray 4 passes through quite a limited amount. Since the geometric perfection shown for the left-hand jaw is never attained in practice—for one thing the focal spot is never a perfect point source—it is usual to place strips, a centimetre or so wide, of copper-tungsten alloy on the inner faces of the jaws. This alloy, often called 'heavy alloy', because of its great density, is superior to lead as an attenuator and the 'facing' gives a greater attenuation for any rays, like ray 4, which try to pass through the jaws in a direction which is not strictly radial.

Another reason why movable diaphragms rather than applicators are used with megavoltage radiations is that with such diaphragms no solid material is introduced into the beam, so that the collimation does not interfere with the 'build-up' of dose below the surface of the irradiated material or the 'skin-sparing' effect which is an advantage of these high-energy radiations. (*See*, for example, CHAPTER XXXIII.) This feature of moving diaphragms is often quoted as the main reason for their use: in fact, it is a minor advantage which, as will be shown later in this chapter, is often forgone for important reasons. The main reason why this form of collimation is used is because applicators would be too heavy to handle.

A major disadvantage of this arrangement is that it gives no immediate indication of the size or shape of the beam, nor of its position on the skin, neither does it provide any method of ensuring that the patient is at the correct distance from the tube—

that is to say, that the correct S.S.D. is being used. It is also unable to provide compression, which is a useful contribution of the applicator.

The handles used for opening and closing the jaws usually have dials attached to them and these indicate the field size at the normal working S.S.D. However, a more useful indication of the field size and, at the same time, of its position on the skin, is provided by a light beam shining through the jaw system. A lamp is placed to one side of the collimating system and by means of a mirror a beam of light is reflected through the collimation, as shown in *Fig.* 365. The distance from the lamp to the mirror is made to be effectively equal to the distance from the X-ray focus to the mirror, so that the size and shape of the light patch on any surface indicate the size and shape of the X-ray beam there.

Protruding from the left-hand side of the body of the X-ray tube in *Fig.* 365 is an arm carrying a rod, a device usually called the 'front pointer'. This arm, as indicated in the diagram, can be swung round into the path of the X-ray beam and its purpose is to indicate when the correct S.S.D. is being used. It is usually so arranged that, with the rod in its lowest position and the ball end just touching the skin, the patient is at the normal S.S.D. Greater distances can be measured by using a longer rod; shorter distances by retracting the rod whose side is scaled to indicate the distances being used. The arm and rod are swung out of the beam before treatment commences.

When it is possible that the distance set may not be maintained during the treatment because of patient movement, or where 'compression' is called for, a perspex or other plastic material applicator box is often attached to the tube end. This does not, of course, play any part in collimation, being bigger than the beam size in use, but merely acts as a distance piece and possibly a compressor. Though the thin end of such a device—it need not be more than 1 or 2 mm.—does increase the skin dose to some extent, the effect is not large, and the benefits gained outweigh the loss.

The Penumbra.—The object of collimation is to produce a beam of some required size and shape, and a desirable feature of such a beam is that it should have as sharp an edge as possible—i.e., the smallest possible penumbra. In practice, there will always be some penumbra, firstly because there is inevitably some leakage of radiation through the collimators (as explained in earlier chapters, it is impossible to stop completely any beam attenuated according to the exponential law), and secondly because of geometric factors. General 'leakage' penumbra is reduced by using adequately thick collimating blocks and is usually less than 0·1 to 1 per cent of the Exposure rate of the main beam. However, there is also the leakage through the edges of the collimating blocks, as illustrated in *Fig.* 366; this, too, can be reduced by using greater thicknesses, but also by proper collimator edge design, as the diagram shows, and also, in some cases, by 'facing' the blocks with an especially good attenuator, like heavy copper-tungsten alloy.

The geometric situation is illustrated in *Fig.* 367, for the purposes of which it is assumed that no diaphragm leakage occurs. The left-hand side of the diagram shows what happens with a point source (an ideal collimator)—there is no penumbra, the beam having a sharp edge. Such a situation never occurs in practice, for the radiation source always has a finite size, and a more practical situation is shown on the right-hand side of the diagram. From this, and the accompanying formula, it will be seen that the size of the penumbra (P) depends first of all on the size of the source (S): quite simply, the bigger the source the greater the penumbra. In addition, the penumbral size depends on the ratio of the distances of the diaphragm from the plane of interest and the source. Broadly speaking, the nearer the diaphragm is to the plane of interest, the smaller the penumbra there. For any diaphragm position, the further away one goes the greater the penumbra.

The minimum penumbra in radiotherapy is obtained when the final diaphragm is on the skin. As far as the skin is concerned, then H = 0 and there is no penumbra at the skin. From this point of view the applicator, with its final defining material within a centimetre or so of the surface, is superior to the movable diaphragm. In turn, that

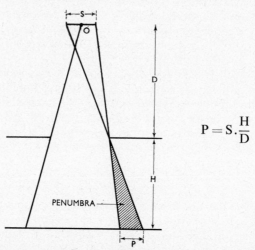

$$P = S \cdot \frac{H}{D}$$

Fig. 367.—The production of penumbra. Left-hand side—point source. Right-hand side—extended source.

device is best placed as close to the skin as possible—usually not closer than 15 cm. with megavoltage radiations if 'build up' is to be preserved—and will be more efficient with large units (D larger) than smaller ones.

Two other points arise from this geometrical analysis. The first is that the beam edge defined by the jaws illustrated in *Fig.* 335 will have a larger penumbra than the edge defined by the pair at right-angles, which are closer to the surface and further from the source. The second point is more important, and is that no matter what collimating system is used, there will always be some penumbra below the skin, and the magnitude of this will increase with increasing depth. But like any other penumbra, it will be smaller the closer the diaphragms are to the skin and the smaller the source size.

Beam Size.—The usual statement of beam size refers to its dimensions on the entrance surface or, more strictly, its dimensions on a plane at right-angles to the central ray at the usual S.S.D. In the case of an applicator this is easy to determine since it is the inside dimensions of the box which finally define the beam dimensions.

With movable diaphragms, at a distance from the skin, the situation is much more difficult since, in this case, there may be considerable penumbra at the skin level. Where, then, is the beam edge? Because it is ill-defined, a number of different conventions have been suggested—for example, that the position of the 80, 85, or 90 per cent isodose line should be used to mark the edge—but that likely to be most generally adopted is the geometrical definition recommended by the International Commission on Radiological Units. This runs as follows: 'The geometrical field size is the geometric projection on a plane perpendicular to the central axis, of the distal end (i.e., the end nearest the patient) of the limited diaphragm as seen from the centre of the front surface of the source'. Should this seem rather pedantic, and difficult to understand, it is hoped that *Fig.* 368 will make the principle clear.

In this diagram the source is assumed to be a cylinder of some radioactive material, and the diaphragm a rectangular hole in a sheet of lead. As required by the definition,

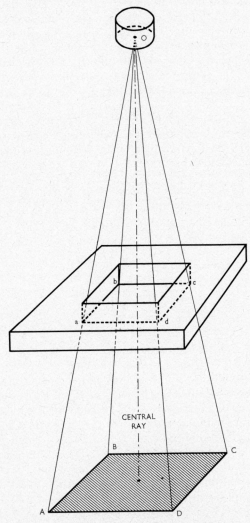

Fig. 368.—The geometric definition of field size.

the geometrical beam size ABCD is defined by lines from the source face centre O, and the corners abcd of the lower edge of the hole. The edge, so defined, is roughly in the middle of the penumbra and roughly at the 50 per cent isodose line but outside the 80 or 90 per cent lines, which are generally regarded as being the limits of the useful beam. Therefore the geometrical beam is greater than the useful or 'physical beam'.

The difference is negligible for beams with applicators where the last diaphragm is at or near the skin, and also for linear accelerators or betatrons where the focal spot is very small and the source to diaphragm distance quite large. For radioactive isotope telecurie units, however, where the source may be 2 cm. in diameter, the skin penumbra is quite large and the useful beam may be as much as 1 cm. smaller each way than the geometric beam.

So far attention has been directed to skin fields—beneath the skin there is always penumbra, no matter what collimating system is used, and therefore the beam size at any depth becomes increasingly less certain. The beam diverges as depth increases, but if it is accepted that the width of the useful beam is the distance between the points at which the dose has fallen to 90 per cent of the central value at that depth, then the useful beam width remains practically constant at all depths. However, this is only an approximation to the truth and the only completely satisfactory guide to beam width anywhere is the appropriate isodose curve.

BEAM DIRECTION

In order to reduce to a minimum the unnecessary irradiation of a patient, the beam sizes chosen for a treatment should be the minimum needed to cover the desired treatment zone. This implies that such beams must be accurately aimed towards the

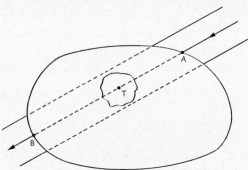

Fig. 369.—Entrance and exit points of a beam.

zone: a relatively small misdirection will result in the underdosage of some parts and the consequent failure of treatment. The most uniform and best conceived treatment plans are of little value unless they can be achieved on the patient. Accurate aiming of X-ray beams is easier with applicators than with movable diaphragms because the box of the applicator gives some indication of the beam's direction. This is not, however, very accurate since quite small angular positional errors produce quite big movements at, say, 10 cm. deep. For example, for that depth a beam edge displacement of nearly 4 mm. results from an angle error of a mere 2°. This is more than can be accepted in accurate work, which therefore calls for the use of beam-directing devices, the two principal of which will be described. For each it will be assumed that the position of the zone to be treated is accurately known; the methods by which this knowledge is acquired, however, are outside the scope of this book.

The Front and Back Pointers Method.—Any line can be defined by two points and this method of beam direction requires the identification and marking, on the patient's surface, of two points lying on a line passing through the tumour centre. Such points are usually established with the aid of radiography, and if it can be arranged that the central ray of the beam enters through one of these points A (the entrance point) and leaves through the second B (the exit point), then, as *Fig.* 369 shows, the ray must pass through the tumour centre T. This is achieved by using front and back, or entrance and exit, 'pointers'.

The simplest and most readily available front pointer for kilovoltage radiation is the treatment applicator which usually carries a small nipple in the centre of its end-plate and this can be brought in contact with A to define the entrance point of the central ray. (The nipple can be removed if the applicator is used for compression in other treatments.) Where no applicator is used (as in the case of megavoltage radiations) the movable distance indicator already described above and illustrated in *Fig.* 365 serves as the front pointer. It is designed so that its adjustable rod lies in the

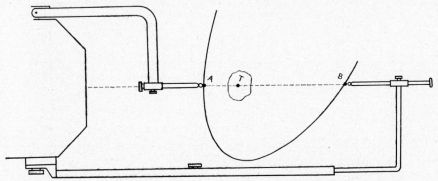

Fig. 370.—Front and back pointers being used to define the direction of a beam.

central axis of the beam and its role in beam direction is exactly the same as that of the applicator. *Fig.* 370 shows it in position, ensuring that the central ray enters through A. It is, of course, drawn aside out of the beam during treatment, though the back pointer can remain in position.

That the central ray enters through A does not guarantee that it passes through T—unless it is known to pass through B; it is to ensure this that the back pointer is used, as shown in *Fig.* 370.

A typical design of this most valuable of beam-direction devices is shown in *Fig.* 371, which also shows an applicator, carrying the nipple N, in position on the tube. Two rigid metal rods (R) are connected together at one end by a plate (A) through a hole in which runs a third rod (B) connected to a simple carriage (C) which can slide along R and be clamped in any position by means of the screw (D). The other end of B carries a metal sleeve (E) through which another rod (F) can be slid backwards and forwards, and locked in any position by the screw (G). The rod (F) is arranged to lie accurately on the central ray of the beam when the whole device is firmly attached to the tube body at M.

This combination of front and back pointers provides the most accurate method of beam direction easily available, provided the points A and B can be accurately determined and their positions maintained.

The Entrance and Exit Points.—In this discussion so far, it has been tacitly assumed that the entrance and exit points, A and B, were marked on the patient's skin. This would be neither very satisfactory in the long run nor accurate at any time. Marks of this sort might easily be removed between treatments—by washing, etc.—and be inaccurately replaced—but much more important is the fact that the skin moves very easily over the underlying tissues and therefore the position of skin marks relative to the tumour centre could well be altered during the positioning of a patient and the whole accuracy of set-up thereby destroyed. It is, therefore, normal to make for the patient a 'shell' of some plastic material which fits, very closely and accurately, the part being treated and can be put on and taken off quite easily. This shell then carries the marks for the entrance and exit points, usually of all the beams used in the treatment. Examples of two such shells are shown in *Fig.* 372. That on the left is for

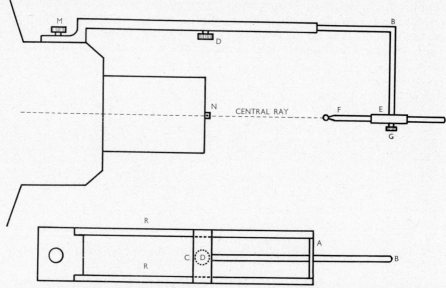

Fig. 371.—Detail of one form of back pointer.

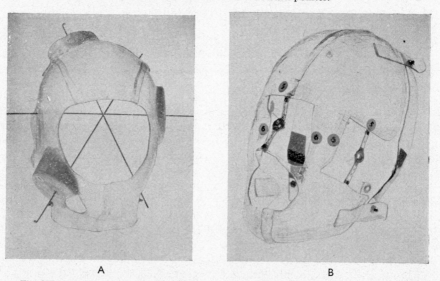

A   B

Fig. 372.—Two beam-direction 'shells'. **A**, For kilovoltage therapy, showing obliquity-compensating wax blocks. Note also intersection of the central rays as shown by the wires. **B**, For megavoltage therapy, showing as much material as possible removed from entrance points of beam. Note the entrance and exit points of the central rays.

kilovoltage radiation, and not only carries the entrance and exit marks for the fields being used but also blocks of wax, to compensate, as described in CHAPTER XXXIII, for the obliquity with which the beam enters the patient and for the curvature of the surface. The right-hand 'shell' is for use with a megavoltage beam and it will be noted that most of the plastic material near the entrance point has been cut away, in order to preserve, as much as possible, the 'build-up' and 'skin-sparing' features of megavoltage beams.

Because of the unreliability of the skin to carry marks, and the general mobility of abdominal tissues, the back pointer method is normally used for sites above the diaphragm and on limbs—that is to say, when there are bony structures over which reproducible 'anchorage' of the shell can be obtained. It should be noted that the back pointer method is unsuitable for treatment where compression is used.

Reproducibility.—As it has been described, the system is accurately reproducible from day to day especially if the shell is accurately made of material that does not warp or distort—perspex or cellulose acetate in sheet form is very acceptable. However, it is very important that the back pointer and either the applicator nipple or the front pointer should remain on the central axis. Even the most rigid device may be distorted in use, so that great care is called for in handling this equipment and the correctness of its alinement must be frequently checked. How this may be done will be described in CHAPTER XXXIX.

The 'Pin and Arc'.—Like the front and back pointer method, this widely used aid to accurate beam direction was first developed by Dr. J. L. Dobbie at the Christie Hospital, Manchester. It is particularly used when the treatment of lesions in the trunk of a recumbent patient requires beams whose exit points may be inaccessible to the back pointer, and also where some degree of compression is being used. For palliative work it is useful for a quick set-up in situations where the tumour position is only approximately known. The 'pin and arc' is most widely used for abdominal tumours, such as those of the bladder or uterine cervix, but there are lung tumours which are also appropriately treated with the aid of this device.

Fig. 373 illustrates the main features of the device. A ruler-like scaled bar, R, is firmly fastened to the X-ray tube housing and along it slides a frame S to which is equally firmly fastened an annular strip of metal, 'the arc', T, which is part of the arc of a circle whose centre lies on the central axis of the beam. On this strip another carriage, U, can move freely or can be clamped in any position. This carriage carries a tubular sleeve in which runs, or can be clamped in any position, the rod or 'pin', V, whose length is such that when it is at its lowest position its lower end is on the central axis and at O, the centre of curvature of T. The pin is usually scaled in centimetres and half-centimetres so that the amount (d) by which its end is moved away from the centre can be read off, as shown in the dotted part of *Fig.* 373, which shows the carriage moved along T, and V withdrawn d cm. It should also be noted that the distance (D) from O to the applicator end is indicated by the reading on bar R. Another scale, not shown on this diagram because it is on the back face of T, enables the angle between the pin V and the central axis to be read off.

How the 'pin and arc' is used, and the geometry underlying this use, is shown in *Fig.* 374. By some means of localization the depth, d, of the tumour centre, O, below some surface mark or feature, M, has been determined. It should be noted that O need not be on the midline of the patient, as it happens to be in this case—the device and method are applicable to any site. The pin is withdrawn the required distance d, and its lower end brought in contact with the surface mark known to be vertically above O. Now, so long as the pin is vertical the rest of the equipment, and especially the applicator, will rotate about O, the arc running through the stationary carriage. At the same time the central ray will always pass through O; thus, keeping the pin vertical and in contact with M, any particular angle θ can be selected.

The pin carriage is then clamped and kept stationary whilst the applicator is moved towards, or away from, O until the desired position is obtained—with

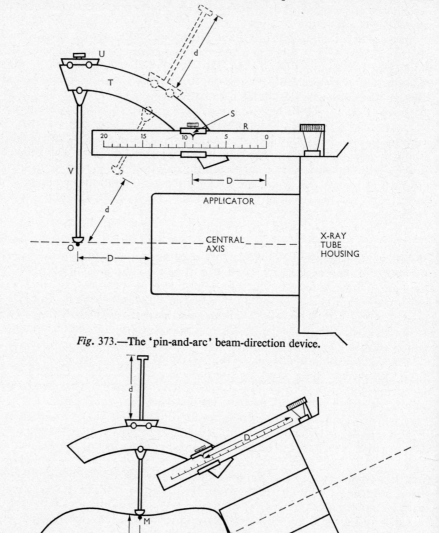

Fig. 373.—The 'pin-and-arc' beam-direction device.

Fig. 374.—The geometrical principles of the use of the 'pin and arc'.

compression if desired. The distance D can be read off the scale or the bar: this distance is, of course, important for dose computation purposes because it is the depth of the tumour in the particular field being directed.

The Isocentric Mounting and 'Pin and Arc'.—One important advance in X-ray tube, or radioactive isotope telecurie source, mounting design is the isocentric mounting, first used by Flanders and Newbery of the Hammersmith Hospital for the early linear accelerators. In this, as shown in *Fig.* 375, the X-ray tube or telecurie source moves in an arc around the patient about an axis which (in the case of the linear accelerator) is 100 cm. from the focal spot. This means that the central ray is always directed towards the same point in space, on this axis. At the same time the

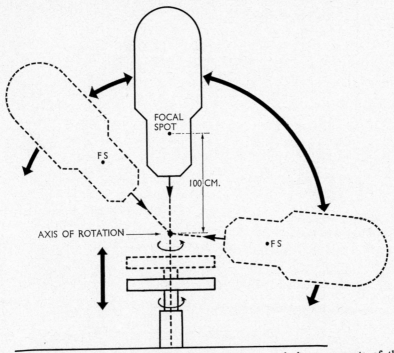

Fig. 375.—The isocentric mounting of a radiation source and the movements of the associated treatment table.

treatment table—which is an integral part of the equipment when this type of mounting is used—is designed to rise and fall, and also to rotate, about a vertical axis which passes through this point—the isocentre (or same centre) for rotations and movements.

Not only does this type of source mounting make the positioning of the patient ('set-up') much easier in practice, but the arrangement lends itself very readily to a variation on the 'pin and arc' techniques, as *Fig.* 376 will help to demonstrate. As before, it can be assumed that the depth at which the tumour centre lies vertically below some skin mark is known. If this tumour centre can be placed at the centre of rotation of the tube—the isocentre—then the central ray will always pass through it, no matter at what angle the tube points.

The procedure to get the tumour centre at the isocentre is quite simple when it is remembered that when the front pointer (*see Fig.* 365) is at its lowest position, its end defines the normal S.S.D., that is to say, it is at the isocentre. The first move, therefore, is with the tube pointing vertically downwards and the front pointer drawn back a distance equal to the depth of the tumour centre, to raise the patient on the table until the front pointer just touches the skin mark. This means that the tumour centre is at the isocentre (*Fig.* 376 A). Movement of the tube to any other position does not alter the passage of the central ray through the tumour centre, and so with the patient remaining in the same position, beams in any desired number of different directions can be accurately aimed at the tumour. The depth of the tumour below the skin for

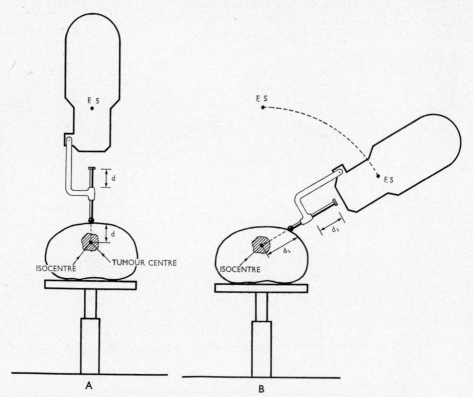

Fig. 376.—The use of the isocentric-type mounting as a 'pin-and-arc' beam director.

each beam direction is readily found by observing the amount that the front pointer has to be drawn back for each direction (*Fig.* 376 B).

    General.—The beam-direction devices and methods that have been described are, in spite of their relative simplicity and low cost, a most important part of modern radiotherapy. Accuracy is a vital ingredient of this treatment agent, and it is no great exaggeration to say that it is better to use kilovoltage beams with careful beam direction than megavoltage beams without it. Happily the choice between these two alternatives does not have to be made, for beam-direction methods are equally as applicable to megavoltage radiations as to those of lower energy. To neglect the extra accuracy that can be gained by beam direction is to throw away much of the value of the powerful and expensive apparatus now in use in radiotherapy.

CHAPTER XXXVI

THE TREATMENT PRESCRIPTION

THE treatment prescription is essentially the instruction from the radiotherapist to the radiographer which, when carried out, will produce inside the patient the desired pattern and magnitude of dose. The prescription must specify the number, size, position, direction, and orientation of the beams to be used as well as the quality of the radiation, the source–skin distance, and the fractionation régime. In addition the magnitude of the Exposure to be delivered on each beam must be given. For example, in the case of the three-field treatment discussed in CHAPTER XXXII (*Fig.* 329), and using the values calculated on p. 486, the remainder of the prescription can be written:

4-MV. X-rays Field	S.S.D.	Beam Size	Given Dose	Percentage Depth Dose at Centre	T.D.	
Anterior	100	8 × 10	2820	70	1974 ⎫	
Left posterior	100	8 × 10	4580	44	2015 ⎬ 6004
Right posterior	100	8 × 10	4580	44	2015 ⎭	

From this information it is usual for the radiographer to calculate the daily exposure required on each field. For example, if the prescription required this dose to be delivered in an overall time of 4 weeks by giving 20 daily exposures on each field and if previous measurement has shown that the X-ray machine output for this beam size and S.S.D. is 185 rad (in soft tissue) per monitor unit at the field reference point (100 per cent point of percentage depth dose curve) we can calculate:

Field	Given Dose	Given Dose per Day	Output	Monitor Units per Day
Anterior	2820	141	185	76
Left posterior	4580	229	185	124
Right posterior	4580	229	185	124

As indicated on p. 575 it is now common practice to use a dose monitor to control the treatment exposure and this is very necessary if the X-ray machine does not have a steady output. If, however, the output is steady, as, for example, on a telecobalt unit, the output may be stated in terms of rad per minute. In these circumstances the daily exposure will be expressed in minutes (and seconds) instead of in monitor units.

The purpose of this chapter is to demonstrate how the prescription is formulated by the radiotherapist for fixed-field treatments and to point out the various features of the dose distribution that are under his control. Most of the necessary information has already been presented in earlier chapters but it is considered profitable to summarize the subject as a whole here.

Volume Irradiated.—The volume to be irradiated to a high dose is either a whole section of the patient, for example the pelvic cavity, or a localized, much smaller volume, such as the larynx or the bladder. The former type of treatment is most usually obtained by employing one or two pairs of parallel opposed beams whilst the smaller, localized volume is achieved by employing two or more beams suitably directed with respect to each other and the tumour as shown in *Fig.* 377. In both cases the dose pattern within the irradiated zone needs to be as nearly uniform as possible, whilst the dose outside the irradiated zone needs to be as low as possible.

It is convenient to consider these two types of treatment separately and first the achievement of a localized uniformly irradiated high-dose zone will be dealt with. This kind of technique is, for obvious reasons, sometimes referred to as 'Multiple Beam Directed Technique'.

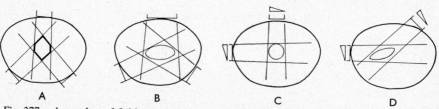

Fig. 377.—A number of field arrangements leading to high-dose volumes of different shapes and sizes.

Multiple Beam Directed Technique.—

Beam Width.—For techniques employing two or three (or more) small beams the high dose is, in general, confined to the region over which the beams overlap. For this reason the beam central axes are normally directed through a common point, T (*see*, e.g., *Fig.* 379) and are co-planar. In this kind of technique it is usual to have rectangular beams and it is conventional to refer to the dimension of the beam in the plane in which the beam central axes lie as the *width*. The other dimension is, of course, the *length* and is at right-angles to the width. It may happen that the width is longer than the length! The size of the high-dose zone is controlled by the widths of the beams, and the shape of the high-dose zone by the relative beam widths and angles between the central axes. The choice of the position and direction of the beams is also governed by: (*a*) the need to avoid nearby 'sensitive' structures which it is desired not to irradiate, and (*b*) the need to choose directions such that the depth of the tumour along the central ray is minimal and therefore the percentage depth dose as large as possible. For several reasons, the inherent curvature of the single beam isodose lines being one, the high-dose zone is not exactly the straight-sided rectangle or hexagon suggested in *Fig.* 377 A. In practice the corners are rounded, yielding circles or ellipses, as shown in *Fig.* 377 B, C, and D.

Beam Length.—It is important to remember that although dose patterns are usually presented in two dimensions, i.e., on a piece of paper (e.g., *Fig.* 331) they are, in fact, intended as a representation of a three-dimensional volume. To this extent they are therefore incomplete. Fortunately the size of the volume in the missing third dimension is simply controlled by, although not necessarily equal to, the length of the beams, which are usually equal to each other. The variation in dose in this direction can easily be read off the appropriate ('long axis') isodose chart, the points at which the dose has fallen, to, say, 90 per cent of the central value are usually considered to define the length of the treated volume: in practice it is 1–2 cm. smaller than the length of the beams.

Number of Beams.—The number of beams which need to be used depends on the depth below the skin surface of the centre of the tissue to be irradiated, as well as on the penetrating power of the radiation. If the depth is small and/or the penetrating power high, the number of beams needed is small and an adequately high dose to the isolated volume achieved using only two or three beams. If the depth is larger or the penetrating power lower then four or five and even six beams may be required. The number of beams needed depends on how much higher than the maximum dose elsewhere the high dose to the treated zone is required to be. If the requirement is, for example, a dose to the tumour which is 150 per cent for a maximum given dose of 100 per cent then the average percentage depth dose at the tumour from each beam can be calculated. This is shown in column 2 of *Table XLIV*. For example if three beams are to be used the average percentage depth dose at the tumour will be $150 \div 3 = 50$ per cent.

Table XLIV.—DEPTH IN CM. OF REQUIRED PERCENTAGE DEPTH DOSE BY DIFFERENT NUMBERS OF FIELDS AND FOR VARIOUS RADIATION QUALITIES

No. OF BEAMS	PERCENTAGE DEPTH DOSE PER FIELD	DEPTH IN CM. FOR REQUIRED PERCENTAGE DEPTH DOSE				
		2 mm. Cu H.V.L.	^{60}Co γ-rays	4 MV.	8 MV.	20 MV.
2	75	3½	5½	6½	9	12
3	50	6¾	10½	13½	17	22
5	30	10½	17½	20½	27	35

The third and following columns of *Table XLIV* give the depth (in cm.) at which the percentage depth dose listed in column 2 occurs for various commonly used radiation qualities. In the head and neck region of the body the depth of the centre of the volume to be irradiated is often in the range 5–7 cm., especially if the lesion is asymmetrically placed and if the treatment is all delivered from the homolateral side. It is clear from *Table XLIV* that in such circumstances a satisfactory dosage can be achieved using only two beams if cobalt-60 gamma rays and megavoltage X-rays are used. As has been indicated on p. 498 such a two-beam technique demands the use of 'wedged' beams: hence their importance in megavoltage techniques. If 2·0-mm. H.V.L. radiation is to be used then for most sites at least three beams are required. Similarly three beams of megavoltage radiation are often enough for the treatment of a bladder in a not too large patient. For larger patients five beams may be required. Five beams are always required if 2·0-mm. Cu H.V.L. radiations are to be used. There are very few situations where more than three beams of 10- or 20-MV. radiation are needed. In practice, of course, the radiotherapist will know from his own previous experience (and at least from that of others) the number of beams likely to be needed for an individual case.

Beam Edge.—Often the radiotherapist is faced with a need to irradiate adequately a certain volume and, simultaneously, to avoid irradiating a nearby (even an immediately adjacent) structure. This is clearly a very difficult situation and one in which a compromise has often to be made. As indicated earlier in this chapter, the need to avoid structures is one of the factors which determine the radiotherapist's choice of beam position and direction. It is helpful to remember that, for most photon beams, the most rapid change of dose with distance occurs at the beam edge, when the dose can fall from say 70 per cent to about 5 per cent over a distance of a few millimetres (*see*, e.g., *Fig.* 360). The magnitude of the change is controlled by the position and design of the collimators, the source size, and the source–skin distance. It is, therefore, often advantageous to ensure that the edge of at least one of the beams passes between the high-dose zone and the structure to be spared. Even if only one edge can be so positioned the differential in dose can approach a factor of two, even though one of the other beams unavoidably passes through the structure. For example the dose pattern along the line PP of the two-wedge beam treatment illustrated in *Fig.* 378 A is shown in *Fig.* 378 B. It can be seen that the dose to point Q is very much less than that to T, 36 per cent of it in fact. The dose to points, such as R, outside both beams is negligible. Even though one of the beams passes through S before it reaches the tumour region the dose to S is still only 62 per cent, simply because it is not irradiated by the other beam. In a three or more beam arrangement points such as S would be even more spared.

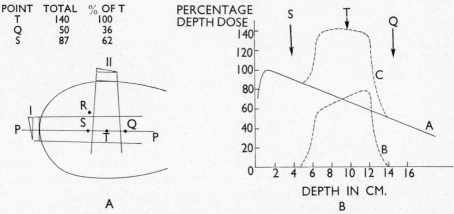

POINT	TOTAL	% OF T
T	140	100
Q	50	36
S	87	62

Fig. 378.—Dose levels inside and outside the high-dose zone. A, The treatment arrangement. B, The variation of dose along PP for: (A) beam I, (B) beam II, (C) beams I and II.

Individual Treatments.—From the above it can be seen that to a large extent the radiotherapist has, by means of his choice of beam size, position, and direction, control over the size, shape, and position of the high-dose zone resulting from a treatment. The number of beams used will also have an effect on the shape of the high-dose zone but is used principally (as discussed *above*) to control the level of dose to the high-dose zone. The radiotherapist is also able, by suitable positioning of the beams, to avoid delivering unnecessary and unwanted radiation to nearby 'sensitive' structures.

In so far as tumour sizes and positions or the sizes and shapes of patients are more alike than they are different, there is, in practice, a limited number of possible general beam configurations and, therefore, treatment techniques. This is not, however, to be taken as implying that the treatment need not be designed specifically for the patient. Although the type of technique used may be the same as that used for other similar patients with similar lesions, the treatment details must be properly individualized for each patient.

Uniformity of Dose.—So far little has been stated about the pattern of dose within the irradiated zone. For reasons which are outside the scope of this text it is required that the dose at all points within the irradiated volume shall be within about ± 5 per cent of the specified value (tumour dose), i.e., it is required that the pattern shall be uniform. It is the main concern of this chapter to discuss how this uniformity is achieved. Two facilities are available. The first is to select appropriately the relative exposures to be delivered on each beam. This is known as 'beam balancing' and in principle is always required even if, in practice, the answer sometimes may be to give equal exposure in each beam! The second facility is the use of suitable wedge filters in addition to 'beam balancing'. Examples of the more common arrangements will now be described.

Three-beam Treatment. (i) Symmetrical Arrangement.—The simplest arrangement of three beams is shown in *Fig.* 379. The angle between each beam and its neighbours is 120°; the central axes intersect at a common central point T at an equal depth below the surface. The dose within the volume where the beams intersect will be substantially higher than that elsewhere provided the percentage depth dose from each beam at central point T is greater than 40 or 50 per cent. If it is not, then more than three beams, say five, are required in order to achieve a satisfactory dose pattern. Remembering that the dose within the high-dose zone should be as uniform as possible, it follows that the total dose at each of the typical points A, B, X, Y, and T (*Fig.* 379) should be as nearly equal to each other as possible.

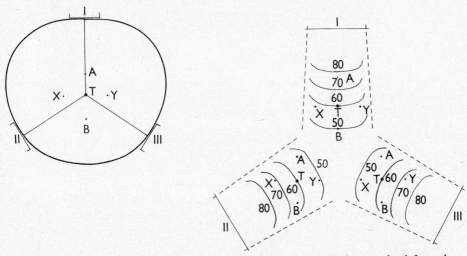

Fig. 379.—A, Three beams at 120° to each other, with the tumour at the same depth for each. The positions of the dose reference points relative to each beam are shown on the right.

The method of achieving this is set out below. It turns out that we can usually make the dose at X equal the dose at Y and that at A equal to that at B. Because of the shape of the isodose lines and the central axis depth dose curve the dose at T may be a little larger than the dose at the other four points. It also often happens that the dose at X and Y is a little different from that at A and B. Fortunately, especially for megavoltage radiation, the differences in these doses are sufficiently small to be negligible and the dose may be considered uniform.

Consider the doses at the points X and Y. Because of their symmetrical position with respect to beam I its contribution is the same to each point and, of course, this remains true no matter what Exposure is given on beam I. The points X and Y are also symmetrical with respect to the beams II and III in the sense that:

Dose from beam II to X = Dose from beam III to Y

and

Dose from beam III to X = Dose from beam II to Y.

Therefore

Total dose from beams II and III to X = Total dose from beams II and III to Y,

provided that the same Exposure is given on beam II as on beam III but no matter what magnitude this Exposure is.

It is clear therefore that the total doses at X and Y arising from all these beams are equal to each other. This equality of dose at points X and Y is inherent in the symmetry of the arrangement; the only condition is that equal exposures are given on beams II and III.

Consider now the doses at points A and B. From beam I the dose at A is larger than that at B (*Fig.* 379 B). The dose at point A from beam II is the same as that from beam III and similarly for point B. The total dose at B from beams II and III is larger than the total dose at A from beams II and III: the opposite of the effect of beam I. The data listed below are those which obtain in an actual case.

BEAM	A		B	X	Y	T
I	74 → (25)	←	49	58	58	60
II	53 → (12·5)	←	65·5	71	51	60
III	53 → (12·5)	←	65·5	51	71	60
II+III	106 → (25)	←	131	122	122	120
I+II+III	180		180	180	180	180

It can be seen that the total dose at A from all three beams is equal to that at B. This arises because the difference in the dose at the points A and B from beam I is exactly balanced by the difference in the dose at points B and A from the two beams II and III combined.

The reason for this convenient result can be seen by reference to *Fig.* 379 right-hand diagram. For the two beams II and III the points A and B lie on a line inclined at an angle of 60° to the central axis. The difference in dose from each of the two beams II and III to the two points is, therefore, rather less than is the case for beam I for which the points A and B lie on the central axis. In fact, since $\cos 60° = \frac{1}{2}$ the former difference is exactly one-half the latter, thus although there are two beams (II and III) contributing to the higher dose at B compared with that at A these are balanced by the contributions from beam I.

In the above example the general level of dose is 180 units and this results from a given dose of 100 units to the reference point of each of the three beams I, II, and III. If it has been decided that the tumour dose shall be 5500 rad delivered in an overall period of 3 weeks, during which each beam will be given 15 equal daily exposures, the daily exposure can be calculated as follows:

$$180 \text{ units correspond to } 5500 \text{ rad}$$

hence

$$100 \text{ units correspond to } 3060 \text{ rad}$$

and the daily given dose is

$$3060/15 = 204 \text{ rad.}$$

If the previously measured dose rate at the reference point, for specified operating conditions of the X-ray equipment, is known to be 68·5 rad/min. the daily exposure time will need to be:

$$204/68·5 = 2·98 \text{ min.}$$

$$= 2 \text{ min. } 59 \text{ sec.}$$

(ii) **Simple Non-symmetrical Arrangement.**—Let us now consider the situation illustrated in *Fig.* 380 which is rather more usual in practice than the completely symmetrical arrangement first discussed. A typical example is a bladder treatment.

Here, whilst the angles between the beams remain equal to each other, the depths of the point T for the two posterior beams (II and III) are different from the depth for the anterior beam (I) although still equal to each other.

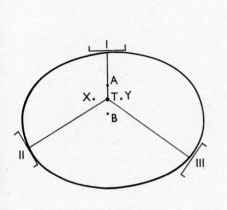

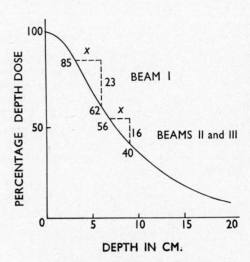

Fig. 380.—Three beams at 120° to each other but for one beam the tumour is less deep than for the other two.

Fig. 381.—The difference in dose at two points *x* cm. apart decreases as the depths of the points increases.

The comments made above concerning the doses to points X and Y from the three beams (I, II, and III) remain valid and the doses at these two points will be identical provided only that the same exposure is given on beams II or III. It is when the doses to points A and B are considered that the difference from the earlier example arises. *Fig.* 381 illustrates that the difference in dose between two points, A and B, a fixed distance (*x*) apart, decreases as the depth of A and B increases. As before, the fact that there are two beams (II and III) contributing a higher dose to B compared with that at A compensates for the fact that A and B lie on a line inclined at 60° (cos 60° = ½) to the central axis. In such a circumstance therefore the difference in doses at A and B from beam I is not balanced by the difference in combined doses from beams II and III.

The various percentage depth doses obtaining in a particular case are:

Beam		Given Dose	A	B	X	Y	T
1.	I	100	85 → (23) ← 62		70	70	72
2.	II	100	44	52	57	43	50
3.	III	100	44	52	43	57	50
4.	II+III		88 → (16) ← 104				
5.	I+II+III		173 → (7) ← 166		170	170	172

In this example the combined doses (line 5), from the three beams, at A and B differ by 7 units. In practice they always differ to a certain extent, sometimes by more than this. Fortunately it is very easy to arrange that the doses at A and B are identical. This is done by increasing the exposure on the two posterior beams (II and III) so as to increase the difference (i.e., 16 units) in *their* combined contributions to points A and B so that it gives the same difference (i.e., 23 units) due to beam I. In this example the given dose on each of beams II and III needs to be increased to $(100 \times 23/16 = 144)$. The revised doses are then:

Beam	Given Dose	A	B	X	Y	T
6. I	100	$85 \to (23) \leftarrow 62$		70	70	72
7. II	144	63·5	75	82	62	72
8. III	144	63·5	75	62	82	72
9. II+III		$127 \to (23) \leftarrow 150$		144	144	144
10. I+II+III		212	212	214	214	216

Lines 7 and 8 show the relative doses resulting from a given dose of 144 units on beams I and II and are obtained by multiplying the values in lines 2 and 3 by the factor $144/100 = 1\cdot44$. It can be seen that a balance has been obtained, the total dose at A being the same as that at B. Although not precisely uniform, the pattern is symmetrical about T, at which the dose is 1 per cent above the general level of 214 units, which can be taken as corresponding to the tumour dose. If, for example, this is desired to be 5500 rad then the given doses on each of the fields are calculated by simple proportion:

Tumour dose = 214 units equivalent to 5500 rad.

Given dose on beam I = 100 units equivalent to $5500 \times 100/214 = 2570$ rad.

Given dose on beam II = 144 units equivalent to $5500 \times 144/214 = 3700$ rad.

Given dose on beam III = 144 units equivalent to $5300 \times 144/214 = 3700$ rad.

From these values the appropriate daily exposure can be calculated as for the previous example once the fractionation régime is decided and X-ray machine output is known. It is worth noting that the given dose on the more distant beams (II and III) is very much more than on the closer beam (I). It can happen that the given doses required on the more distant beams exceed that which can be tolerated. In such cases the radiotherapist must either accept a (small) non-uniformity to the dose pattern or employ extra beams.

After designing a treatment it is worth while calculating the dose to the tumour centre (T), as a check on the arithmetic, using the expression:

Tumour dose = Sum of (given dose × percentage depth dose) for each field, viz.:

Beam I $2570 \times 0\cdot72 = 1850$

Beam II $3700 \times 0\cdot50 = 1850$

Beam III $3700 \times 0\cdot50 = 1850$

_____

5550

This corresponds to 216 units in the table above from which the tumour dose was taken to be 214. On this basis the tumour dose = $5550 \times 214/216 = 5500$ rad, which is the desired value.

It is interesting to note that each beam contributes the same dose to the central point (T). This is a consequence of the angular symmetry (120°) and points to a very easy method of calculation for such cases. Each beam needs to contribute one-third of the total dose to T, hence the required given dose is obtained by:

$$\text{Given dose} = \frac{\text{Tumour centre dose}}{3} \times \frac{100}{\text{Percentage depth dose}},$$

where percentage depth dose is that appropriate for each beam separately.

(iii). Asymmetrical Arrangement.—In practice all the depths and the angles between the beams may be different, as in *Fig.* 382. For such circumstances the same method of beam balancing is employed, but it is, necessarily, a little more complex. First, the total dose to X and Y from beams II and III is made equal by balancing the relative given doses on beams II and III. Secondly, the total dose to points A and B from all three beams are made equal by balancing the relative given doses on beams I, II, and III: the relative given doses on beams II and III being maintained as already calculated.

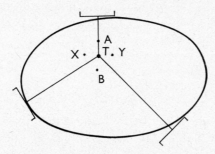

Fig. 382.—A general three-beam treatment.

It is convenient to set out the calculations as in the following example:

Beam	Given Dose	A	B	X	Y	T
1. I	100	86 → (23) ← 63		72	72	74
2. II	100	45	52	57 → (14) ← 43		50
3. III	100	34	41	33 → (10) ← 43		38
Increase given dose on beam III to 100×14/10 = 140:						
4. III	140	48	57	46 → (14) ← 60		53
Then adding lines 2 and 4:						
5. II+III	100+140	93 → (16) ← 109		103	103	103
Decrease given dose on beam I to 100×16/23 = 69·5:						
6. I	69·5	60 → (16) ← 44		50	50	51·5
Then adding lines 5 and 6:						
7. I+II+III		153	153	153	153	154·5

Hence given doses of 69·5, 100, and 140 units on beams I, II, and III respectively, will result in a uniform dose of about 153 units. If a tumour dose of 5250 rad is required, the actual given doses would be:

$$\text{Beam I} \quad 5250 \times 69\cdot5/153 = 2380 \text{ rad,}$$
$$\text{Beam II} \quad 5250 \times 100/153 = 3430 \text{ rad,}$$
$$\text{Beam III} \quad 5250 \times 140/153 = 4800 \text{ rad.}$$

In this example we see that complete uniformity is obtained at the price of a rather too high given dose on beam III. The therapist will need to decide whether to accept this; whether to reduce it and to compensate by increasing the given dose on beam I or beam III, thereby also accepting a small degree of non-uniformity of dose; or whether to employ additional beams.

Two Beams with Wedges.—The properties and the need for the use of wedge filters have been discussed in an earlier chapter (*see* pp. 498–502), where the relationship between the wedge angle and the angle between the beam central axes (the hinge angle) was given. This relationship would seem to imply that a very large number of different wedges (of different angles) are necessary. It turns out, in practice, as will be demonstrated below, that only a few different wedges are required. This is fortunate since a need for a large number of wedge filters would have the serious disadvantages that:

1. There would be an increased possibility of using the wrong wedge. In any case it is usually considered necessary to have some system of interlocks which ensures that the correct wedge is being used, and that it is the correct way round. This is possible if there are only a few wedges but would be impracticable for a large number.

2. A large amount of effort, time, and, therefore, money would have to be spent in designing, making, testing the 'wedges', and measuring the associated isodose charts.

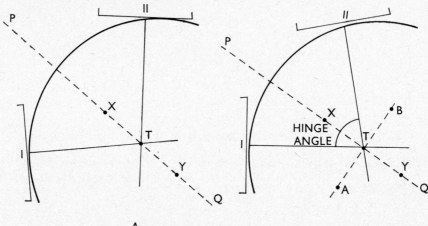

Fig. 383.—Choosing the wedge angle and the field position.

Consider now the arrangement shown in *Fig.* 383 A, which shows the positioning of two wedge fields chosen by the radiotherapist because it gives the desired shape and position of the high-dose zone (the region where the beams overlap). The beams to be used are those for which the wedge angle (*WA*) is as nearly as possible to the value given by:

$$WA = 90 - HA/2 \quad (see \text{ p. } 501)$$

where *HA* is the hinge angle—in this case the angle between the central axes. For dose balancing draw a line PQ through T bisecting the angle between the axes and mark on it the two points X and Y. Using the isodose chart for the chosen wedge beam read off the contributions to X and Y from beam I—in general they will not be identical. Therefore reposition the beam central axis, by rotation about T, until a position is found for which the doses at X and Y are identical. If the dose at X was initially less than that at Y decrease the hinge angle, whilst if it was initially greater increase the angle. This is the final position of the beam and is shown in *Fig.* 383 B. A similar procedure is now carried out for beam II.

If the radiotherapist considers that the amount of movement, and therefore the final position of the beams, is unacceptable in the sense that it changes the size and shape of the high-dose zone significantly then it will be necessary to start again with a different wedge angle beam (lower if the hinge angle needs to be increased and vice versa) and repeat the procedure. Once an acceptable arrangement (*Fig.* 383 B) is obtained, a line is drawn through T at right-angles to PQ and the doses to points A and B considered. Since the beams' positioning and the wedge angle ensure that the doses at X and Y are identical separately for each of the two beams, the relative Exposure on these two beams can be 'balanced' so as to achieve equal doses at the points A and B. The data given below refer to the circumstances of *Fig*. 383. In writing down the various percentage depth doses due cognizance has been taken of any effects of oblique incidence. In so far as the final pattern (in this plane) is uniform the wedge is acting also as a compensator (p. 495).

Beam	Given Dose	X	Y	A		B	T
1. I	100	79	79	104 → (47) ←		57	81
2. II	100	83	83	60 → (52) ←		112	85
Increase given dose on beam I to $100 \times 52/47 = 111$:							
3. I	111	87	87	115		63	90
Add lines 2 and 3:							
4. I+II		170	170	175		175	175

The mean tumour dose can be taken as 173 units and the given doses calculated as before; if the tumour dose is to be 5500 rad, then:—

Beam I   Given dose $= 5500 \times 111/173 = 3530$ rad,

Beam II   Given dose $= 5500 \times 100/173 = 3180$ rad.

It may happen that it is not possible to move a beam, say beam I, in the way described, its position being fixed by the need to avoid some sensitive structures (*Fig*. 384). When this occurs, the position of two points X and Y, at which the doses from beam I are equal, are identified. The angle of the second beam (II) is then adjusted until the doses from it to the points X and Y are also equal to each other. The relative given doses of the two beams are now balanced as previously in order to make the total doses at A and B equal.

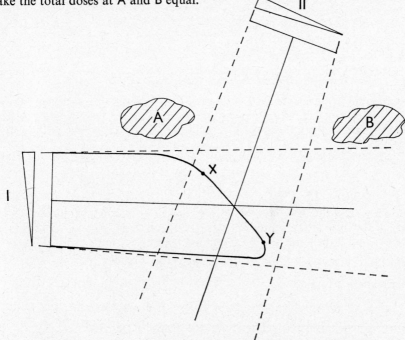

Fig. 384.—Positioning a field to avoid the irradiation of zones A and B.

Parallel Opposed Beams.—The most simple use of two beams is illustrated in *Fig.* 385 in which the central axes of the two opposed beams are coincident. Such an arrangement is used when it is desired to irradiate a *whole region* of the patient to a reasonably uniform dose. The two beams of radiation are not, of course, directed at the patient simultaneously but alternately from each beam (*Fig.* 385 B). The distance (RL) between the two beam entry points is referred to as the 'interfield distance'. When calculating the doses for such a treatment it is usually assumed that the spaces between the applicator surface and the skin as well as those to the side and behind the patient are filled with bolus material during each treatment (*Fig.* 385 B). The standard percentage depth dose values and isodose charts are therefore applicable.

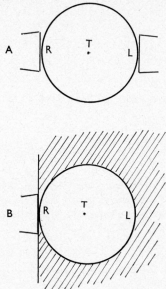

Fig. 385.—Treatment by parallel opposed beams. A, General arrangement. B, Treatment arrangement with spaces around the part filled with bolus material.

For example, consider the case where the interfield distance is 12 cm., the beam size is 15×10, the S.S.D. 50 cm., and the radiation quality 2·0 mm. Cu H.V.L. The relevant percentage depth dose values obtained from tables are:

Beam	Given Dose	R	T	L
I	100	100	58·3	26·6
II	100	26·6	58·3	100
I+II		126·6	116·6	126·6

In this example the dose is lower at the centre (T) than it is at either of the two surfaces. If the dose at the centre T is to be 3500 rad, from equal given doses on the two beams I and II the value of that given dose will be

$$\text{Given dose} = 3500 \times 100/116\cdot6 = 3000 \text{ rad.}$$

The corresponding total dose on the skin surface (the maximum skin dose) is:

$$\text{Maximum skin dose} = 3000 \times 1\cdot266 = 3800 \text{ rad,}$$

alternatively this could be calculated from the central dose, viz.:

$$\text{Maximum skin dose} = 3500 \times 126\cdot6/116\cdot6 = 3800 \text{ rad.}$$

The daily exposure on each beam is now easily calculated as the earlier examples. In this example it will be seen that the minimum central axis dose occurs at the centre of the patient whilst the maximum occurs at the skin surface. The exact pattern produced depends on the interfield distance, the radiation quality, and, to a lesser extent, the beam size. The graphs of *Fig.* 386 show the variation of dose along the

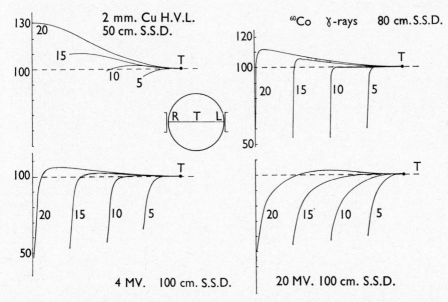

Fig. 386.—Variation of dose as percentage of dose at T along the common axis of a parallel opposed beams treatment. The interfield distance RL is indicated against each curve; 20 × 20 cm. fields in each case.

common central axis line (R.T.L.) for a range of interfield distance and radiation qualities. It can be seen how at the small interfield distances and/or high radiation qualities the centre is the maximum dose whereas for the larger interfield distance and/or lower radiation qualities the centre is a minimum. For the megavoltage radiation where the 'build-up' effect serves to reduce the incident surface dose, the surface dose is always the minimum but there can be a maximum at about the 'build-up' depth. The latter is often referred to as the 'subcutaneous dose'. It is clear from *Fig.* 386 that an acceptable degree of uniformity can be obtained with 2·0 mm. Cu H.V.L. radiation only for small interfield distances. Hence, nowadays, it is usual to restrict the use of this technique to megavoltage radiations. *Fig.* 386 shows that with 20-MV. X-rays only the centre of the patient is 'uniformly' irradiated because of the substantial 'build-up' depth associated with this radiation energy. If the low dose in these superficial layers is undesirable it can be removed by the use of 'build-up' bolus material applied to the patient during treatment.

When using a parallel opposed pair of beams the thickness of the patient may vary considerably over the area of the beam. A common example of this is in the treatment of the head, neck, and upper mediastinum (*Fig.* 387). In such a circumstance one of two policies can be adopted. The first is to 'bolus' up the patient so that the effective thickness is constant and approximately equal to the greatest thickness. Inevitably this has the disadvantage that the central dose is lowered (larger interfield distance) and any 'skin sparing', due to 'build-up', lost.

The second possibility is to accept the range of thickness and to calculate the resultant dose pattern in order to check that the maximum and minimum doses are within acceptable limits. The dose will be maximal in the thinnest section and minimal in the thickest ones. A simple method of working, which applies for megavoltage radiation at an S.S.D. of 80 cm. or larger, is to assume that the patient is of uniform thickness given by:

$$\text{Thickness} = \frac{a + b + c}{3},$$

where a, b, and c are the maximum, minimum, and central thicknesses. The required given doses are calculated as before as the basis of their thickness. The use of this method ensures that the dose within the irradiated volume is within ± 10 per cent of that calculated for the 'parallel' patient of thickness t.

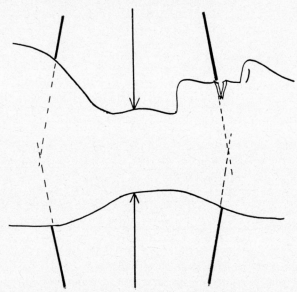

Fig. 387.—Parallel opposed beam treatment of a part of variable thickness.

Other Arrangements.—Many arrangements of beams other than those described above are used in practice but this is not the place to attempt a complete catalogue. It is useful, however, to describe very briefly three examples.

1. *Wedge Parallel Opposed Pair Plus Plain Beam.*—As shown in *Fig.* 388 A the treatment consists of a parallel pair of beams both of which are 'wedged' plus a single plain (unwedged) beam at right-angles. The wedged pair gives a uniform irradiation across the patient but with a higher dose at A than at B. This difference in dose at A and B is balanced by the corresponding but opposite difference from the plain beam, the given doses being balanced appropriately. A uniform dosage is thus achieved in the region over which the beams overlap.

The attraction of this method is that the high-dose zone may easily be positioned anywhere within the patient section by a suitable choice of beam position (*Fig.* 388 B and C).

2. *Inclined Wedge Pair Plus Plain Beam.*—The arrangement is as shown in *Fig.* 389 and is often used for the treatment of, say, a bladder. Its advantage is that all the

beams enter from the same side of the patient and avoid irradiating the underlying regions. The relative given doses are chosen to balance the difference in dose at the points A and B resulting from the wedge pair by the opposite difference resulting from the plain beam.

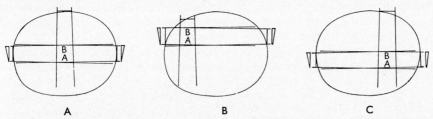

Fig. 388.—Examples of treatment by a parallel opposed pair of wedge beams plus a plain beam.

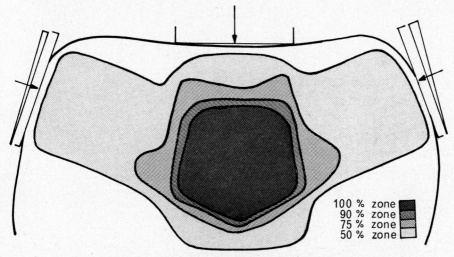

100 % zone
90 % zone
75 % zone
50 % zone

Fig. 389.—A bladder treatment using an inclined wedge pair and a plain beam.

3. *Double Wedge Pair.*—If the tumour depth is greater than that shown for *Fig.* 389 three beams may not be sufficient and the arrangement of *Fig.* 390 is preferred. It has the same advantage as the immediately preceding example. The beam pair (I and II) yield a uniform (but not sufficiently high) dose to the tumour region and are balanced in the usual way. Beams III and IV form an identical pair and again give a uniform (but not sufficiently high) dose to the tumour region. The summated doses in the tumour region from the two pairs is, however, sufficiently larger than the dose elsewhere for the treatment to be acceptable.

As indicated above, many other beam arrangements can be used. Of course the arrangements adopted for any particular patient will be, at least to a certain extent, unique. In all cases, however, an acceptably uniform dose within the region where the various beams overlap is sought, and usually achieved, by a suitable choice of relative given doses and wedges appropriate to the number of beams used and the angles between their central axes as well as to the depth of the central point from each beam. Of course it will not always be possible to design a treatment which has a perfectly uniform dose within the tumour region without there being unacceptable defects; for example, a too high given dose on one or more beams; an unacceptable direction for one or more of the beams; or the use of an unavailable wedge. In these circumstances a compromise appropriate to the individual situation needs to be made.

Single Beam Treatment.—So far nothing has been stated about the most simple of all radiotherapy treatments, namely the single beam. Clearly, apart from choosing the radiation quality, the S.S.D., and the beam size, the radiotherapist has no control over the pattern of dose or the size and shape of the volume of tissue irradiated. The main use of the single beam arises in two groups of circumstances:

a. Superficial Lesions.—The maximum dose of radiation from a single beam is at or near the surface. The single beam is therefore useful if the lesion is such that the highest dose is required over the superficial few mm. or cm. If the radiation quality is low (e.g., 1–2 mm. Al H.V.L.) and the S.S.D. small (10–20 cm.) the dose falls off rapidly with depth. In a sense therefore the high dose is limited to the region near the surface, the deeper, underlying structures receiving an acceptably low dose.

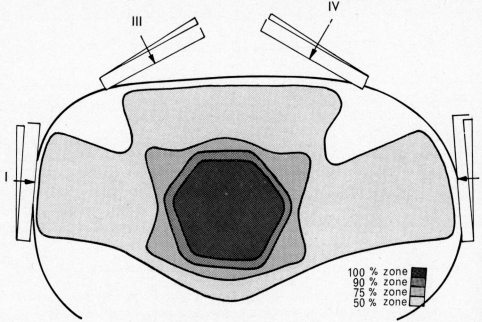

100 % zone
90 % zone
75 % zone
50 % zone

Fig. 390.—A bladder treatment using a double wedge pair.

In a later chapter it will be shown that for a beam of not too high energy (2–5 MeV.) electrons the dose is fairly constant from the surface down to a certain depth (controlled by the electron energy) beyond which the dose falls off very rapidly. Single beams of such electrons are therefore very useful for the irradiation of superficial lesions. Unfortunately as the electron energy, and therefore the depth to which the more and less uniform dose extends, is increased, the rate of fall-off beyond this depth becomes less rapid (*Fig.* 438). In such circumstances the cut-off of dose at a depth is no better and usually not as good as that which can be obtained by using the admittedly rather more complex technique of two beams of well-collimated photons.

b. Palliative Treatments.—It is sometimes necessary to deliver a dose of radiation for example to a spinal metastasis or an upper mediastinal obstruction, in order to relieve distressing symptoms without there being any intention—because of its impossibility—of effecting a cure. For such treatments, where the patient may be very ill, what is required is a quickly delivered, simple treatment which does not demand the more elaborate setting-up and preparation (and therefore, to some extent inevitable delay) of a planned multibeam treatment. Fortunately it is not usually necessary, or possible, to deliver the high dose needed for a radical treatment and the need to confine the high dose to a limited volume of tissue is, therefore, not so critically important. Very often the simplicity, speed, and convenience of a single beam of penetrating radiation (^{60}Co gamma rays, 4-MV. and 300-kV. X-rays) more than compensate for the deficiencies of dose pattern, and yield the best compromise.

CHAPTER XXXVII

SOME SPECIAL TECHNIQUES

1. ROTATION THERAPY

ROTATION therapy is often said to be the logical extension of multi-field teletherapy treatments. Because the absorbed dose rate in an X-ray beam decreases with depth beyond the reference point, more than one beam has to be directed towards any deep-seated tumour if that tumour is to receive an adequate treatment dose without excessive irradiation elsewhere. Generally, a radiotherapist aims at delivering, to the tumour zone, a dose which is about 50 per cent higher than that at, or near to, the skin, and in this way marked reactions are generally confined to the tumour zone.

Fig. 391 and its accompanying table show how the tumour dose is built up, relative to the skin dose, when increasing numbers of fields are used to treat a bladder

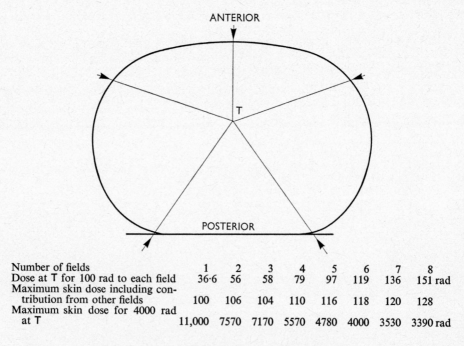

Number of fields	1	2	3	4	5	6	7	8
Dose at T for 100 rad to each field	36·6	56	58	79	97	119	136	151 rad
Maximum skin dose including contribution from other fields	100	106	104	110	116	118	120	128
Maximum skin dose for 4000 rad at T	11,000	7570	7170	5570	4780	4000	3530	3390 rad

Fig. 391.—Multi-field treatments. How the tumour and skin doses change when the same dose is delivered to different numbers of fields.

tumour in an average-sized patient whose body outline is shown in the diagram. In each case the fields used are uniformly spaced out, with one field aimed directly at the tumour T in the AP direction. The diagram shows how five fields would be

536

.arranged. Whilst not necessarily using the best therapeutic arrangements, the series uses quite satisfactory field positions and serves to illustrate how the tumour dose increases relative to the skin dose as more and more fields are used. Looked at in another way, this means that, for any desired tumour dose, the skin dose steadily decreases the more fields used.

In passing, it should be noted that the increase in the tumour dose in this case— which is typical of many in practice—is not as rapid as the increase in the number of fields might suggest. This is because the distance from some fields to the tumour is inevitably greater than that of others. For example, the depth of the tumour for the AP field is 8 cm. and that field contributes 36·6 to the tumour for every 100 at its reference point. When two fields are used—in this case the AP and the PA fields—the PA field is 12 cm. from T to which it contributes 19·4. The total contribution is thus 56·0, which is considerably less than $2 \times 36·6$.

Another factor that must be remembered is that the skin receives dose contributions from other fields, either by direct transmission or by scattering. This contribution increases as the number of fields increases, and is worst when fields are opposite one another, so that one contributes directly to the other.

Nevertheless these minor disadvantages, though worthy of note for what follows, do not affect the general observation that the more fields that are used the lower the dose to the skin, and the more the dose is concentrated in the tumour zone. The logical outcome of such an observation is to increase the number of fields as much as possible: to use not 5 or 6 fields but as many fields as the periphery of the patient will accommodate side by side. This, in effect, is achieved by using rotation therapy, in which the beam is stationary and the patient rotated, or the patient is stationary whilst the source rotates about the tumour centre, at which the beam always points. It is often said that rotation therapy is equivalent to multi-stationary field therapy using an infinite number of fields. Whilst this is true in one sense, in the important practical sense of the depth dose achieved, rotation therapy is more equivalent to using that number of stationary fields which can be accommodated around the periphery.

This is no new technique: the first attempts at rotation therapy were made in the late 1920's and much work on the subject was carried on in the fourth and fifth decades of the century. Before the ready availability of megavoltage radiations that we enjoy today, rotation therapy seemed to offer the best method of achieving high tumour and low skin dosage. Many ingenious rotation devices for X-ray tubes or treatment tables and chairs were developed, but today the large majority of rotation therapy is carried out with the patient stationary (and thus generally more accurately placed), and a telecurie cobalt-60 gamma-ray source rotating around the long axis of the patient (*Fig.* 392). Radioactive isotope gamma-ray sources, it should be said, are particularly suitable for rotation therapy because they have no high-tension cables to get entangled during rotation. Although the principles are the same whatever the source, it is the rotating cobalt-60 source which will be in mind in the description that follows.

Dosemetry in Rotation Therapy.—Although simple and elegant in principle, rotation therapy presents a number of difficulties in practice. One of these is the ensuring that the axis of rotation not only passes through the tumour centre, but lies in the axis of the tumour itself, otherwise the usually cylindrical (or cigar-shaped) high-dose zone produced by the rotation will not encompass the tumour. A second and more difficult problem is that of dosemetry, which involves lengthy and laborious calculations (unless some form of computer is available to remove the drudgery) and some simplifying assumptions. The first of these is that the rotation treatment can be represented by a large number of stationary fields at equal intervals around the rotation circle. Usually 18 such fields are assumed, at 20° intervals to one another.

In fixed-field therapy the S.S.D. is usually fixed and the beam size at the surface is constant for each application or each setting of the beam-defining 'jaws', so that isodose charts may be prepared for each beam and the dose at any point in the patient read off, as has been described in CHAPTER XXXII. As is shown in *Fig.* 393, the situation is much more complex in rotation therapy in which the distance S.A.D.

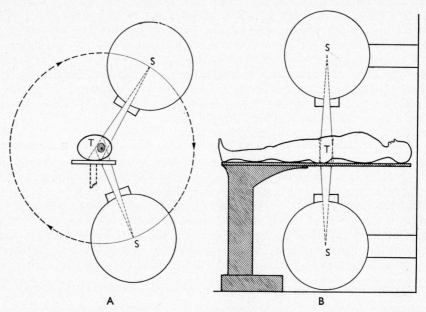

Fig. 392.—Rotation therapy. A shows two positions of the radiation source (S) as it rotates around the tumour centre (T). B shows that complete rotation calls for a treatment table supported at one end only.

(Source–Axis Distance) from the source to the axis of rotation T, and the field size, B, at that level, remain constant, whilst the S.S.D. (remember this is Source–Skin Distance), the surface area of the field, and the surface dose rate change with each position of the beam. Conventional output and depth dose data are, therefore, of little value in this work since different sets of values would have to be available for each S.S.D. and field area. Instead, dosage data are usually based upon the centre of rotation, and this enables the dose at that point (which, being at the tumour centre, is in the region where an accurate knowledge of dosage is most important) to be determined most accurately and quite easily. Doses at other points are rather more difficult to assess and, in general, the accuracy with which they are known decreases the further they are from the centre.

The Dose at the Centre of Rotation.—The most widely used approach to obtaining this is through the Tissue–Air Ratio, which is the ratio of the Exposure rate at T in the patient for any particular size of the beam to the Exposure rate at that point 'in air', that is, when no patient is in position. The point in the beam is the same, the conditions of attenuation and scattering are different. Values of the Tissue–Air Ratio (T.A.R.) for a range of thicknesses of overlying tissue have been tabulated for various

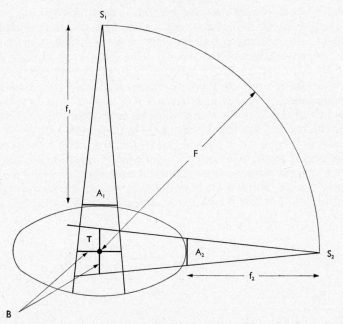

Fig. 393.—In rotation therapy the source–axis distance (F) and the field size (B) at the axis of rotation (T) remain constant, whereas the source–skin distance (f) and the skin field size vary.

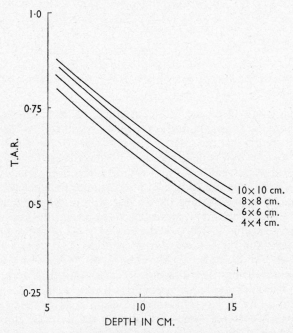

Fig. 394.—Variation of T.A.R. with depth for several field sizes. Cobalt-60 gamma radiation.

radiation qualities and beam sizes and it is found that, for depths of main interest in radiotherapy, i.e., about 8 to 15 cm., the T.A.R. increases with radiation energy and also with field size. It decreases with the depth of the point but, perhaps somewhat unexpectedly, is independent of the S.A.D. This last fact is because distance from source mainly controls the primary radiation contribution and therefore influences the 'in air' and 'in tissue' doses to the same extent, and hence does not alter their ratio.

Dose Calculation.—*Fig.* 394 gives some T.A.R. values for a cobalt-60 gamma-ray telecurie unit and indicates the sort of differences produced by field size (at the axis of rotation, of course), and depth, changes. Values of this sort can now be used to assess the axis dose when a patient is treated by rotation therapy—assuming, of course, that the patient is made of unit-density material. Correction for lungs or bone is possible but here the simpler case will first be dealt with.

For any position of the beam the Exposure rate at the tumour centre is found by multiplying the T.A.R. for that particular depth by the 'in air' Exposure rate at

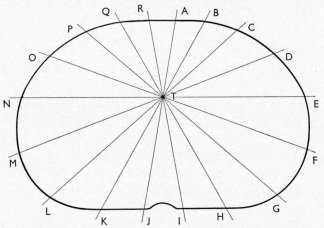

Fig. 395.—A body-section outline, with tumour–skin distances at 20° intervals.

the centre. The latter, of course, is a constant for a particular field size, whilst the T.A.R., and hence the Exposure rate at the tumour, will vary as the beam goes round. However, by assuming that the rotation treatment can be represented by a fairly large number of stationary fields equally spaced around the circle of rotation, the Exposure per rotation can be calculated. A fairly common practice is to calculate for 18 fields at 20° intervals and to assume that each field operates for one-eighteenth of the time per revolution. As detailed below, the average tumour-centre Exposure rate can thus be assessed and hence the total treatment time to deliver the desired dose.

As a first stage in this, a full-scale drawing is made of the outline of the body at the treatment level and the tumour centre is marked on it. Lines are then drawn (as shown in *Fig.* 395) at intervals, in this instance, of 20° to represent the central rays of the 18 stationary fields. The distances TA, TB, TC, etc., from the tumour centre to the skin are then measured and entered into a table such as *Table XLV*, into which are also entered the T.A.R. corresponding to each depth for the beam size being used —in this case an 8 × 10 cm. beam. Because in the example chosen—of a bladder tumour—the centre of rotation lies on the midline, and as the body section is symmetrical about that line, only half the fields have to be dealt with.

Table XLV.—T.A.R. VALUES FOR CENTRE OF RADIATION. COBALT-60 GAMMA-RADIATION

DIRECTION OF BEAM	SURFACE TO CENTRE DISTANCE (cm.)	T.A.R.
AT	8·2	0·755
BT	9·1	0·719
CT	10·5	0·665
DT	13·0	0·579
ET	15·5	0·502
FT	16·8	0·466
GT	16·8	0·466
HT	13·8	0·552
IT	12·0	0·612
	Mean value 12·9	Mean value 0·590

The calculation proceeds as follows:

Suppose Exposure rate 'in air' at centre of rotation T = 62 R per min.

Average T.A.R. from *Table XLV* = 0·590

∴ Average Exposure rate at tumour T = 62 × 0·590 R per min.

and, since 0·965 is the roentgen-rad factor for ^{60}Co gamma rays,

Average absorbed dose rate at T = 62 × 0·590 × 0·965

= 35·3 rad per min.

If the total treatment is required to deliver 5000 rad to the tumour centre in 15 separate treatments (3 weeks) then:

Time for 5000 rad = 5000/35·3 = 141 min.

and Time for treatment = 9·4 min. = 9 min. 24 sec.

It is tacitly assumed in this calculation that, during any treatment session, the source makes an integral number of rotations. Some types of equipment are provided with a variable-speed drive which can be adjusted to achieve this. However, this is not an essential refinement, for the total treatment will certainly involve a considerable number of sessions, and uniformity can be achieved simply by noting the position at which the source is stopped at the end of one day's treatment, and starting the next day's treatment at that place. Thus no particular segment of the body is under- or over-treated.

The Dose at any Other Point.—Much more difficult to calculate is the dose at any other point since, strictly speaking, a different isodose curve is needed for each beam for every different S.S.D. that might be used in a rotation treatment. For instance, in the example dealt with above, the depth of the tumour varied from about 8 to 17 cm., depending upon the direction in which the beam is pointing, and therefore the S.S.D. changed from 75 − 8 = 67 cm. to 75 − 17 = 58 cm., with corresponding changes in the surface area of the beam.

Fortunately with cobalt-60 gamma rays, as with all other megavoltage radiations, some simplification is possible because of the small amount of scattered radiation, so that it is possible to prepare an isodose curve at one S.S.D. for each beam (for each setting of the collimating 'jaws') and apply simple corrections to allow for S.S.D. changes.

An average tumour depth in the body is about 10 cm., so that it is not unreasonable to prepare an isodose curve with an S.S.D. which is 10 cm. less than the distance

F from the source to the axis of rotation of the machine being used. For example, if $F = 75$ cm., isodose curves, for each jaw setting likely to be used, would be made for an S.S.D. of 65 cm. These are then used in the standard fashion to read off the dose at any point, though corrections have to be applied, as an example may make clear.

Consider the treatment of the patient whose outline has already been used in *Fig.* 395, and especially the dose at a point P, 3 cm. posterior to the centre of rotation T. A point on the midline has been chosen to reduce by half the number of values that have to be entered in the table, a saving of space and some of the authors'

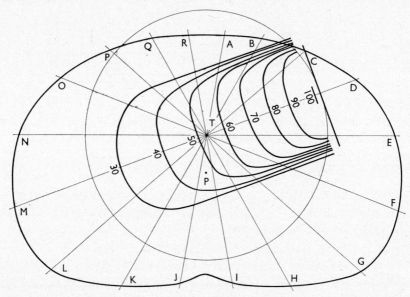

Fig. 396.—The estimation of the dose contribution at two points T and P. Note the 10-cm. diameter circle and the fact that the isodose chart for the field position chosen for illustration lies inside the body-section outline. The actual contributions at T and P will therefore be *less* than indicated by the chart (52 per cent at T and 46 per cent at P) because of the extra thickness traversed by the beam.

patience! The method is equally applicable to any point. As previously, it will be assumed that the rotation treatment can be represented by 18 stationary fields equally spaced around the centre of rotation, and as with any other dosage computation with isodose curves, the full-scale outline is first drawn on squared paper and the position of the fields marked on it, as is shown in *Fig.* 396. For convenience a circle 10 cm. in diameter may also be drawn with its centre at the axis of rotation T. The appropriate isodose curve is then laid on the diagram with its central axis along one of the radial lines, and its 65-cm. S.S.D. mark (its surface level under normal use) laid on the circle which, it will be realized, is 65 cm. from the source. Readings of the percentage depth doses at P and also at T can then be made—and, of course, at any other point at which it is desired to know the dose. The readings (46 at P and 52 at T) obviously do not represent the true percentage depth doses at the points concerned, since in order to reach those points the radiation has to pass through greater thicknesses of tissue than it had to under the conditions under which the isodose chart was made. (They would apply to the circular cross-section.) For P the value is less than that indicated because of the extra thickness t_p whilst for T the extra thickness is t_T. Because of the small amounts of scattered radiation involved, correction for these extra thicknesses is simply made by allowing for their extra attenuation. In other words, the readings are multiplied by $e^{-\mu d}$ where μ is the attenuation coefficient for the radiation involved. The value of this coefficient is obtained from the slope of the central percentage depth dose curve and so is not the 'narrow beam' coefficient which would be obtained from, for example, half-value layer measurements. Rather, it represents the penetrating power of the actual beam being used, and takes some account of the scattered radiation. For the beam used in this example—that is, with a 10×8 cm. beam of cobalt-60 gamma rays, the value of μ is 0·048 cm.$^{-1}$.

For some of the fixed beams, of course, the skin is inside the 10-cm. circle and the isodose curve position is further away from the tumour than is necessary, as a second beam position given in *Fig.* 397 shows. In such a case, the readings taken from the

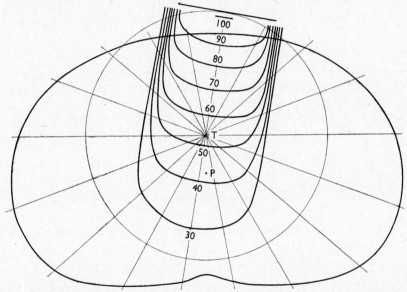

Fig. 397.—The estimation of the dose contribution at T and P for a beam position for which the 10-cm. circle lies outside the outline. In this case the contributions at T and P will be *greater* than the chart readings (52 per cent and 42 per cent respectively).

chart underestimate the values actually being received, because the beam suffers less attenuation in the patient than it did in the phantom when the chart was being measured. Allowance must be made for this *missing* tissue by multiplying by $e^{+\mu d}$, μ and d having the same meanings as before.

Thus the true values at P and T from the field in position D (*Fig.* 396) are $46e^{-\mu l_P}$ which equals 37·7, and $52e^{-\mu l_T}$ which equals 44·8. The total effects at P and T, as for any other points, may be obtained in like manner by placing the isodose curve in each beam position in turn, and adding up the corrected contributions, as shown in *Table XLVI*. For point T—the axis of rotation—the reading before correction will always be the same, of course.

For a point not on the midline it would, of course, be necessary to read off the contributions from all 18 fields, but here the total can be found for both T and P

Table XLVI.—THE DOSE CONTRIBUTION AT T AND P. COBALT-60 GAMMA RAYS
$$\mu = 0.048 \text{ cm}^{-1}$$

| | | POINT T | | | | POINT P | | |
FIELD	READING	t_T	$e^{-\mu t_T}$	CORRECTED VALUE	READING	t_P	$e^{-\mu t_P}$	CORRECTED VALUE
A	52	−1·8	1·09	56·7	42	−2·1	1·11	46·7
B	52	−0·9	1·04	54·1	43	−0·4	1·02	43·8
C	52	+0·5	0·98	51·0	43	+1·6	0·93	40·0
D	52	+3·0	0·86	44·8	46	+4·0	0·82	37·7
E	52	+5·5	0·77	40·0	50	+6·0	0·75	37·5
F	52	+6·8	0·72	37·4	54	+6·7	0·72	38·9
G	52	+6·8	0·72	37·4	60	+5·0	0·79	47·4
H	52	+3·8	0·83	43·1	63	+3·1	0·86	54·2
I	52	+2·0	0·91	47·3	65	+2·0	0·91	59·1
				411·8				405·3

by multiplying the effect of half the fields by two. Since the actual dose at T is known from the T.A.R. it is normal to take the summated contribution at T as 100 per cent and to express all other summated depth doses as percentages of this.

Thus the percentage depth dose at P from the complete rotation would be

$$\frac{\text{Summated value for P}}{\text{Summated value for T}} \times 100$$

or, using values from *Table XLVI*,

$$\frac{405 \cdot 3}{411 \cdot 8} \times 100 = 98 \cdot 4 \text{ per cent.}$$

If the absorbed dose at T, as assumed in the example earlier in this chapter, is 5000 rad, then the absorbed dose at P would be

$$98 \cdot 4 \times 5000 = 4920 \text{ rad.}$$

In this way the percentage depth dose, or total dose at any point in the body, can be calculated and, though relatively straightforward, it will be obvious that the acquiring of information to obtain a complete dose distribution is much more laborious than with fixed fields, using the method described in CHAPTER XXXII. Also it must be acknowledged that the method is less accurate since the approximations and corrections are not strictly right at points near the surface. Fortunately, the accuracy is satisfactory in the centre—the tumour region—where a knowledge of the dose is most necessary. It should also be mentioned that the method outlined is not the only one that can be used. A number of others have been described in the radiological literature, each making slightly different assumptions, or corrections, each having advantages and disadvantages over the others, and all giving very similar final answers in the region of main interest.

Because of the labour involved in obtaining the complete dose pattern by this method, more and more recourse is being made to using computing machines to undertake the calculations, and it is in this sphere of activity that the computer is at present of most value in radiotherapy treatment planning. Where neither a computer nor labour to undertake full investigations of every case is available, it is usual to follow standard methods that have been fully investigated elsewhere, and only determine the T.A.R. for the individual case. A wide range of isodose charts for standard rotation treatments is now available from the International Atomic Energy Agency in Vienna.

Factors affecting the Dose Distribution.—The general pattern of the dose distribution produced by rotation therapy is of a central, relatively circular high-dose zone

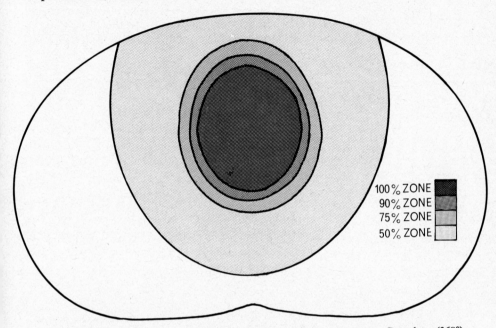

100% ZONE
90% ZONE
75% ZONE
50% ZONE

Fig. 398.—Dose pattern produced by rotation therapy treatment. Complete (360°) rotation with ⁶⁰Co beam unit. Note that the high-dose zone is elliptical with its long axis at right-angles to the long axis of the body section, which is roughly elliptical.

falling off fairly rapidly to a low-dose level throughout the rest of the body section being irradiated. A typical pattern is shown in *Fig.* 398. In any particular case the detailed pattern depends on a number of factors.

    1. *Width of Beam.*—With any given quality of radiation and any given patient, by far the most important variable factor is the beam width. It will be recalled from the discussion of the tumour dose that is built up with increasing numbers of stationary fields, that the ratio of tumour to skin dose (the effective percentage depth dose of the treatment) increases as the number of fields is increased. Now it was also stated that a rotation therapy treatment produces almost the same percentage depth dose as is given by using that number of fields which will just fit round the periphery. Obviously the smaller the beam width the greater the number of fields that can be used, and though smaller fields have smaller percentage depth doses than larger fields, the reduction is by no means proportional to the reduction in size. From this it follows that the smaller the beam width the greater the tumour percentage depth dose. Or stated in another way, for a given tumour dose, the larger the beam width the greater the peripheral and skin doses.

2. *Radiation Energy* (*Quality*).—With multi-fixed-field therapy the greater
the percentage depth dose values for the individual field, the greater the
final tumour-to-skin dose ratio. Similarly with rotation therapy. Megavoltage radiations give a much higher tumour-to-skin dose ratio than do
kilovoltage beams, because of their superior penetration, so much so
that for this, and for other reasons which will be mentioned later, kilovoltage radiation rotation therapy is seldom used today.

3. *Angle of Rotation.*—Up to this point it has been assumed that the patient
was irradiated from all directions (complete rotation), though, of course,

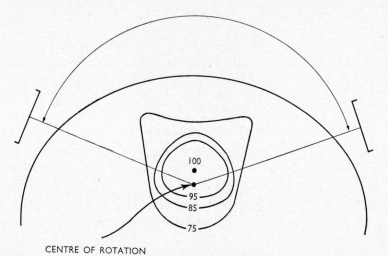

CENTRE OF ROTATION

Fig. 399.—Partial rotation. The centre of the high-dose zone is displaced from the centre
of rotation towards the skin.

this is not essential and in fact there are situations in which it is advantageous to use partial rotation. For example, it might be desired to avoid
irradiating through the spine, or some other important structure. The
chief effect of using partial rotation, other than that it reduces the ratio
of the tumour dose to the skin dose, is to displace the high-dose zone
towards the surface proximal to the rotating source, as illustrated in
Fig. 399. As the angle of rotation is decreased, the more this zone
approaches the surface.

4. *Size of Patient.*—With any given field size and for a given dose at the
axis of rotation, the dose in the peripheral regions will be greater in the
larger patients than in smaller people. The effect is not as great as might
at first be expected, however, since the larger the periphery the greater
the number of stationary fields that could be fitted round (this is the
simple equivalent to the rotation case). This increase in field number
tends to increase the tumour-to-skin ratio and therefore to offset to
some extent the decrease in contribution to the tumour which is produced
by increasing its depth.

5. *Penumbra.*—This may be an important factor when radioactive isotope
sources, such as cobalt 60, are used. These are relatively large and
produce quite a large penumbra which will to a certain extent increase

the field width and produce a zone of higher dose than desired outside the zone being treated.

6. *Tissue Heterogeneity.*—The method by which the radiation is delivered, for example whether by fixed or moving beams, in no way affects its attenuation in the material through which it is passing. Therefore tissue inhomogeneities have the same effect on the radiation in rotation as in fixed-field therapy. Lungs or cavities transmit more radiation than the corresponding thickness of soft tissue, whilst bone 'shadows' the tissues beyond it because of its greater attenuating power.

As for fixed-field work, the effect of bone 'shielding' is very small in rotation therapy with cobalt-60 gamma rays and may be neglected without introducing great inaccuracy. Lungs and cavities have a greater effect and provided their dimensions are known they can be allowed for in the same way as allowance is made in fixed-field work. That part of the rotation cycle in which the beam traverses lung or a cavity before reaching the tumour will contribute more radiation to the tumour than might be expected from uncorrected distributions—a general rule is that the presence of a zone of lower density pulls out the high-dose zone in that direction.

7. *The Treatment Table or Couch.*—A most desirable feature of any radiotherapy treatment is that the patient should remain still during the exposure to radiation, otherwise the desired treatment zone will be neither uniformly nor adequately treated. For this reason many treatments, and especially those using rotation, are carried out with the patient lying horizontally on a couch or treatment table. With fixed-field therapy it is usually possible to avoid having to fire the beam through the support, but with rotation therapy, except over very limited arcs, it is clearly impossible to avoid having the beam passing through the table for at least a part of the total treatment.

For this reason the table top must be as uniform in thickness as possible and have as small an attenuation as possible. Heavy metal supports down each side, or down the centre of the underside of the table, for example, cannot be permitted because of the considerable 'shadows' that they would cast. These are not, it must be confessed, easy conditions to fulfil if the table is also to be strong, and successful tables are products of skilful and ingenious design.

Then, of course, allowance has to be made for attenuation of any radiation passing through the table before reaching the patient, for this reduces the dose values at any point from what they would have been had the patient been suspended in air, an impractical method of treatment(!) which was tacitly assumed in the readings which led to *Table XLVI*. The normal method of making the required allowance is to modify the patient outline by adding to it in the appropriate directions thicknesses which would produce the same attenuation as the table and mattress. An example of this is given in *Fig.* 400.

Rotation Therapy versus Fixed-field Therapy.—There has been much debate concerning the relative merits of fixed-field and rotation therapy and no conclusive answer is yet forthcoming. Nor is one likely to be, since each method has its advantages and disadvantages: in some circumstances one is to be preferred; in some, the other.

With rotation therapy the skin dose is usually markedly lower than it would be, for the same tumour dose, in fixed-field therapy, and the high-dose zone is more regular in shape, being circular or slightly elliptical. Furthermore, for any given apparatus the fall-off of dose outside the treated zone is more rapid in rotation work.

On the other hand, all the skin is irradiated, and the whole body section receives noteworthy irradiation in rotation therapy, whereas only limited skin areas are

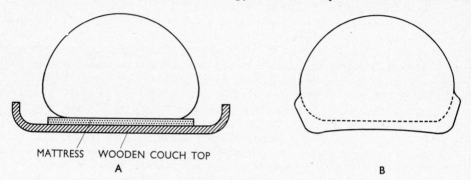

MATTRESS   WOODEN COUCH TOP
A   B

Fig. 400.—A, The patient on the table and mattress. B, The modified body outline to allow for the effects of the table and mattress.

dosed, and some parts of the section receive practically nothing, with fixed fields. This complete sparing of some tissues may be clinically very important—for example, if lungs are being irradiated—whilst the smaller integral dose with fixed fields is an additional, if minor, advantage.

However, the main advantage of fixed-field therapy lies in its possibilities for more accurate treatment. There is no doubt that the accuracy with which a high-dose zone can be produced, and known, around a tumour, whose axis may not lie in any practicable axis of rotation, is greater when fixed fields are used with the sort of beam-direction devices already described.

A not unreasonable conclusion seems to be that where the available apparatus cannot treat a particular tumour adequately with three fields, rotation therapy can be valuable. When the percentage depth dose values are great enough to give the desired tumour dose, and an acceptably small skin dose, with three fields, fixed-field treatments should be chosen. In practical terms, rotation therapy is sometimes very valuable with cobalt-60 telecurie units: it is almost always unnecessary with linear accelerators working at 4 MV. or more.

Before leaving the subject it might be useful to consider why rotation therapy at 250 kV. was rather brusquely passed over earlier in this chapter. Rotation therapy seemed an answer to the difficulty arising because the percentage depth dose values obtained with kilovoltage beams are rather inadequate for the treatment of the centrally placed tumour in the trunk. For head tumours and trunk tumours in the smaller patients the method was acceptable but for central tumours in large patients even rotation therapy was inadequate. Furthermore, with kilovoltage beams the shape, position, and dosage homogeneity of the high-dose zone depend, to a more marked extent than with higher energy radiations, on patient size and shape, the position of the axis of rotation, and the angle of rotation. With these lower energy radiations it is more difficult to prescribe, obtain, and evaluate the required dose. The availability of cobalt-60 units, making the problem so much simpler, virtually brought the end to kilovoltage rotation therapy.

CHAPTER XXXVIII

TELETHERAPY SOURCES

THE factors involved in teletherapy treatments having been discussed, it is now appropriate to consider the X-ray tube or the telecurie gamma-ray source needed to carry them out. As in previous chapters, it is convenient to consider radiations generated at below 1 million volts (and in practice this means the 'deep-therapy' or 'orthovoltage' radiations which are usually generated at up to 300 kV.) separately from megavoltage radiations. The basic principles of X-ray production have been described in CHAPTER V. Electrons from a heated filament are accelerated across an evacuated tube by a high voltage and produce X-rays when they impinge upon the target. A high-voltage generator is required to supply the appropriate voltage and current, whilst the X-ray tube must be designed to withstand that voltage and to cope with the cooling problems arising from heat production associated with the X-ray production. Furthermore, the equipment must be capable of easy movement and accurate positioning in relation to the patient. CHAPTER XXII described the salient features of tubes used in diagnostic radiology, and many of their features are equally applicable to therapy tubes. In fact there is little essential difference between a stationary anode diagnostic tube and a 200-kV. therapy tube.

KILOVOLTAGE THERAPY EQUIPMENT

Radiotherapy, generally, aims at delivering a dose of a few hundreds of rads to a point deep inside a patient in a few minutes. Up to about 1950 most radiotherapy equipment used voltages of 200–300 kV. to achieve the desired penetration, and tube currents of between 10 and 20 mA. to give outputs commensurate with reasonable treatment times without creating insuperable cooling problems. Much equipment of this type is still in use. The working subject–source distance (S.S.D.) is usually 50 cm., and represents a compromise between the desire for large S.S.D. values, and hence greater percentage depth doses, and the desire for high output which calls for smaller S.S.D.

Fig. 401 shows a cross-section of a typical X-ray therapy tube designed to work at 250 kV. The general similarity with the stationary anode tube (*Fig.* 191, p. 277) will be clear: the main points of difference are:

1. *Length.*—Because of the much higher voltage that is going to be used (say 250 kV. compared with not more than 150 kV. in diagnostic radiology) the tube is longer so that no spark can pass from one high-tension electrode to the other. Whereas a length of about 25 cm. is adequate in the diagnostic tube almost twice that length is needed for the radiotherapy tube.

2. *Cooling.*—In diagnostic radiology currents often of upwards of 200 mA. are used for fractions of a second, and the limiting factor is the amount of 'instantaneous' heat that the target metal can tolerate. To a large extent this depends on the target material. In radiotherapy the exposure is usually of the order of minutes, but the current is seldom more than 20 mA., and here the controlling factor is the rate at which heat can be

removed from the target material—which means that the conductivity of the anode assembly and its cooling are the factors of greatest importance. This cooling is often achieved by flowing oil over the back of the

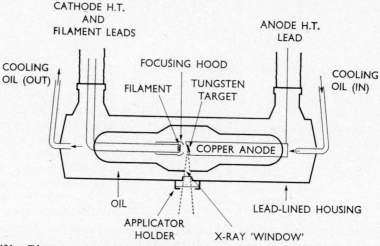

Fig. 401.—Diagrammatic cross-section of a typical 250-kV. radiotherapy X-ray tube in oil-filled housing.

anode and passing it from the tube housing into some cooling radiator in which it gives up its heat to the surrounding air, or even is cooled by water. Very efficient cooling can be achieved by the use of a jet of water spraying the back of the target as shown in *Fig.* 402. This is only possible,

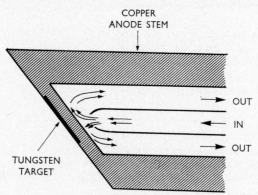

Fig. 402.—The water cooling of an earthed target.

however, if the target is at earth potential—otherwise the water, which is a conductor, albeit a poor one, would short-circuit the anode potential to earth, unless an elaborate insulated cooling system were provided. The use of earthed targets will be discussed later.

3. *Focal Spot Size.*—For radiography, where a sharp shadow is needed, the aim is to use as small a focal spot as possible, and frequently focal spots measuring 1 mm. × 1 mm. or less are used—*see* CHAPTER XXII,

for instance. Although the size of the focal spot of a therapy unit influences the size of the geometric penumbra (CHAPTER XXXV) the situation is nothing like so critical and focal spots of 1 cm. diameter are quite common. This, of course, makes it easier for the target surface to withstand continuous high loading.

4. *Target Angle.*—As described in CHAPTER XVIII the target surface in the diagnostic tube is inclined at an angle of about 17° in order to get an acceptably small effective focal spot and yet have the heat spread over an area several times larger. Such a large inclination automatically limits the angular size of the beam that can be used without gross interference from the 'heel' effect (CHAPTER XVIII). However, at the 100-cm. (or so) source–film distance usually used in radiography there is no difficulty in obtaining uniform beams of adequate size. A very different situation obtains in radiotherapy using 50-cm. source–subject distance. At that distance the maximum uniform field would be too small for much practical work. Therefore, and because that angle gives the most uniform beam, it is usual to use a 30° target.

Centre-earthed and Target-earthed Tubes.—*Fig.* 401 shows the so-called 'centre-earthed' tube, in which both the filament (negative) and the target (positive) are at high voltage. The advantage of this arrangement is that for any given potential difference between the two electrodes the maximum potential difference with respect to earth is only half that value. For example, for a 250-kV. generating voltage the filament will be at −125 kV. and the target at +125 kV., and the cables, etc., only have to be insulated to withstand 125 kV.

A disadvantage of this method of electrical connexion has already been pointed out—it is difficult, if not impossible, to use water cooling, whilst the presence of cables at both ends of the housing tend to impede its movement and to make the accurate application of the tube to the patient more difficult.

An alternative electrical connexion is to earth the target and to have the filament at a high negative voltage. In such a case any cable or other part of the electrical supply has to be insulated to withstand the full voltage applied across the tube, in other words double that of the 'centre-earthed' case. Offsetting this obvious and important disadvantage is the fact that target cooling can be done by using water, direct from the mains if desired, and also that the earthed target can be at one end of a relatively small-diameter tube and therefore provide greater access to the patient for the accurate positioning of the tube and hence directing of the beam.

HIGH-TENSION GENERATORS

The general principles of the operation of the components of circuits providing high voltage for X-ray tubes, along with the appropriate control equipment, have been discussed in CHAPTER XXIII and much of what was said there applies equally to radiotherapy equipment. In this chapter attention will be fixed upon the type of circuit most suitable for therapy purposes, for which, it must be recalled, as high an output and as hard a beam, as is practicable, are wanted.

Bearing in mind the factors which control radiation output and quality (*see* CHAPTER V), it will be clear that, though any of the voltage supplies described in CHAPTER XXIII can be used to generate X-rays for radiotherapy, a circuit giving as constant and as continuous a voltage as possible is desirable. A full-wave rectifying circuit is better than a half-wave circuit or self-rectification, but a constant voltage supply is better than either and is much to be preferred. This is often provided by means of a Greinacher circuit.

The Greinacher Circuit.—This is not only a constant potential, but also a voltage-doubling circuit, its nearly constant voltage output to the X-ray tube being at almost twice the peak voltage supplied by the transformer. The basic circuit is shown in *Fig.* 403. Each condenser is charged to the full potential of the transformer during alternate half-cycles of the voltage wave. When the upper end (in the diagram) of

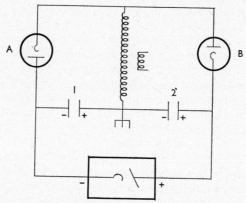

Fig. 403.—The Greinacher circuit.

the transformer is negative, valve A will conduct and condenser 1 is charged up, whilst when the transformer polarity is reversed current will pass through valve B and condenser 2 is charged. These condensers are in series and once fully charged they act as the voltage supply to the tube, the voltage across which will be roughly twice the transformer peak voltage.

The tube current (the mA.) passing through the tube is supplied by the partial discharging of the condensers, and their voltages consequently fall, each being 'topped up' again on alternate half-cycles, as illustrated in *Fig.* 404. In that diagram the voltage supply to each condenser is shown, as is the variation of the voltage across the condensers as the tube draws current from them. For example, at P condenser 1 is charged to full voltage, and as current flows out of it, during the exposure, its voltage falls progressively until Q is reached, when the rising transformer voltage applied to the condenser through the valve 'tops up' the condenser voltage to the peak voltage of the transformer, at P_1, after which the pattern is repeated. A similar state of affairs obtains with condenser 2 on the alternate half-cycles. The voltage across the tube is the sum of the potentials across the two condensers—for example, the values indicated by V_1, V_2, etc. As will be seen from the upper curve, this tube voltage is constant (except for a 'ripple' of a few per cent, at a frequency twice that of the voltage supply) and is a little less than twice the peak voltage of the transformer. The magnitude of the 'ripple' is controlled by the current through the tube—the greater the mA. the greater the ripple—and by the capacity of the condensers—the greater the capacity the smaller the ripple. Usually the capacities are chosen so that the 'ripple' at maximum tube current is about 5 per cent, i.e., the voltage applied to the tube varies, say, between 240 and 250 kV.

The Resonant Transformer.—Although the Greinacher circuit best fulfils the requirements that were laid down initially, it is very heavy and bulky. The generator has thus to be separate from the tube, to which it has generally to be connected by cables. It is not possible to incorporate tube and generator in one tank, so eliminating the need for cables, which tend to impede accurate application to the patient. Therefore, during the last decade or so, a different type of generator, first developed for 1-MV. and 2-MV. machines, has been used very successfully at lower voltages. It is called the *resonant transformer.*

Although, using ordinary frequency supplies, a transformer needs a heavy iron core if it is to function properly, this core can be dispensed with if a fairly high-frequency supply is used, provided the secondary coils of the transformer are 'tuned'

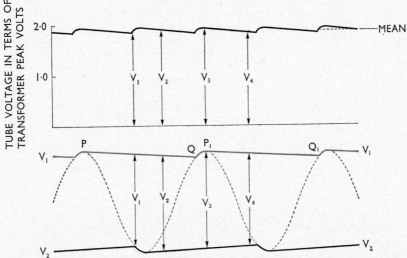

Fig. 404.—The operation of the Greinacher circuit. The lower diagram shows the transformer voltage (dotted), and the voltage across condenser 1 ($V_1 V_1$) and condenser 2 ($V_2 V_2$) when the X-ray tube is working. The upper diagram shows how the voltage of the tube varies.

to that frequency (i.e., will 'resonate' with it). This is not difficult, in practice, with 1000 cycles per sec. supplies (the normal mains frequency is 50 cycles per sec.), though exactly how it is done is beyond the scope of this book. Suffice it to say that using this technique the X-ray tube can be placed down the centre of the resonant (or tuned) transformer coils, where the core would normally be, a direct connexion made from one end of the transformer secondary to the tube filament, and the whole enclosed in a relatively small tank. *Fig.* 405 shows, diagrammatically, the arrangements inside the tank. Several important features should be noted. First, that this approach is readily adapted to the earthed-target connexion, and secondly, that self-rectification is used. This, for a given peak voltage, gives a rather softer beam than would be given by a constant potential unit, but this disadvantage is more than offset by the compactness of the complete unit and the greater ease with which it may be used in accurate treatments. In any case the lost quality can be regained by a relatively small increase in kilovoltage (300 kVp against 250 kV. constant potential, for example), which has the additional advantage that it gives a greater output for a given tube current. Since the target-earthed arrangement allows of better target cooling, higher tube currents can also be used, so that the resonant transformer X-ray unit is generally a higher output machine than its constant-potential counterpart.

Superficial Therapy Equipment.—For dermatological and other treatments where the tissues to be treated are close to the surface, it is not only unnecessary but actually undesirable to have beams of high-penetrating power. Therefore relatively low-generating voltages and short S.S.D. are used—typically, for example, 100 kV. and

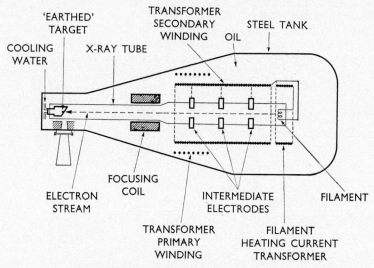

Fig. 405.—A resonant transformer X-ray unit.

15-cm. S.S.D. The tubes are therefore smaller than those using higher voltages, and usually a half-wave rectified generator is used. The tube construction and the associated electrical circuits are almost identical to those used for the stationary anode diagnostic tube, apart from the fact that the target angle is not so steep and the oil surrounding the tube is itself cooled by a coil of copper tubing through which water flows.

MEGAVOLTAGE EQUIPMENT

For reasons that have been set out in CHAPTER XXXIII, high-energy X-rays, and especially those generated at voltages in excess of 1 million volts, have important advantages from the therapeutic point of view, compared with those generated at 200 or 300 kV. Therefore the past twenty years or so have witnessed great efforts to devise machines suitable for radiotherapy, and capable of producing these radiations.

For kilovoltage machines the electrons have been accelerated to the high energy required for X-ray production by a high voltage generated in a transformer and applied directly between the filament and the target of the tube. There is, however, an upper limit to the voltage that can be applied in this way, the limit being set, mainly by insulation problems, at about 2 million volts. For X-rays of higher energy than this, indirect methods of electron acceleration have to be found, and two, in particular, have been used. The first is the linear accelerator, usually used for the equivalent of from 4 to 10 million volts, and the second is the betatron, used for therapeutic purposes in the range 20–35 million volts.

The Linear Accelerator.—To avoid vague generalizations an accelerator designed to accelerate electrons to an energy of 4 MeV. (and hence to serve as a 4-million-volt

X-ray tube) will be described, though it must be stressed that the same principles apply to all versions of this machine.

The basic principle involved is that radio-waves, like all other electromagnetic radiations, are alternating electric and magnetic fields travelling through space. Since an electric field applies a force to a charge particle placed in it, it follows that, if an electron is injected into a beam of radio-waves at an appropriate place and time, it will be acted upon by the force and tend to be carried along by the waves.

In broad terms what happens is very similar to what happens to a surf bather when he is carried along by a wave. If he launches himself into the wave at the correct moment, he will rush along at the speed of the wave, always provided, of course, that the wave is big enough and powerful enough to carry him.

Similarly the radio-waves must have enough power to be able to 'carry' the electrons along. In practice it is not possible to provide this power continuously: it can only be generated in short bursts, or 'pulses', by a special thermionic valve called a magnetron. This was developed during the Second World War for radar work, and can produce several hundred pulses per second, each pulse lasting for a few microseconds (millionths of a second).

Acceleration of the electrons to the required energy (4 MeV. in this case) takes place in what is called a corrugated wave-guide, which is a cylindrical tube across which are placed, at varying intervals along its length, metal disks with small central holes, which make them very similar to the iris diaphragm of a camera. *Fig.* 406 A gives a diagrammatic idea of the guide's construction.

Although radio-waves, in common with all other electromagnetic radiations, travel with the same, constant, velocity in free space (i.e., with the 'speed of light'),

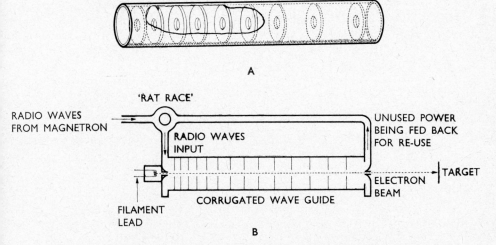

Fig. 406.—A, An impression of the construction of a corrugated wave-guide, showing the iris diaphragms and their spacing. B, The wave-guide as an electron accelerator.

they can travel more slowly in special circumstances, such as when passing along a wave-guide. In such circumstances the exact velocity depends on the spacing of the disks as well as the size of the holes in them. Thus, it is possible to arrange for the waves to be travelling at about 0·4 times the velocity of light at the beginning of the guide but to have speeded up to about 0·99 of that velocity by the time they reach the other end. Since the guide also directs the electric field of the waves along the axis of the tube, electrons can be carried along with the waves and, in a corrugated guide 1 metre long, will acquire the same energy as they would have acquired had a potential difference of 4 million volts been applied across the tube.

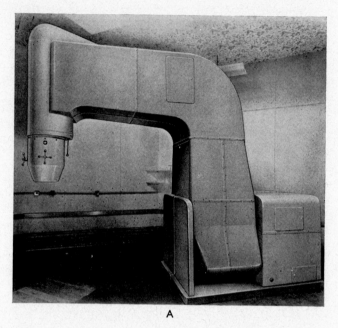

A

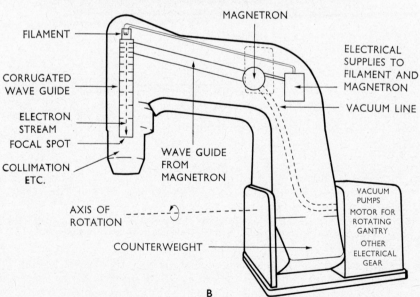

B

Fig. 407.—A, An isocentrically mounted 4-million-volt linear accelerator. B, The main features of the accelerator and where the components are housed.

Fig. 406 B shows the general layout of the components of the accelerating system. Radio pulses (the wavelength is 10 cm.) pass down a plain guide into the corrugated guide. As the pulses start down this guide electrons are shot into them from a heated filament, which is at a negative potential of 40 kV. The electrons have the same speed as the waves and are carried along, accelerating with the waves, to the end of the guide and on to the target where 4-MV. X-rays are generated. The precise energy acquired depends on the details of the wave-guide design and especially upon its length—the longer the guide the greater the energy acquired.

From the end of the wave-guide the electrons travel a short distance to the thin target, which closes the end of the vacuum vessel which encloses the corrugated wave-guide. (Like every X-ray tube, and for the same reasons, the linear accelerator's acceleration section is highly evacuated.) The target is made of a tungsten–copper alloy (which has good thermal conductivity as well as high atomic number) and is about 1 mm. thick. For reasons already given in CHAPTER V a 'transmission target' is used, most of the X-rays generated travelling in a forward direction. Because of the high efficiency of X-ray production by megavoltage electrons (*see*, for example, *Table V*, p. 54) relatively little heat is produced, in marked contrast to the situation in the kilovoltage range, so that target cooling presents very little difficulty. In the 4-MV. accelerator water flowing through a small pipe fastened round the periphery of the target disk is sufficient to carry away any heat generated. Another advantage of the high efficiency of X-ray production is that a small focal spot may be used without danger of overheating and melting the target centre. A 6-mm. diameter spot is quite usual, and therefore no great geometric penumbra results even when the beam-defining diaphragms are at some distance from the patient.

Successful generation of high-energy radiation does not, in itself, guarantee successful therapeutic application, the mounting of the X-ray tube being, in some ways, almost as important as the tube itself. One of the reasons why linear accelerators have proved so good is the excellence, for radiotherapy, of their 'isocentric' mounting, which has already been described and discussed in CHAPTER XXXV. One form of 4-MV. accelerator, with this form of mounting, is shown in *Fig.* 407 A, on the 'key' (*Fig.* 407 B) to which the positions of the main features and components are indicated.

As already stated, the corrugated wave-guide is 1 metre long and the cylinder which houses that guide, the electron gun, the collimators, and other auxiliary gear is 180 cm. long. This length means that the tube cannot readily be rotated to point in all directions. The machine shown in *Fig.* 407 can be rotated, about the horizontal axis, from pointing vertically downwards, to a position in which the beam points upwards to an angle of 20° to the horizontal. Any further rotation would cause the apparatus to strike the floor, unless a special retractable floor, or a pit, is provided. Complete rotation is impracticable in a machine of this size.

Since many radiotherapists wish to do rotation therapy or to be able to treat from any direction so that the patient does not have to be moved between the application of each field, accelerators now being made have been designed to have a horizontal accelerating guide, the high-energy electrons from which are turned through a right-angle by their being passed through an intense magnetic field.* A much more compact machine, capable of complete rotation about its horizontal axis, is thus produced, as can be seen from the picture of an 8-million-volt accelerator shown in *Fig.* 408.

---

* It will be recalled that the electric motor is based upon the fact that a wire carrying a current moves when placed in a magnetic field. A stream of electrons constitutes an electric current and behaves in a similar way to a current-carrying wire; in a magnetic field they follow a curved path.

In spite of its complex components the linear accelerator has proved a most reliable machine and in countries where good technical help is available it is probably the best machine for X-ray therapy.

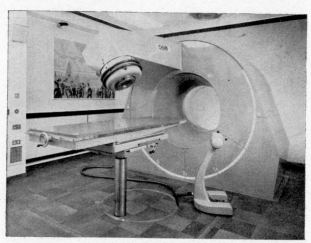

Fig. 408.—An 8-million-volt linear accelerator, isocentrically mounted and capable of rotation through 360°.

The Betatron.—Provided that its corrugated wave-guide is long enough, there is really no limit to the electron energy (and, therefore, the X-ray energy) that the linear accelerator can produce. However, for energies above about 10 MeV. the machine becomes too bulky for convenient clinical use and, where higher energies are desired, it is more usual to employ a betatron. This machine, though by no means small, is, for energies of 20 MeV. and upwards, much more compact than a linear accelerator. It works on the same principle as the high-tension transformer and is best described with the aid of diagrams, such as *Figs.* 409 and 410.

The electrons from a heated filament are accelerated to high energies inside a highly evacuated ring-shaped vessel, which is usually referred to as a 'doughnut' ('donut' is the American spelling), because of the similarity of its shape to that of the confection of the same name. This vessel is placed between the poles of a powerful electromagnet, which is energized by an alternating current passing through magnetizing coils, and thus providing a fluctuating magnetic field through the 'doughnut'.

Electrons are shot into the 'doughnut' (by applying a negative voltage of about 20 kV. to the heated filament), while the magnetizing current, and therefore the magnetic field, are small (at point *S* in *Fig.* 410 A), and are pulled into a circular orbit by this magnetic field. Part *A* of the line in *Fig.* 410 B shows the track followed by the electrons from the filament into the circular orbit.

Now the magnetic field has two separate, though related, functions. First, it keeps the electrons moving in a circular orbit, and secondly, it accelerates them to high energies. It will be recalled that, if a changing magnetic field passes through a coil of wire, a voltage is induced in that coil. This is the principle of the transformer. In like manner an electron moving in a circular orbit, through which a magnetic field is changing, will gain as much energy per revolution as it would have gained from the voltage that would have been induced in a single turn of wire, of the same diameter as in the orbit, in the same changing magnetic field. Each revolution that the electron makes increases its speed and its energy, the total energy acquired depending on the number of revolutions that it makes whilst the magnetic field is building up to the maximum value corresponding to current M.

As its speed increases the electron tends to swing out on a wider orbit, like that indicated by B in *Fig.* 410 B. However, it must be remembered that the curvature of the path, followed by a charged particle in a magnetic field, increases as the magnetic

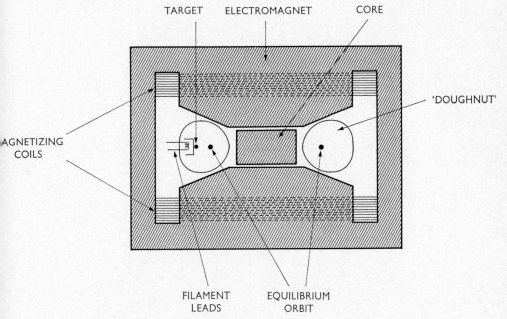

Fig. 409.—A diagrammatic section through a betatron.

field increases (the radius of the orbit decreases). Now, in the betatron, not only is the magnetic field through the orbit increasing (and so accelerating the electron) but so also is the magnetic field at the orbit. This increase tends to make the electrons follow an orbit of smaller radius (as C in *Fig.* 410 B). By careful design of the pole pieces of the betatron magnet, and by some concentration of the magnetic field by the core (*Fig.* 409), the orbit-increasing effort of the changing magnetic field through the orbit (the transformer effect) is precisely balanced by the orbit-shrinking effect of the increasing field at the orbit, throughout the current-increasing period S to M. All this time the electron is gaining energy and moving in exactly the same orbit.

When M is reached, a potential is suddenly applied to the subsidiary electrode E so that the electrons leave the equilibrium orbit and spiral outwards as shown by D in *Fig.* 410 C. They either hit a small target T, which is part of the filament housing, and then produce X-rays, or it can be arranged that they miss the target and escape through a window (W) in the side of the 'doughnut' and emerge as a beam of high-energy electrons. In practice W and the place of emergence of the X-ray beam are close together: they are separated in the diagram to avoid confusion.

For the high-energy (usually 20-MV. or upwards) electrons produced in the betatron, no target cooling is necessary because of the high efficiency of X-ray production (*see* CHAPTER V), whilst the beam itself is relatively narrow and in the 'forward' direction indicated.

The above is, of course, a greatly simplified account of some very complicated phenomena, and it gives no impression of the great technical achievement that the successful working of the betatron represents. Some idea of the difficulties can be gained from the fact that, in each quarter-cycle of the magnet's excitation—$\frac{1}{600}$ sec. with the 150 cycles per second supply that is usually used—the electrons make some

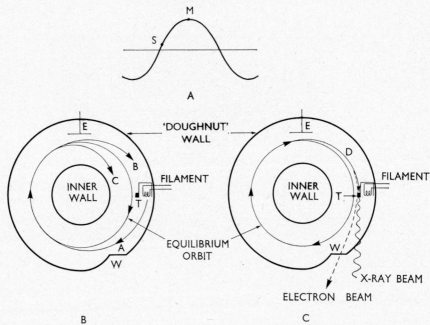

Fig. 410.—How a betatron works. **A**, The variation of the magnetizing current. **B**, The equilibrium orbit and alternatives. **C**, The production of X-rays or an electron beam.

400,000 revolutions, travel about 300 miles and yet do not stray out of the equilibrium orbit until forced to do so at the end of the acceleration period.

Though initially used to generate high-energy X-ray beams, betatrons, as far as radiotherapy is concerned, are now mostly used to generate high-energy electron beams, usually with energies up to about 35 MeV.

Gamma-ray Beam Units.—An alternative to producing high-energy photon beams by the acceleration and stopping of electrons (i.e., using an X-ray tube) is to use the high-energy gamma rays emitted by some radioactive materials. Of the hundreds of isotopes that emit gamma rays there are, however, a mere handful that are suitable for this form of radiotherapy. The required features include a long half-life (so that the source does not have to be changed too often); a high specific activity—curies of radioactivity per gramme of material (so that the source may be small, for a reason to be given later); and, of course, high-energy gamma rays. Initially, before artificial radioactive isotopes were available, radium 228 was used, but because of its scarcity and high price, sources were limited to a maximum of about 10 curies. Modern gamma-ray beam units, in contrast, contain thousands of curies of either cobalt 60 or, less frequently, caesium 137. Cobalt 60 has a half-life of about 5·3 years and emits gamma rays of 1·17- and 1·33-MeV. energy, which means that the beam has roughly the same penetrating power as a 3-million-volt X-ray beam. Caesium 137, on the other hand, has a longer half-life (about 30 years) but emits a lower energy gamma ray (662 keV.) and, for reasons which will be given later, is less widely used than cobalt 60. Iridium 192 has also been used because it is readily available, but its 74 days' half-life is too short to commend this isotope for general use.

Cobalt-60 Beam, or Telecurie, Units.—In general design all radioactive isotope gamma-ray beam units are very similar—a lead-filled steel container or 'head', near to the centre of which there is a radioactive source of considerable strength. This source can be moved (usually by an electric motor) so that it comes opposite to an opening in the container through which the gamma rays emerge to form the treatment beam. At the end of the treatment exposure the source is moved back into its original protected place.

One of the great advantages of this type of radiation source is, of course, its constancy of output (apart from the slow, predictable reduction as the source decays), and this is also one of its great disadvantages! It not only means a completely steady and known output rate free from the inevitable, even though small, short-term fluctuations of any X-ray source, but also a source that can never be switched off! Therefore adequate protection must be afforded so that the radiographic staff may work safely in the treatment room, setting the patient in position, and so on. In the early beam units, using radium, the source was stored in a lead-lined safe, which could be outside the treatment room. The radium source was then transferred pneumatically to and from the treatment head through a flexible tube in much the same way as cash is conveyed between customer and accounts department in a large store. This sort of method is not, however, acceptable for modern kilocurie sources since even with small transport times, quite a large and undesired whole body dose would be given to the patient as the source flashed forwards and backwards at the beginning and end of a treatment period. Furthermore, the radiation hazard to the staff if the source stuck in the transport pipe is too great to be accepted, in spite of the advantages of the smaller head that can be used if the source is only in it during treatment.

Construction.—A typical cobalt-60 beam unit, suitable for a source containing up to about 4500 curies (4·5 kCi), is shown diagrammatically in *Fig.* 411. Basically it is made up of two lead-filled steel spheres which merge into one another. The larger sphere, at the centre of which the source rests when not in use (i.e., when it is in the 'safe' position), has a diameter of about 2 ft., and the smaller sphere is just over 1 ft. across. Centrally pivoted on the common axis of the spheres is a rather flat drum (lead filled) near to the edge of which the source is placed. This drum can be rotated electrically, and the source moved from the centre of the large sphere ('safe') to the centre of the smaller sphere. In this latter position it is opposite the beam port, through which the gamma rays emerge through the collimators to give the treatment beam. In all other directions the rays are effectively cut off by the surrounding lead. At the end of treatment the source returns to its 'safe' position when the Exposure rate on the surface of the machine is low enough to present no hazard to staff working in the room. It will be noted, in *Fig.* 411, that copper-tungsten (often called 'heavy') alloy has been used in some places. This alloy is a better attenuator than lead, for high-energy radiations, because of its greater density but is too expensive for general use. It is, therefore, mainly used where space is at a premium and the maximum protection has to be obtained in the available space. Thus it is used to compensate for lead that has been removed to accommodate the collimation system, and also for the master collimator.

Source Design.—The radiation output of a cobalt-60 machine depends on the shape and size of the source as well as upon the amount of radioactive isotope that it contains. Usually the source is cylindrical in shape, its length being about the same as its diameter. In order to reduce geometric penumbra to a minimum the

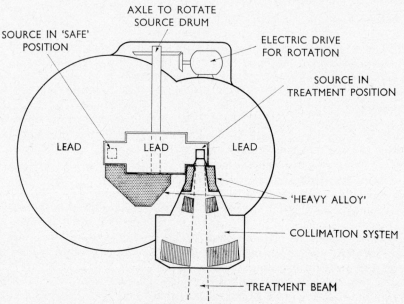

Fig. 411.—A diagrammatic section through a cobalt-60 beam unit.

source diameter must be kept as small as possible (*see* CHAPTER XXXV). This reduces the amount of radioactive material in the source unless the length is correspondingly increased. Unfortunately, this solution is not acceptable, for even if the volume of radioactive material were kept constant the radiation output would not, because radiation coming from the back of the source would be increasingly attenuated, as the source length increased, by the source material in front of it (often known as 'self-attenuation'). Therefore the source is seldom more than 2 cm. long and has about the same diameter. This is considerably greater than the 6-mm. focal spot of the linear accelerator, or the even smaller focal spot of the betatron. With the cobalt-60 unit, therefore, there is inevitably a much greater geometric penumbra, which constitutes something of a disadvantage compared with the X-ray machines.

Some idea of the design of the actual source may be gleaned from *Fig.* 412, which indicates that it consists of a double-walled stainless-steel container into the inner compartment of which the radioactive cobalt is sealed. Both inner and outer containers are sealed by welding or high-temperature brazing, this precaution being necessary because radioactive cobalt, though it has no gaseous product which might leak, is dusty, and these precautions have to be taken to ensure that none of the dust escapes to contaminate the apparatus. Although the risk of a leak is extremely small, it is advisable that periodic 'wipe' tests should be made around the treatment head, and especially the collimating system. Surfaces are wiped over with damp cotton-wool which is then tested for radioactivity.

The radioactive cobalt in the source is in the form of thin disks (each about 2·5 mm. thick), as shown in the diagram, or, increasingly nowadays, of tiny cobalt cylinders each about 1 mm. long and 1 mm. in diameter. The latter are 'packed by vigorous agitation of the capsule'.

Therapy Apparatus.—Because it requires only simple low-voltage electrical supplies—to move the source, and light the beam-indicating lamp—and needs no

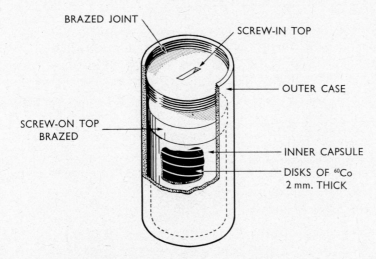

Fig. 412.—A telecurie cobalt-60 source, made up of a number of disks of the radioactive material, inside a carefully sealed container.

electrical power for radiation generation, this type of gamma-ray source, having no complicating heavy supply cables, is especially suitable for rotation therapy, and the majority of cobalt-60 telecurie units offer this facility. *Fig.* 413 shows one such unit, in which the treatment head is attached to a large annulus, which is driven around the horizontal axis by an electric motor. When loaded with about 4000 curies of cobalt 60 this machine gives about 100 R per minute at a S.S.D. of 75 cm.

Caesium 137 as a Beam Source.—Parameters of importance in deciding which of a selection of possible sources is preferable, include half-life, gamma-ray energy, Γ factor, and availability, and when caesium 137 is compared with cobalt 60 it is found that some of its features are more desirable, and some are less.

Half-life.—As already stated, the half-life of caesium 137 is over 30 years compared with 5·3 years for cobalt 60, which means that caesium 137 decays about 2 per cent per year against 1 per cent per month for the shorter-lived material. In practical terms cobalt sources usually have to be replaced every 3 or 4 years, whereas a caesium-137 source will serve for 20 or so years before its output falls too low to be acceptable therapeutically.

Radiation Energy.—The gamma rays from caesium 137 have an energy of just over 660 keV. and are thus equivalent to a 1·5-million-volt X-ray beam, whilst the 1·17- and 1·33-MeV. rays from cobalt 60 are like a 3-million-volt beam. Therein lie advantages and disadvantages. Being of higher energy the cobalt-60 gamma rays will be more penetrating and, for otherwise equal conditions (field size, F.S.D., etc.), give better percentage depth doses in a phantom or a patient than would caesium-137 beams. This advantage is not great: for example, the dose delivered to a point 10 cm. deep from a 100-cm.² cobalt-60 beam at 50-cm. S.S.D. is about 10 per cent greater than that from a caesium-137 beam under the same conditions.

Against this the lower-energy caesium-137 gamma rays suffer considerably more attenuation in the high atomic number materials used for the treatment heads, so that a caesium-137 unit can be much smaller, and therefore more easily used than a cobalt-60 unit. The latter may be 2 ft. or more in diameter against 1 ft. for the caesium-137 machine, their weights being roughly in the ratio of 10 : 1.

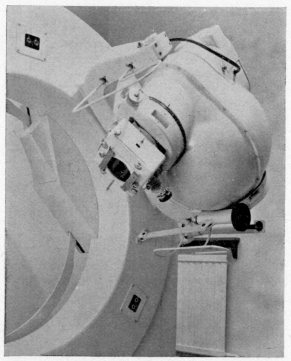

Fig. 413.—A kilocurie cobalt-60 radiotherapy unit for rotation as well as fixed-field treatments. Part of the rotating annulus can be seen to the left of the treatment head.

Gamma-ray Constant.—As far as radiation output is concerned the advantage is very much with cobalt 60 whose gamma-ray constant (Exposure rate at 1 cm. in R per hr. per millicurie) is about 13 compared with 3·3 for caesium 137. This advantage is further enhanced by cobalt's 8 : 3 density advantage. For any given volume of source there will be nearly three times as much cobalt as caesium.

Availability and Source Size.—An unbiased appraisal of the facts so far set out would, probably, lead to the conclusion that caesium 137 is a better material, for beam units, than is cobalt 60. In fact cobalt 60 is much more widely used and is to be preferred. The reason for this lies in availability and source size. Cobalt 60 is produced by the irradiation of cobalt 59 in the nuclear reactor, as the result of an n–γ reaction. For this reason the amount of radioactive cobalt in a source of any given size depends on the length of time for which the irradiation is carried on, and upon the flux density (neutrons per ml. per sec.) in the part of the pile into which the cobalt is placed. With heavy water as a moderator, high flux densities are possible and sources containing 4000 or 5000 curies, in cylinders whose height and diameter are 2 cm., can be obtained.

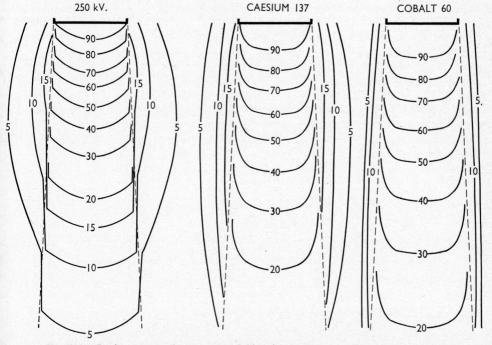

Fig. 414.—Isodose curves for 5×5 cm. fields with 250-kV., caesium-137, and cobalt-60 radiation beams. Note the superiority of cobalt 60 both as regard percentage depth dose and scattered radiation outside the beam. Caesium 137 gives better depth doses than 250 kV. but roughly the same amount of radiation outside the main beam.

With caesium 137 the situation is quite different. This isotope is obtained from uranium fission products from which it can be extracted along with non-radioactive caesium 133 and a shorter-lived radioactive isotope caesium 134. The specific activity (curies of caesium 137 per gramme of caesium) is thus fixed at about 25 curies per gramme (compared with about 150 curies per gramme for cobalt 60) and variation of source strength can only be achieved by variation in source size. For greater radiation output larger volumes of caesium must be used. There is, however, a limit to the source size that is acceptable for radiotherapy. Too large a diameter gives large penumbra, whilst increasing the source length does not achieve proportionate output increase because of the self-absorption already discussed. The usual compromise results in a source which is very similar in outer appearance to that used for cobalt 60, is about 2·7 cm. diameter and about 4 cm. long, and which contains about 2000 curies of caesium 137. Such a source gives about 6 or 7 R per min. at 1-metre S.S.D., and therefore for therapeutic purposes caesium-137 telecurie units normally are used at an S.S.D. of 30 or 40 cm., at which a reasonable output is obtained.

Even so the geometric penumbra produced by a caesium-137 unit is not small, and is far greater than that from a cobalt-60 unit. As a result of the enforced rather small S.S.D., as well as, though to a lesser extent, the lower energy of the radiation the percentage depth doses from a caesium-137 unit are much inferior to those from a cobalt-60 machine. In fact the caesium-137 beam is more comparable with a kilovoltage beam (say 2·5 mm. Cu H.V.L.) at about 50-cm. S.S.D. both in percentage depth dose values and also in penumbra. In the X-ray case the 'penumbra' is scattered radiation rather than of geometric origin, but the fact remains that the general appearance of caesium-137 beam isodose curves is very similar to that from a 250-kV. machine, and not so much like that from cobalt 60 as *Fig.* 414 reveals.

It is now generally agreed that caesium 137 is not an alternative to cobalt 60 as a rival to megavoltage X-ray sources, but rather a possible substitute for kilovoltage (say 250-kV.) machines with the great advantage of a steady—if rather small—output and very little electrical equipment to give trouble. Even these advantages, however, are offset by the relatively low output, the fact that it is not easy to achieve large field sizes and 'flat' isodose curves, and the bulkier and heavier shielding that has to be used.

CHAPTER XXXIX

ACCEPTANCE TESTS AND CALIBRATION

WHEN a new X-ray set or telecurie gamma-ray beam unit is installed there are a number of tests that have to be carried out on it before it is put into any kind of service. Subsequently there are a whole range of measurements that have to be made to establish its radiation characteristics for treatment purposes, and finally there are tests and measurements that are carried out periodically and regularly to ensure that the working of the machine remains constant. Not all these tests and measurements will be carried out by the same person but all are concerned with the safety of the staff and patients, and with the accuracy of treatment, so that they are very much the concern of the radiographer and radiologist.

COMMISSIONING TESTS

Initial Mechanical Tests.—The first tests that have to be carried out are simple and purely mechanical. Though modern equipment is very carefully designed, made, and assembled, mistakes can occur and it is 'better to be sure than sorry'. Therefore, before any attempt is made to get radiation from the set, each brake should be carefully released, in turn, to ensure that any counterweighting is satisfactory, and that the tube head does not rush up, or down, or rotate violently, as has happened in the authors' experience. With its brake released each movement should be free and smooth running and be able to be stopped at will when the brake is reapplied. Precisely what tests of this sort have to be made will depend on the details of the equipment. The main point will, however, be clear: all mechanical features must be known to be working properly.

Radiation Protection.—A description of the methods for protecting people from radiation hazards, and of the methods of measurement which are used to check the efficiency of protective measures, will be given in CHAPTERS XLIII, XLIV, and XLV. Suffice it to say at this stage that the radiation protection for any new installation must be thoroughly surveyed and shown to be effective, before any further work is done with the equipment. This protection includes the protective walls, doors, windows, and so on, and also any protection incorporated in the machine itself.

Further Mechanical Tests.—In radiotherapy it is essential to know the precise direction of the radiation beam, and since it cannot be seen, its position, or at least the direction of its central ray, is usually indicated by some mechanical devices, such as the front and back pointers (*see Fig.* 370, p. 513). Often, also, provision is made for a light beam to simulate the treatment beam as *Fig.* 365 (p. 507) shows. It is, of course, vital that the axis of the beam should lie along the axis of the mechanical devices and that so also should the axis of the light beam.

The relevant parts of the system are the radiation source (i.e., focal spot of an X-ray tube or the radioactive material in a telecurie unit), the collimating system (i.e., applicator or movable diaphragms or 'jaws'), and the beam-direction device,

567

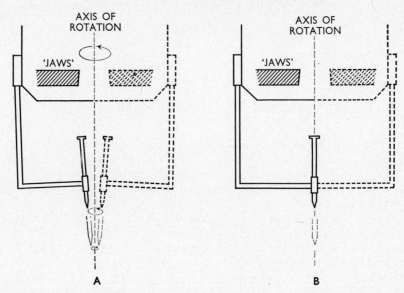

Fig. 415.—Alinement of front pointer on to axis of rotation of 'jaws'. A, Pointer mis-placed describes circle around axis when system is rotated. B, Correctly alined pointer remains stationary during rotation.

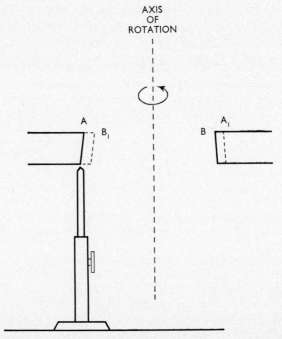

Fig. 416.—Check the symmetry of the collimator 'jaws'. The adjustable pointer is brought close to the edge of 'jaw' A. The 'jaws' are then rotated through 180° to the positions shown dotted. The edge of 'jaw' B is not close to the pointer, indicating that the 'jaws' are not spaced equally on either side of the axis.

be it front and back pointers, light beam, or any other system. When the unit is in correct adjustment the following conditions are fulfilled:

1. The front and back pointers are on the axis of rotation of the collimation system at all treating distances.
2. The collimator 'jaws' are symmetrically placed in relation to this axis, and move symmetrically about it.
3. The light source is effectively on the axis. It is not usually actually on the axis but to one side as *Fig.* 365 (p. 507) shows.
4. The radiation source must be centred on the axis.

That these conditions hold for any piece of equipment cannot be assumed: a series of relatively simple tests will reveal whether they do, or enable appropriate alterations to be made. Precise details of the tests depend on the type of equipment and its design. Taking the case of a cobalt-60 gamma-ray beam unit as an example, the tests are as follows:

1. First of all the front and back pointers have to be adjusted so that when the collimators and pointer mounting are rotated the tips of the pointers remain stationary at all treating distances. This can only happen if they lie on the axis of rotation.

   The test is illustrated by *Fig.* 415, in which, for the sake of clarity, only the front pointer is shown. It should be noted that in this diagram, as in the four which follow it, the misplacement is grossly exaggerated, for ease of illustration, compared with what may be met in practice. In section (A) the front pointer is both displaced sideways from the axis and is at an angle to it. The tip of the pointer will, therefore, describe a small circle around the axis when the jaws and pointer are rotated. The size of the circle varies, as shown, with the position of the rod, and it is possible, in a case like that illustrated, for the tip to remain stationary for one position of the rod, and yet the pointer be wrongly mounted. Only when the rod lies on the axis of rotation, as shown in (B), does the point remain stationary for all rotations.

2. Next the collimator jaws have to be tested to see whether they are placed symmetrically with respect to their rotation axis. A simple way of doing this is to set up a pointer, as shown in *Fig.* 416, so that it just touches the edge of one of the jaws being tested. The collimator is then rotated through 180°, and only if the jaws are correctly placed will the second jaw just touch the pointer. *Fig.* 416 also shows what happens when symmetry is not achieved.

   This test should be carried out for each pair of jaws and for settings of each pair, and furthermore it should be done with the machine in various positions. When the machine is pointing vertically downwards, or upwards, for example, gravity will tend to pull the jaws into symmetry, whereas if the beam is being fired horizontally one set of jaws may flop downwards somewhat, and therefore no longer remain symmetrical about the axis. Hence it is not sufficient to carry out this test with the machine in just one position.

3. If a light-beam indicator is provided, it must be adjusted by altering the position of the lamp or mirror until the light patch for any field is symmetrical around the front pointer. *Fig.* 417 A shows a badly adjusted light beam passing asymmetrically through the 'jaws' because its axis

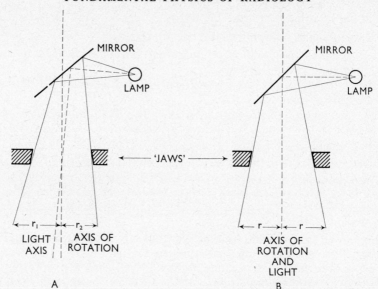

Fig. 417.—The position of lamp and mirror system. A, The adjustment is faulty so that the beam of light does not pass symmetrically through the jaws, and the illuminated area (which should indicate the size of the gamma-ray beam) is not symmetrical with the axis of rotation. The distance r_1 is greater than r_2. B, Here, by tilting the mirror, correct positioning has been achieved and the lighted area is equal on each side of the axis.

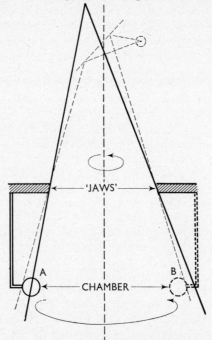

Fig. 418.—The 'off-axis' source. The chamber is firmly attached to one jaw and Exposure rate readings taken in position A and, after rotation through 180°, in position B. Because of the source position the amount of beam passing through the chamber is different in the two positions. The light beam—already adjusted as described—shown dotted indicates the desired beam position in which both positions would be equally irradiated.

is not coincident with the axis of rotation. In *Fig.* 417 B the mirror has been tilted and the desired symmetry achieved.

4. Next it has to be established that the source is positioned so that its centre lies on the rotation axis. *Fig.* 418 illustrates the situation where this condition is not fulfilled and also the test that has to be carried out.

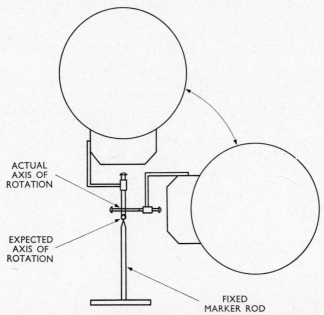

ACTUAL
AXIS OF
ROTATION

EXPECTED
AXIS OF
ROTATION

FIXED
MARKER ROD

Fig. 419.—Test for accuracy of indication of axis of rotation. If axis is at distance indicated by front pointer, the tip of that pointer will remain in contact with the fixed rod for all positions of the apparatus.

For that test an ionization chamber is firmly fixed, as shown, to one of the jaws, and placed so as to be close to the edge of the beam, as indicated for instance by the light beam. An Exposure-rate reading is taken and then the jaws rotated through 180° and the reading repeated. If the source is not properly centred the two readings will differ, for reasons that will be clear from *Fig.* 418. There the chamber is actually only half in the beam in position A, even though it is fully inside the light beam, whereas it is well inside in position B. The reading at B will be greater than that at A. This test is quite critical provided the chamber can be placed near the beam edge, small movements of which will bring about quite big changes in reading.

5. Finally, if the machine can be used for rotation therapy, the accuracy of its rotation must be checked. (Up to now the word 'rotation' has been used in connexion with the turning of some part of the apparatus —here it is used for the movement of the whole.) This again can be done simply. As shown in *Fig.* 419 a pointer is set up and brought in contact with the front pointer which has been adjusted so that its end is at the source to axis-of-rotation distance. The machine is then rotated and the two should remain in contact. If they do not—as shown in

exaggerated fashion in the diagram—the axis of rotation is not being properly indicated by the pointer and the source may be at the wrong distance.

Other Equipment.—Tests of the type described apply equally well, of course, to the linear accelerator or any other equipment using movable 'jaw' collimation. In

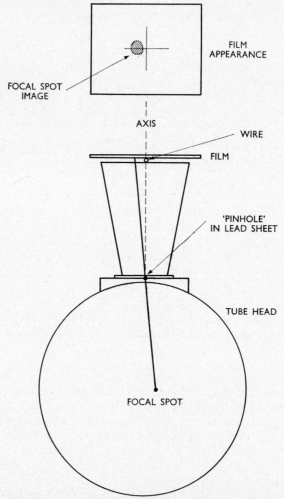

Fig. 420.—The 'off-axis' focal spot test with an applicator. In the upper part of the diagram the film appearance shows that the focal spot image is to one side of the cross, meaning that the focal spot is not on the axis. The lower diagram shows how this image is produced.

principle they apply to all apparatus though where applicators are used for beam definition slightly different, but equally simple, tests have to be used.

Whether or not the axis of the back pointer lies on the axis of rotation of the applicator can be tested as described above. To find out whether the focal spot also lies on this axis, a sheet of lead with a small ('pin-') hole through its centre is fixed to a rectangular applicator the end of which goes into the slide, whilst two pieces of wire, in the form of a cross, are fastened along the long and short axes at the other end. The 'pin-hole' is carefully centred on the applicator, and, with the beam firing vertically upwards (for convenience), a wrapped X-ray film is placed on the applicator end, as shown in *Fig.* 420, and an exposure made. On the developed film will be found a 'pin-hole' picture of the focal spot and a shadow of, at least part of, the wire cross. The intersection of the wires and the centre of the focal spot image should coincide. If they do not, as shown in *Fig.* 420, the centring is faulty and the direction of adjustment can be deduced from the radiograph.

A further test that must be carried out on each application is to make sure that the X-ray field that it produces is of the size and shape expected. For this each applicator is fitted to the tube in turn, a wrapped film placed on its end as above (but now, of course, there are no cross-wires and no lead sheet and 'pin-hole') and a short X-ray exposure made. The developed film will show a blackened area indicating the beam size and shape which can be checked for correctness very simply. Errors of the type being looked for here are very rare but sometimes occur when the lead diaphragm in the applicator is of the wrong size, or when lead lining used in the wall in some designs of applicator becomes displaced.

RADIATION TESTS

The equipment may now be said to have been shown to be mechanically satisfactory, and to be safe to use. Final decisions about working conditions, i.e., which generating voltages, and which filters, should be used, have now to be made, and then radiation tests and full calibration carried out. On the subject of working conditions it is important to remember that, generally, a choice of operating voltage is usually practicable only in the kilovoltage range, and it is only in this range that change of filtration is likely to have any very worth-while effect. *Table XV* (p. 153) shows that quite heavy filtration of the 1-MV. beam produces relatively little change in its penetrating power. So little are the advantages to be gained from the quality changes likely to be possible with any particular X-ray machine, and so considerable are the dangers of wrong exposure arising from the use of the wrong voltage setting or filter, that the most advisable policy is to have but one set of working conditions with each tube. In general this will be the highest kilovoltage and that filter which gives the hardest beam commensurate with a reasonable radiation output. This chapter assumes 'one tube, one set of working conditions'.

'Pin-hole' Pictures.—For X-ray tubes working at up to about 300 kV. a valuable initial radiation test is the taking of a 'pin-hole' picture of the focal spot. The method has already been described in CHAPTER XVIII. As time goes on and the tube is used, the focal spot pattern may change, and it is desirable to be able to compare its appearance with what it looked like initially. Any change and especially non-uniformities can give important clues about the condition of the filament and of the target surface. Changes of X-ray output may be explained, or incipient tube failure predicted, on such evidence. 'Pin-hole' pictures cannot readily be obtained with megavoltage X-ray apparatus, and are not necessary with radioactive isotope machines.

Half-value Layer.—The X-ray apparatus when delivered may, or may not, have the desired filtration incorporated. Half-value layer measurements have to be made in either case to ensure that the finally used filtration is adequate but not excessive. It will be recalled from CHAPTER XIII, for example, that beyond a certain thickness additional filtration does not produce further 'hardening' of the beam, but simply reduces output.

When the half-value layer is known, the appropriate depth dose data and isodose curves may be selected from the large published range. A small problem arises when the half-value layer achieved does not coincide with the values for which data are available (1·0, 1·5, 2·0, 2·5, or 3·0 mm. Cu, for example). Two courses are open: the operating kilovoltage or the filter may be altered to give a half-value layer for which data are available, or advantage is taken of the fact that the percentage depth dose values change very slowly with change of quality. This means that data for any quality may be obtained quite easily and accurately by interpolation from standard data.

Treatment Timing Problems.—Many X- and gamma-ray treatments are given on the basis of a known Exposure rate for a certain length of time. For example, if an Exposure of 250 R is called for from a machine giving 60 R per min., the treatment time would be 4 min. 10 sec. (250 sec.). Accuracy in such treatments, therefore, calls for an accurately known, and maintained, output rate, and for accurate timing.

Treatment times are usually controlled by an electrically driven timer which is started by the switching on of the beam, and which ends the exposure at some pre-set time. Its accuracy, which should be tested before any output calibrations are made, is easily checked with the aid of a stop-watch.

Methods of measuring output have already been discussed in CHAPTER XXXII and will be reviewed again later. Whichever method is used, it should be remembered that the method of switching the beam on and off may introduce errors.

In some apparatus the treatment is controlled by a shutter which is opened and closed electrically; in some X-ray equipment the output builds up from zero to

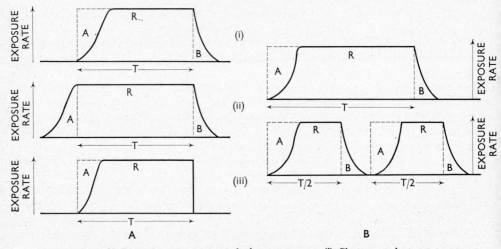

Fig. 421.—A, Exposure-rate patterns during treatment: (i) Shutter or isotope source moves from start of timer. (ii) Timer starts when shutter fully open or source in position. (iii) Kilovoltage builds up from start of timer. Output ceases as timer cuts off kV. B, The determination of the magnitude of the 'end-effects'.

its full value as the generating voltage builds up in the first few seconds of the treatment; in telecurie units the source usually has to be moved into position at the start of treatment and removed at the end. For this sort of reason the Exposure rate is not likely to be constant throughout the exposure period. It may not attain its full value immediately, or, where the timer only starts timing when the shutter is fully open, some radiation may be delivered before the treatment 'officially' starts. Similarly, the irradiation may continue after the timer has apparently ended the treatment, because the shutter takes a little while to close, or the isotope source to move back into its safe position. Some of these variations are shown in *Fig.* 421A.

Thus during any exposure there will be a period of irradiation at the full rate plus some 'end-effects', and any single measurement designed to measure the true dose rate may give a false idea because it assumes that the rate has been constant throughout. If it were, the reading D would be equal to the Exposure rate (R) multiplied by the time T. In fact in the three examples shown in *Fig.* 421 A the reading would be: (i) $R \times T - A + B$, (ii) $RT + A + B$, and (iii) $RT - A$. Which of these three applies in any particular case, and what are the relative values of A and B, will not be readily clear. A single measurement will not indicate the true value of R: two measurements can do so.

The best method is illustrated in *Fig.* 421 B. A value of D is obtained for an exposure of T and then again for two periods of $T/2$. In the first instance there will be one set of end-effects, whilst in the second measurement there will be two such sets. Any differences between the two readings will be due to one lot of end-effects, and so the correction to be applied can be established. For example:

Reading for 1-min. exposure 58 R   Reading for two $\frac{1}{2}$-min. exposures 56 R
∴ One 'end-effect' reduces reading by 2 R
∴ True 1-min. reading $= 58 + 2 = 60$ R
or   True Exposure rate $= 60$ R per min.

The 'end-effect' will be present in any exposure but can generally be ignored for actual treatments. If the Exposure to be used were 250 R then the 'end-effect' error would still be 2 R, which is less than 1 per cent. On the other hand, to have ignored it in the calibration would have introduced an error of more than 4 per cent.

Radiation Distribution 'in Air'.—For reasons outlined previously (inverse-square law, 'heel' effect, and oblique passage of rays through the tube wall and filters) the primary radiation Exposure rate, at any distance from the tube, will fall off on either side of the central axis. Measurements of this Exposure rate must therefore be made along and parallel to and perpendicular to the tube axis, to reveal the extent of this falling-off, and to determine whether or not the field is symmetrical about the central axis. Lack of symmetry may be corrected by special filters, as may the falling-off, especially with megavoltage machines for which, as already described, 'beam-flattening' filters are commonly used. Some fall-off is usually tolerated with kilovoltage beams, and the maximum field size is usually set for a drop of between 10 and 15 per cent.

OUTPUT CALIBRATION

Having ascertained that the beam is satisfactory, calibration for treatment purposes may be carried out. This involves determining the output, at some reference point, for each applicator or, if movable jaw collimators are used, for a range of field shapes and sizes. Details of the methods that can be used have been given in CHAPTER XXXII, and it may be reiterated that, in the authors' opinion, that based on measurements at 5 cm. deep is to be preferred.

Monitor Ionization Chamber.—If the source output is steady, as it is of course from radioactive material, accurate dosage can be achieved from a knowledge of the radiation output and the treatment time. The output of most X-ray tubes, however, is subject to some fluctuation, and nowadays it is normal to monitor the treatment beam by means of an ionization chamber that goes right across the beam, and is positioned as shown in *Fig*. 422. This means that the chamber volume is quite large, and since it is also at a place of fairly high output, the electronic amplifier associated

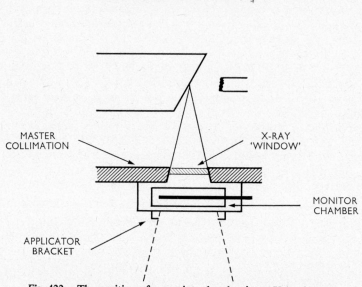

Fig. 422.—The position of a monitor chamber in an X-ray beam.

with it may be relatively simple, but very stable and reliable. A further, and equally important, reason why the chamber extends right across the beam is that thereby it affects all parts of the beam equally and does not cast a local shadow, as did the thimble ionization chambers which were once used placed centrally in the beam.

It must be remembered that this monitor chamber measures the primary radiation only and at a distance away from the patient. Its reading is proportional to the radiation being received by the patient, the factor relating the two varying with the field size and having to be taken into account in the calibration of the monitor.

If the monitor indicates Exposure rate the output of each beam shape and size is measured for a fixed reading on the meter, and then, during treatment, it is the radiographer's responsibility to keep the output steady at this value.

Alternatively, the monitor may be of an integrating type and add up the Exposure being delivered to the patient. In this case the treatment may be terminated manually, or automatically when a certain reading, known to correspond to the desired Exposure to the patient, from the field being used, is reached.

PERIODIC CHECKS

An X- or gamma-ray beam unit, like a car or any other mechanical device, should be routinely 'serviced' to ensure smooth and safe operation. Inspection to ensure mechanical and electrical safety and the accuracy of mechanical devices like front and back pointers should be carried out at least monthly, whilst radiation tests should be carried out at shorter, or longer, intervals according to their importance. 'In air' distribution checks, for example, should be carried out at least annually and at the same time it is useful to take a 'pin-hole' picture of the focal spot. On the other hand, checks for the constancy of the output are much more important and should be carried out very frequently. Where there is no radiation monitor, and treatments are done on the basis of kV., mA., and time, at least one field output should be checked every day. Where there is a monitor its accuracy should be tested at least once a week, if not more frequently. Whenever there has been any alteration, or major adjustment, to any apparatus, detailed rechecking must be undertaken.

Even this degree of care does not, however, guarantee safety. A fault may develop immediately after checking has been carried out. Since the consequences of dosage errors can be so serious, a considerable responsibility rests with the radiographer, who must, at all times, be on the alert for signs and symptoms in the running of the apparatus which suggest faulty performance, and should immediately report suspicions to those responsible for the maintenance of the equipment. Better a dozen reports which prove to call for no action than one fault overlooked. One of the reasons why a study of physics is included in the training of radiographers is that they may have some understanding of how the apparatus works, of the importance of the various factors involved, and of the possible effects of changes in these factors. In radiography the price of safety is eternal vigilance.

CHAPTER XL

GAMMA-RAY SOURCES FOR PLESIOTHERAPY

ALTHOUGH, nowadays, much of the radiotherapy of cancer is carried out with beams of X- or gamma rays (teletherapy), it has not always been so. For many years after their discovery, X-rays were little used for treatment purposes, except for superficial lesions, because the penetrating power of the radiations available was inadequate for the successful treatment of lesions inside the body. Up to the early 1930s, generating voltages above 150 kV. were rare.

On the other hand, the decay products of radium (and radon) emit gamma rays of average energy about 1 MeV., and from quite soon after the discovery of radium these radiations were used for treatment purposes. For several decades, in fact, radium—or Curie—therapy constituted a major part of radiotherapy.

Because the amounts of radium and radon available to individual hospitals were small, sources had to be placed close to the part being treated if adequate treatments were to be given and three main approaches to this short-distance, or 'plesio', therapy were developed. These were:

1. 'Mould' or 'plaque' treatments, in which the gamma-ray sources are mounted on some carrying materials, nowadays often one of the light plastics. The sources are thus maintained at some desired distance from the tissues to be treated. That distance is seldom greater than 2 cm. and is usually 0·5 cm. or 1·0 cm.
2. 'Implant' treatments, in which the sources are inserted directly into the tissue in or around the zone to be treated.
3. Intracavitary treatments, in which the sources in suitable containers are inserted into body cavities for the treatment of the tissues immediately surrounding those cavities.

The effectively very short treating distances in these types of treatment mean that the Exposure rate falls off rapidly with increasing distance from the sources (in other words, poor percentage depth doses) in spite of the high energy of the radiation, because of the dominant role of the inverse-square law. Though it might normally be regarded as a disadvantage, this property can be put to good effect. When coupled with the ability to arrange sources close to or around the diseased tissues, it means that treatment doses can largely be confined to those diseased tissues with relatively small doses elsewhere; and this with radiation possessing the desirable features (such as low selective bone dosage and high bone-penetration) associated with high-energy photons. In some situations, therefore, this type of treatment is superior to any other at present available.

Until the 1950s, radium and radon were the only available gamma-ray sources suitable for plesiotherapy but since then, and especially in the past decade or so, caesium 137 has increasingly replaced radium whilst radon has been almost completely superseded by gold 198. Cobalt 60 (as a radium replacement), iridium 192, and tantalum 182 have also been used.

Radium and Radon as Gamma-ray Sources.—Radium is the sixth member of the radioactive series which starts with uranium and ends in lead. Radium 'decays', with the emission of an alpha particle, into the inert gas radon. Some details of the series from radium onwards are shown in *Fig.* 423 which reveals a number of important facts. The first is that neither radium nor radon emits the desired gamma rays. Why, therefore, are radium and radon used as sources when the desired gamma rays come from radium B and radium C, and mainly from the latter? Why not use these substances alone? The answer lies in the half-lives of the various members of the radium series. From *Fig.* 423 it will be seen that the half-lives of Ra A, B, and C are approximately 3, 27, and 20 minutes respectively—all of which are very short in comparison

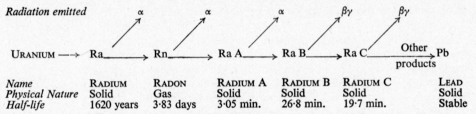

Fig. 423.—The radium 'family' showing the radiations emitted, the nature of the products, and their half-lives.

with the 1620 years half-life of radium or even with the approximately 3½ days of radon. A source of Ra B or C could easily be prepared but it would decay far too rapidly to be of any practical use. Within about 20 min. half would have gone, whilst in about 4 hours it would be down to one-thousandth of its starting strength.

To be of any practical value the Ra C must be continuously replenished, and it is for this reason that radium or radon were used. For better understanding of this, an analogy may be useful. Consider the water supply to a house. There is the internal plumbing to the taps, a storage tank of relatively small capacity somewhere up in the top of the house, and then a reservoir usually miles away (the distances and positions are immaterial to the analogy).

If only the water in the house pipes is available, the water pressure at the tap falls rapidly and the supply is quickly used up. In like manner the supply of gamma rays

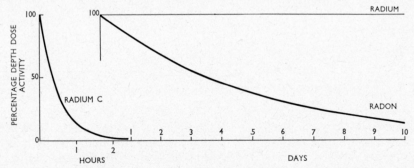

Fig. 424.—The 'decay' curves for radium, radon, and radium C. Note the change in time scale.

from Ra B and C alone would be rapidly exhausted, the activity (and therefore the radiation output) quickly falling as shown in *Fig.* 424. However, if an initially full storage tank is connected to the system, water would be available for much longer and the pressure would fall more slowly. Finally, connexion to the reservoir ensures an almost indefinite supply of water at a constant pressure. These later systems are closely parallel to the emission of gamma rays from sealed radon or radium sources. The presence of radon ensures the replacement of the rapidly decaying Ra B and C so that the gamma-ray output is maintained over a longer period, decaying according to the half-life of radon, i.e., falling to half in just over $3\frac{1}{2}$ days (*see Fig.* 424). Radium, in contrast, provides an almost constant source, akin to the reservoir compared with the house-tank role of radon. It continually replenishes the decaying stocks of radon and hence of Ra B and C so that the gamma-ray activity of a *sealed* source containing radium is effectively constant. With a half-life of 1620 years it loses about 0·03 per cent of its strength every year, or about 1 per cent every 30 years!

Radium B and C—and hence sealed sources containing radium or radon—emit gamma rays of a number of different energies, the most important of which are at approximately 0·6, 1·1, 1·8, and 2·2 MeV. The overall average energy can be taken as being about 1·0 MeV., or not very different from the energy of the gamma rays from cobalt 60 (approx. 1·2 MeV.). Ra B emits beta rays of 0·65 MeV. maximum energy, whilst those from Ra C have a maximum energy of 3·17 MeV.

Radium Tubes and Needles.—*Fig.* 425 A illustrates the construction of a typical radium tube, such as would be used in 'mould' or in intracavitary treatments, and of a

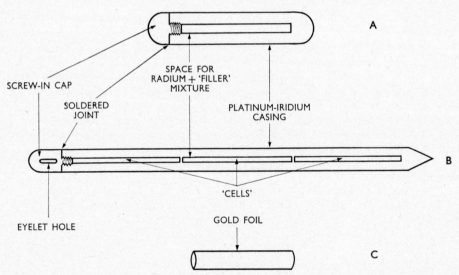

SCREW-IN CAP

SPACE FOR RADIUM + 'FILLER' MIXTURE

SOLDERED JOINT

PLATINUM-IRIDIUM CASING

'CELLS'

EYELET HOLE

GOLD FOIL

Fig. 425.—The construction of: A, A radium tube, and B, A radium needle; C, Shows a gold foil cell.

typical radium needle, which would be used in a radium 'implant'. Basically the design of each is the same, differing only in so far as the needle has a point whereas both ends of the tube are rounded, and in so far as the needle is much more slender, being made as thin as possible to reduce the trauma produced when it is implanted into the tissues. Both needle and tube are containers for potentially dangerous material and have to fulfil a number of requirements.

The Outer Case.—The radium needle (*see Fig.* 425 B) consists of a narrow-bore tube of platinum, alloyed with 10 per cent iridium to increase its hardness and strength. (Henceforth, any reference to 'platinum' in the context of radium and other radio-active material containers should be understood to mean this platinum–iridium alloy.) One end is closed with a solid point, whilst the other, after loading, is closed with a solid cap, which is pierced by an eyelet hole. The cap is screwed into the needle tube and finally soldered in place, not only to guard against its becoming unscrewed during use (and thus allowing the needle contents to spill out) but more specifically to render the needle gas-tight.

A gas-tight container is essential, not only because radon is a danger to health if breathed, but also because if radon leaked out then Ra B and C, the sources of the required gamma rays, would not be completely retained inside the needle or tube. Some would be deposited in many places outside the needle. Such places would hence become radioactively contaminated and therefore present a potential health hazard. Furthermore, the needle's gamma-ray activity would be reduced. Regular tests, such as will be described below, have to be made on all radium needles and tubes to determine whether any are leaking radon, and if they are, they must be taken out of service.

The Wall Thickness.—The metal of the needle is not only a container for the radium and its decay products, it also acts as a filter, removing the unwanted alpha and beta radiation. Like gamma rays, these particle radiations produce biological effects, but because of their poor penetrating powers their effects will be within a millimetre or so of the source and they will contribute nothing at any greater distance. Alpha particles are stopped by very thin layers of solid material (a sheet of paper, for instance) whereas beta particles are more penetrating, at least 1 mm. of lead or 0·5 mm. of platinum or gold being needed to stop the beta particles from Ra C. Therefore, the minimum thickness of the needle wall (the minimum *filtration* as it is usually termed) is 0·5 mm. of platinum–iridium alloy. In practice, slightly thicker needle walls are used (0·6 or 0·65 mm.) because of the extra strength, especially against bending, gained thereby. For radium tubes, when there is no question of insertion into tissues, walls 1·0 mm. thick are commonly used.

Although these wall thicknesses are small, the high atomic number and density of platinum mean that their effect on the gamma rays, especially those passing through obliquely, is not insignificant. In some cases account has to be taken of it.

The Filling.—Pure radium, a soft putty-like material rather like sodium, could only be loaded into the narrow bore of the needle with great difficulty. Therefore, since radioactivity (a nuclear phenomenon) is unaffected by chemical combination, radium needles and tubes are loaded not with the pure element but with one of its crystalline compounds, usually either radium sulphate or chloride. The quantity of radium salt to be used in any source, however, is much smaller in volume than the cylindrical hole into which it is to be placed. Therefore, to ensure that radioactive material is spread as uniformly as possible along the whole internal length of the container (the so-called 'active length'), it is usual to mix some inactive chemical with the radium salt to act as a 'filler'. Originally magnesium oxide was used but nowadays barium sulphate has replaced it.

Originally, too, the radium salt and filler were loaded directly into the needle cavity, but nowadays 'cell' loading is generally adopted. With this technique the radioactive mixture is loaded into sealed cylindrical cells about 1 cm. long, made of gold foil which is usually 0·1–0·2 mm. thick. Dependent upon the needle length required, one, two, or three of these cells are inserted in to the needle cavity: *Fig.* 426 shows a three-cell loading.

In addition to giving certain manufacturing advantages, cell loading offers important user benefits. The first of these is that more uniform loading can be achieved. The space available for the radioactive material in any needle is very small (about 0·05 cm.[3]) and it is very difficult to judge just the right volume of material to fill it.

Therefore there is the possibility that the powder used will 'pack down' and, if direct loading is use, produce the effect shown in *Fig.* 426 A, where the 'active length' (the length over which the radium is spread) is shorter than it should be. With cell loading similar packing would occur but the total effect would be shared between the cells and the much more acceptable distribution, shown in *Fig.* 426 B, results.

Another potential advantage of cell loading is that it would reduce the danger of spillage of radioactive material should the needle become cracked or, worse still, fractured. In such a case the cell itself may well not break, but even if it did only one-

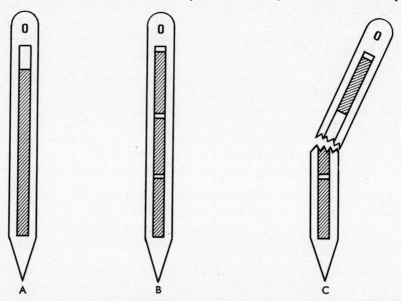

Fig. 426.—The advantages of 'cell loading'. **A**, Shows 'packing' effect when volume of radium salt and 'filler' is less than the total volume available, in a directly loaded needle. **B**, Shows similar 'packing' in three cells but a much more uniform distribution over the whole needle length. **C**, Shows reduction of spillage in the case of a broken needle. Two cells remain intact.

third of the total needle content, in the case of a three-cell needle, would be liable to spill out (*Fig.* 426 C).

The Care and Custody of Radium Containers.—Except that it usually has rounded ends instead of having a point and may not have an eyelet hole, the construction of a radium tube is the same as that of the needle. Once either has been manufactured, for example at the Radiochemical Centre, Amersham, England, and *never* in a hospital, a needle or tube can be used over and over again for many years. However, when first received and periodically thereafter (usually annually or when some specific damage is suspected) sources should be tested to determine whether the distribution of the radioactive material is satisfactory and to check that no radon is leaking out of the container. Both tests are simple to carry out.

Uniformity and Leakage Tests.—To test the uniformity of the radioactive material within the source, the needle—or more usually a batch of needles—is laid on an X-ray film (still in its envelope) for a minute or two. The gamma rays affect the film so that when it is developed there are blackened patterns upon it, such as those shown in *Fig.* 427. Because of the effect of the inverse-square law and the closeness of the needle to the film, the blackening at any point is almost entirely due to the radium nearest that point, so that like variation in blackness, along the needle length, is a good indication of the distribution of the radium within the needle. In *Fig.* 427, for example, the small gaps between the cells of the cell-loaded needle can be seen in both patterns. The greater blackening at the end of the right-hand pattern indicates a greater amount of radium in the lowest cell than in the others. In this case the non-uniformity of cell loading is deliberate, but the example shows how any non-uniformity, including the unintentional, could be revealed. This test is an example of an *autoradiograph*, the needles producing their own photographs by their gamma radiation.

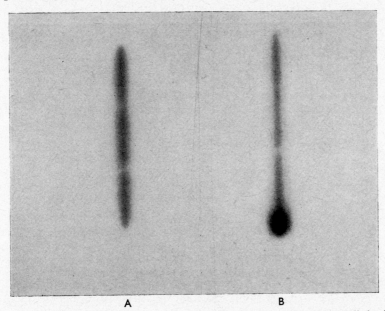

A   B

Fig. 427.—Autoradiographs of: A, A three-cell needle, and B, A cell-loaded needle having an extra strong cell at one (the point) end—an 'Indian club' needle.

The test for radium leakage is equally simple. For this test the radium tube or needle (or again often a batch of sources) is placed in a test-tube along with some cotton-wool. The tube is corked and left for several hours (usually overnight). If a source is leaking then Ra A, B, and C will be deposited on the cotton-wool which, at the end of the test, is removed from the tube and checked for radioactivity with a suitable radiation detector (usually nowadays a scintillation counter). Evidence of any radiation from the wool shows that a source is leaking. If a batch has been tested, each individual source must then be checked in the same way until the culprit or culprits are found and carefully sealed in a suitable container for return to the makers or suppliers for repair or replacement. Leaking sources should never be retained by a department.

The Handling of Radium Containers.—Radium containers are potentially danger-ous first, because of the radiations they emit, and secondly, because radon and radium salt, which have leaked out because of damage, are highly dangerous if they get into the body. Fortunately radium sources can be used perfectly safely provided simple precautions are taken. Some aspects of the problem are discussed in CHAPTER XLIV, whilst for further detail the reader is referred to Chapter 31 of *The Treatment of Malignant Disease by Radiotherapy*, 2nd ed., by Ralston Paterson (London: Arnold). A few simple general rules here, however, could be useful.

The hazard from the gamma radiation can be reduced by attenuation or by distance or by both. Wherever possible radium should be stored or handled in or behind blocks of lead or steel. When this is not possible, for example when it is being inserted into or is in a patient, workers should keep as far away as possible. Radium containers must *never* be touched with the fingers or any other part of the body.

Damage to radium containers and, hence, the risk of radon leak or radium salt escape can be averted by careful handling. Inevitably, however, from time to time a radium needle will become bent while being used. No attempt should be made to straighten it, except by experienced staff and then only if the bend is slight. If the bend is greater than a few degrees the needle should be sealed up (in case it is leaking) and returned to the suppliers. When local straightening is carried out the needle must then be tested for radon leakage. Details of this are given in *Guidance on the Testing of Sealed Sources of Radio-isotopes for Leakage and Surface Contamination* (HPA Report Series No. 1, 1970). Great care should be taken to ensure that radium sources are not mislaid. Not only are they valuable but also they would constitute a radiation hazard if left lying around. In addition, there is then a danger of their being damaged or getting into refuse and hence into the hospital incinerator. All hospital refuse should be carefully tested with a radiation detector before being removed by the public refuse-removal service or before being incinerated in the hospital system.

Then there is the question of sterilization of sources before use and cleaning after use, and here it must be realized that application of heat to a radium container may be dangerous. Helium gas accumulates inside radium containers (the alpha particles are helium nuclei), the amount increasing steadily as time goes on. If there were any traces of water inside the container—most unlikely in modern sources but possible in older ones—this water would be disintegrated into hydrogen and oxygen by alpha-particle bombardment, thus increasing the gas accumulation. At ordinary room temperatures the gas pressure is unlikely to be high, partly because there is always some space for it but more importantly because it will be 'occluded' into the container metal and contents, rather like a sponge holds water. If, however, the needle is heated, gas is driven out of the metal and, of course, tries to expand as well. Quite high pressures may thus be generated if the temperature is raised too much—pressures high enough to blow out the end of a needle or tube and scatter its dangerous contents all around. Therefore, there is a general rule that no radium source should ever be heated to more than 100° C. They can be placed in open sterilizers or a water-bath and brought up to the temperature of boiling water but they should never be subjected to superheated steam sterilization or heated up in water in a dish over, say, a Bunsen burner. There is always a danger that this water will boil dry whilst unattended and the source be subjected to the full burner flame temperature. At least once this has happened in a British hospital causing a tube to explode with serious consequences to property but, fortunately, none to people.

Caesium 137 as a Gamma-ray Source.—Radium is a relatively rare material, produced by complex chemical extraction processes from uranium and, therefore, very expensive. Caesium 137, as pointed out in CHAPTER IV, is one of the most abundant of the 'fission products' resulting from the operation of a nuclear reactor. Its extraction is relatively simple and, though its encapsulation into tubes and needles costs roughly the same as the encapsulation of radium, the smaller overall cost of caesium 137 sources was their first attraction as replacements for radium in gamma-ray plesiotherapy.

Caesium 137 decays into stable barium 137 with the emission of beta particles of maximum energy 0·51 MeV. accompanied by 0·66 MeV. gamma rays. In these basic physical properties lie its important advantages as an alternative to radium as a gamma ray source for radiotherapy.

On the debit side is the fact that, whilst radium provides an essentially constant source of gamma rays over many years, the 30 years' half-life of caesium 137 means that sources will probably have to be renewed every 15–20 years and a strength correction of between 2 and 2·5 per cent applied every year.

From the treatment point of view, the lower-energy gamma radiation (0·66 MeV. compared with about 1·0 MeV. average for radium) is no disadvantage since the inverse square law almost entirely controls the exposure-rate pattern in the tissues of the treatment zone for this type of therapy. The energy is high enough to retain much of the bone penetration and lower bone dosage advantages of megavoltage radiation, and yet being lower than that for radium gamma rays (which have a 2·2-MeV. component), has a positive advantage in the matter of the thickness required for adequate protection for barriers and storage boxes. Barriers for caesium 137 can be about half the thickness of those required for comparable amounts of radium: a considerable saving in weight and cash.

However, the main advantages of caesium 137 are that the daughter product (^{131}Ba) is non-gaseous and stable and that its beta particles have relatively low energy (0·51 MeV. against 3·2 for Ra C). The solid daughter product means that there is no leak hazard, a major bugbear in the case of radium sources, whilst the lower-energy beta particles are much more easily removed. Taken together, these two facts mean that the containers for caesium 137 do not have to be meticulously gas-tight and it is not essential to use platinum as the container material. The use of some other material, especially one of lower atomic number, would be financially advantageous and have the physical advantage of reduced gamma-ray attenuation, especially of the obliquely travelling rays. On the other hand, platinum–iridium alloy is strong, does not tarnish, and is completely tolerated by body tissues.

Caesium 137 Source Construction.—In practice, because they are used as alternatives to radium sources, caesium 137 needles and tubes appear almost identical to standard radium sources. A chemically stable, insoluble caesium 137 compound is loaded into platinum–iridium containers of total wall-thickness 0·5 mm. that are sealed by brazing. Before being put into service each container undergoes wipe and immersion tests to ensure that the surface is free from contamination and the source is properly sealed.

Source strengths are expressed either as the radium equivalent (in the milligrammes of a radium point source filtered with 0·5 mm. Pt, which would give the same Exposure rate as the caesium 137 source at a distance of 25 cm. away), or as the equivalent caesium 137 activity (in the activity of a caesium 137 point source giving the same Exposure rate). As will be seen in the next chapter the former method of strength statement has important practical advantages.

Radon and Gold 198.—Although long half-life is generally a desirable feature for gamma-ray sources for plesiotherapy, there are circumstances under which it is advantageous to implant sources permanently into the tissues. For example, such a technique obviates a second surgical opening of the bladder (for source removal) if used in the treatment of bladder cancer. In cases of this sort a short half-life is essential and initially radon was the source providing it. As *Fig*. 423 shows, radon has a half-life of 3·83 days and is a source of exactly the same gamma radiation as radium (in passing it should be recalled that the Exposure rate from 1 mg. of radium equals the Exposure rate from 1 mCi of radon). Radon is a gas which can be extracted by a rather complex purification process from the mixed gases (which include hydrogen, oxygen, and helium) which accumulate over a solution of radium chloride. The pure gas can be pushed into an evacuated length of gold capillary tube (whose wall would be 0·5 mm. thick). This tube would be cut into lengths of 5 mm. or so by means of a blunt-edged cutter. Gold is a fairly soft metal which, like lead, 'flows' when squeezed, so that the cutting process sealed the radon into the short lengths of gold tube, which were usually called 'seeds'.

This preparation presented fairly considerable radiation hazards as well as dangers of radon leakages. Therefore, radon has now been almost completely superseded by the solid gold 198 which is prepared by the neutron irradiation of stable gold 197 in a nuclear reactor. It has a half-life of 2·7 days and, in decaying to stable mercury 198, it emits beta rays whose maximum energy is 0·96 MeV., and 0·412 MeV. gamma rays. These gamma rays are a little lower in energy than might be wished from the clinical point of view, but on the other hand, the lower energy makes it much easier than for radon to incorporate worth-while radiation protection into the introducers ('guns') used to insert sources into the tissues. Removal of the unwanted beta particles is achieved by encasing the small gold 198 sources (about 3–5 mm. long and 1 mm. in diameter and usually called 'grains') in little sheaths of platinum 0·15 mm. thick.

Gamma-ray Output and Specific Gamma-ray Constant.—From the radiotherapeutic point of view the important feature of any radioactive source is the amount of radiation coming from it in unit time. This depends upon the amount of radioactive material present, the size of the source, the thickness and material of the container wall, and the specific gamma-ray constant (Γ) formerly called the 'k factor' for the material. This constant, for any gamma-ray emitting isotope, is the Exposure rate in roentgens per hour at 1 cm. from a 1 mCi point source of the material. In the case of radium and radon the value quoted is for 0·5 mm. platinum filtration. In the more recently introduced S.I. unit, this constant, stated in terms of roentgens per hour from 1 Curie at 1 metre, is therefore numerically different by a factor of $\frac{1}{10}$, e.g., the old 'k' factor for cobalt 60 is 13·4 R per hour per mCi at 1 cm., whereas the specific gamma-ray constant in the new units is 1·34 R per hour per Ci at 1 m.

CHAPTER XLI

PLESIOTHERAPY DOSAGE CALCULATIONS

IN plesiotherapy (i.e., mould, implant, or intracavitary treatments) the distance between the gamma-ray sources and the tissues being treated is small, being a few centimetres at the most. The variation of Exposure or Exposure rate from point to point is, therefore, controlled mainly by the inverse-square law. If, for example, a point source of some gamma-ray emitter is 1 cm. from the skin, the percentage depth dose at 1 cm. below the skin (and 2 cm. from the source) cannot be more than 25, even if the intervening material has no effect. In fact, it has been experimentally verified that for gamma rays of energy 0·4 MeV. (from gold 198) up to 1·24 MeV. (from tantalum 182), a range which includes the gamma rays from caesium 137 and the majority of those from radium sources, the effect of the material through which the radiation has to pass can be ignored in plesiotherapy. The radiation loss by attenuation is almost exactly compensated for by radiation gain by scattering by the surrounding tissues.

In the case of radium gamma-rays there is an overall tissue effect of a reduction of about 1·5 per cent per cm. At first sight this might be expected to have a not inconsiderable effect in some of the moulds and implants to be discussed later, in which some sources are several centimetres from parts of the area being treated. However, it must not be forgotten that the bulk of the radiation reaching any point comes from sources near to that point and consequently suffers little attenuation. Radiation from a source 5 cm. away will, admittedly, suffer something like a 7·5 per cent reduction, but since the magnitude of its contribution to the total Exposure is relatively small the overall effect is negligible. Hence the straightforward use of the inverse-square law alone—a great simplification—never results in errors (usually over-estimations) of more than 4 or 5 per cent, and usually much less.

SOME DOSAGE CALCULATIONS

For some simple sources and points near to them, Exposure-rate computations are straightforward, as the examples below will show. For many of the source arrangements used clinically, however, the computations are, at least, very laborious and can be complex. In such cases individual calculations are replaced by the use of an already established system such as that devised by Paterson and Parker, which is based on large numbers of inverse-square law calculations.

1. *A Point Source.*—This is the simplest possible case. The Exposure rate (R) at a point d cm. from a point source containing M mCi of a radio-isotope, whose specific gamma-ray constant Γ is given by:

$$R = \frac{\Gamma \cdot M}{d^2} \text{ roentgens per hour.}$$

In the case of a radium source whose Γ value refers to a filtration of 0·5 mm. platinum a 'filtration correction' must be applied to allow for any extra attenuation by the excess filtration over this standard 0·5 mm. Assuming that the total filtration is *t* mm., then the formula becomes:

$$R = \frac{\Gamma . M}{d^2} e^{-\mu(t-0.5)/10}.$$

Note that the excess thickness $(t-0.5)$ mm. is divided by 10. Filtration is always stated in millimetres whereas the linear attenuation coefficient μ refers to attenuation per centimetre. To make the thickness appropriate for the calculation it too must be in centimetres and hence the divisor 10. For practical purposes the attenuation correction factor can be stated in a simple form. μ for platinum for the gamma rays from a radium tube may be taken as 2·0 cm.$^{-1}$ and, using this value, the corrector can be calculated to be very nearly 2 per cent for each 0·1 mm. of filtration *in excess of* 0·5 mm. The error involved in using this simple rule rather than evaluating the exponential function is never more than 0·6 per cent for filtration up to 1·0 mm., the maximum normally used.

2. *A 'Line' Source.*—Whilst the simple point source calculation can always be used for radium 'seeds' or gold 198 'grains', they are not valid for points close to a relatively long radium or caesium needle. Take, for example, a 1-mg. radium needle whose 'active length' (that is the length over which the radium salt is packed) is 3 cm. and whose filtration is 0·5 mm. platinum. At a point (P) 1 cm. from its centre (*see Fig.* 428 B) the Exposure rate would be 5·5 *R* per hour (it is assumed that $\Gamma = 8.4$ *R* per hour per mg.), whereas at 1 cm. from a 1-mg. point source the value would be 8·4 *R* per hour.

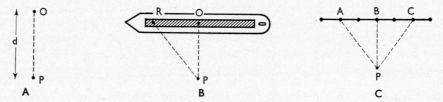

Fig. 428.—Point and line sources.

This quite considerable difference is due to the fact (revealed in *Fig.* 428 B) that almost all of the radium is at a greater distance than 1 cm. from P. Allowance for this can be made by dividing the 'line' of radium into a number of shorter lengths and assuming that the radium in each length is concentrated in a point source at its centre. *Fig.* 428 C shows the 3-cm. 'active length' needle divided into three 1-cm. pieces and $\frac{1}{3}$-mg. assumed to be concentrated at *A*, *B*, and *C*.

For each of these sources the value of $\Gamma . M/d^2$ can be calculated and added together to give the total effect. Such a computation yields an answer of 5·6 *R* per hour. Had the 3-cm. needle been divided into five parts rather than three, the calculated Exposure rate would have been 5·5$_3$ *R* per hour—less than 1 per cent different from the 5·5 *R* per hour quoted above which was obtained by the use of a more exact formula involving the calculus.

The alternative approach, using the inverse-square law, has been given at some length to illustrate that quite simple methods can yield acceptably accurate results.

Had the needle been shorter or the point P further away agreement would have been closer, and one is led to ask how large may a source be and yet still be regarded, for calculation purposes, as a point source. The answer depends on the distance from the point of interest. A simple rule is that if the distance from point to source (OP in *Fig.* 428 B) is five or more times the length of the source, then that source can be regarded as a point. The error introduced by this assumption is less than 1 per cent.

3. *A Ring Source.*—If radium or any other gamma-ray sources are arranged around the circumference of a ring of diameter D (*see Fig.* 429), the Exposure rate along the central axis AB is easily calculated since a point P is at the same distance from all points on the ring (PQ, for instance, equals PR). As far as Exposures along the central axis are concerned, the radioactive material could be concentrated at one point (say Q) on the ring and the Exposure rate (*R*) at P will simply be given by the point source formula

$$R = \frac{\Gamma.M}{PQ^2} = \frac{\Gamma.M}{(D/2)^2 + h^2},$$

where *M* is the source strength in millicuries and *h* is the distance of the point P below the plane of the ring (i.e., *h* = OP).

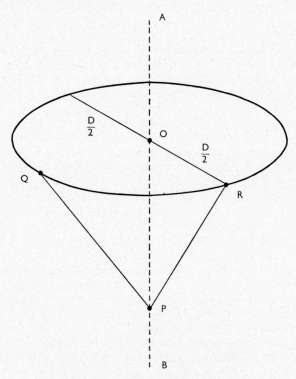

Fig. 429.—The ring source and its central axis.

For points not lying on the central axis the precise computation of the Exposure rate involves the use of calculus-based formulae which are beyond the scope of this book. Reasonably accurate results could be obtained, as in the case of the line source, by dividing the ring into a number of small parts, finding the distance from each part to the point in question, and hence calculating the individual contributions with the aid of the inverse-square law. Summing their individual contributions gives the total Exposure rate at this point. Such computations are extremely time-consuming and can involve quite complex geometric or trigonometric calculations in the establishment of the distances. Therefore, Exposure rates for 'off-axis' points are seldom worked out individually. As in the case of other source configurations, 'point-by-point' calculations are seldom undertaken; instead, required Exposure-rate information is generally obtained with the aid of an established 'Dosage' system.

THE MANCHESTER DOSAGE SYSTEM

As pointed out on p. 424, radiotherapy generally aims to deliver a dose of radiation of known magnitude as uniformly as possible to the tissues being treated. In the 1930s a great step towards the achievement of these aims, as far as radium treatments were concerned, came through the work of Ralston Paterson and Herbert M. Parker and some of their colleagues at the Holt Radium Institute, Manchester. In what is now generally known as the 'Manchester system' they placed gamma-ray plesiotherapy on a rational basis. A major innovation was their adoption of the roentgen (at that time almost exclusively used for X-rays, its validity for gamma rays being in dispute) as their unit of dosage. They formulated rules indicating how gamma-ray sources are to be arranged to produce the desired uniformity in irradiation in a wide variety of circumstances, and provided tabulated data which enable the amount of radioactive material (originally radium or radon) required to deliver the required Exposure in some stated time to be calculated. The coming of megavoltage teletherapy has greatly reduced the use of gamma-ray plesiotherapy and therefore only techniques in fairly frequent use will be discussed, namely the single planar mould, single plane and volume implants, and the intracavitary system for the treatment of cancer of the uterine cervix. Readers interested in the double mould, the cylinder mould, or the line source system should consult *Radium Dosage: the Manchester System*, published by E. & S. Livingstone of Edinburgh, or Ralston Paterson's *Treatment of Malignant Disease by Radiotherapy*, which has already been referred to.

Though differing in detail, which will best be understood if described separately under each heading, all parts of the system are based on inverse-square law calculations, no allowance being made for attenuation or scattering. The other basic assumption was that the gamma-ray constant (Γ) for radium is 8·4 R per hour and on this rate all the dosage data given below are based. Their adoption for use with other gamma-ray emitters, the problem of conversion of the Exposure to absorbed dose in rads and the problem of the use of more up-to-date values of Γ factor will be discussed at the end of the chapter. With this in mind, for the sake of simplicity, the systems will be presented as originally intended, for use with radium.

Single Planar Moulds.—The word 'planar' implies that the radium sources are mounted on a flat or curved surface parallel to that being treated, the curved surface being less than a semi-cylinder. As with each of the other systems, the planar mould system sets out answers to two questions:
1. How much radium is required?
2. How should it be arranged?
What Exposure is needed, to what area or volume of tissue, and in what time, are questions that have to be decided by the radiotherapist.

In the case of the planar mould the amount of radium required depends mainly on the value of the desired Exposure, the area being treated, and the 'treating distance' (h). The latter is the distance from the surface carrying the radium to the surface being treated. The clinical working unit was taken as 1000 roentgens (the systems were all devised long before the introduction of the rad) and *Table XLVII* below shows the number of milligramme-hours of radium required to deliver 1000 R for different areas and treating distances. The tables assume radium filtered by 0·5 mm. Pt. If this is not so in practice, then correction by the 2 per cent rule already stated is applied *to the radium being used*. For example, a mould is loaded with one 2·5 mg. tube (Radio-chemical Centre type RAC E3) filtered by 0·5 mm. Pt. The extra filtration on the latter tubes is (1·0–0·5) = 0·5 mm. and hence the extra attenuation is 5 × 2 per cent = 10 per cent. The equivalent activity (at 0·5 mm. Pt. filtration) of the 5 mg. tube is therefore 5 × 0·9 = 4·5 mg. and the total effective radium on the mould is:

$$1 \times 2\cdot5 + 8 \times 4\cdot5 = 2\cdot5 + 36\cdot0 = 38\cdot5 \text{ mg.}$$

When considering the distribution rules the originators were faced with a need for compromise. Absolute uniformity of irradiation can probably be achieved over any surface but the price would be complexity of distribution rules too great for practical purposes. Balancing simplicity of rule against reduced uniformity, it was decided that a radiation field could be described as uniform if the variation is not more than ± 10 per cent. This enabled quite simple rules to be presented and, in fact, if they are strictly followed the variation very seldom exceeds ± 5 per cent.

Table XLVII.—Milligramme Hours per 1000 *R* for Moulds of Different Areas and Treating Distances

Area (cm.²)	Treating Distance (cm.)				
	0·5	1·0	1·5	2·0	2·5
0	30	119	268	476	744
2	97	213	375	598	865
4	141	278	462	698	970
6	177	333	536	782	1066
8	206	384	599	855	1155
10	235	433	655	923	1235
12	261	480	710	990	1312
14	288	524	764	1053	1386
16	315	566	814	1113	1460
18	342	605	863	1170	1525
20	368	641	910	1225	1588
22	393	674	960	1280	1650
24	417	707	1008	1335	1712
26	442	737	1056	1388	1768
28	466	767	1100	1438	1826
30	490	795	1142	1487	1880
32	513	823	1185	1537	1936
34	537	854	1226	1587	1992
36	558	879	1268	1638	2048
38	581	909	1308	1685	2100
40	603	934	1346	1732	2152
44	644	990	1420	1825	2255
48	685	1043	1490	1915	2354
52	725	1098	1554	2004	2450
56	762	1152	1618	2092	2548
60	800	1206	1682	2180	2646
65	846	1272	1755	2282	2759
70	890	1340	1827	2380	2875
75	936	1407	1901	2472	2990
80	981	1473	1966	2562	3103
85	1025	1536	2034	2647	3214
90	1070	1596	2102	2732	3327
95	1114	1656	2172	2813	3437
100	1155	1716	2238	2890	3545

Distribution Rules.—The amount of radium needed is determined—for the area, treating distance, total Exposure and treatment time decided—with the aid of *Table XLVII*, and is then arranged according to the rules. For example, if an area of 20 cm.² is to receive 6000 R over 50 hours from a mould for which $h = 1\cdot0$ cm., we have (from *Table XLVII*):

the milligramme hours (mgh.) per 1000 R for 20 cm.² and $h = 1$ are 641.

∴ For 6000 R: 641 × 6 = 3846 mgh. will be needed.

∴ Radium required for 50-hr. treament will be 3846/50 or 76·9 mg.

Whilst any shape of area can be used, the tables strictly apply to circles and squares (and to rectangles with simple correction), and it is these shapes that are almost always used.

Circles: The distribution of radium depends on the value D/h, D being the diameter of the area being treated, or the radium sources on the mould—which are equal for flat moulds but different for curved surfaces (*see Fig. 430*—and h being the treating distance. If D/h is less than 3, a single circle of radium sources will produce uniform irradiation over the treated surface—within the definition of 'uniformity' given above. The most uniform situation is achieved when $D/h = 2\sqrt{2}$ (i.e., just over 2·8). For this 'ideal circle' the central and peripheral doses are equal and the variation elsewhere across the circle is minimal. For increasing values of D/h (i.e., the circle diameter increases relative to the treating distance) the central dose progressively falls relative to the peripheral dose. At first satisfactory uniformity is restored by placing some radium at the centre of the circle, as a 'centre spot'. However, for even greater values of D/h the radiation between periphery and centre dips unacceptably, so that in addition to the outer ring and centre spot an inner ring at half diameter has to be used. The distribution of the radium being used between the three possible locations, i.e., outer ring, inner ring and centre spot, for different values of D/h is given in *Table XLVIII*.

Table XLVIII.—RADIUM DISTRIBUTION FOR CIRCULAR PLANAR MOULDS

PERCENTAGE RADIUM	D/h				
	LESS THAN 3	3 TO LESS THAN 6	6 TO LESS THAN 7·5	7·5 TO LESS THAN 10	10
In outer circle	100	95	80	75	70
In inner circle	—	—	17	22	27
In centre spot	—	5	3	3	3

In every case the radium should be distributed as uniformly as possible around the prescribed circles using as many radioactive foci as possible. A circular arrangement may be considered as being achieved if a minimum of six containers is used and the space between the active ends of adjacent sources does not exceed the treating distance.

Squares and Rectangles: For square and rectangular moulds the general pattern of sources is to have some around the periphery and possibly some in lines (usually called 'bars') parallel to a side (the longer side in the case of a rectangle). The number of 'bars' is such that the area is divided into strips of width not greater than twice the treating distance (i.e., 2h). Radium should be so arranged around the periphery that the linear density (i.e., the number of milligrammes per centimetre) is constant. So, too, should be the (different) linear density in the 'bars'.

How the available radium is divided between periphery and 'bars' depends on the number of the latter. If one 'bar' suffices, its linear density should be half of that in the periphery, whereas if two or more 'bars' are needed, the linear density goes up to two-thirds of the peripheral value. Whilst an attempt should be made to have active radium along the whole length of any line of a mould, a satisfactory arrangement is achieved if, as in the case of circles, the space between the active ends of adjacent sources does not exceed the treating distance.

As already stated, the figures in *Table XLVII* apply strictly to circles and squares. For rectangles the reading of milligramme hours should be increased by a small factor dependent upon the elongation (i.e., the ratio of longer to shorter sides) of the rectangle. Values of this factor are given in *Table XLIX*.

*Table XLIX.—*ELONGATION CORRECTION FACTORS FOR RECTANGULAR MOULDS

Ratio of sides of rectangle	1·5 : 1	2·0 : 1	3·0 : 1	4·0 : 1
Multiply mgh. per 1000 R by	1·025	1·05	1·09	1·12

Curved Surfaces: The distribution rules and dosage tables apply strictly to flat areas, i.e., where the radium-bearing and the treated areas are equal. They may still be used for curved areas (not greater than semi-cylinders or hemi-spheres) subject to the following modifications.

    *a. Convex Areas.—*Where the area being treated is convex the amount of radium is ascertained for *the area being treated* but is spread over the larger but corresponding area on the mould (*Fig.* 430 A).

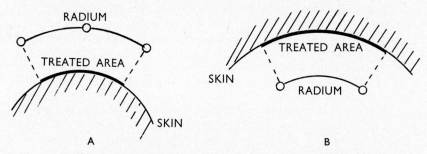

Fig. 430.—Curved moulds to treat A, Convex and B, Concave areas.

    *b. Concave Areas.—*In these cases the area used for computation purposes is the (smaller) *area of the applicator* (*Fig.* 430 B). It will be noted that, in each case, it is the smaller of the two areas (treated area and mould area) that is used for finding the milligramme hours per 1000 R. Furthermore, it is the dimensions and shape of that area which determine the *distribution* of the radium. For example, if a convex treated area 3 × 3 cm. is of such curvature that the mould area is 3 × 6 cm., no elongation correction would be needed because the basic area is square and, in addition, equal amounts of radium would be loaded along each side rather than amounts in the 2:1 ratio of the mould sides.

20

Some Examples of Applications of the System.—In the examples given below the radium tubes specified are mainly chosen from one series (the 'F' series) of sources approved for use in British hospitals and available from the Radiochemical Centre, Amersham, England. Their principal physical characteristics are:

Tube	Content	Overall length	Active length	Filtration
F1	1·5 mg.	7·5 mm.	5 mm.	
F2	2·5 mg.	12·5 mm.	10 mm.	0·5 mm. Pt
F3	3 mg.	7·5 mm.	5 mm.	
F4	5 mg.	10 mm.	10 mm.	

1. *Circular Mould at 1-cm. Treating Distance.*—A flat mould is to treat a circular area 5 cm. in diameter and deliver 6000 R over a period of 8 days. The mould is to be worn for about 10 hours daily.

Area 19·6 cm.^{2}; $h = 1·0$ cm.; mgh per 1000 R (from *Table XLVII* by interpolation) = 634.

∴ 634 × 6 = 3804 mgh. for 6000 R or about 47·5 mg. for 80 hours.

Distribution: $D/h = 5/1 = 5$, therefore a 5 per cent 'centre spot' is needed. There are 47·5 mg to be distributed and hence the 'centre spot' should contain 0·05 × 47·5 or 2·375 mg., whilst the remainder (45·125 mg.) would be distributed as evenly as possible around the periphery.

Such loadings are seldom exactly attainable in practice since radium sources are only available in a limited series of strengths. Therefore, the problem is usually that of finding an acceptable compromise. In seeking this it should be remembered that the treatment time for a mould may be increased or decreased quite considerably without affecting the efficacy of the treatment since the biological effect of a given Exposure depends upon the overall treatment time and very little upon the duration of the daily fraction. However, it must also be emphasized that, as far as possible, the *relative* amounts in the 'centre spot' and periphery should not be altered since it is the ratio that controls the uniformity (or otherwise) of the irradiation. For example, if the 'centre spot' has to be greater than the calculated figure the peripheral loading must be increased proportionately to maintain the ratio, and the treatment time reduced to allow for the greater amount of radium being used.

For the mould under discussion the 'centre spot' would be the 2·5-mg. tube (F2), and to match this the peripheral radium would have to be 47·5 mg. (2·5 is 5 per cent of a total of 50) at the same filtration. This quantity would be achieved by using 19 type-F2 tubes, but since each has a total length of 1·25 cm. they could not be fitted on to the 15·7-cm. long periphery. A solution slightly less acceptable numerically is to use 16 type-F3 tubes, totalling 48 mg. and a total overall length of 12 cm. These, as shown in *Fig.* 431 A, fit easily into the available space. The total active length is 8 cm. and, therefore, each of the 16 gaps between the adjacent active ends will be $(15·7 - 8)/16$ which, being less than 1 cm., satisfies the spacing proviso. Thus the loaded radium (all at 0·5 mm. Pt filtration) is

$$2·5 + 16 × 3 = 50·5 \text{ mg.}$$

of which the 'centre spot' represents a very acceptable 4·95 per cent. The total, however, is rather more than the 47·5 mg. associated with an

80-hour treatment time, so that the treatment time must be reassessed. The required milligramme hours are 3804 and therefore the treatment time with 50·5 mg. will be 3804/50·5 = 75·5 hours. Assuming that the treatment is to be fractionated and delivered in an overall time of 10 days, the mould would be worn for a total of 7 hours 33 minutes each day. In such a situation the radiological safety of visitors, staff, and of the patient will be helped by the mould not being worn during times when such persons are in the near vicinity.

2. *Circular Mould at* 0·5 *cm. Treating Distance.*—Had the treating distance for the mould discussed above been 0·5 cm., the radium used and its distribution would have been as follows:

Area 19·6 cm.²; $h = 0·5$ cm.;   mgh per 1000 R (by interpolation) = 363

∴363 × 6 = 2178 mgh. for 6000 R or about 27 mg. for 80 hours.

Distribution: $D/h = 50/0·5 = 10$, therefore a 'centre spot' (3 per cent), an inner ring (27 per cent), and an outer ring (70 per cent) are needed. The division of 27 mg. into these fractions is given below but its practical realization raises a difficulty since the 'centre spot' needs a source smaller than any radium tube available. A solution is to use a standard 'seed' needle—a radium needle (type C1) whose active length is 3 mm.—containing 1 mg. at 0·5 mm. Pt filtration, and to scale up the other loadings appropriately. The higher loadings can then be achieved by using type-F1 tubes as shown below and illustrated in *Fig.* 431 B.

	Per cent	Of 27 mg.	Alternative	In practice
'Centre spot'	3	0·8	1	1 mg. (C1)
Inner ring	27	7·3	9	9 mg. (6 type F1)
Outer ring	70	18·9	23·3	24 mg. (16 type F1)

This distribution satisfies practically all the criteria laid down, with the exception that gaps between the active ends on the inner ring are rather

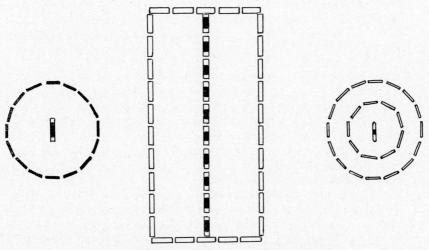

Fig. 431.—Examples of source distribution on moulds.

greater than the treating distance, though not seriously so. The point of main importance is the substantial increase in the radium used over that specified, a total of 34 mg. instead of 27 mg. The treatment time, therefore, would be 2178/34 = 64 hours instead of the planned 80 hours, a change which, however, is acceptable for a fractionated treatment.

3. *Rectangular Mould at* 1·5 *cm. Treating Distance.*—A mould 12 × 6 cm. at a treating distance of 1·5 cm. is to be used to deliver 5000 R in 50 hours spread over 8 days.

Area 72 cm.²; $h = 1·5$ cm.;   mgh per 1000 R = 1857 + 5 per cent correction for 2:1 elongation.

∴1857 × 1·05 × 5 = 9749 mgh. for 5000 R or 195 mg. for 50 hours.

Distribution: The area has to be divided into strips not more than 2h (i.e., 3 cm. in this case) wide, and therefore a single 'bar' is needed parallel to the 12-cm. sides. It will have half as much radium per centimeter (half the linear density) as the periphery. If there are ρ milligrammes per centimetre in the periphery and $\rho/2$ in the 'bar' the total radium will be $\rho (12 + 12 + 6 + 6) + 12\rho/2 = 42\rho$.

$$42\rho = 195 \quad \text{or} \quad \rho = 4·7 \text{ mg. per cm.}$$

Thus, each long side should carry 12 × 4·7 or about 56 mg., each short side, 6 × 4·7 or 28 mg., and the 'bar' should have (4·7/2) × 12 or 28 mg.

The following practical loadings seem to be the most appropriate with the radium sources already described:

Long side 10 type-F4 sources, i.e., 10 × 5 mg. each side
Short side   5 type-F4 sources, i.e., 5 × 5 mg. each side
'Bar'   10 type-F2 sources, i.e., 10 × 2·5 mg.

The total loaded radium is, therefore,

$$(50 + 50 + 25 + 25) + 25 = 175 \text{ mg.,}$$

rather less than originally required and requiring the increased treatment time of 9749/175 or 55·7 hours, which is perfectly acceptable.

Two points must still be made about this mould. In the first place, the total length of the radium tubes selected for both the periphery and the 'bar' is greater, in each case, than the available length. For example 10 type-F4 tubes have a total length of 12·5 cm. and therefore cannot fit into the available 12-cm. side length. In loading the mould, therefore, a certain amount of overlapping of sources is necessary (as indicated in *Fig.* 431C). This is commonly necessary and, though it makes loading somewhat more difficult practically, it has the advantage of reducing the between-radium gaps. The second point is more general and important. It will be noted that the amount of radium used on this mould is very considerably greater than in the other two examples, in spite of the fact that the treatment Exposure is smaller. The increase is, of course, due to the greater area being treated and to the greater treating distance being used (the latter probably to achieve rather greater percentage depth doses). In this sort of case the (unwanted) dose to surrounding and more distant tissues, for the same dose to the treated area, will be much greater as will be the hazard to staff dealing with the mould or the patient. For this reason, among others, such heavily loaded moulds are seldom used since the arrival of megavoltage therapy. But the method of calculation also illustrated by the example is equally applicable to smaller rectangular moulds which still have a place in modern radiotherapy.

Dose below the Treated Surface.—In the discussions and illustrative examples given above attention has been concentrated on the value and uniformity of the dose on the surface at the treating distance (h cm.) from the plane of the mould. Although the tumours treated by this technique may be quite thin they do have a finite thickness and and may penetrate several millimetres below the surface. It is, therefore, relevant to consider what are the doses at various depths (d cm.) below the surface. These doses may be calculated quite easily using the information on milligramme hours per 1000 R given in the tables.

By way of example let us return to the case of the 12×6 cm. rectangle for which it was calculated that for a surface dose of 5000 R at a treating distance of 1·5 cm. a loading of 9749 mgh. was required. The tissues at a depth of 0·5 cm. are at a total distance of 2·0 cm. ($= h + d = 1·5 + 0·5$) for which the mgh. per 1000 s value, including the 5 per cent elongation correction, is 2541 ($= 2420 + 5$ per cent). Hence the dose at a depth of 0·5 cm. is given by

$$\frac{\text{mgh. used}}{\text{mgh. per 1000 R}} \times 1000 = \frac{9749}{2541} \times 1000 = 3837 \text{ R.}$$

Alternatively we can express the dose at a depth as a percentage depth dose—the dose at the surface being 100 per cent.

$$\text{Percentage depth dose} = \frac{\text{mgh. per 1000 R at distance } h}{\text{mgh. per 1000 R at distance } h + d} \times 100.$$

In the present example this is:

$$\frac{1857 \times 1·05}{2420 \times 1·05} \times 100 = 76·7 \text{ per cent}$$

and for a surface dose of 5000 R the dose at 0·5 cm. deep is therefore:

$$5000 \times \frac{76·7}{100} = 3837 \text{ R.}$$

as before.

Calculations similar to this demonstrate that the percentage depth dose, and, therefore, dose at a depth, increases as the treating distance increases. In this branch of radiotherapy small values of treating distances are chosen so as to ensure that the main dose is confined to the immediate vicinity of the surface and that the underlying tissues are not over-dosed. However, care must be taken in the case of infiltrating tumours that too small a treating distance is not used. *Table L* shows how the percentage depth dose at 0·5 cm. deep varies with treating distance for a 12×6 cm. area.

In practice it is rare for treating distances greater than 2·0 cm. to be used. Not only is a very large activity of radioactive material likely to be involved if greater distances are used but the need for high percentage depth dose is probably better satisfied using other methods of treatment, e.g., an X-ray beam. Of course, since the radium (or other material) will have been distributed so as to result in a uniform dose at the treating distance, the dose at a depth will not be so uniform. At the larger distance the dose in the centre will be greater and the dose towards the edges of the area will be smaller than that calculated using the method just described.

Table L.—VARIATION OF PERCENTAGE DEPTH DOSE WITH MOULD TREATING DISTANCE

For mould area 12 × 6 cm.

Treating distance (h cm.)	0·5	1·0	1·5	2·0
Percentage depth dose at 5 cm. deep	66·4	73·6	76·7	82·8

Interstitial Treatments—Planar and Volume Implants.—Because of their very short treating distances gamma-ray moulds can only treat adequately lesions of limited depth, i.e., those which are close to a surface. X-ray therapy, even before the coming of megavoltage sources, could provide greatly superior percentage depth doses, but for lesions in sites in close proximity to or mainly surrounded by bone this advantage was completely offset by the much greater bone dosage, and bone-shielding effects of the kilovoltage radiations (*see* CHAPTER XXXIII and especially pp. 476–481). Therefore, until megavoltage teletherapy was available, lesions in the mouth, for example, were almost exclusively treated with gamma-ray plesiotherapy and usually by implants, in which radium (or radon) sources were implanted directly into or around the tissues being treated. Although interstitial treatments are much less used today than they were 25 years ago they still have considerable value in cases where a very localized treatment using high-energy photons is required. There is one essential difference between moulds and any form of interstitial treatment from the physical point of view. Whereas, in the mould, it is theoretically possible to achieve absolute uniformity of irradiation over the treated surface, this is never possible in an implant because of the intensely high, though very localized zone of irradiation immediately around each implanted source. It is, therefore, necessary to have a modified conception of 'uniform irradiation' for application to interstitial work. By 'uniform irradiation' in implants is meant that over an area or throughout a volume of tissue the irradiation does not vary by more than ± 10 per cent, *except* for the localized high spots immediately around the sources. On this basis dosage tables and distribution rules have been drawn up for planar and for 'volume' implants.

Planar Implants.—The planar implant is a direct development of the planar mould with $h = 0.5$ cm. Instead of the sources being mounted on some mould material 0·5 cm. outside the surface to be treated, they are implanted into the tissues in a plane to produce 'uniform' irradiation of planes at a distance of 0·5 cm. on either side. The milligramme hours per 1000 R for various areas are thus identical with those for planar moulds at $h = 0.5$ cm., as comparison between *Table LI* and the 0·5-cm. column of *Table XLVII* will reveal. The same distribution rules would be appropriate but for reasons given below simplified versions are usually applied to implants.

This form of treatment is usually regarded as treating a slab of tissue 1 cm. thick with the implant in the centre, as shown in *Fig.* 432. The stated Exposure refers to the faces ABCD and A′B′C′D′ and is effectively the minimum Exposure value for the slab, in which (if we ignore the 'hot spots' immediately round each source) Exposures of up to about 30 per cent higher than the stated exposure will occur.

Thus, and inevitably, variations of Exposure in an interstitial treatment are greater than those from a mould. For this reason, as well as because the range of sources available for implantation is usually more limited, and also because some source arrangements used in moulds (lines of several separate tubes as in *Fig*. 431 C, for example) are impractical in implants, the planar implant distribution rules are considerably simpler than those for moulds. However, it must be emphasized that the latter should be applied wherever possible since they yield better distributions.

Distribution Rule for Single Plane Implants:—Some sources should be arranged around the periphery and the remainder spread as evenly as possible over the area itself. The proportion of the radium used on the periphery depends on the implant areas as follows:

Area	Under 25 cm.²	25–100 cm.²	Over 100 cm.²
Peripheral fraction	$\frac{2}{3}$	$\frac{1}{2}$	$\frac{1}{3}$

Some Practical Points: Commonly implants are rectangular, consisting of peripheral needles outlining the area with a row of parallel needles (usually of weaker strength) across it as shown in *Fig*. 432. The parallel needles should not be more than

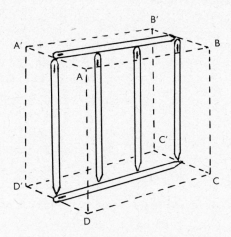

Fig. 432.—Dosage planes of radium implant.

1 cm. apart nor should their active ends be more than 1 cm. (preferably no more than 0·5 cm.) from the needles at right-angles to them, which are usually called the 'crossing' needles. In those implants where short sources—such as radon 'seeds' or gold-198 'grains' are used—their spacing should not exceed 1 cm. In some clinical situations it may not be possible to insert one or even both 'crossings'. For example, in a single plane implant of the tongue a 'crossing' at the lower (deeper) end of the implant has usually to be omitted. The geometric area of these implants is the width multiplied by either the distance from the top crossing to the distant active ends, in the case of a single 'crossing', or by the active length of the needles where no 'crossing' is inserted. For dosage calculations purposes, however, the value of the area used to find the appropriate milligramme hours per 1000 R is that geometric area less 10 per cent in the case of one 'uncrossed' end, and less 20 per cent in the case of both ends being 'uncrossed'.

Volume Implants.—Whereas the planar implant is a direct development of the planar mould, the volume implant is based on quite different considerations. It stems

Table LI.—Planar Implant Table
(Filtration 0·5 mm. Pt)

Area (cm.²)	0	2	4	6	8	10	12	14	16	18	20	22	24	26	28	30	32
Mgh. per 1000 R	30	97	141	177	206	235	261	288	315	342	368	393	417	442	466	490	513
Area (cm.²)	34	36	38	40	44	48	52	56	60	65	70	75	80	85	90	95	100
Mgh. per 1000 R	537	558	581	603	644	685	725	762	800	846	890	936	981	1025	1070	1114	1155

Table LII.—Volume Implant Table
(Filtration 0·5 mm. Pt)

Volume (cm.³)	1	2	3	4	5	10	15	20	25	30	40	50	60	70	80	90	100	110
Mgh. per 1000 R	34	54	71	86	100	158	207	251	292	329	399	463	523	579	633	685	735	783
Volume (cm.³)	120	140	160	180	200	220	240	260	280	300	320	340	360	380	400			
Mgh. per 1000 R	830	920	1005	1087	1166	1243	1317	1390	1460	1529	1595	1662	1726	1788	1851			

ELONGATION	f (per cent)
1·5 : 1	+ 3
2 : 1	+ 6
2·5 : 1	+ 10

from mathematical considerations of dosage distributions in variously shaped volumes uniformly filled with a hypothetical gamma-ray-emitting liquid and then of the effect on these distributions of the liquid being condensed into discrete sources like radium needles or radon 'seeds'. Spheres, cylinders, or cuboids (brick-shaped) can all be dealt with but, in practice, the method is seldom used for other than cylindrical volumes of roughly circular cross-section, and it is this type which will be considered.

Clinically the volume implant is used in situations where sources can be implanted throughout the tissues to be treated, completely surrounding and impaling them. In this case the basic question 'How much radium?' can be answered by the formula:

$$M = 34 \cdot 1 V^{\frac{2}{3}} \times f,$$

where M is the number of milligramme hours per 1000 R, V is the implanted volume in cubic centimetres and f is a correction factor, seldom very different from $1 \cdot 0$ which allows for any elongation (elongation is the ratio of the longest to the shortest axis) of the volume. Values of M against V when f is taken as $1 \cdot 0$ (no elongation) are presented in *Table LII*, which also includes some values of f.

Distribution Rules for Cylindrical Volume Implants: For distribution purposes a volume implant can be considered to have two components, the outer surface or 'rind' and the 'core', which is, in fact, the whole volume to be irradiated. In the case of the cylindrical implant the 'rind' consists of the 'belt' or curved surface of the cylinder and two flat ends. With this in mind the required radium is distributed according to the following rules:

1. The radium is divided into 8 parts, of which 4 parts go into the 'belt', 2 parts into the core, and 1 part into each end.

2. The belt should contain not less than 8 needles and the core not less than 4. The core radium should be distributed as uniformly as possible throughout the volume and not concentrated at the centre. Furthermore, the number of needles used should, if at all possible, be such as to ensure not more than $1 \cdot 0$–$1 \cdot 5$ cm. of tissue separating any needle from its nearest neighbour.

3. Where it is impracticable to close one, or both, 'ends' of the cylindrical volume, the geometric volume of the implant (i.e., the area of cross-section or times the active length of the active length of the belt and core needles for one or two 'uncrossed' ends respectively) must be reduced for dosage computation purposes by $7\frac{1}{2}$ per cent for each 'open' end, and the radium divided into either 4 parts to the belt, 2 to the core, and 1 to the end, or 4 parts to the belt and 2 parts to the core.

4. The 'crossing' needles should be inserted at the level of the active ends of the belt and core needles. When it is desired to place them at the level of the tips of the needles the 'crossing' strength increases so that the division of radium is as follows. With both ends 'crossed', 4 parts to the belt, 2 to the core and 2 to each end; with one end 'crossed', 4 parts to the belt, 2 to the core, and 2 to the end.

If these rules are obeyed the Exposure throughout the treated volume will never fall by more than 10 per cent below the stated Exposure nor rise to more than about 15 per cent above it, except in the localized high-Exposure zones immediately around each needle.

Some Examples of the Application of the Implants Systems.—As in the mould examples, those following illustrate the use of radium sources (in this case needles) approved for British hospitals in practical needles selected from the following set:

Needle	Content in mg.	Overall length in cm.	Active length in cm.	Filters
A1	0·5	2·5	1·5	0·6 mm. Pt
A2	1·0	4·2	3·0	0·6 mm. Pt
A3	1·5	5·8	4·5	0·65 mm. Pt
B1	1·0	2·5	1·5	0·6 mm. Pt
B2	2·0	4·2	3·0	0·6 mm. Pt
B3	3·0	5·8	4·5	0·65 mm.

1. *Rectangular Planar Implant.*—Such as might be used for a relatively thin lesion on a fairly flat surface. The area to be treated is 4×5 cm. and the Exposure 6500 R delivered in about 7 days.

Area 20 cm. (no elongation correction);　mgh per 1000 R (from *Table LI*)
$$= 368.$$
$$\therefore 368 \times 6·5 = 2392 \text{ mgh. for } 6500 \; R \text{ or about 14 mg. in 168 hours.}$$

The area being less than 25 cm.^{2}, two-thirds of the radium (or about 10 mg.) should be arranged as uniformly as possible around the periphery and one-third (or roughly 5 mg.) spread over the area. An appropriate arrangement is shown in *Fig.* 433 A, each long (5-cm.) side being a 3-mg. (type-B3) needle. Five 1-mg. (type-A2) needles satisfactorily provide the sources to be spread over the area. The total radium rather exceeds the 14 mg. originally estimated and, therefore, the treatment time must be re-assessed, cognizance being taken of the fact that the needles used all have filtration greater than 0·5 mm. Pt. A 3 per cent radiation must be applied to the 3-mg. needles and 2 per cent to the others.

$$\therefore \text{Total radium} = 2 \times 3 \times 0·97 + 2 \times 2 \times 0·98 + 5 \times 1 \times 0·98$$
$$= 14·6 \text{ mg.}$$
$$\therefore \text{Treatment time} = 2393/14·6 = 164 \text{ hours.}$$

It should be noted that in implants, where the treatment is continuous, there is not the same latitude of time variation that there is with fractionated treatments like moulds. The biological effect of any treatment depends on the overall treatment time and any marked reduction in it would increase the biological effect of a given Exposure and vice versa. Small changes such as the above (which is less than 3 per cent) are quite acceptable.

2. *Rectangular Planar Implant with an 'Uncrossed' End.*—Detailed discussion of the need for implants with 'uncrossed' ends is beyond the scope of this book, but they are useful, for example, in the treatment of fairly superficial lesions on the side of the tongue. Because the 'uncrossed' end means a falling off of Exposure towards that end of the implant (the stated Exposure applies to a little more than the 'top' half of the implant area) the needles chosen are normally longer than the area to be treated to ensure uniformity over it. In this case the implant area is to be 4 cm. wide and about 3·5 cm. long and is to deliver 6000 R, again in about 7 days. To meet these requirements type-B1 and -B2 needles (total length

4·2 cm., active length 3·0 cm.) are suitable, giving a length of implant (from 'crossing' to lower active ends) of 3·6 cm.

Area = 4·0 × 3·6 less 10 per cent for one 'uncrossed' end = 13 cm.²; mgh. per 1000 R = 274

∴274 × 6 = 1644 mgh. for 6000 R or about 10 mg. in 168 hours.

Since the area is less than 25 cm.², about 6·6 mg. would be needed round the periphery and 3·3 mg. over the area. The most suitable arrangement, to approximate the required amount of radium and to maintain the required ratio of peripheral to area radium, is shown in *Fig.* 433 B. Three 2-mg. (Type-B2) needles go on three sides of the periphery and three 1-mg. (type-B1) needles are spread over the area. The treatment time will, therefore, be found as follows (the 0·98 factor corrects for the radium filtrating being 0·6 mm. Pt):

∴ Total radium = $(3 \times 2 + 3 \times 1) \times 0.98 = 8.8_2$ mg.

∴ Treatment time = $274 \times 6/8.8_2$ mgh. or 187 hours.

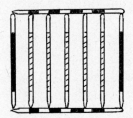
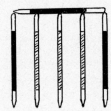
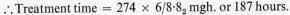

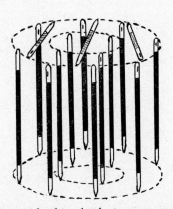

Fig. 433.—Planar and volume implant source arrangements.

3. *Cylindrical Volume Implant with the 'Uncrossed' End.*—Such treatments are used in the mouth and the axilla for example. A cylindrical volume implant of circular cross-section of 4 cm. diameter is to be carried out with needles of total length 4·2 cm. and active length 3·5 cm., again chosen to carry radium well beyond the bottom of the volume to be treated to compensate for the 'uncrossed' end. The upper end is to be 'crossed' at the tips of the other needles. Thus the implant length is 3·6 cm. and its geometrical volume $\frac{1}{4}\pi \times 4.0^2 \times 3.6$. Because of the 'uncrossed' end the

'effective' volume is $\frac{1}{4}\pi \times 4\cdot0^2 \times 3\cdot6 \times 0\cdot925$ or 41 cm.^{3}. Hence, from *Table LII* by interpolation, the mgh. per 1000 R will be 405. For 6500 R the (required Exposure in 7 days) $405 \times 6\cdot5 = 2633$ mgh. will be needed. For a 168-hour treatment, 2633/168 or nearly 16 mg. should be used.

For one 'uncrossed' end and one 'crossing' at the needle ends the division of the radium would be 8 mg. (4 parts) to the belt, 4 mg. (2 parts) to the core, and 4 mg. (2 parts) to the end. This can be achieved, as indicated in *Fig.* 433 C by 8 1-mg. (type-A2) needles round the belt with 4 1-mg. (type-A2) needles in the core. The end could be two 2-mg. (type-B2) needles but a better arrangement, as shown, is to have one 2-mg. needle plus two of the shorter (type-B1) 1-mg. needles.

$\therefore$ 'equivalent' radium (allowing for filtration) $= 12 \times 1 \times 0\cdot98 + 1 \times$
$$2 \times 0\cdot98 + 2 \times 1 \times 0\cdot98 = 15\cdot7 \text{ mg.}$$

$\therefore$ Treatment time $= 2633/15\cdot7$ mgh. or 168 hours.

Intracavitary System for Cancer of the Uterine Cervix.—The only site regularly treated by gamma-ray plesiotherapy to which the above methods cannot be applied is the uterine cervix. This is mainly because of the special shape of the zone to be treated and because, the treatment being of the intracavitary type (inevitably leading to a falling dose through the treatment zone from within outwards), the concepts of dose uniformity described above cannot be applied. The shape of the volume to be treated is not symmetrical around the sources, as will be described, and there is a very considerable variation in the size and shape of the organs concerned.

Suspended in the centre of the pelvis by ligaments, the uterus normally lies in the midline of the body and is anteverted so that it is at right-angles to the vagina, into the top of which the cervix (the 'neck' of the womb) protrudes. *Fig.* 434 A shows the situation diagrammatically, indicating the position of the bladder anterior to the uterus with the rectum lying immediately behind the uterus and the vagina.

The initial spread of a tumour arising in the uterine cervix is laterally into the tissues of the suspensory ligaments and seldom forwards into the bladder or backwards into the rectum. It is the object of the treatment, therefore, to raise to as high a dose as can be tolerated a relatively thin 'triangle' of tissue (called the paracervical triangle), shown shaded in *Fig.* 434 B. Through this zone run the important uterine arteries and the ureters and it was demonstrated many years ago that the initial lesion of radiation necrosis in this type of treatment would be due to high dose effects in the medial edge of the broad ligament, where the uterine vessels cross the ureter, rather than due to direct effects on the rectum or bladder. Radiation tolerance in this 'triangle', therefore, is the limiting factor in the treatment of the uterine cervix.

Dosage statement in this type of treatment presents difficulties, and the first problem to be solved was the choice of some point or points at which dosage may be calculated and stated. Such a point must be anatomically comparable from patient to patient; should be one at which dosage is not highly sensitive to small, clinically unimportant alterations in source positions; and should be in the region of limiting radio-sensitivity. The point selected, which fulfils these criteria, is at or very near to the place where the uterine artery crosses the ureter. Designated 'Point A', it is defined as being a point 2 cm. lateral to the centre of the uterine canal and 2 cm. from the mucous membrane of the lateral fornix of the vagina in the plane of the uterus. *Fig.* 435 shows its position in addition to that of the second defined dosage point, Point B. The dosage at this second point gives an indication of the rate of fall-off of dosage laterally, information of importance, for example, when supplementary X-ray treatment is given. Point B is at the same level as Point A but 5 cm. from the midline and is chosen because of its proximity to the important obturator gland.

Having selected and defined the dosage statement points, the next aim of the system was to design applicators, in which radium would be placed, to fit the range of

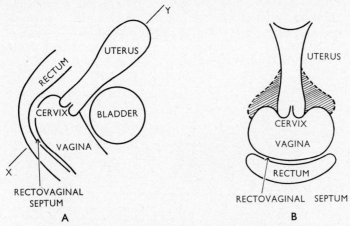

Fig. 434.—Anatomical relationships (diagrammatic) of the uterine cervix and neighbouring structures. A, Sagittal section. B, Plan in plane XY of A.

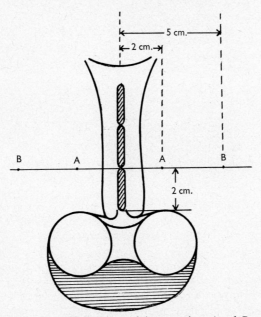

Fig. 435.—The positions of dosage points *A* and *B*.

vaginal and uterine sizes met in practice and then to devise loadings to enable the same Exposure rate to be attained, at Point A, regardless of which applicators are used.

Ovoids and Intra-uterine Tubes.—In this type of treatment some radium sources are placed in the vagina and some in the uterus. For the former the 'Manchester' system uses special containers made of hard rubber or plastic and usually called 'ovoids'.

Their shape is based on the isodose curves around a radium tube of 1·5 cm. active length and they are available with diameter 2·0, 2·5, or 3·0 cm. Normally they are used in pairs, inserted across the vagina one in each lateral fornix at the level of the cervix, as shown in *Fig.* 435. They are locked in position either by a 'spacer' which fixes them 1 cm. apart or by a 'washer' which allows them to lie almost in contact. At least 1·5 cm. of gauze 'packing' is used behind the ovoids to prevent their movement during the treatment period and also to hold away the rectovaginal septum.

Because it is considered important, from the clinical point of view, to avoid dilatation of the cervix (which has the attendant risk of tearing open a way for sepsis or for

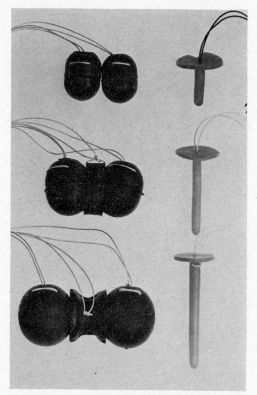

Fig. 436.—The 'Manchester' cervix applicators.

disseminating malignant cells), thin rubber is used for the intra-uterine tubes. These are closed at one end and have a flange at the other to ensure that when the tube is inserted and packed into position it does not slip out. Tubes are available in three different lengths, capable of taking in line either one, two, or three radium tubes of about 2 cm. overall length. Examples of all these applicators are shown in *Fig.* 436.

The Loading of the Applicators.—The roughly triangular-shaped treatment zone is produced by distributing radium in the uterus and in the vaginal ovoids, and the loading of each size of applicator is devised so that, whichever combination is used, the Exposure rate at Point A is, within a few per cent, the same. In selecting the loadings, however, an additional limitation has to be met. Although high, the tolerance of the vaginal mucosa is not unlimited and experience has shown that not more than about a third of the total Exposure rate at Point A should be delivered from the vaginal radium. With this in mind the relative loadings shown in *Table LIII* may be used to achieve the desired constancy of Exposure rate at Point A.

Table LIII.—Loading in Terms of 'Units'

		(*Figures indicate loading from cervix to fundus*)
Intra-uterine applicators		
Long applicator	3 radium tubes	4–4–6 'units'
Medium applicator	2 radium tubes	4–6 'units'
Short applicator	1 radium tube	10 'units'
Vaginal ovoids		
Large ovoids	9 'units' in each	
Medium ovoids	8 'units' in each	
Small ovoids	7 'units' in each	

Non-standard Insertions.—Before looking at an appropriate magnitude for the 'unit' referred to in *Table LIII*, two valuable practical modifications of the standard system deserve mention. The use of the single (short) intra-uterine tube is relatively infrequent and is confined to the treatment of 'stump' carcinoma or to the rare cases where the uterine canal cannot be found and the intra-uterine applicator is placed in a cavity lined with tumour. For both types of case, experience has shown that it is undesirable to use the full loading specified above for the short tube which, in practice, is 'under-loaded' with 8 units and a reduced Exposure rate at Point A accepted.

When the vagina is narrow, or where a tumour is spreading down the vaginal wall, an alternative, 'tandem', arrangement of the ovoids is valuable. They are placed one below the other in the vagina, with the upper ovoid having its centre at the level of the intra-uterine tube, and are oriented so that the radium tubes are parallel to the vaginal axis. Again the Exposure rate at Point A will be reduced—by about 7 per cent compared with that for the transverse ovoids.

The Size of the Unit.—The number of milligrammes of radium which constitute the 'unit' depends on the Exposure rate required, and this in turn depends on the total Exposure to be used and the total treatment time. Opinions will differ on these matters but in the example given below of one operation of the system it is assumed that 8000 R have to be delivered to Point A in 144 hours (which is usually divided into two roughly equal periods separated by several days). The desired Exposure rate is, therefore, of the order of 55·5 R per hour, which can be achieved if the 'unit' referred to in *Table LIII* is 2·5 mg. filtered with 1·0 mm. Pt (a normal filter for this type of work).

Table LIV shows the details of this 'ideal' loading and the Exposure rates at Point A due to each intra-uterine tube and ovoid pair. In the case of the short tube the 'under-loading' already referred to is used. From the figures for the Exposure rates the very satisfactory constancy of Exposure rate at Point A from each standard type of intra-uterine tube and each ovoid pair arrangement can be seen. The maximum range of Exposure rate over all standard arrangements of intra-uterine tubes and vaginal ovoid pairs is the remarkably small 1·6 per cent (57·6 R per hour with a long intra-uterine tube, plus medium or small ovoids and washer, to 56·7 R per hour from a medium tube used with large ovoids and spacer).

Practical Loading.—In general the G-type radium tubes available from the Radiochemical Centre at Amersham, England, are very suitable for the loadings proposed in *Table LIV*. The intra-uterine loadings can be fulfilled exactly by using the G2, G3 and G4 tubes for the 10-, 15- and 20-mg. sources, respectively. With the ovoid loading there is a little more difficulty. The 20-mg (G4) tube is exactly right for the medium ovoid, but no available single tube is exactly right for the large or the small ovoids. The desired loadings in these cases can be achieved in one of two ways. The first uses

Table LIV.—'IDEAL' AND PRACTICAL LOADINGS AND EXPOSURE RATES AT POINT A

APPLICATOR	IDEAL		PRACTICAL	
	Loading in mg.	R per hour at A	Loading	R per hour at A
Intra-uterine				
Long	10–10–15	37·1	G2–G2–G3	37·1
Medium	10–15	36·9	G2–G3	36·9
Short	20	29·5	G4	29·5
Each ovoid				
Large	22·5	With washer 20·4	G1 + 2 G2	20·4
		With spacer 19·8		19·8
Medium	20	With washer 20·5	G4	20·5
		With spacer 20·3		20·3
	18·5	With washer 20·5	2 G1 + G2	21·1
		With spacer 20·4		21·0

Practical Exposure rate for standard arrangements: 57·5 ± 0·8 R per hour or about 140 hours for 8000 R at Point A.

Practical Exposure rate for short intra-uterine tube and any standard ovoid pair: 50 R per hour or 13 per cent down.

For the tandem position of the ovoids the Exposure rate with either standard intra-uterine tube is 53·1 R per hour or 8 per cent down.

different strength tubes in the ovoids in the first and second insertions (which, of course, must be of equal duration). For example, each large ovoid would hold a 25-mg. (G5) tube at the first insertion and a 20-mg. tube (G4) at the second, whilst each small ovoid would correspondingly have a 20-mg. tube first with a 15-mg. tube at the second insertion. These loadings would be the equivalent of the 22·5 mg. needed for the large and the 17·5 mg. needed for the small ovoids, respectively, for the whole treatment. A neat solution but carrying a hazard that erroneous loadings might be used or ovoids prepared for, say, a second insertion for one patient may be used for the first for another and vice versa.

The alternative approach is to make use of the fact that if these tubes are bunched together there will be considerable extra filtration in many directions and the effective content of a bunch of three G-type tubes is about 10 per cent less than their stated total content. One 5-mg. (G1) and two 10-mg. (G2) tubes have, thus, an effective content of 25 − 10 per cent = 22·5 mg., which makes them suitable for large ovoids, whilst two 5-mg. (G1) and one 10-mg. (G2) tubes are equivalent to 18 mg. and hence appropriate for small ovoids. Though there will be small uncertainties about Exposure rate in some directions, 'bunched' tubes are usually preferred to the altered loading and it is therefore the former that is given in *Table LIV*. From this table it will be quite clear that the same total Exposure can be delivered to Point A in the same treatment time for all combinations of standard applicators. For the short intra-uterine tube and the 'tandem' positioning of the ovoids this is not so: the reduced Exposure rate in each case would mean a larger treatment time for the same total Exposure. However, this longer treatment time brings the danger of overstepping mucosal tolerance and, therefore, the same treatment time is used for the non-standard arrangements and lower total Exposures at Point A are accepted.

Dosage at Other Points.—The system described fulfils the requirements concerning Point A, which is the most important reference point being representative of the para-cervical triangle. But what of Exposures at the other points? Point B is out near the pelvic wall and the Exposure it receives gives a useful indication of the 'throw' of radiation laterally. Being at some distance from the sources, its Exposure rate depends little on the distribution of the radium and almost entirely upon the total amount being used. The following generalization is valid for all combinations of applicators used in the system. Milligramme hours per 1000 R at Point B (filtration 1·0 mm. Pt) = 4000. Thus, for example, if two medium ovoids and spacer, plus a medium length intra-uterine tube are used to deliver 8000 R at Point A, requiring 140 hours of treatment, then the Exposure at Point B will be found as follows:

$$\text{Mg. for 140 hours} = 2 \times 20 + 10 + 15 = 65.$$
$$\therefore \text{Mgh.} = 65 \times 140.$$
$$\therefore \text{Exposure} = \frac{65 \times 140}{4000} \times 1000 = 2275 \text{ R.}$$

A region, not so far mentioned, which is vulnerable to high dosage is the recto-vaginal septum at the level of the cervix. It is generally accepted that the dose there should not exceed that at Point A, which can be assured by careful arrangement of the gauze packing used to hold the ovoids in position. At least 1·5 cm. of well-packed gauze should be between the ovoids and the septum; if, with the chosen ovoids, there is insufficient space for this thickness to be inserted, smaller ovoids are recommended.

Exposure and Absorbed Dose.—The above description of the 'Manchester System' has been in terms of Exposure and roentgens because this is in keeping with the original description and, more important, it is in that form that the basic data are presented. Conversion of Exposure in roentgens into absorbed dose in rads is quite simple with the formula given (p. 131) namely:

$$\text{Absorbed dose in rad} = \text{Exposure in roentgens} \times f.$$

For soft tissue and for radium gamma rays (or for the gamma rays from any other sources likely to be used) the value of f may be taken as 0·957. If desired, *Tables LXVII, LI,* and *LII* may be converted to indicate milligramme hours per 1000 rads instead of per 1000 R simply by dividing each number by 0·957.

Alternative Gamma-ray Sources.—Although the mould and implant systems were designed for use with radium (and radon) they are equally valid, with appropriate numerical modification, for any other gamma-ray emitter, provided the gamma-ray energy is more than about 0·2 MeV. and provided that due allowance is made for the different specific gamma-ray constant and half-life of the radio-isotope to be used. Conveniently, gamma-ray sources may be divided into two classes. First, there are those, sometimes called 'radium substitutes', whose half-life is so long compared with the individual treatment time (say, at least 100 times greater) that they may be re-garded as being constant sources during any treatment. Then in the second category there are those radio-isotopes which have been called 'radon substitutes', with short half-lives (usually a few days), which are used because their relatively rapid decay allows of their being permanently implanted into the tissues without the delivery of excessively high doses.

Factor Allowance.—For both the above classes allowance has to be made for the fact that the specific gamma-ray constant (Γ) of any other radio-isotope is likely to be different from the 8·4 assumed for radium. This can be done quite simply. Assuming a specific gamma-ray constant of Γ then, if M milligramme hours of radium are required for some treatment, $M \times 8\cdot4/\Gamma$ millicurie-hours of the isotope in question will be needed. For example, a mould of area 15 cm.² at a treating distance of 0·5 cm. needs 302 mgh. per 1000 R according to *Table XLVII*. If caesium 137, for which the Γ-factor is 3·1, is to be used instead of radium, then $302 \times 8\cdot4/3\cdot1$ or 818 millicurie hours would be needed.

Decay Allowances.—Whilst the Γ-factor allowance applies equally to both long- and short-lived isotopes, the allowance that has to be made for decay is different in the two cases.

Long Half-life Sources: During any individual treatment these sources can be considered to be of constant strength but correction may be necessary for their continuing decay over longer periods of time. For example, cobalt 60 decays about 1 per cent per month and caesium 137 about 2 per cent per year, so that it is convenient to make a revaluation of stated source strengths every 3 months or every 2 years respectively.

Short Half-life Sources: Because of their short half-lives this type of source is almost always used once only, so that no question of long-term decay has to be considered. The source strength at the beginning of the treatment is readily calculated on the basis of the stated source strength at some stated time previously. With these sources account must be taken of the decay during the course of the treatment time. With a source which may be considered constant over the period, the number of milli- curies needed for a treatment is found by dividing the millicurie hours by the proposed treatment time. This approach is not valid when the source decays markedly during the treatment period so that, for example, the Exposure delivered in the first hour will be considerably more than that in the last when the source will be much weakened. The activity needed in this type of case is found by dividing the millicurie hours by a parameter called the 'equivalent hours' for the proposed treatment time. This para- meter is the equivalent time in which a *constant* source, having an activity equal to the initial activity of the used isotope, would give the same Exposure as the used isotope gives in the chosen treatment time.

It will, of course, be shorter than the chosen treatment time with the result that the number of millicuries required will be greater than had the source not decayed—as one would expect. How the value of this parameter is calculated may best be seen by con- sidering two types of treatment, (*a*) permanent implantation, where the source decays completely whilst in the tissues into which it is implanted and gives up all its radiation to them, and (*b*) treatments where sources are used for a limited time, as in the case of a mould worn continuously for several days.

a. Permanent Implantation—Complete Decay: In this case the parameter 'equivalent hours' is what is also known as the *average life* of the isotope, which is numerically the half-life divided by 0·693. In other words, the effective number of hours (H_E), as far as the calculation is concerned and for the complete decay of an isotope of half-life T, is given by

$$H_E = T/0\cdot693.$$

Thus, if a gamma-ray emitter whose specific gamma-ray constant is Γ and whose half-life is T is permanently implanted to deliver an Exposure calling for M mgh. of radium according to the tables, the initial activity (C) to be used will be given by:

$$C = \frac{M \times 8\cdot4/\Gamma}{H_E}$$
$$= (M \times 8\cdot4/\Gamma)\,(0\cdot693/T).$$

If, for example, gold 198 ($\Gamma = 2\cdot3$, $T = 2\cdot7$ days) is to be permanently implanted (in the form of 'grains') as a 2-cm. diameter circle to deliver a total of 6000 R, the initial activity needed will be found as follows:

Area $3\cdot1$cm.^{2}; Mgh. per 1000 R (from *Table LI*) $= 122$.

$\therefore$ Mgh. needed $= 122 \times 6$.

$\therefore$ Required activity of gold 198 will be
$$C = (122 \times 6 \times 8\cdot4/2\cdot3) (0\cdot693/2\cdot7 \times 24)$$
$$= 28\cdot6 \text{ mCi.}$$

b. *Partial Decay:* Sources are sometimes used for a limited period of continuous irradiation. The computation of C given above has, therefore, to be modified. This is quite straightforward when it is remembered that the Exposure resulting from the decay of an isotope from 3 mCi to 2 mCi is exactly the same as from the complete decay of 1 mCi. In each case, it is said, we have 1 *millicurie destroyed*.

Consider, for example, a treatment over t hours using an isotope of half-life T. For every millicurie at the beginning there will be $1 \times e^{-\lambda t}$ or $e^{-0\cdot693t/T}$ at the end of the treatment. In other words $(1 - e^{-0\cdot693t/T})$ mCi will have decayed completely. The 'effective millicurie hours' H_E is therefore modified from that above, by this factor, and thus we have:

$$H_E = (T/0\cdot693)(1 - e^{-0\cdot693t/T})$$

and it is this modified value that is used in the calculation of the required millicuries. In other words, if M mgh. of radium are needed for a particular treatment then the number of millicuries (C) required for a treatment lasting t hours will be given by:

$$C = \frac{M \times 8\cdot4/\Gamma}{H_E}$$
$$= (M \times 8\cdot4/\Gamma)(0\cdot693/T)/(1 - e^{-0\cdot693t/T}).$$

By way of example of the use of this formula assume that an area of 8 cm.^{2} is to be treated to an Exposure of 5000 R in 6 days by a continuously worn mould ($h = 0\cdot5$ cm.) loaded with gold 198 'grains'. From the 'mould' table it will be found that 206×5 or 1030 mgh. are needed. Since the half-life of gold 198 is $2\cdot7$ days and the treatment time (t) is 6 days then:

$$1 - e^{-0\cdot693t/T} = (1 - e^{-0\cdot693\times6\times24/2\cdot7\times24}) = 0\cdot786.$$

Hence the required activity will be:

$$(1030 \times 8\cdot4/2\cdot3)(0\cdot693/2\cdot7 \times 24)/0\cdot786 = 51\cdot2 \text{ mC.}$$

Practical Cases.—With the aid of one or other of the formulae given above any emitter of gamma rays of appropriate energy could be used in the 'Manchester system', provided its half-life and Γ-factor are known. In passing it should be pointed out that the formula

$$C = (M \times 8\cdot4/\Gamma)(0\cdot693/T)/(1 - e^{-0\cdot693t/T}) = M(8\cdot4/\Gamma)(1/H_E)$$

is completely general and applies to all situations. The other formulae—for long-life isotopes and for permanent implantation, for example—are simply special cases of it.

Unfortunately, Γ factors are not always known very accurately, especially for conditions of clinical use. For example, the Γ-factor for caesium 137 is usually quoted as 3·32, but this is for an unfiltered source: the value for a caesium-137 needle or tube will be less than this and will depend upon the chemical form of the powder used in the source as well as upon the thickness and material of the container.

In practice the situation is simplified by the strength of caesium-137 sources being stated in terms of 'milligrammes radium equivalent'. This is the amount of radium (at 0·5 mm. Pt filtration) which would give the same Exposure rate as the caesium-137 source at the same distance. Therefore, caesium-137 sources may be used in the system precisely as if they were radium—no formula of any kind has to be applied except for the occasional correction to the source strength to allow for decay.

The use of short-level isotopes is also rather simpler than the somewhat fearsome formula above might suggest. Gold 198 is the only such material in any general use in plesiotherapy and therefore it is worth while to tabulate some of the factors in the formula as has been done in *Table LV*. The computation of the required activity thus reduces to table reading and simple multiplication.

Table LV.—Factors for the Calculation of the Decay of Gold 198 and the Activities needed for Different Treatment Times

$$C = M(8·4/\Gamma)[0·693/T(1 - e^{-0·693t/T})]$$
$$= M(8·4/\Gamma)(1/H_E).$$

Assuming that $T = 2·7$ days and $\Gamma = 2·3$.

t (days)	1	$1\frac{1}{2}$	2	$2\frac{1}{2}$	3	$3\frac{1}{2}$	4	$4\frac{1}{2}$	5
$e^{-0·693t/T}$	$0·77_4$	$0·68_1$	$0·59_3$	$0·52_6$	$0·46_3$	$0·40_7$	$0·35_8$	$0·31_5$	$0·27_7$
$(8·4/\Gamma)(1/H_E)$	0·172	0·122	0·096	0·082	0·073	0·066	0·061	0·057	0·054
t (days)	$5\frac{1}{2}$	6	$6\frac{1}{2}$	7	$7\frac{1}{2}$	8	9	10	∞
$e^{-0·693t/T}$	$0·24_4$	$0·21_4$	$0·18_8$	$0·16_5$	$0·14_6$	$0·12_8$	$0·09_9$	$0·07_7$	0
$(8·4/\Gamma)(1/H_E)$	0·052	0·050	0·048	0·047	0·046	0·045	0·043	0·042	0·039

A Minor Complication.—Throughout the description of the Manchester Dosage System mention has been made, from time to time, of the radium Γ factor upon which it is based, namely 8·4. This value was chosen in 1932 and now proves to be slightly though remarkably little, in error according to the best modern measurements which give 8·25. This means that the Exposures actually delivered are slightly less than those stated. The difference (less than 2 per cent) is probably too small to be clinically important and is, therefore, generally ignored in clinics where in any case tumour doses and tissue tolerance have been established on the basis of the published system. However, if it were decided to change the tables to refer directly to rads rather than to roentgens there is every reason why the small error in the originally chosen factor should also be allowed for:

$$\text{mgh. per 1000 rads} = \text{mgh. per 1000 R} \times \frac{8.4}{8·25} \times \frac{1}{0·957},$$

where 'mgh. per 1000 R' is the value obtained from the original tables based on the 8·4 value.

It should be noted that this error does not apply when alternative gamma-ray sources are being used together with the formulae given on pp. 588 and 589, since the 'erroneous' 8·4 is replaced by the (hopefully!) correct Γ-factor for the material being used. However, it does apply to caesium-137 sources used on the basis of equivalent milligrammes.

CHAPTER XLII

PARTICLE RADIATIONS IN RADIOTHERAPY

OVER the past twenty years as machines capable of accelerating charged particles to high energy have become more widely available in general physics, considerable attention has been focused on the possibilities of using particle beams as therapeutic agents. The pattern of ionization produced by high-energy particles may be different from that produced by photons and it is possible that they may have different biological effects, and in some way be more efficient agents for the treatment of cancer. High-energy protons, electrons, and neutrons have all been used clinically in beam therapy whilst the possibilities of negative π-mesons have been discussed and some radio-biological work has been carried out with them. Since three of the particles are charged and one is uncharged it is convenient to consider them separately under these headings.

CHARGED PARTICLES

The first feature of the ionization pattern of charged particles that could be of therapeutic advantage has already been discussed in CHAPTER III and illustrated in *Fig.* 12 (p. 26). Unlike photons these particles have a very definite range. Further-more, the ionization they produce is mostly concentrated at the end of their track (Bragg effect). Because of these properties there is the possibility that a stream of charged particles might give very little absorbed dose near the surface, a concentration of dose at some depth, and no effects beyond this. In other words, the radiotherapists' aim of having radiation absorbed dose only in the tumour zone from a single beam would seem close to realization. Unfortunately, as will be shown in subsequent pages, the Bragg effect does not occur for some particle *beams* and when it does occur it is a very real disadvantage.

Charged particles might also produce ionization differently spaced along their tracks and hence have a different Ionization Density—or in modern parlance—give a different Linear Energy Transfer. This latter term, usually abbreviated to L.E.T., indicates the amount of energy delivered by an ionizing particle per unit length of its track. It is known that L.E.T. differences are associated with differences in Relative Biological Effectiveness (R.B.E.); the greater the L.E.T. the more effective the radiation at producing biological results. Thus, since charged particles may well differ in L.E.T. from X-rays, different R.B.E's are to be expected, though whether the therapeutic ratio will be changed is not known. Probably it will not be.

Apart from having potentially desirable ionization patterns, any charged particle must have sufficient penetrating power to reach deep-seated tumours if it is to be a serious alternative to high-energy X-rays or gamma rays. This may call for very large accelerating equipment which may have the disadvantages not only of being very expensive, but even more important, being relatively, if not completely, immobile in the sense that the beam is either fixed in space or very difficult to apply accurately to the patient. Furthermore, with these large complex machines reliability and stable beams are difficult to attain. π-Mesons, for example, have to be produced by a very large cyclotron. Because this machine is too large to be moved, treatments have to be carried out with a fixed direction beam, the patient being moved to achieve the desirable directions of the beam relative to the body—not a very satisfactory method.

Protons.—High-energy protons (it will be recalled that these particles are hydrogen nuclei and hence have unit mass and charge) travel in straight lines through matter, and with an energy of 100 MeV. have a range in tissue of about 10 cm. Their ionization pattern is shown in curve A of *Fig.* 437 which clearly shows the steep increase in dose at the track end, and no effect beyond. However, it will also be observed that the width of the 'Bragg peak', that is to say the width of the high-dose zone, is very small. Taking the maximum value as 100 per cent, the ionization has fallen to 50 per

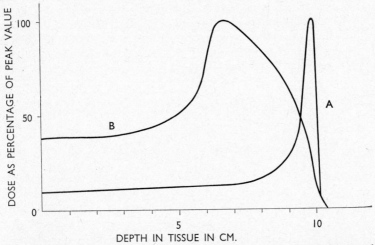

Fig. 437.—Depth dose patterns for 100-MeV. protons. A, The unmodified beam, showing a very narrow high-dose zone; B, The pattern resulting from the described treatment through a series of wax blocks.

cent in less than 0·5 cm. in either side of the maximum, so that the beam, in this form at least, is quite unsuitable for cancer therapy where tumours several centimetres thick have to be uniformly dosed.

It has been suggested that this difficulty can be surmounted by carrying out some of the treatment through different thicknesses of unit-density wax placed on the skin. Each such thickness would 'pull' the peak towards the surface by an amount equal to the wax thickness being used, and the resultant beam would be the sum of the individual parts. In particular a wider high-dose zone would be expected. Curve B of *Fig.* 437 shows what would happen if the treatment were given in 30 equal parts with wax thicknesses ranging from 0 to 5·8 in steps of 0·2 cm., on the skin. The high-dose zone is considerably widened, now being 4·5 cm. between the 50 per cent levels instead of the previous 1 cm., but the dose across this zone is still far too inhomogeneous to be acceptable for cancer therapy. Furthermore, the skin dose has been considerably increased—practically to the same extent as the high-dose zone has been widened. By giving decreasing exposures as the wax block thickness is increased a rather better, though still far from excellent, distribution can be achieved. Even with this sort of complexity the looked-for advantage of the Bragg curve has not materialized and in fact, on closer examination, it would appear that this shape is a real disadvantage since proton beams cannot be made acceptably uniform for the treatment of tumours of the sizes likely to be met in practice.

Another point that must be remembered is that high-energy proton beams, because of the method of their production, are also narrow and therefore that field size required in cancer work can only be obtained by 'scanning' the beam backwards and forwards across the area being treated in much the same way as the electron spot 'scans' across the television screen to give the picture. Having to do this certainly complicates treatments and when it is remembered that the L.E.T. of high-energy protons is very similar to that of X-rays, so that their biological effects are very similar, it will be realized that the advantages of protons over photons are much smaller than hoped, if indeed they exist at all.

Up to the present, high-energy proton beams have only been used for very special irradiations to destroy small parts of the brain without having recourse to surgery, and where the exact dose and the uniformity of the dose are not of great importance. These attempts have apparently been successful but, even so, it is unlikely that these

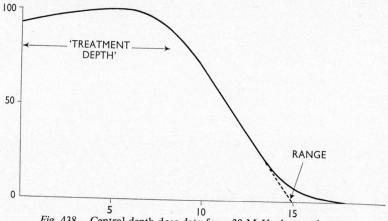

Fig. 438.—Central depth dose data for a 30-MeV. electron beam.

particles, the production of which calls for a large cyclotron, will ever become widely used cancer therapy agents.

Electrons.—These very light particles, with their single negative charge, have the considerable advantage over the much heavier protons that, for the same energy, their range is much greater. It is therefore much easier to attain penetrating powers adequate for radiotherapy. For example, 20-MeV. electrons have a range of about 10 cm. in unit-density material and this would seem to be adequate for reaching the majority of tumours. Unfortunately, however, electrons are easily scattered so that, unlike protons which travel along straight tracks, they follow very tortuous paths. As a consequence their average penetration into a phantom or a patient is usually only about a half of their actual range, i.e., the distance they travel before coming to rest.

For this reason also the ionization pattern produced by a *beam* of electrons is very different from that shown by the Bragg curve. As *Fig.* 438 shows, the absorbed dose curve shows a plateau of almost constant value from the surface to a depth equal to about half the range, followed by a fairly rapid falling off to *almost* zero dose at a depth equal to the range.

An interesting feature of the absorbed dose curve, from the physics point of view, is the small but not insignificant dose beyond the range of any electron. How can this arise? It is due to *Bremsstrahlung*, the 'braking' X-radiation which is produced when electrons are slowed down by any material (*see* p. 46). Because of the low atomic number of the soft tissues X-ray production in them is very much less efficient than it would be in the high atomic number target of the X-ray tube. Nevertheless, enough is produced to provide a noticeable, and in this case unwanted, contribution to the dosage of the patient.

As in the case of the proton beam modified by wax 'filters', the dosage pattern in the electron beam does not readily lend itself to the planning of good treatments of deep-seated tumours. However, a single electron beam might be useful in providing a high-dose zone around a more superficial tumour, with very much less dose beyond than would be given by X-ray beams. If the 'useful dose' is defined as the dose which is not less than 90 per cent of the maximum then a simple rule gives the depth at which this occurs—what might be termed the 'treatment depth' of the beam (*see Fig.* 438). This depth, in centimetres, is approximately a quarter of the accelerating voltage in megavolts. For example, for 20-MeV. electrons 90 per cent of the maximum occurs 5 cm. from the surface, so that 5 cm. is the 'treatment depth'. By this token 35- or 50-MeV. electrons would be needed if central trunk lesions are to be treated in some large people.

Any radiation beyond the 'treatment depth' is unwanted radiation, so that the more rapidly the dose falls off beyond that depth (that is the greater the slope of the curve of dose depth) the better the treatment. For 2–5-MeV. electrons the falling off is very steep so that although electrons with these energies have only small penetrating powers and therefore are suitable for the treatment of only superficial lesions, the cut-off of dose beyond the lesion is very rapid. These electrons are therefore potentially very valuable for widespread superficial lesions like mycosis fungoides, any X-ray treatment of which would involve the irradiation of undesirably large volumes of tissue because X-ray beams do not have this rapid cut-off. As the electron energy increases, however the slope decreases, and with it the amount of unwanted irradiation increases. In practice this means that electron beams which are energetic enough to treat deep-seated tumours are no better than X-rays which, however, can be generated at much lower energies for the same effective treatment depths (4-MV. X-rays are equivalent to 29 or more MeV. electrons).

Unlike X-ray beams for which the percentage depth dose values increase with S.S.D., the distance from source to surface has little effect on electron beam depth dose values, which are controlled almost entirely by the electron range. The only effect of S.S.D. is that short values produce more divergent beams. Electron beam depth dose values depend almost entirely upon the density of the material through which they are passing, and therefore cavities, or zones of low-density material such as the lungs, have a much greater effect upon the dose pattern for electrons than they do for X-rays. As *Fig.* 339 shows, there is greater transmission of X-rays through the lower density lung than through soft tissue and therefore greater dose in the lung and beyond it than there would be in soft tissue. The increase, however, is tempered by the effect of the inverse square law. With electrons the situation is quite different, as *Fig.* 439 shows. In the left-hand diagram a somewhat idealized depth dose curve for electrons in soft tissue is shown, whilst the right-hand diagram shows what happened when some of the soft tissue is replaced by lung (here assumed to have a density of one-third). Because of this reduced density the distance scale is increased by a factor of three, the total range increased considerably and a considerable volume of lung, and possibly tissues beyond it, raised to high dose.

Another important difference between X-ray and electron beams is in their absorbed dose rates, those attainable with electrons being hundreds of times greater than those from X-ray tubes. Whilst this could have some clinical advantage, there can be no doubt that it is also a dangerous feature unless the utmost care is taken in treatment timing and dose control. With treatment times of a few seconds or even less, serious dosage errors, and therefore possibly serious injury to the patient, could result unless the monitoring systems are both accurate and reliable and are used with greatest care.

As with protons, the electron beam emerging from the generator is usually fairly small in cross-sectional area (about 0·5 cm. diameter is common) and can only be useful for radiotherapy if the electrons are spread over a much wider area. This might

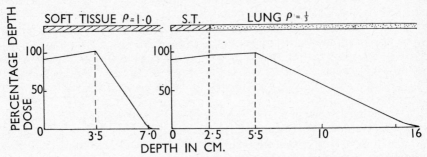

Fig. 439.—Penetration of electrons through (A) soft tissue, and (B) 2·5 cm. of soft tissue followed by lung tissue.

be done by 'scanning' as already suggested for protons. More usually, however, the larger beams can be produced by passing the electrons through some scattering material. The choice of material is not critical but it is usually aluminium, copper, or tin. Since electrons are very easily scattered reasonable beams can only be obtained by having the collimator come right down to the skin just like an X-ray 'applicator'. This means that there is negligible geometric penumbra at the surface and very little at depths of many centimetres. However, as *Fig.* 440 shows, there is considerable radiation outside the geometric limits of the beam especially at the greater depths. This is due to scattering in the phantom or patient and this scattering also accounts for the curvature of the isodose curves being considerably greater than those obtained with a 4-MV. X-ray beam (*see*, e.g., *Fig.* 326). In this connexion it is interesting to compare what might be called the 'treatment width' of the electron beam with that of a 4-MV. X-ray beam. By 'treatment width' in this context is meant the distance, at any depth, between the points at which the percentage depth dose is 90 per cent of the central percentage depth dose *at that depth*. For a typical 4-MV. beam (6×6 cm. at 100-cm. S.S.D.) this width remains practically constant at 5·7 cm. from the level of the 100 per cent central percentage depth dose to the level of 30 per cent. On the other hand, for an electron beam field of the same size the width at the peak dose level is 6 cm., yet only 2·4 cm. at the 30 per cent level. Hence, in spite of the beam divergence and the spread of electron doses over much wider areas, the useful beam width (i.e., that over which the intensity only varies by 10 per cent) progressively diminishes, which can only be a considerable impediment to the successful use of electrons in radiotherapy.

A minor point to be considered in the use of electron beams is that because scattering has to be used to produce adequately wide beams, X-rays will be produced (*Bremsstrahlung*) just as they are in an X-ray tube target and they will contribute to the beam, superimposing upon the electron pattern a typical X-ray depth dose pattern. Using aluminium or even copper or tin, however, as scatterer the efficiency of X-ray production will be low and these rays never constitute more than 2 or 3 per cent of the total beam.

Whether or not electron-beam therapy is of great value in radiotherapy has yet to be decided. The L.E.T. of electrons is very similar to that associated with X-rays (which produce their effects by photo, Compton, and pair-production electrons) so that their biological effects are unlikely to be different. Their dosage pattern in phantom or patient is generally less favourable though the fall-off of dose beyond the treatment depth may be useful, especially in superficial treatments. The value of

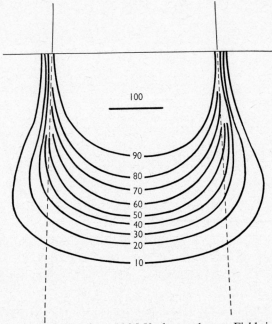

Fig. 440.—An isodose chart for a 15-MeV. electron beam. Field size 6 × 8 cm.
S.S.D. 90 cm.

electron beams of energies up to 35 MeV. for cancer treatment is now under serious investigation in a number of centres.

Negative π-Mesons.—When matter is bombarded by extremely high-energy protons or photons a number of species of short-lived sub-atomic particles are produced; among them are negatively charged particles about 250 times as heavy as the electron; these are called negative π-mesons. In very large cyclotrons large numbers of these particles can be produced with energies high enough to enable them to penetrate many centimetres into soft tissue. For example, a 50-MeV. negative π-meson has a range of almost 10 cm. in unit-density material, and since π-mesons are relatively heavy they will suffer relatively little scattering. They are eventually brought to rest by being captured by a nucleus of the irradiated material, which then emits alpha particles and protons. Since these particles have a short range there will be a zone of very intense ionization around the end of the particles' range. Within this zone there will be a very high L.E.T. and hence the possibility of enhanced biological effects. Furthermore, as will be described in the section below in which neutrons are discussed, very high L.E.T. radiations have an advantage in that this effect is not dependent on oxygen being present. For this reason negative π-mesons have been strongly advocated in some quarters for cancer therapy.

Fig. 441 shows the pattern of ionization produced by a beam of negative π-mesons as they penetrate into unit-density material and it will immediately be apparent that the clinical use of the beam presents the same sort of difficulties as high-energy protons—the high dose peak is much too narrow for the treatment of normally occurring cancers and it is most unlikely that it can ever be adapted for this purpose. An additional disadvantage of these particles is that they are only produced by very

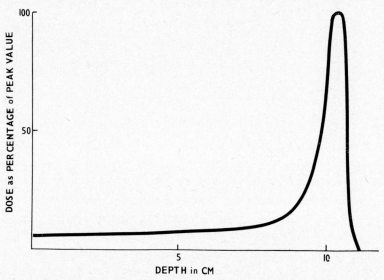

Fig. 441.—Depth dose pattern for a beam of 50-MeV. negative π-mesons.

large cyclotrons and almost inevitably would have to be used in the clinically unsatisfactory fixed-beam way. In spite of their radiological attractions it is unlikely that negative π-mesons will ever be of great use in radiotherapy. For one thing they are too expensive to produce and are likely to remain so.

UNCHARGED PARTICLES

Charged particles ionize the atoms close to which they pass and hence transfer energy to the material, because of the interaction (repulsion or attraction) between their charges and those on the electrons in the atoms. Uncharged particles exert no such electrostatic effect and therefore they can pass right through matter completely unaffected by its presence until they come into direct 'contact' with a nucleus. The first consequence of this property is that uncharged particles have much greater penetration into tissue (or any other material) than have charged particles of the same energy. For example, the almost exponential penetration of 14 MeV. neutrons results in significant doses extending to depths well below the finite range of 14 MeV. protons. The second consequence is that any ionization arising from neutron irradiation is due to nuclei that, having been hit by neutrons, are given sufficient energy to become ionizing particles. In tissue the most likely nuclei to do this are the protons in the hydrogen, so that a large part of the energy transfixed from the neutrons to the tissue is to these 'recoil' protons. About 30 per cent of the neutron energy is transferred to other recoiling nuclei such as carbon and oxygen and also to helium nuclei ejected from nuclei in nuclear reactions. These particles will have small velocities and, having multiple charges, will produce very densely ionized tracks, i.e., will have very high L.E.T. values.

Neutrons.—These are the only uncharged particles likely to be of any radio-therapeutic interest, and they were used for the treatment of a long series of patients in San Francisco in the 1940's. In that instance the neutrons were produced by means of a cyclotron. For a number of reasons this work was not regarded as being successful and was abandoned, but recent work in radiobiology has revived interest in the use of neutrons for treatment purposes and suggests that they may have important advantages over photon radiations.

This is because experimental work has shown that the magnitude of the effect of X-rays on biological material depends upon the degree of oxygenation of the irradiated materials. Living cells irradiated in the absence of oxygen, for example, suffer less damage than they would if given the same dose in an atmosphere of air or oxygen. Now in a tumour there are probably many cells which are not getting an adequate blood-supply, possibly because the growth impedes it, and which are, therefore, less well oxygenated than other tumour cells and their normal fellows. Cells which are 'starved' of oxygen will be less damaged by radiation—they will be more radio-resistant. Hence a number of tumour cells will not be destroyed and the result is a failure of treatment.

One approach that has been made to overcome this difficulty is to try to increase the oxygen supply to the 'starved' cells by enriching the oxygen content of all the blood in the hope that even the limited supply of this enriched blood will provide enough oxygen to restore the radiosensitivity of the cells. This is achieved by placing the patient, during radiotherapy treatment, in a tank filled with oxygen at 2 or 3 atmospheres' pressure.

An alternative approach, now giving encouraging results in the development stage, attempts to exploit the relatively recently discovered fact for experimental systems that the biological effects of neutrons (in sharp distinction to those of X-rays) do not depend to any great extent on the presence or absence of oxygen. Neutrons are said to have a small 'oxygen enhancement ratio'. If this sort of result, which seems to depend on the fact that the ionization density (ionization per unit length of track) and therefore the L.E.T. for neutrons is much higher than for X-rays, could be obtained in human tissue it might have a most important bearing on our ability to cure cancer.

In broad terms three types of neutrons are available to us—classified in terms of their energy: (1) slow or low energy; (2) medium speed and energy; (3) fast or high energy. Slow neutrons are available in very great numbers in the nuclear reactor but their collimation into usable beams is impossible, and though their biological effect is almost completely independent of the amount of oxygen present (they show no 'oxygen effect') they also have no worth-while penetration power. For the production of artificial radioactive isotopes, as already described, they are excellent: for beam therapy they are useless.

Optimum Neutron Energy for Radiotherapy.—The penetrating power of a neutron beam generally increases as the neutron energy increases, so that, in this respect, the higher the neutron energy the better for radiotherapy. However, it must not be forgotten that the low oxygen enhancement ratio (O.E.R.), from which therapeutic advantage may accrue, is associated with high L.E.T. Since L.E.T. tends to decrease with increasing energy it is necessary to consider if and how L.E.T. (and O.E.R.) vary with neutron energy.

In the irradiation of biological material with neutrons whose energy is 1 or 2 MeV., most of the energy absorbed goes to recoil protons whose mean energy increases (and, therefore, whose L.E.T. decreases) with increasing neutron energy. Above 5 MeV., however, neutron interactions resulting in the disintegration of carbon, nitrogen, or oxygen nuclei take up an increasing fraction of the available energy, so that by 15 MeV. these interactions take 30 per cent of the absorbed energy. A product of these interactions is alpha particles, whose L.E.T. is much greater than that of recoil

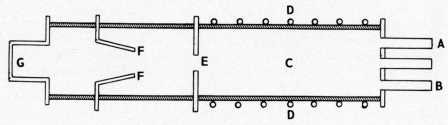

Fig. 442.—D–T reaction discharge tube.

protons. Thus the decrease in the L.E.T. of the recoil protons, which results from increased neutron energy, is, to a considerable extent, offset by the increasing pro-duction of heavier, charged (and higher L.E.T.) particles, so that the O.E.R. associated with fast neutron irradiation increases only slightly with increasing neutron energy up to 15–20 MeV. For neutron energies above this range information on their physical and biological effects is sparse so that prediction on trends at higher energies is difficult.

Compromising to obtain as great a penetration as possible whilst retaining as low as possible an O.E.R., most clinical work has been undertaken with neutrons in the 6–15 MeV. range. At the lower end there is sufficient penetration for many treatments, whilst at the upper, the O.E.R. is still significantly lower than that for X-rays of energies that can be used in radiotherapy to make this adequately penetrating radiation an exciting radiotherapy prospect. Neutrons in this energy range can be produced by a relatively small and probably adequately movable cyclotron, but the total output would probably be too low for treatment purposes. Fortunately, neutrons can be produced by a simpler and much smaller piece of equipment.

A Neutron Generator for Radiotherapy.—If deuterons (deuterium-^{2}H-nuclei) with an energy of about 200 keV. are made to bombard tritium nuclei (tritium is the hydro-gen isotope of mass 3) 14-MeV. neutrons are produced in what is usually called the D–T reaction. *Fig.* 442 shows diagrammatically the 40 cm. long tube in which this reaction can take place for the production of neutrons for therapeutic purposes. It contains a mixture of tritium and deuterium at low pressure, and an electrical discharge is produced in this gas mixture in section C by passing a radio-frequency electrical current through the surrounding coil D. Positively charged ions from this discharge diffuse through the hole in the electrode E and are accelerated on to the target G by the high tension of 200 kV. applied between E and G. F is an electrode which is at about 500 V. negative with respect to the target and is used to prevent any electrons, which may be liberated when the ions strike the target, from being accelerated back down the tube. The surface of the target G is covered with the element erbium on to which tritium atoms are chemically bound. When these tritium atoms are bombarded by the deuterium ions (deuterons) in the ion beam striking the target, 14-MeV. neutrons are given out. An ingenious feature of the operation of the tube is that because the gas is a mixture of deuterium and tritium, the target is continuously replenished with tritium by the tritium ions in the beam and therefore target life is increased. The tube A at the right-hand end of the main tube contains material containing deuterium and tritium which, when heated electrically, gives off these gases to replace those used up in the running of the tube. The gas pressure is measured by a gauge in B.

That the penetrating power of the 14-MeV. neutrons is quite adequate for radiotherapy can be seen from *Fig.* 443, which shows that the percentage depth doses in a

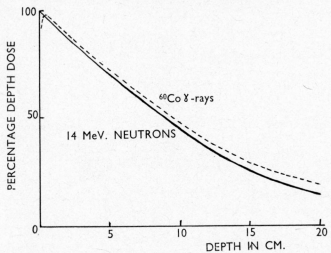

Fig. 443.—Central axis percentage depth dose curves of cobalt-60 gamma rays and 14-MeV. neutrons; 75 cm. S.S.D.; 10 × 8 cm. field.

phantom irradiated by these neutrons are very comparable with those obtained with cobalt-60 gamma rays. The main problem with this type of generator is that its output and running life are not yet as large as are desirable for radiotherapy. Neutrons are emitted equally in all directions from the target and a production of 10^{12} neutrons per sec. must be regarded as the minimum that is clinically acceptable, with a tube running life of several hundred hours. Currently, tubes of acceptably long life are available but the output is as yet only about a half of that called for. There is little doubt, however, that, as experience accumulates, tubes with the desirable output and life will be produced.

To use the source for treatment purposes it is necessary to produce well-defined beams of various sizes and shapes. As the neutrons are emitted equally in all directions (isotropically) the source tube must be housed in a protective housing and a variable collimation system provided. Because the distance between the source and patient cannot be great owing to the limited tube output (75 cm. is a likely figure) and because it is undesirable to make the equipment so bulky that it is immobile, the choice of protective and collimating material to give the greatest attenuation in the available space presents a considerable problem. *Fig.* 444 shows details of the protection provided in one therapy machine. The tube itself is housed in an oil-filled tank for insulation purposes, and the main shielding is of iron surrounded by polythene containing about 2 per cent of boron, the latter being very effective in capturing the slow neutrons which have escaped through the iron. The whole is enclosed in a lead and steel outer casing. Collimation is by removable applicators made of boron-loaded polythene and steel; these applicators fit into a conical hole through the main protective cover, and a number are available to give the different fields needed by the radiotherapists.

Even with quite thick collimators (each is about 50 cm. long) there is a larger penumbra of radiation around the main beam than there is, say, around a cobalt-60

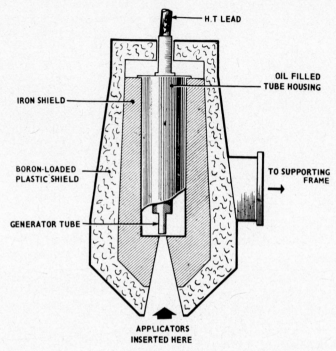

Fig. 444.—Protective shielding for a 14-MeV. neutron therapy machine.

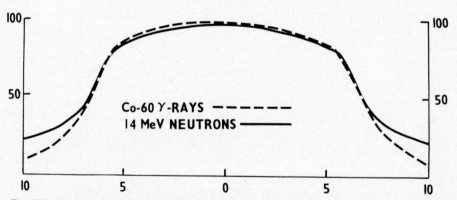

Fig. 445.—Variation of radiation across the field at about 10 cm. deep in a phantom irradiated (a) with cobalt-60 gamma rays and (b) with 14-MeV. neutrons.

beam as *Fig.* 445 shows, and since this means unwanted irradiation and tissue damage it is a disadvantage of the neutron beam. However, as *Fig.* 446 shows, the amount of radiation outside the main beam is little different from that produced by scattering in a kilovoltage beam as a comparison with *Fig.* 316 on p. 444 will reveal.

In general the use of neutron beams in radiotherapy presents the same problems as those already met in X- and gamma-ray beam therapy: in one particular, however, neutrons are unique. This is because neutrons may induce radioactivity in materials they irradiate (*see* pp. 31 and 32). Thus the patient, the collimators, and any objects

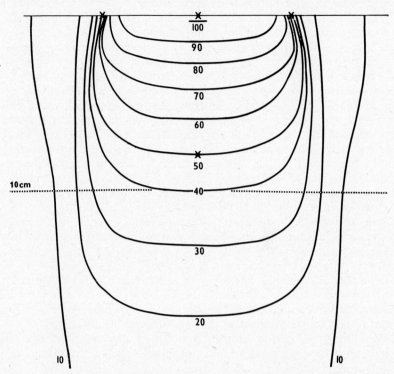

Fig. 446.—Isodose curves for a 10×10 cm. 14-MeV. neutron beam; 75 cm. S.S.D.

in, or part of, the room may become radioactive, and the amount must be considered and if necessary taken into account when the treatment is being planned or equipment designed. Fortunately, any radioactivity induced in the patient is both too small in quantity or in half-life to present any problem of extra dosage to the patient or of unwanted irradiation of the staff caring for the patient. As for the collimators, however, the end closest to the target will be in a very high neutron flux and will become sufficiently radioactive to make hazardous the handling of the collimator by staff. Mechanical devices will therefore have to be provided for the positioning and removal of collimators. Of the other irradiated objects the treatment table, the floor, and the walls present the biggest problem since large areas of these may be irradiated at each treatment. Careful choice of materials fortunately reduces the hazard to small proportions. For instance, since silicon is more readily activated than calcium, limestone rather than sand has to be used as the basis of the concrete used in any part of the building which might be irradiated by the neutron beam.

X-rays and other Beam Sources—A Summary.—The aim of radiotherapy is to deliver a uniform dose of radiation of adequate magnitude to all tumour cells and as little possible elsewhere. Our ability to achieve this depends upon geometric factors, which largely control the dose distribution, and upon the details of the interaction

21

of the radiation with matter and in particular with normal and with malignant tissue. Each radiation that has been used, or suggested, for radiotherapy has features which might be exploited to advantage as well as less desirable features, and the final choice as to which is the best radiation to use must, inevitably, be based on a compromise balancing these features for optimum result.

From the geometric point of view well-defined beams are obviously desirable, and thus megavoltage beams arising from a small focal spot and suffering little scattering have an advantage over kilovoltage beams with their relatively large amount of scattered radiation outside the geometric beam (compare *Figs*. 316, p. 444 and 326, p. 456) and also over radioactive isotope teletherapy beams with their relatively large geometric penumbra due to the larger source diameter. Equally X-rays have advantage over the readily scattered electrons and neutrons which are so difficult to collimate. Were it possible to obtain a beam of protons or π-mesons with a suitably wide 'Bragg peak', they would have an important geometric advantage over X-rays because they suffer little scattering. However, as has been shown, acceptable distributions are unlikely to be available, and so from the point of view of dose distribution megavoltage X-rays appear to have considerable advantages over most of their rivals and are likely to remain the radiation of choice unless another radiation can be shown to have major interaction advantages.

In passing through the body radiation has to traverse a variety of different tissues and any excessive interaction with one type may be a disadvantage. For example, the much greater attenuation and absorption of lower-energy X-rays in bone compared with soft tissue is one of the reasons why megavoltage X-rays are preferred. Charged particle radiations are generally unaffected by the atomic number of materials, their interaction depending mainly on density, so that they show no major shielding or absorbed dose differences in bone, whilst neutrons tend to pass more readily through bone than through soft tissue because of the smaller hydrogen content of the bone. Fat, on the other hand, having a higher hydrogen content absorbs neutron energy more readily than does soft tissue and the possibility of higher fat doses must not be overlooked in neutron therapy.

Long experience has taught radiotherapists that X-ray therapy is more effective if the treatment is carried out with a number of doses spread over several days than if one large dose is given. When using any other radiation it must not be assumed that the fractionation pattern suitable for X-rays will be suitable for another radiation. There is some radiobiological evidence, for example, that a single neutron treatment may be more effective than a fractionated treatment, though it must be recognized that the treatment of a human tumour involves a far more complex system than those usually involved in radiobiological experiments, the results of which, though suggestive, are no substitute for carefully planned clinical tests. For each radiation considerable investigation will have to be undertaken to establish the optimum régime. At this juncture there is no evidence of special advantage for any particular system.

As pointed out on p. 425, the fact that one radiation is biologically more effective than another (produces the same effect for smaller absorbed dose, or a greater effect per rad) does not, of itself, mean that it is a more effective radiotherapeutic agent, since in radiotherapy it is the magnitude of the effect on malignant tissue compared with that on normal tissue that is of prime importance. Neutrons have, for example, compared with cobalt-60 gamma rays, an R.B.E. of 3 or more but if this applies to both normal and malignant tissues no therapeutic advantage accrues from it. A difference in effect on the two types of tissue is needed and, in this respect, much more important than R.B.E. is the influence that oxygen has upon the biological effect of any radiation, since oxygen content is one factor that may be different in malignant and normal tissues. A low 'oxygen enhancement ratio' could be advantageous since the radiation would not suffer the X-ray impediment of being less effective against the anoxic cells (those lacking oxygen) which may form part of malignant tumours.

On balance it would appear that the factors of greatest importance in radiotherapy are the geometric and oxygen factors. Megavoltage X-rays, closely followed by cobalt-60 gamma rays, have a considerable geometric advantage over the rest and are only likely to be superseded as the main radiotherapeutic agents by a radiation whose independence of oxygen more than offsets its geometric disadvantage. Of all the radiations cited neutrons look the most likely to play this role. Whether they will replace X-rays only time can tell—and a good number of years may have to elapse before a verdict can be given. At the present time it seems safe to say that they are 'the radiation most likely to succeed', but even then probably only in those cases where there is an important absence of oxygen. These may represent a small fraction of the total, so that X-rays and neutrons are more likely to be complementary than competitive.

Californium 252.—A very interesting and quite different source of neutrons is californium 252, which has an atomic number of 98. It is one of the so-called 'trans-uranic elements' which have been produced as a result of atomic energy and uranium fission studies, and is produced by the bombardment of plutonium with very intense neutron fluxes. Though very difficult to make, usable quantities are now being produced in the United States of America and are being made available to selected radiotherapy departments throughout the world for clinical trial.

Californium 252 decays with a half-life of about $2\frac{1}{2}$ years and, unlike any other radioactive substance which we have discussed, its rather complex decay scheme includes the emission of neutrons. About 97 per cent of the nuclei emit alpha particles which are absorbed by the container and are not used, whilst the other 3 per cent undergo spontaneous fission, each fission producing about four neutrons as well as gamma rays. The absorbed dose rate (in rads per hour) due to the neutrons at, say, 1 cm. from a californium-252 source is about 1·7 times the gamma-ray absorbed dose rate, though as time goes on the proportion of gamma rays to the total radiation increases. This is because some of the fission products are gamma-ray emitters so that as the californium-252 decay proceeds and quantities of these products build up they add increasing amounts of gamma radiation to the total emission.

In assessing the biologically effective radiation output of a californium-252 source allowance has to be made for the greater biological effectiveness of neutrons compared with X- or gamma rays. If the neutrons' contribution is increased by the accepted R.B.E. factor of 3, the total effective radiation output of 1 μg. of californium 252 is a little less than the output of 1 mg. of radium. (When mixed radiations with different R.B.E. are concerned the dosage unit is the rem, which is discussed later on p. 632.)

Unlike the D–T reaction, which yields mono-energetic (14 MeV.) neutrons, californium 252 gives a continuous spectrum of neutron energies from about 6 MeV. downwards, the average neutron energy being about 2–4 MeV. For this reason mainly, though also because the quantities of californium 252 available are not likely to be great enough, this nuclide is not likely to be used as a source of neutron beams for radiotherapy. However, it has interesting possibilities for use in the way radium is used, in needles and tubes, in interstitial and intra-cavitary work. For this purpose californium-252 hydride is electro-deposited on to a platinum–iridium wire, and after heating to increase the adherence of the deposit, the wire is sealed in platinum–iridium needles or tubes in the same way as has been described for radium.

Whether neutrons' independence on oxygen can be exploited in plesiotherapy techniques remains to be seen: certainly the material offers interesting possibilities though its relative scarcity and its relatively short half-life vitiate against its very widespread use.

SECTION IV. RADIATION PROTECTION

CHAPTER XLIII

GENERAL PRINCIPLES AND MATERIALS

THE medical use of ionizing radiations, whether for diagnosis or therapy, not only results in the irradiation of the patient but may also result in some degree of exposure of radiologists, radiographers, X-ray department porters and orderlies, and even office, or other, workers in rooms around the X-ray department. All these people are, therefore, subject to some degree of radiation hazard and it is the object, of what is usually called 'Radiological Protection', to ensure that the doses received are as small as possible, so that the consequent damage never constitutes a significant hazard to the health of the irradiated person.

Radiological protection is a large subject and much of it is beyond the scope of this book. Nevertheless, a knowledge of its basic facts and principles is necessary to all working in the field and can conveniently be presented as answers to a series of questions:

1. Why is protection against radiation necessary?
2. What dose levels can be allowed?
3. What measures can be taken or materials used to provide protection?
4. How are these used in specific instances?
5. How can the success of protection measures be confirmed?
6. What about protection of the patient?

THE BIOLOGICAL EFFECTS OF RADIATION

As has already been said on several occasions, ionizing radiations damage all living material to some extent and this may constitute a hazard to health. For those who wish to have detailed accounts of these biological effects there are many books available, but the lucid and succinct descriptions in the 1956 and 1960 reports of the British Medical Research Council on *The Hazards to Man of Nuclear and Allied Radiations* are especially recommended. In this chapter the briefest summary must suffice.

Though, naturally, there is no distinct line of demarcation between any of the radiation effects, they can, quite conveniently, be considered under three headings:

1. Prompt personal effects.
2. Delayed personal effects.
3. Racial effects.

Prompt Personal Effects.—Except when very large doses indeed are received, ionizing radiations produce no visible effects during or immediately after the exposure, but within a few hours or days marked effects may appear. For example, an absorbed dose of 1000 rad of X-rays delivered to a limited area of skin, in an exposure lasting a few minutes, will produce, within a few days, a reddening of the skin (an erythema) which disappears fairly quickly. There would be no other effect. On the other hand, a dose of 100 rad to the whole body in a similarly short time would probably cause more dramatic results, such as severe vomiting and diarrhoea, within 24 hours.

At this dose level recovery is fairly rapid. For higher doses the effects are greater and more prolonged. A single whole-body dose of 500 rad could result in death.

The relative magnitude of the doses quoted above should be noted. It offers a good example of the importance, in determining general radiation effects, of the volume of tissue that is irradiated. A small irradiated volume can tolerate a much larger absorbed dose in rads than a large volume can.

Delayed Personal Effects.—Lower doses do not produce the effects mentioned but may have different effects which take much longer to appear. The larger doses may also have these delayed effects. There may well be a latent period of as much as 20 years between the exposure and the appearance of any damage. This is especially so where there has been chronic low-dose irradiation over a considerable period, rather than a single exposure, or a few exposures giving a high dose.

The most common site of local over-irradiation is the hands, where scaly, warty growths or even skin cancer may develop. Many of the early X-ray and radium workers (often called the 'X-ray martyrs'), who unwittingly received fairly large doses over long periods, suffered terrible injuries and ultimate death from this type of local irradiation. Excessive irradiation of the eyes, especially by neutrons, can lead to cataract formation.

When large sections of the body are irradiated ('whole-body' irradiation is a useful general term) the main damage is to the blood-forming organs, and especially to the bone-marrow. Such damage may lead to severe, and sometimes fatal, anaemia, or even to the development of a blood cancer—leukaemia.

Racial Effects.—The prompt, and the delayed, effects would be suffered by the irradiated person and no one else. However, there are other changes produced by radiation which do not affect the health of the irradiated person in the slightest degree, and yet which in the long run may be far more important than any purely personal injury. These are the changes that radiation can produce in our hereditary material whenever male or female gonads are irradiated.

To understand what happens, a simplified description of the hereditary process is needed. The fertilized ovum, from which every human being develops, contains in its nucleus two sets of rod-like structures called **chromosomes,** each set consisting of one each of 23 different types of chromosomes. One set comes from the father and the other from the mother. Chromosomes themselves are made up of large numbers of sub-microscopical particles called **genes,** which are responsible for all our inherited characteristicss—eye and hair colour, facial features, intelligence, and so on. Since there are two sets of chromosomes and genes, which work together, our inherited characteristics are a mixture of those of our parents.

In our turn each of us can hand on one set of chromosomes, and genes, to our offspring, and the individual genes of that set will normally be identical with one or other of those received from our parents. It is unlikely that we shall hand on the complete set donated by either parent, rather we hand on some from one set and some from another—but they are normally identical with those received. In other words, we usually hand on characteristics that we inherited.

Occasionally, however, a gene undergoes a change—it **mutates**—and a new characteristic, not previously present in the family line, may appear. Changes of this sort may be beneficial—they may result in good looks or high intelligence where those desirable characteristics have notably been lacking. Much more likely, however, the mutations will be harmful—or deleterious as they are usually described. It may seem arrogant to suggest that any change to the human race can only be for the worst, but the fact is that natural selection has weeded out many weak characteristics and any gene change may well reintroduce them. The result of gene mutations, therefore, may be an offspring physically or mentally handicapped, and for this reason the changes must be regarded as being generally undesirable. Now many mutations occur 'spontaneously'—that is to say, uncontrollably and for unknown reasons. However, it is known that ionizing radiation can induce mutations, and therefore it is desirable to keep to a minimum the irradiation of the gonads where the ova, or the sperm, with their sets of chromosomes are produced and stored.

Gene mutations obviously do not affect the irradiated person: they only affect some future generation. Nor do they necessarily affect the next generation, nor the one after that. Many genetic effects only operate when the two genes producing them are identical, which means that a harmful effect may lie dormant for generations before it is matched in some child both of whose parents have a gene of that type. Nevertheless, increasing the numbers of mutations undoubtedly increases the risk of producing such physical or mental weaknesses in future generations, so that it is vital that there should be no unnecessary irradiation of the gonads.

PERMISSIBLE DOSES

Though not all the harmful effects of radiation have been mentioned, the picture presented is a forbidding one: ionizing radiations must seem thoroughly dangerous. In spite of the fact that they can serve many useful purposes, such as curing cancer or revealing T.B. or fractured limbs, or many forms of disease, is their use on human beings permissible? In considering this question it should be recalled that many other useful things are also potentially dangerous or even lethal. Circular saws and carving knives can easily maim or kill, yet they can be used quite safely (provided due precautions are taken) for (respectively) sawing up trees or carving the Sunday joint. Safe working conditions have been devised for these tools and equally safe conditions have been devised for the use of ionizing radiations. Far from being hazardous, radiology carried on in the excellent working conditions of a modern hospital is probably one of the safest of modern occupations.

Little has been said, so far, about the dose levels needed to produce the injuries described, and nothing about the fact that the body can repair damage produced by radiation just as it can repair damage produced by saws or knives, provided, in each case, that the damage is not too great. Since the effects of ionizing radiations are proportional to the dose received, safe working conditions are achieved if the doses received are such that the damage they produce is readily wiped out by the body's defences. In such a case the hazard from radiation exposure is acceptably small. It should be noted, however, that radiation-induced gene mutations cannot be reversed, or repaired, which constitutes a powerful reason why doses to the gonads, in particular, must be kept as low as possible.

Whilst many early workers suffered great injury or even death due to over-exposure, the magnitude of the doses they received was unknown and therefore their fate, whilst a terrible warning, did not provide much quantitative information on which to base safe working conditions. Most of our information comes from animal experiments or is deduced from radiotherapy where large doses are deliberately used on patients for the cure of disease. Because of this lack of direct evidence the now generally accepted permissible levels of dose certainly contain a considerable 'factor of safety'.

The Dose Levels.—Having taken into account all the available information, the International Commission on Radiological Protection (I.C.R.P.) has recommended a series of maximum permissible doses (M.P.D.) for different body tissues, for radiation workers, and has also indicated the 'Dose Limit'—as they term it—for members of the general public. It should be noted, and stressed, that the quoted values are *maxima*—every effort must be made to keep doses received to an absolute minimum. In fact the great majority of radiation workers receive doses well below the M.P.D.

The values quoted for radiation workers are such that the hazard that the doses represent to health is small compared with the ordinary hazards of life. A radiation worker is, for example, far more likely to be involved in a motor-car accident than to suffer ill-effects from radiation, even if receiving the M.P.D. Genetic changes will, inevitably, be produced but their effect on future generations will be small because of the relatively small number of people involved. It is for this, genetic, reason that the Dose Limit for the general population is set at a much lower level than the M.P.D. for radiation workers.

Full details of the accepted values of the M.P.D. for a variety of situations can be found in the *Recommendations of the International Commission on Radiological Protection* (I.C.R.P.), Publication 9 (1966), published by Pergamon Press, and a few of the more important examples are given below. Before quoting them, however, it is necessary to look at the problem of how effective doses of more than one radiation can be added together.

R.B.E., Dose Equivalent, and the Rem.—As already pointed out on p. 424, because the biological effectiveness of one radiation may be different from that of another, equal absorbed doses (rad) of different radiations do not necessarily produce biological effects of the same magnitude. Radiations with a high L.E.T. (*see* p. 614) have a greater biological effectiveness than those with a low L.E.T. The difference is usually expressed by the R.B.E. (p. 424) which, it must be emphasized, is not necessarily a constant for the two radiations concerned. It may, for example, depend on the rate at which the radiations are delivered, and may also depend upon the biological effect being observed. Take, for example, the R.B.E. for fast neutrons compared with ^{60}Co gamma rays. It is considerably greater for production of cataract of the eye than it is for the production of skin erythema. Similarly it is greater for very low dose rates (chronic irradiation) than for the higher dose rates used in radiotherapy.

Whenever beams of mixed radiations have to be measured and their combined biological effects assessed the differences in their biological effectiveness have to be taken into account, and this is done by multiplying the absorbed dose of each radiation by its appropriate R.B.E. and adding all these together to arrive at what might be termed the 'biologically effective dose'. In radiological protection work where, among other things, M.P.D. must be legally prescribed, the use of a series of factors each of which depends on a number of variables, as R.B.E. does, would, to say the least, be both inconvenient and confusing. A modified approach is therefore used.

Protection regulations must assume the worst; if there is any uncertainty they must always err on the side of safety. Therefore for each radiation (or strictly for ranges of L.E.T. values) a *quality factor* (Q.F.) is laid down. This is, essentially, the upper limit of the R.B.E. for the particular radiation (or L.E.T. range) compared with ^{60}Co gamma rays, for the most important biological effect produced by that radiation in the body. Values of the quality factor for radiations likely to be encountered in radiology are given in *Table LVI*, from which it will be seen that for the radiations usually employed in diagnostic radiology or X-ray and gamma-ray therapy the value is unity.

The sum of the products of the absorbed dose in rads and the quality factor for each radiation is called the dose equivalent, the unit of which is the *rem*. Thus

Dose equivalent in rem = (Dose in rad × Q.F.) + (dose in rad × Q.F.).
                              Radiation 1   Radiation 2

The rem is, therefore, the quantity of any radiation which will produce the same biological effect as 1 rad of ^{60}Co gamma rays (for which the Q.F. is 1). An example might help to make the method of use clear.

Example.—
Assume that outside a treatment room which houses a 14-MeV. neutron generator there are 0·3 mrad per hour of gamma rays (Q.F. = 1), 0·6 mrad per hour of slow (or thermal) neutrons (Q.F. = 3), and 0·1 mrad per hour of fast neutrons (Q.F. = 10), what is the total dose equivalent rate?

$$
\begin{aligned}
\text{Gamma rays } 0·3 \times 1·0 &= 0·3 \text{ mrem per hour,} \\
\text{Thermal neutron } 0·6 \times 3·0 &= 1·8 \text{ mrem per hour,} \\
\text{Fast neutrons } 0·1 \times 10 &= 1·0 \text{ mrem per hour,} \\
\text{Dose equivalent } &= 3·1 \text{ mrem per hour.}
\end{aligned}
$$

*Table LVI.—*QUALITY FACTORS

Radiation	Quality Factor
X-rays and gamma rays	1·0
Electron (including beta rays) of energy more than 30 kV.	1·0
Thermal (slow) neutrons	3
Fast neutrons	10
Protons	10

Maximum Permissible Doses and Body Burdens.—The maximum permissible doses which are of particular interest to radiological workers are.—
1. When the whole body is fairly uniformly irradiated—5 rem in a year.
2. For the skin, thyroid gland, or bone—30 rem in a year.
3. For the hands and forearms, feet and ankles—75 rem in a year.

Behind these recommendations is a general assumption that the doses are spread fairly uniformly over the year (the average rate for whole-body irradiation would be roughly 100 mrem, that is 100 mrad for X-ray workers, per week). However, it is acceptable if up to a half of the total is received in a quarter of the year.

For members of the general public the annual dose limits are set at one-tenth of the M.P.D. for the corresponding tissues.

Protection against external radiation sources is relatively straightforward as the following pages will show. However, those people working with radioactive materials are subjected to an additional hazard, namely the possibility of these materials entering the body and constituting an internal radiation source. Measures to prevent, or minimize, this are also described below but for the planning of such measures it is necessary to have some idea of the amount of any particular isotope which constitutes a hazard.

For this purpose the I.C.R.P. have recommended maximum values ('body burdens') for the amounts of different radioactive isotopes which can be deposited in the body without constituting a hazard. In arriving at these amounts it is necessary to know what is likely to happen to the ingested material in the body—whether it is uniformly distributed or whether it is concentrated in some organ—and also something about the speed with which it is likely to be eliminated from the body, i.e., its biological half-life. Where the isotope is likely to be uniformly distributed the maximum permissible amount is that which will produce a whole-body dose of 100 mrem per week (5 rem per year). In those cases in which the isotope is concentrated in a particular organ (for example, iodine in the thyroid) the amount is that which will produce the M.P.D. for that organ (30 rem per year in the case of the thyroid). Some examples of maximum permissible body burdens are given in *Table LVII.*

Table LVII.—MAXIMUM PERMISSIBLE BODY BURDENS FOR SOME IMPORTANT RADIOACTIVE ISOTOPES

Radioactive Isotope	Maximum Permissible Body Burden in μCi
Hydrogen 3 (tritium)	1000
Carbon 14	300
Phosphorus 32	6
Iron 59	20
Strontium 90	2
Iodine 131	0·7
Radium 226	0·1
Californium 252	0·01

PROTECTIVE MEASURES AND MATERIALS

A very good dictum for X-ray protection is 'Keep out of the Beam', and, at first sight, this may seem relatively easy in diagnostic radiology, where only during fluoroscopy may the worker have to place himself in the direct line of the beam. However, it must not be forgotten that the beam has to be aimed towards other rooms in which people may be working, and that, quite inadvertently, they may be 'in the beam'. Furthermore, how far this instruction can be obeyed depends upon what is meant by 'the beam'. The geometric primary beam is not the only radiation in the X-ray room, for every irradiated object (such as the X-ray table, or the patient) is a source of scattered rays, and a much wider zone than the 'useful' beam receives radiation.

Since radiation sources differ so much, and are used in so many different ways, it is quite impossible to describe the protective measures used in every case. Rather an attempt will be made to outline the general principles involved, and to illustrate their practical application by reference to a few of the more important situations.

General Principles.—For any given radiation source the amount of radiation at any point in the beam depends upon the distance from point to source (effect of inverse-square law) and the thickness and nature of any material through which the radiation has to pass (exponential attenuation). Most protection schemes depend upon both distance and barriers: the greater the distance and/or the thickness and atomic number of the barrier, the smaller the Exposure rate. Some simple examples will illustrate these points. In each of these examples the aim will be to reduce the Exposure rate at the point of interest to 1 milliroentgen per hour. (A worker subjected to this rate for every hour of his or her working time would receive less than 40 per cent of the M.P.D.)

Before dealing with specific examples, however, the formula or formulae involved must be considered. The basic data are illustrated in *Fig.* 447, in which S is the source of radiation and P the point at which the Exposure rate is to be determined. The distance from S to P is D cm. and there may be a barrier (B) between them. This barrier is t cm. thick and the linear attenuation coefficient (the 'broad beam' coefficient in this sort of case—*see* p. 152) of its material is μ cm.$^{-1}$ The 'output' of the source is X_c R per hour at a distance D_c cm.

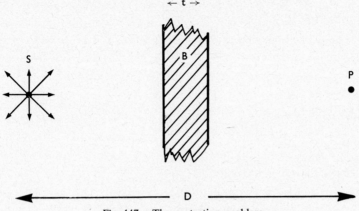

Fig. 447.—The protection problem.

First the influence of the inverse square law (p. 10) has to be considered. According to that law X_c is inversely proportional to D_c^2, i,e.,

$$X_c = k/D_c^2,$$

where k is an arbitrary constant. Similarly X_1 the Exposure rate at P is inversely proportional to D, i.e.,

$$X_1 = k/D^2.$$

Hence

$$X_1/X_c = D_c^2/D^2 \quad \text{or} \quad X_1 = X_c D_c^2/D^2.$$

If the barrier is in position the amount of radiation reaching P will be reduced by attenuation according to the exponential law (p. 60), which says that the rate (I_0) with no barrier is related to the rate (I) with a barrier t cm. thick by

$$I = I_0 e^{-\mu t}.$$

In the case illustrated by *Fig.* 447 the Exposure rate with no barrier is X_1, hence the exposure rate (X) with the barrier in place is

$$X = X_1 e^{-\mu t} = X_c(D_c^2/D^2) e^{-\mu t}$$

and this is the equation which will be used in the examples below. In those cases where there is no barrier (inverse square law alone) $t = 0$ and $e^{-\mu t} = e^{-0} = 1$ the formula reduces to

$$X = X_c(D_c^2/D^2).$$

Examples.—
1. A small radium source gives 10 R per hour at 1 cm.
    a. At what distance will the Exposure rate be down to 1 mR per hour?
    b. What thickness of lead ($\mu = 1 \cdot 0$ per cm. for this radiation) is needed for a storage box for this source if workers are to be allowed to remain at up to 10 cm. of the source?

a. $X_c = 10$ R per hour; $D_c = 1$ cm.; $X = 10^{-3}$ R per hour. In this case $t = 0$,

$$\therefore X = X_c(D_c^2/D^2) \quad \text{or} \quad D^2 = X_c D_c^2/X,$$

$$D^2 = 10 \times 1^2/10^{-3} = 10^4 \quad \text{or} \quad D = 100 \text{ cm.,}$$

i.e., at 1 metre from the source the Exposure rate will be down to 1 mR per hour.

b. $X_c = 10$ R per hour; $D_c = 1$ cm.; $D = 10$ cm.; $X = 10^{-3}$ R per hour; $\mu = 1$ cm.$^{-1}$ In this case t has to be found and the full formula used:

$$X = X_c(D_c{}^2/D^2)\,e^{-\mu t} \quad \text{or} \quad 10(1^2/10^2)\,e^{-1\cdot 0t} = 10^{-3}$$

$$\text{or} \quad e^{-t} = 10^{-2}.$$

From tables of e^{-x} it will be found that $e^{-4\cdot 6} = 10^{-2}\star$ so that

$$e^{-t} = 10^{-2} = e^{-4\cdot 6} \quad \text{or} \quad t = 4\cdot 6 \text{ cm.}$$

In other words the required protection is achieved by using 4·6 cm., or rather less than 2 in. of lead.

2. A beam of 200-kV. X-rays is directed horizontally across a room. Assuming that there is no attenuation in the air (which is tacitly assumed in all this work) at what distance will the Exposure rate be down to 1 mR per hour, if it is 80 R per min. at 50 cm.?

No barrier is involved ($t = 0$) so that the simpler formula is used:

$X_c = 80$ R per min. $= 80 \times 60$ R per hour; $X = 10^{-3}$ R per hour; $D_c = 50$ cm.

$$X = X_c D_c{}^2/D^2 \quad \text{or} \quad D^2 = X_c D_c{}^2/X.$$

Hence

$$D^2 = 80 \times 60 \times 50^2/10^{-3} = 1\cdot 2 \times 10^{10}$$

or

$$D = \sqrt{(1\cdot 2 \times 10^{10})} = \text{approximately } 1\cdot 1 \times 10^5 \text{ cm. or about 1100 metres.}$$

This distance (almost three-quarters of a mile) is considerably greater than the length of any X-ray room, or of most hospitals for that matter! Safe working conditions, in the direction of the beam, can only be achieved by the provision of some kind of attenuating barrier between workers and source. The required thickness of such a barrier is the subject of the next example.

3. Assuming that the X-ray beam in the last example is directed towards a room in which a worker has to spend most of his working day, how thick must the intervening wall be (a) if it is made of concrete ($\mu = 0\cdot 38$ cm.$^{-1}$ for this beam) and (b) if it is made of lead ($\mu = 25$ cm.$^{-1}$)? The work place is 500 cm. from the source.

$X_c = 80 \times 60$ R per hour; $X = 10^{-3}$ R per hour; $D_c = 50$ cm.; $D = 500$ cm.

$$X = X_c(D_c{}^2/D^2)\,e^{-\mu t} \quad \text{or} \quad 10^{-3} = 4800\,(50^2/500^2)\,e^{-\mu t}$$

or

$$e^{\mu t} = 10^{-3}/48 = 2\cdot 083 \times 10^{-5}.$$

From tables of e^{-x} it will be found that $e^{-10\cdot 78} = 2\cdot 083 \times 10^{-5}$ so that

$$\mu t = 10\cdot 78.$$

$\star$ A method of finding values of μt when tables of exponential functions are not available is given in APPENDIX II.

So far, in the calculation, no mention has been made of the wall material. The required protection is achieved by a combination of attenuation coefficient and thickness such that their product is 10·8. If concrete is the material used then, since the 'broad beam' linear attenuation coefficient for this radiation is 0·38 cm.$^{-1}$, the thickness needed would be given by

$$\mu t = 0.38t = 10.78 \quad \text{or} \quad t = 28.0 \text{ cm. or about 11 in.}$$

A concrete wall 11 in. thick would therefore have to be built (it would probably be made 1 ft. thick to be on the safe side!) to give adequate protection under the circumstances described. This is quite a substantial wall and sometimes the available space does not allow such thick barriers to be used. In such a case a more efficient attenuation (a substance with a larger μ) is called for. Lead is such a material, and with lead ($\mu = 25$ cm.$^{-1}$ in this case) the required thickness would be given by

$$25 t = 10.78 \quad \text{or} \quad t = 0.431 \text{ cm. or about } 4\tfrac{1}{2} \text{ mm.}$$

Lead's greater efficiency for this radiation is immediately apparent (less than one-sixtieth of the thickness of concrete). It stems, of course, from its greater density and atomic number.

4. If the X-ray equipment quoted in *Example* 3 were replaced by equipment producing radiation of the same quality but with twice the output (160 R per minute at 50 cm.), (*a*) what would be the effect on the Exposure rate at the work place, assuming that the lead barrier specified above was being used, and (*b*) what lead barrier would be needed to restore the Exposure rate at the work place to the desired value of 1 mR per hour?

a. $X_c = 160 \times 60 = 9600$ R per hour; $D_c = 50$ cm.; $D = 500$ cm.; $t = 0.432$ cm. and $\mu = 25$ cm.$^{-1}$.

$$X = X_c(D_c{}^2/D^2)\, e^{-\mu t} = 9600(50^2/500^2)\, e^{-10.8} = 2 \times 10^{-3} \text{ R per hour.}$$

This, of course, is exactly what would be expected. Double the amount of radiation being produced and the amount being transmitted will be doubled. To restore the position a thicker barrier must be used.

b. $X_c = 9600$ R per hour; $D_c = 50$ cm.; $D = 500$ cm.; $X = 10^{-3}$ R per hour; $\mu = 25$ cm.$^{-1}$.

$$X = X_c(D_c{}^2/D^2)\, e^{-\mu t} \quad \text{or} \quad 10^{-3} = 9600(1/100)\, e^{-\mu t},$$
$$e^{-\mu t} = 10^{-3}/96 = 1.04_2 \times 10^{-5} = e^{-11.47},$$
$$\mu t = 11.47 \quad \text{or} \quad t = 11.47/25 = 0.459 \text{ cm.}$$

Thus an extra 0·028 cm. or 0·28 mm. of lead would be needed to cope with the increased output. In passing it should be noted that the extra lead is equal in thickness to the half-value in lead for this radiation (H.V.L. = $0.693/\mu = 0.693/25 = 0.028$ cm.). This illustrates the rule that a particular added thickness always reduces the beam by the same fraction. In this case the added half-value layer reduces the beam emerging from the original barrier by a half and so exactly compensates for the increased output.

5. Finally, what would happen if a cobalt-60 beam unit with the same output as in *Example* 4 (i.e., 160 R per min. at 50 cm.) were to replace the

X-ray equipment? For cobalt-60 gamma rays the broad beam linear attentuation coefficient for lead may be taken as $0 \cdot 92$ cm.$^{-1}$.

$$X_c = 9600 \text{ R per hour}; \quad D_c = 50 \text{ cm.}; \quad D = 500 \text{ cm.}; \quad \mu = 0 \cdot 92 \text{ cm.}^{-1}$$

and $t = 0 \cdot 459$ cm.

$$X = X_c(D_c{}^2/D^2)\, e^{-\mu t} = 9600(50^2/500^2)\, e^{-0 \cdot 92} \times 0 \cdot 459$$

$$= 9600 \times 0 \cdot 01 \times e^{-0 \cdot 423} = 96 \times 0 \cdot 655$$

$$= 72 \cdot 9 \text{ R per hour.}$$

Over 1 R per min. will be reaching the work point, and of course this is far too great an Exposure rate for safe working. Much more protection is needed. It will be noted from *Example* (4b) that in order to achieve the required Exposure rate of 10^{-3} R per hour with a beam of the same 'output' as here, the product μt had to be $11 \cdot 47$. The same is true here so that the required thickness of lead would be given by

$$\mu t = 11 \cdot 47 = 0 \cdot 92t$$

$$\therefore \quad t = 11 \cdot 47/0 \cdot 92 = 12 \cdot 3 \text{ cm.}$$

Nearly 5 in. of lead would be needed in this case—or an equivalent thickness in some other material. A very thick barrier is needed for this very penetrating radiation whenever the beam can be directed towards an occupied space. Whenever possible this is avoided in the design of the treatment rooms.

Primary and Secondary Barriers.—From these examples it will be seen that the amount of radiation reaching any place depends not only on the distance of that place from the radiation source, the nature and thickness of any interposed barrier, but also upon the quantity and quality of radiation leaving the source. The higher the energy of the radiation (the 'harder' its quality), the more that will pass through any barrier: the 'softer' the quality the more effective the barrier will be as a protector.

The protection problem in most X-ray rooms is illustrated in *Fig.* 448. Not only is there the primary radiation (P) of the relatively narrow useful beam, but there is also leakage radiation (L) emerging through the shield of the X-ray tube, and scattered radiation (S) from all irradiated objects and especially the patient. The two former (P and L) are of about the same quality, though the leakage radiation Exposure rate from a modern tube will only be about $0 \cdot 1$ per cent of the primary Exposure rate. Scattered radiation (S) will be 'softer' than the other two and considerably lower in Exposure rate than the primary beam.

Barriers to provide protection against the primary beam are usually called *Primary Barriers* and must be incorporated in any part of the floor, walls, and ceiling of the X-ray room at which the primary beam can be fired. Any surfaces at which the primary beam cannot be fired, but which may receive scattered radiation or leakage radiation, need only be *Secondary Barriers*. Because some of the radiation to which they are exposed is less penetrating than the primary beam, and because the Exposure rate is much smaller, secondary barriers are usually only about half as thick as primary barriers. A very substantial saving in building costs may, therefore, be achieved if the direction of firing of the primary beam can be restricted. This is especially the case with radiotherapeutic equipment for which primary barriers are often of considerable thickness. It may be added that considerable restriction may be applied to source movement without any noticeable effect on the ease of using the apparatus. Since protection devices always 'play safe', it is usual, in practice, to make primary barriers 15 or 30 cm. wider all round than the area on

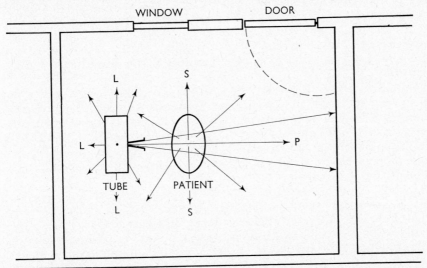

Fig. 448.—Primary (P), scattered (S), and leakage (L) radiation during an X-ray exposure.

to which the primary beam can fall. As a general rule, doors and windows should be so sited that they never need to be primary barriers.

Materials.—The attenuating effect of any barrier depends on the product μd since:

$$I = I_0 e^{-\mu d}.$$

Therefore whilst it is usual to employ a material with a large linear attenuation coefficient, should this material be unsuitable for any reason (which may include price) a thicker layer of less attenuating material can be used.

Lead is the most commonly used protective material, having the double advantage of high density and high atomic number, which means that it has a higher linear attenuation coefficient at all radiation energies than any other commonly available material. (Uranium is denser and has a higher Z value and hence a higher value of μ, but it is hardly commonly available!) For comparison purposes, therefore, lead is generally accepted as the standard material against which all other materials are measured through the concept of the 'Lead Equivalent'. This is the thickness of lead which provides the same degree of protection as the barrier being discussed, for the radiation in question. For instance in the third example above 28·4 cm. of concrete and 4·3 mm. of lead both reduced the Exposure rate, at the point in question, to 1·0 × 10⁻³ R per hour. Therefore, the 'lead equivalent' of that particular concrete wall (28·4 cm.) is 4·3 mm. of lead.

In many cases lead is not a suitable material for protection purposes and alternatives have to be sought. For example, it cannot be used in a viewing window (!), neither is it suitable for the protective gloves and aprons worn by those who may have to work in radiation beams. When a large area of wall has to be protected, lead sheet is not always convenient, and it may be too expensive. Which alternatives are used depends upon the circumstances (*see*, for instance, *Example* 3 above).

For example, viewing windows are often needed in X-ray rooms and though they can be made of thick plate glass, when increase of thickness (d) compensates for the smaller attenuation coefficient (μ), it is more usual to use 'lead glass'. This is made by adding lead salts to the silicates used in the manufacture of glass. It is acceptably transparent and being denser and of higher average atomic number is a better protective material than ordinary glass. In a similar manner lead salts, or even metallic lead, may be added to rubber or plastics, to give 'lead rubber' or 'lead-loaded' plastics, from which protective gloves or aprons of satisfactory flexibility can be made.

For walls, even lead sandwiched between layers of wood, to form 'lead plywood', is often inconvenient or too expensive and yet ordinary brickwork or concrete may be inadequate except in greater thicknesses than are desirable. In such circumstances 'barium plaster' or 'barium concrete' may be extremely useful. These are plaster and concrete mixtures containing a high proportion of barium sulphate which, because of its high density and the high atomic number of barium, greatly increases the attenuation of the mixture.

Barrier Thickness and Radiation Energy.—For most radiations used in radiology, the linear attenuation coefficient falls steadily with increasing radiation energy for all materials, as has been described in CHAPTER VII. This means that the higher the generating voltage the thicker the barrier needed to give a specified degree of protection. *Table LVIII* illustrates this by showing the thicknesses of lead and of concrete

Table LVIII.—THICKNESSES OF LEAD OR CONCRETE NEEDED TO REDUCE EACH BEAM TO 0·01 PER CENT OF THE INITIAL VALUE

Generating voltage	50 kV.	75 kV.	100 kV.	200 kV.	250 kV.	300 kV.	400 kV.	500 kV.	1 MV.	2 MV.	3 MV.
Lead (in mm.)	0·5	1·3	2·4	4·6	6·5	11	21	40	100	155	185
Concrete (in cm.)	6·4	10·4	15·2	30	32	36	41	56	69	91	102

required to produce the same percentage reduction in Exposure rate for beams generated from 50 kV. up to 3 MV. The increased thicknesses at the higher voltages are clearly seen: a barrier of lead 200 times as thick at 1 MV. as at 50 kV., for instance. Also the superiority of lead will be apparent; at 50 kV., for example, the required layer of concrete is 120 times as thick as the lead barrier (64 mm. as opposed to 0·5 mm.). However, it will also be seen that the difference between lead and concrete, though still considerable, is not as great at the higher energies as it is at the lower.

Lead Equivalent and Radiation Energy.—This change in the ratio of the required thickness of lead and concrete is important and is shown in more detail in *Table LIX*

Table LIX.—THE LEAD EQUIVALENT OF 150 mm. OF CONCRETE FOR BEAMS OF DIFFERENT ENERGIES

Generating voltage	50 kV.	75 kV.	100 kV.	200 kV.	250 kV.	300 kV.	400 kV.	500 kV.	1 MV.	2 MV.	3 MV.
Lead equivalent (in mm.)	1·4	2·0	2·4	2·3	3·0	3·8	5·4	7·1	13·0	22·0	26·0

which gives the lead equivalent, at each generating voltage, of the same thickness of concrete (in this case 150 mm.). Note the difference from *Table LVIII* which shows thicknesses of material for the same degree of protection—this table says nothing about the protection afforded but merely how much lead is needed to do what the concrete would do. It illustrates very clearly the changing efficiency of lead as an attenuator. Lead is relatively much more effective at low energies than at high energies —remember, the more efficient the attenuator the smaller the thickness for given attenuation.

The reason for this trend has already been discussed in CHAPTER VII. With low-energy radiations lead enjoys a double advantage over other commonly used protective materials, like concrete, brick, steel, and 'barium' concrete or plasters. It is denser than any of them and because of its higher atomic number will have a much greater photo-electric effect ($\propto Z^3$). Small thicknesses of lead will, therefore, be equivalent to much greater thicknesses of other materials. At the higher energies, however, the photo-electric effect is relatively unimportant and the Compton process (independent of Z) is mainly responsible for the attenuation, and therefore lead has only a single superiority—that of higher density. For the higher energies, therefore, greater thicknesses of lead are needed. Note that lead is roughly five times as dense as concrete, and with 3-MV. radiation the ratio of the required thicknesses is just over five to one.

In between the two extremes of *Table LIX*, the lead equivalent gradually increases, because the photo-electric effect diminishes in importance. One minor point of possible interest should, however, be mentioned. This is the small break in the continuous increase in lead equivalent that occurs in the 100-kV.–250-kV. region. The lead equivalent at 200 kV. is slightly less than that at 100 kV., which is contrary to the general trend. This is due to there being an 'absorption edge' in the lead attenuation pattern at about 80 keV. (radiation of this energy is very prominent in the spectrum of radiation generated at 200 kV.) and it means that radiation of energy rather greater than 80 keV. will suffer more attenuation than will radiations of rather lower energies. Over a small part of the energy range, therefore, lead attenuates the higher energies rather more efficiently than the lower, and this is reflected in the small check to the steady increase in lead equivalent due to the general decrease of attenuating power with increasing energy. It must be confessed, however, that this phenomenon is of greater academic than practical interest.

Protective Barriers at High Energies.—*Fig.* 449 shows how the *mass* attenuation coefficients (essentially the radiation removed per unit mass of material) for a number of different substances, including some used in protective barriers, vary with radiation energy. Immediately a very striking fact is revealed: over quite a large range of radiation energies the attenuation per gramme is practically independent of the material. This is because, as stressed in CHAPTER VI, the Compton effect, which is the major contributor to attenuation in the high-energy range, is independent of atomic number and depends only on electron density, which practically is the same for all substances except those containing hydrogen.

Thus, for radiations in this range of mass attenuation coefficient equality (roughly for radiation generated between about 1 and 4 MV.) it is not the material of which the wall is made that is of prime importance but rather the weight of material in the wall. An example may help to make this clear. Assume that a wall 2·5 m. high and 3·5 m. long is being built to provide protection against 2-MV. radiation and that it is to be made of concrete 90 cm. thick. The weight of such a wall would be about 23 tonnes. If instead of concrete the wall was made of lead, or of steel, and in each case weighed 23 tonnes, the protection provided would be the same in each case. The lead wall would be thinnest (about 18 cm.) compared with the steel (about 25 cm.) and the concrete (90 cm.) but weight for weight the protection would be the same. In the high-energy range, therefore, the choice of material for a particular protective purpose will depend on characteristics other than its attenuation properties.

For example, because lead is very expensive and a soft material unsuitable for building into large walls, it is seldom used in the protection of megavoltage X-ray rooms, when concrete is usually the material of choice. Similarly, steel is more

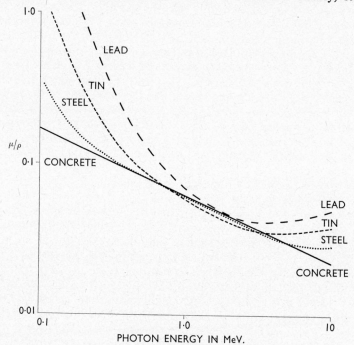

Fig. 449.—The variation of mass attenuation coefficient with radiation energy for a number of substances.

suitable for protection barriers in radium, or other radio-isotope-handling labora-tories, even though these barriers may have to be half as thick again as they would if made of lead. On the other hand, where it is essential to keep the barrier thickness as small as possible, as for instance in a telecurie radioactive isotope machine, lead is generally used. In special circumstances, however, it is replaced even in this sort of situation. The main collimation of cobalt-60 beam units, for example, is often made of 'heavy alloy'—an alloy of tungsten and copper which is denser than lead —or even uranium which, as already mentioned, has both a greater density and atomic number than lead.

CHAPTER XLIV

DEPARTMENTAL PROTECTION

THE whole object of radiation protection is to ensure that no one is unnecessarily irradiated, and, for the moment, attention will be concentrated upon the protection of those working in and around the radiological department. It must not be forgotten, however, that similar considerations apply to the patient, whose specific protection will be dealt with later.

Details of protection arrangements depend very much on local circumstances as well as upon the radiation source and the radiation it emits. The size of the room,

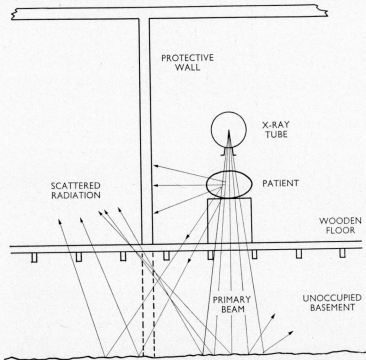

Fig. 450.—Radiation may be scattered in a floor or the space beneath, and reach adjoining rooms as shown. To prevent this the protective wall must be taken below floor level as indicated by the dotted line, or protective material can be incorporated in the floor.

the proximity of other radiation sources, the type of work being carried on in nearby rooms, and the length of time that they are occupied each day, and the amount and type of radiological work being done, will all influence the design of the protective barriers. Only general considerations, therefore, can be usefully discussed here, and these under three headings:

1. The X-ray therapy department.
2. The X-ray diagnostic department.
3. The radioactive isotope department.

643

In the first two of these the hazard is mainly one of whole-body irradiation whilst in the third, though whole-body exposure cannot be ignored, special attention may have to be given to exposure of hands and eyes. In all three there is a dual problem to be solved—that of providing safe working conditions for radiological staff and of the general protection of all people liable to come near the department. This latter,

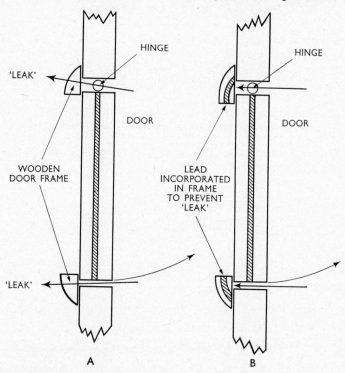

Fig. 451.—Radiation may 'leak' through the inevitable spaces around a fully protective door set in a full protection wall, as shown in A. To prevent this overlapping protective material must be included, as shown in B.

especially, means that as little radiation as possible must be allowed to escape from the room housing the source. In the case of X-ray departments for both diagnosis or therapy it is natural to think of having adequately thick walls, but surprisingly often the need for protective barriers in floors and ceilings is overlooked. Even if the X-ray room is on the ground floor, with no working space below, it must be remembered that although photons travel in straight lines in free space they can be scattered round corners, and, therefore, occupants of adjoining rooms can be irradiated as shown in *Fig.* 450 unless some protection is added to the floor, or the intervening wall carried down as is shown dotted. In like manner, radiation can 'leak' under or around the sides of protective doors unless there is a proper overlap of protective material such as that shown in *Fig.* 451.

In estimating the thicknesses of walls, ceilings, and so on, two factors not previously mentioned have to be taken into account, and these tend to make the problem a little easier than might at first sight be imagined, or to make protection, designed without making allowance for them, more effective. These factors allow for 'work load' and for occupancy. No X-ray set is going to be used all the time—the radiographic exposure or therapy treatment takes up only part of the time for which the patient is actually in the room. Positioning the patient takes a considerable time, and X-rays are being produced, and therefore their hazard exists, for probably no more than one-fifth of the working day. Less protection will be required if this is taken into account than if the thickness is based on tube-output values alone. Similarly, a thinner barrier is permissible if the space beyond is not likely to be permanently occupied: for example, if it is a corridor one can assume that it is only likely to be occupied for about a quarter of the time, and therefore rather thinner walls are acceptable than would be for, say, an office. On the other hand, a film store just outside an X-ray room may need extra shielding because of the sensitivity of the material and the need to prevent its being 'fogged'. Film should, however, be stored, if possible, well away from any radiation sources.

Table LX.—Primary and Secondary Barrier Thicknesses of Typical Diagnostic, 'Deep Therapy', and 'Megavoltage' X-ray Departments

	Primary Barrier in			Secondary Barrier in		
	Lead	Ba Concrete	Concrete	Lead	Ba Concrete	Concrete
100 kV.	2·5 mm.	0·75 in.	6·5 in.	1·0 mm.	0·25 in.	3 in.
250 kV.	12 mm.	6·5 in.	20 in.	7 mm.	3·5 in.	12 in.
4 MV.	26 cm.	3 ft. 6 in.	5 ft.	15 cm.	2 ft.	2·5 ft.

Densities: Lead = 11·4 g./ml. Ba concrete = 3·2 g./ml. Concrete = 2·2 g./ml.

In order to give the reader some idea of the barrier thicknesses required, those that might be used in some typical radiological situations are given in *Table LX*. It must be emphasized that these are average figures and not necessarily applicable to any specific installation.

We now turn to the special problems of the three types of department listed.

1. THE X-RAY THERAPY DEPARTMENT

In the modern X-ray therapy department (and this includes, of course, the department using teletherapy radioactive isotope units) the radiographic staff is always outside the room during a treatment, because the amount and penetrating power of the scattered radiation make it impossible to provide safe working conditions for anyone left in the room during the exposure. A high degree of radiological protection may therefore be provided for radiotherapy staff by the provision of adequately thick walls. However, some awkward problems still remain.

Windows.—For example, because the staff is outside the room it is necessary that they should be able to see the patient, and furthermore that the patient should have the psychological comfort that he is seen and can attract attention should the need arise. Since the window should afford the same degree of protection as the wall in which it is installed, and since it is not easy to provide both protection and transparency, it is obviously desirable that the windows should be so sited, and the tube movements so restricted, that the primary beam cannot fall upon the window, i.e., that it should only have to be a secondary barrier. With kilovoltage radiations lead glass is almost always used and even when only a secondary barrier, it is an expensive part of the installation. With 250-kV. radiation—calling, as *Table LX* has shown, for about 7 mm. of lead as a secondary barrier—the thickness of lead glass would be nearly 1½ in., costing more than £100 for a window only 1 ft. square. In the megavoltage range the thickness of lead glass needed would make the window prohibitively expensive, as well as of very poor transparency. Therefore numerous sheets of plate glass in an oil bath, or a glass-ended tank of water several feet thick, or indirect vision through a periscope of mirrors have been used with ⁶⁰Co telecurie units or linear accelerators. Nowadays the preferred alternatives are either to do

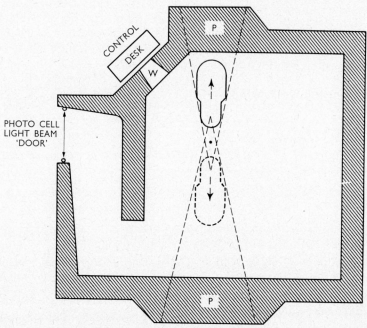

Fig. 452.—Plan of room suitable for megavoltage X-ray unit. The 'maze' entrance will be noted and the position of the light beam, interruption of which cuts off any treatment in progress. Note that the viewing window cannot receive the primary beam—it need only be a secondary barrier. W = Window; P = Primary barriers.

away with the window altogether and use closed-circuit television, or to use a glass-ended tank filled with zinc bromide solution. The latter has the highest density of any transparent liquid. Both methods have advantages and disadvantages, both have their protagonists and opponents, and both fulfil their role very well.

Doors.—As with the viewing window, it is advantageous if doors can be sited so that they need only be secondary barriers. A door, incorporating the 12-mm. lead which constitutes a primary barrier with 250-kV. radiation, would not only be very expensive but it would also be extremely heavy, calling for very special hinges and mounting, and also be fatiguing to have to open and close frequently.

Not only must the door prevent the escape of radiation, but it must also prevent anyone entering the room whilst irradiation is in progress. To this end it must operate electrical switches (or 'interlocks') which cut off the radiation beam as soon as the door is opened a small amount, and which also will not allow the beam to be switched on until the door is fully closed.

For megavoltage radiations a door providing even a secondary barrier would be impossibly heavy to be moved by hand and therefore 'maze' entrances are usually used. With this arrangement, an example of which is given in *Fig*. 452, access to the room is along a short corridor from which radiation only emerges after being scattered several times and, therefore, reduced to quite safe Exposure rate levels. A door is unnecessary with this arrangement except in so far as it prevents inadvertent entry during treatment. However, even this can be very conveniently prevented by having a light beam across the 'maze' entrance and arranging that the interruption of this beam cuts off the treatment.

Machines.—When radiation treatments are terminated by the closing of a shutter, which cuts off the beam from the patient, but the tube remains fully energized all the time, it is vitally important that the shutter mechanism is completely reliable, and furthermore that the protective materials around the tube are adequately thick. Otherwise leakage radiation may lead to staff doses in excess of maximum permissible values. If it is necessary to leave the tube running between treatment sessions, reduction of the applied kilovoltage by about 25 per cent would reduce the hazard by a very considerable factor. With radio-isotope telecurie units it is essential that the source-removal mechanism or the shutter should work on a 'fail–safe' principle—that is to say, any failure of electricity supply mains or any other fault should automatically lead to the movement of the source back to its safe position, or the closing of the shutter. The fact that an exposure is in progress should be indicated by a red light on the control desk and over the room door.

2. THE X-RAY DIAGNOSTIC DEPARTMENT

In contrast to the therapy department the amounts of radiation involved in each exposure are small, and the actual exposure times short. Furthermore, the generating voltages are relatively low, and the penetrating power of the radiation, especially the scattered radiation, is not very great. Assuming, for the moment, that no one has to go into the line of fire of the primary beam, a relatively light screen of lead plywood containing about 1 mm. of lead will provide adequate protection. It is usual for the control desk to be placed behind this screen and for both to be taken as far away from the patient as possible, thus taking full advantage of the effect of the inverse-square law. Behind this screen the radiographer will receive virtually no radiation dose. A useful point to remember, in siting the control desk and screen, is that the patient is the source of radiation (the scattered radiation) against which protection is being sought and therefore that if the irradiated part of the patient can be seen from any point, scattered radiation can reach that point—unless, of course, the patient is seen through a protective window!

In radiography it should *never* be necessary for radiographic staff to be in the primary beam, a very short exposure to which would deliver the maximum dose permissible for several weeks. If a restless patient is being radiographed and someone has to hold him or her (the usual case is the radiography of a young child) this must *never* be done by a radiographer: a relative (the mother in the case of a child) who is unlikely to have to do this office again may quite legitimately be asked to help, but should, of course, wear a lead rubber apron or other appropriate protection.

Before leaving radiography it should be mentioned that use of the smallest field size that will achieve the desired object will not only improve the radiograph but reduce the dose to the patient. Simply because less scatter is generated, the workers' protection is also improved.

Fluoroscopy, with the usual fluorescent screen apparatus described earlier, presents a different situation. Here the radiologist has to stand in the direction of the main beam, and he may have to put his hands into the beam in order to observe the effect of pressure or manipulation on the part being examined. However, the position in which he stands is fully protected by the lead glass backing of the fluorescent screen, and the lead rubber screens that usually hang below it and are appended to its side like wings. As for his hands, these should be shielded with protective gloves if they have to be placed in the beam—if at all possible palpation or manipulation should be carried out with the beam temporarily switched off. An alternative method may be to use wooden or other depressors to apply the required pressure.

The radiographer may not be quite so fortunately placed, and may have to stand to one side to pass films or other required materials to the radiologist. Though out of the line of the main beam she may be at considerably greater risk from the scattered radiation. The patient is the source of radiation to be guarded against. The radiographer must therefore take up a position shielded by the lead rubber screens or must wear a lead rubber apron as protection against the secondary radiation.

3. THE RADIOACTIVE ISOTOPE DEPARTMENT

The protection problems associated with the clinical use of radioactive isotopes are quite different from those which are met in either type of X-ray department. This is because radiation is emitted continuously from radioactive materials—it can never be switched off—and also because the sources have, in one way or another, to be prepared for use, and administered or applied to the patient. As a result, workers have to come fairly close to the sources and problems of irradiation of the hands and eyes, as well as of the whole body, have to be dealt with. Manipulation of sources takes place as much as possible behind shielding barriers, and with the aid of long-handled instruments to take as much advantage as possible of 'distance attenuation' due to the operation of the inverse square law. However, there is a limit to the length of the devices that can be used expeditiously—if a longer instrument reduces the exposure rate at the hand by a factor of two but its use increases the time for a particular operation by a factor of three its contribution to radiation protection is an illusory one! Lead is the most commonly used material for protective barriers in radioactive isotope departments but steel is also widely used. Many isotopes emit high-energy gamma radiations the attenuation of which depends little on atomic number so that, except where space is at a premium and the greater density of lead is advantageous, steel is often preferred since this is a good construction material for barriers, storage boxes, and the like. One further difference between the X-ray departments and the radioactive isotope departments must be noted. The latter cannot be considered as confined to one specific part of the hospital: radioactive materials are used in many places and protection problems occur wherever they go— even into the world at large when a patient who has received certain types of test or treatment leaves hospital.

Though there are common problems associated with both types of radioactive isotope source it will be convenient to consider 'sealed sources' and 'unsealed sources' separately.

Sealed Sources.—This general title is given to those materials which are permanently sealed into suitable containers. Under normal circumstances the radioactive material never leaves the container, so that the hazard they present will be regarded initially as one of radiation only. Usually sealed sources contain radioactive isotopes of long half-life so that they can be used over and over again. They have, therefore, to be stored as well as prepared for use and cleaned after used. All this takes place in a handling laboratory, a general plan of which is shown in *Fig.* 453 A. In the description that follows it is assumed that the sources contain radium, though the procedures apply equally to any other gamma-ray emitting sealed sources, for example caesium 137 or cobalt 60.

The Handling Laboratory.—The philosophy behind the design of the handling laboratory is that the radium and its radiation should be 'contained' behind the protective barrier and in shielded containers as much as possible. Furthermore, the amount of radium taken out of the store and brought on to the bench at any one time must be kept as small as possible, and for this purpose protective storage boxes are provided for the temporary storage of sources. Steel partitions are provided to reduce the amount of radiation reaching one part of the work bench from sources in another.

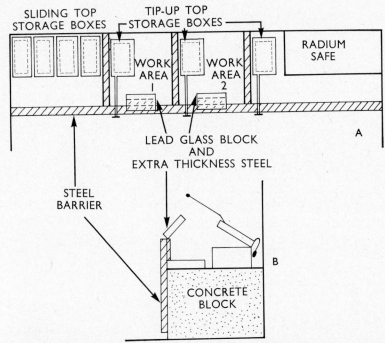

Fig. 453.—A radioactive isotope handling laboratory. A, Plan showing main protective barrier and the separate work and storage areas. B, Section through work area, showing extra protection, eye and head protective glass block, and tip-up top storage box.

The main working surface is a concrete block covered with a non-absorbent continuous sheet material such as P.V.C., along the front of which runs a wall of steel 3 in. thick from almost ground level to 4 ft. 6 in. high, as shown diagrammatically in *Fig.* 453 B. Three-inch thick steel partitions divide the bench into four separate areas, one of which contains the main storage 'safe' (the right-hand area), and one of which (the left-hand area) has a number of sliding-top storage safes in which prepared sources can be held until required for use, or returned sources kept until they can be cleaned and returned to the 'safe'. In between these are two work areas where needles may be 'silked', i.e., have a colour-coded silk thread passed through the eyelet for strength identification, for anchorage in use, and for removal after use, or tubes loaded into applicators for intracavitary therapy or on to 'moulds' for superficial treatments. At either of these places sources are cleaned after use. Because it is at the work areas that a worker will spend most time, the barrier is increased for extra protection by the addition of an extra thickness of steel or lead, whilst on top of the barrier there is a block of lead glass 3–6 in. thick through which the worker can see the source that he is dealing with and yet enjoy a measure of eye protection. This glass block as well as the barrier and the tip-up top storage box are shown in *Fig.* 453 B. The bench is designed so that for work behind it the arms and wrists are rested on the barrier top—which is clad in P.V.C. for comfort—and the sources are manipulated with long-handled tongs or forceps. The hands should never approach within less than about 9 in. of the radiation material.

Details of a simple, typical radium safe are given in *Fig.* 454. It consists of a series of drawers each of which, as the pulled-out drawer shows, is made up of a 1-in.

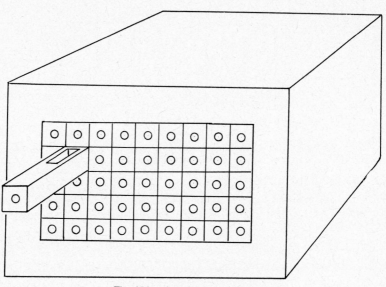

Fig. 454.—A radium storage safe.

square steel tube, about 1 ft. long, and filled with lead except for a small central cavity in which the sources are stored. The number of drawers should be such that each carries only a relatively small amount of radium, so that when a drawer is pulled out for the removal of some sources the worker is not exposed to radiation from more than a few sources and so is not subject to excessive radiation. Around the drawers is a layer of lead 3–6 in. thick (depending on the total amount of radium being stored) and thus when all the drawers are closed all the radium is surrounded by a considerable thickness of lead and the amount of gamma radiation 'leaking out' is acceptably low. This 'safe' provides radiation safety, but not necessarily security against theft or even inquisitive interference, against which the radium 'safe' may be built into a more conventional security safe, which also provides a degree of protection against fire damage. The storage boxes are usually made of 3-in. steel plate with either counterweighted tip-up tops or sliding tops.

Transport, Storage, and Use.—The prepared sources are generally used outside the handling laboratory—in the operating theatre for example—and must be transported hence as quickly as possible to reduce to a minimum the inevitable irradiation of people along the route. A long-handled protected trolley like that shown in *Fig.* 455 is particularly suitable for this purpose. It can incorporate enough protection to safeguard the person pushing it and also people passing by and yet it is sufficiently mobile to be able to be moved quickly without great muscular effort. Some years ago the introduction of the sort of handling laboratory scheme depicted in *Fig.* 453 reduced the whole-body dose to the laboratory staff to half of what it has been with the older type of laboratory protection. The cost was a thousand pounds or so. Later a trolley of the type described was purchased for less than £50 and produced another 50 per cent drop in whole-body dose!

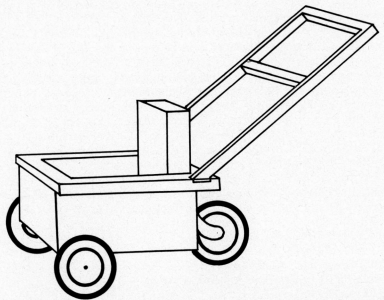

Fig. 455.—A protected trolley for transport of radioactive materials within a hospital.

On arrival at their destination the sources (which will have been brought in a protective carrier) are transferred temporarily to a protective safe or box similar to those in the handling laboratory. Should sterilization be necessary then, as described in CHAPTER XL, this can be done in an open, hot-water sterilizer which is surrounded by about 3 in. of lead. Until the sources are in use in a patient they must be kept in protective containers of one kind or another, so that as little radiation as possible escapes to present a hazard.

Once the sources are in, or on, a patient the use of barriers to protect other patients or nursing staff is seldom very practicable and therefore, in general, as much as possible has to be made of the protection afforded by distance. Patients undergoing treatment with sealed sources are distributed throughout the ward and X-ray therapy patients are interspersed between them. In this way no dangerous radiation zones are set up. Nursing procedures on 'sealed-source' patients are carried out as quickly as possible, the staff keeping as far as practicable from the part of the body being treated; movable screens incorporating several centimetres of steel or lead have been tried in some hospitals to afford a degree of protection but are generally regarded as cumbersome. They slow the work down, so that the decrease in radiation exposure rate is offset by an increase in the exposure time. Screens for this purpose have not found general acceptance: indeed the radiation protection world still awaits the the evolution of a practicable screen.

Records.—Sealed sources, especially if they contain radium, are valuable and, therefore, it is economically necessary that they should not be lost. More important, however, a mislaid sealed source also presents an unpredictable radiation hazard and, even more serious, the possibility of it suffering damage so that its contents leak out not only to contaminate the surroundings but also to be ingested by anyone in the area. One microgram of radium permanently deposited in the body would be a major hazard to health; when it is realized that a 1-mg. needle contains a thousand such hazards the importance of taking every precaution to ensure that no loss, however, temporary, occurs will be apparent.

All manipulations must be carried out quickly (to reduce the dose received) but also carefully, and meticulous records must be kept of all source movements. These records must include the signatures of responsible people into whose care the sources pass in their tour of use, e.g., of the Radium Curator who issues them, of the Theatre Sister, of the implanting Radiotherapist, of the Ward Sister under whose care the patient is nursed, and finally the Radium Curator who receives them back. At each stage the numbers and types of source must be carefully checked; good records not only prevent economic loss, they are part of good radiation protection.

Even the best systems may, however, fail sometimes and defences must be devised to prevent a mislaid source getting into drains or being thrown away with hospital refuse. No patient into whom sealed sources are implanted or inserted should, for the duration of treatment, be allowed to use the normal water-closet facilities. All bed-pans from such patients should be checked for radioactive sources. For the same reason all refuse bins from whatever source in the hospital (office papers, floor sweepings, soiled dressings, food scraps, and so on) must be collected together and checked with a Geiger counter or similar sensitive radiation detector before the contents are disposed of. All laundry leaving the hospital should be similarly checked. Only by measures such as these and the constant vigilance of the staff can a high measure of security be assured.

Damaged Sources.—So far in discussing their handling, it has been assumed that the sources remain sealed, that none of their contents escape, and, therefore, that they present only a gamma-radiation hazard. Faults, however, may develop and some of the radioactive material may leak out to form a contamination and health hazard. 'Leak' tests as described on p. 583 should be carried out regularly on all radium sources, and 'wipe' tests on all other sealed sources. In the latter case the source is wiped over with a small piece of cotton-wool which has been moistened with detergent and is held in long forceps. The wool is then tested for radioactive contamination by a sensitive counter, the type of instrument depending on the type of radiation to be expected from the source material. If a 'leak' or a 'wipe' test is positive the offending source must immediately be taken out of service, sealed into a suitable container, and returned when convenient to its makers for repair or replacement.

Unsealed Sources.—Radioactive materials which in one way or another, for tracer studies or for radiotherapy, are introduced directly into the patient's tissues are often called 'unsealed sources', because in use no container separates them from the tissues. (Unlike sealed sources these radioactive materials are almost always of short half-life, many are pure beta-ray emitters, and the source strengths are generally much less than those for sealed sources, being rarely more than a few millicuries and often only microcuries). Therefore, unsealed sources do not present such big external irradiation problems as far as staff are concerned, the main protection attention being directed towards avoiding the contamination of equipment and workers, and the prevention of ingestion or inhalation (by anyone other than the patient for whom they are intended!) which might lead to radioactive materials being deposited in, and seriously irradiating, important tissues and organs.

The great majority of radioactive materials in clinical use are purchased from commercial undertakings, such as the Radiochemical Centre at Amersham, in a form suitable for almost direct use. However, a certain amount of 'handling' is still necessary in the receiving department before they can be used. Generator 'columns' such as those described on p. 394 have to be eluted and the resulting fluid diluted further; the contents of ampoules have to be withdrawn, usually by a syringe, and also probably diluted; and for some work materials like blood or serum or other fluids have to be 'labelled'. All such work must be carried on behind a protective barrier, using long-handled or remotely controlled devices as far as possible.

In a handling bench for unsealed sources all surfaces should be non-absorbent and easily cleaned, so that any splashed material can be easily removed. Work should also be carried out within, or over, enamel trays lined with absorbent paper, the trays being large enough in area and depth that they would catch and hold all the material being used should the container break. Where there is any risk of radioactive vapours or aerosols being formed the manipulation must be done in chemical fume-hoods— behind appropriate barriers, of course. One small but important point: open containers should be studiously avoided. Quite intense beams of beta rays can emerge, which would be stopped by putting on the lid.

Wherever possible, radioactive materials should be handled in liquid form since their remote handling is much easier than the remote handling of powders or gases. Liquids, however, must never be pipetted by mouth because of the danger of accidental ingestion; for the same reason smoking, eating, or drinking in laboratories where radioactive material is handled is absolutely forbidden. Both to provide some measure of protection against beta radiation, but mainly to protect the hands against splashes of radioactive material, rubber gloves and readily disposable over-gloves should always be worn when handling unsealed sources.

Generally, unsealed sources are administered to the patient as a drink or by injection. In the first case the drink is usually prepared in a waxed paper, or a plastic cup from which the patient sucks the liquid through a straw. When using this method, care must be taken that the radioactive material does not become preferentially attached to the vessel, which appears to be empty yet has radioactive material adhering to its sides—in other words the cup is still radioactive but the patient isn't! The exposure to radiation in this process for patient and staff is minimal. Where a syringe is used, the fingers and hands of the doctor must come close to the radioactive material, so that some protection is desirable. A lead sheath should cut out radiation most efficiently but would make the syringe heavy and rather unwieldy and, of course, it is not transparent so that the doctor cannot see how the injection is proceeding. Compromise is therefore usual: a sheath of Perspex 1 cm. thick allows the liquid to be seen, cuts out practically all beta radiation, and, mainly by the effect of distance, considerably reduces the gamma-ray dose.

Spills.—Should a spill of radioactive material occur, and under this heading must be included urine, etc., from patients given radioactive materials, the decontamination of affected places, equipment, or people must be immediate and thorough. However, action must not be so immediate that it is overhasty and only serves to make matters worse, initially at least. In the case of an accident resulting in radioactive material being spread around, all movement in the area concerned must be stopped except where it is necessary to remove any persons who may be at risk. Then the action to be taken must be planned calmly but quickly. Such emergencies should be anticipated and a drill established to deal with them. In addition, there should be ready for immediate use protective clothing like rubber boots, face masks, waterproof suits (preferably of plastic), and rubber gloves as well as mops, buckets, and general cleaning materials.

When tackling the work, care must be taken not to spread the radioactive material more than has already happened and, when the bulk of the liquid has been carefully mopped up, assiduous washing of the affected places with soap, or detergents, and water should be continued with frequent checks with a radiation detector to determine how the operation is proceeding and to indicate when a satisfactory clearance has been achieved. Anyone splashed with radioactive material should remove all affected clothing, which should be stored in plastic bags until the activity has decayed sufficiently for the clothes to be cleaned or laundered. Any possibly affected areas of the body should be washed in soap and water until the counter indicates an acceptably low level of activity. Where the person is injured, for example with broken glassware, the wound should be very thoroughly cleaned in running water, and mild bleeding encouraged during the washing in the hope that any radioactive contamination will be thereby removed.

Radioactive Waste Disposal.—Earlier the point was made that problems concerning radiation protection in radioactive isotope work are not confined to the rooms in which the material is prepared or administered or even the ward in which the patient may be nursed. Hazards to some extent exist everywhere to which the material is taken to, or in, or from the patient. The 'radioactive' patient is a potential radiation hazard to others and until the radioactivity he carries has fallen below certain accepted values he must be treated with this hazard in mind. (In practice these remarks only apply to a patient undergoing radiotherapy by radioactive isotopes. The amounts used for diagnostic purposes constitute no hazard to the patient let alone his neighbours.) Nursing procedures should be carried out expeditiously and he should not mix freely with fellow patients though he may be quite fit enough to do so. A special aspect of this concerns the sending home of patients by public service vehicle or ambulance soon after the administration of a radioactive isotope. The maximum activity of iodine 131 in a patient being discharged is set at 15 mCi if the patient is to travel by public transport, whilst for gold 198 or phosphorus 32 the level is set at 30 mCi. Three things are taken into account in deciding upon these values. First there is the direct dose to other people with whom the patient may share the transport, and whose interests must be safeguarded; second there will be an effect on any photographic film being carried in the bus or train, and which could be ruined by overexposure; whilst thirdly there is always a chance that the patient might vomit, and hence contaminate with radioactivity places and facilities used by the public.

Should such an accident occur it would be cleaned up as already described in the preceding section but one aspect of the work has not yet been dealt with—the disposal of waste radioactive material. It is continually necessary to stress that the emission of radiation from radioactive materials cannot be controlled in any way—it certainly cannot be switched off—and therefore radioactive material is a potential health hazard and cannot, lightly, be discarded into the environment. The disposal of radioactive wastes therefore has to be very carefully controlled, and comprehensive regulations are in force to ensure this. Sealed sources no longer needed are usually stored until radioactive decay has reduced their activity to negligible levels (*N.B.*—in 10 half-lives the source will decay to a thousandth of its original value, whilst in 20 half-lives it goes down to a millionth of its original value) and then—in the case of radioactive gold, for example—the metal can be returned to the original source for reactivation and reissue. For long half-life materials such as radium, caesium 137, or cobalt 60 special disposal facilities are available from bodies like the British Nuclear Fuels Ltd.

Unused unsealed sources are often also easily stored until decay renders them innocuous and they can then be put into the drains or burned. Radioactive excreta, because of their bulk are difficult, as well as unpleasant, to store. And if stored they could well constitute a source of undesirable irradiation of nurses and other staff. In most cases, however, immediate disposal into the sewage system affords a sufficiently great dilution that there is no hazard to sewage workers. Even so, hospitals and all other organizations using radioactive materials have to abide by regulations laid down by government departments responsible for the environment—and this is very much as it should be.

General.—Because of the magnitude of the subject no attempt has been made to do more than cover the general principles of radiation protection, which are not likely to change. Details of the subject will change as our knowledge, especially of the biological effects of radiation, increases. For up-to-date information reference should be made to publications like the British Ministry of Health's *Code of Practice for the Protection of Persons against Ionising Radiations arising from Medical and Dental Use.* A worker to whom the code applies is required to read the parts of this very complete document 'which affect his work and well-being' and to sign 'a statement that he has understood them'. It is hoped that our general survey will materially help in the achieving of this understanding.

CHAPTER XLV

PROTECTION INSTRUMENTS AND PERSONNEL MONITORING

THE provision of apparently adequate barriers and protective devices does not guarantee the safety of the workers concerned. It could be that the barriers are not adequate through some error in calculation; or they may contain cracks or other errors of construction or design through which radiation can 'leak'; or again, and improperly, new and more powerful equipment may be installed in a room without any change in the protective barriers. On the other hand, workers might fail to take full advantage of the protection provided or even ignore it altogether. Any installation must therefore be thoroughly surveyed with suitable radiation detectors to confirm that the intended protection is provided, whilst each worker should be 'monitored' to ensure that he or she is not being over-irradiated. The instruments and methods used for these two purposes are quite different and will be considered separately.

DEPARTMENTAL SURVEYS

The Exposure rates of the radiation leaking through barriers, or through cracks in barriers, will usually be very small (of the order of milliroentgens per hour), so that ionization chambers of quite large volume are usually used for their measurement. A suitable instrument for general survey work of this nature is shown in

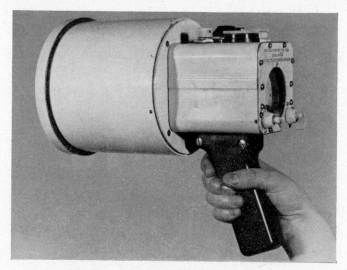

Fig. 456.—A typical radiation survey meter.

Fig. 456. This has an ionization chamber with a volume of about 800 ml. and a robust and fairly sensitive, battery-operated amplifier, which presents the Exposure rate as a reading on a meter. On the most sensitive range the full-scale reading of this sort of instrument will be about 3 mR per hour.

Instruments of this type cannot be used, however, for measurements with exposures of very short duration, such as are common in diagnostic X-ray departments, because the response time of the electrical circuit is about a second, and the Exposure would therefore be concluded before the instrument could fully respond. Neither is the type of device shown suitable for searching for tiny beams arising from cracks or other defects in barriers, since the reading can only be accurate if the whole chamber is irradiated. Some other type of detector is needed. In some cases this is a Geiger-Müller counter, which has high sensitivity and a relatively small volume, but even more useful is the photographic film. A piece of film (in a light-tight wrapping, of course) fastened on to a suspect barrier, or strapped on to an X-ray tube housing thought to be defective, will integrate the effect of many Exposures and reveal quite tiny defects. Where excessive radiation is suspected but its precise origin is doubtful, a direction-indicating film holder may yield useful information. An example of this device is shown in *Fig.* 458 C, p. 669. When this is irradiated from one direction, the metal peg casts a shadow which is revealed on the film after development, and so the direction of the beam can be deduced. A few such devices disposed around a room will usually indicate the origin of the radiation.

PERSONNEL MONITORING

The doses of radiation received by workers are commonly measured either with photographic film or with condenser ionization chambers, such as the B.D.11 type of chamber, shown in *Fig.* 64 (p. 111). Each method has advantages over the other, and disadvantages. Ionization chambers are basically more accurate than film and their response is relatively independent of the radiation energy. On the other hand, they are generally more bulky and fragile; they are liable to electrical leakage due to dampness or to dust, and, above all, they give no indication of the magnitude of an Exposure greater than that required to discharge them (usually about 500 mR). In an attempt to counteract these effects it is customary, when condenser chambers are used, to use them in pairs and to arrange that one has ten times the range of the other.

As already pointed out in CHAPTERS VIII and XVI, the effect of X-rays on photographic film is roughly proportional to the Exposure to which it is subjected, but also is very dependent upon the radiation energy. The sensitivity of a particular type of film may also vary from batch to batch, and the blackening also depends on the conditions of processing. For these reasons the photographic film was found to be an unsuitable basis for standard radiation dosemetry. Provided careful controls are maintained, however, it can be used with an accuracy of probably at least ± 20 per cent, for personnel monitoring purposes. Film is reasonably robust, provides a permanent record of the Exposure, and can cope with Exposures from as little as 10 mR up to Exposures as large as 20 R, a much greater range than is possible with a single ionization chamber. This large range is achieved by using a double-coated film, one coating being of normal sensitivity and the other being relatively insensitive. The first of these is used to measure Exposures of the levels usually received by workers (10 to 40 mR per week). The second coat, on the other hand, only shows measurable blackening for much larger doses, which completely blacken the sensitive coating. The more sensitive coating has to be removed before the estimation of the larger doses is possible.

Even the variation of blackening with radiation energy can be turned to good effect since, as will be described, it enables the film to indicate the quality of the radiation as well as its quantity.

THE FILM 'BADGE'

The variation in sensitivity, with radiation energy, of a typical photographic emulsion used for X-ray monitoring is shown in curve A of *Fig.* 457, from which it will be seen that the blackening of a plain piece of film does not, alone, give a reliable indication of the Exposure to which the film has been subjected. Any given degree of blackening may be produced by a small amount of low-energy radiation or by a

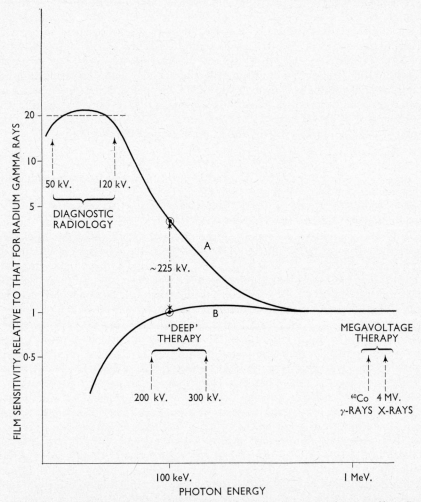

Fig. 457.—Variation of film sensitivity with photon energy. Curve A—open film. Curve B—film sandwiched between two sheets of tin each about 1 mm. thick. Dotted arrows indicate approximately the values that would be obtained for radiation beams generated at the voltages shown.

much larger amount of radiation of higher energy. If, however, the film is 'sandwiched' between two thin sheets of tin, each about 1·0 mm. thick, the blackening per unit Exposure is much more uniform over a wide range of radiation energies, as curve B of *Fig.* 457 shows. What happens, of course, is that the tin has practically no effect on the high-energy radiation, so that the blackening per unit Exposure is practically unaffected by the presence of the tin. On the other hand, the lower-energy radiation is considerably attenuated in the tin, so that the amount of radiation reaching the film, and hence the blackening it produces, are reduced.

If the increase of attenuation with decreasing energy could just match the increase of blackening, the ideal would be achieved—that is to say, the blackening per unit Exposure would be the same at all radiation energies. Though this cannot be done precisely, careful choice of tin thickness enables the ideal to be approached over a

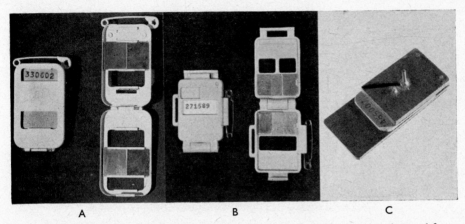

A	B	C

Fig. 458.—Some film 'badges'. A, Simple type with tin filter and 'open' region, and for which the curves shown in *Fig*. 457 would apply.   B, British Radiation Protection Service badge incorporating six filters and an 'open' film.   C, Direction-indicating badge.

wide range of radiation energies, as *Fig*. 457 shows. For radiation generated at 200 kV. and up to about 4 MV., or even more, the blackening per unit Exposure is almost constant under 1·0 mm. tin, and therefore, under these circumstances, film blackening can be used as a dosemeter. This, of course, is the basis of the personnel monitoring film 'badge' dosemeter, some examples of which are shown in *Fig*. 458. Section A of that illustration shows an early form of badge which incorporated a strip of tin across the middle of the film, both behind and in front (X-rays may reach the film from all directions), while section B shows a more complicated 'badge' now in general use in Britain. In the latter a number of different 'filters' are used so that beta rays and neutrons as well as X-rays may be measured. *Fig*. 458 C shows the direction indicator referred to earlier.

Processing, Calibration, and Measurement.—As stressed several times, the film sensitivity varies from type to type and even from batch to batch of the same type. It can only be used as a dosemeter if carefully calibrated and carefully processed. Fortunately, since the sensitivity of the film under the tin is constant over a wide range it is possible to calibrate the film at one energy only. This is most easily done using the hard gamma rays from radium since the Γ factor (Exposure rate at 1 cm. from 1 mg.) is fairly accurately known.

The usual procedure is to expose on a table such as that shown in *Fig*. 459 a number of films, in their 'badges', to known Exposures of gamma rays from radium. In this case the films are left for different lengths of time at a constant distance from the central source: an alternative is to set up a group of films on a similar table with each film at a different distance from the source, and leave them all for the same length of time. In either method films are subjected to Exposures covering the range likely to be met on the films used for monitoring. These specially exposed films are included with the monitoring films for development, and a calibration curve for the batch of films in use can be made. The doses corresponding to the blackenings of the monitoring films are easily read off this curve. *Fig.* 460 shows an example of a typical calibration curve, and the sort of reading that may be made on it.

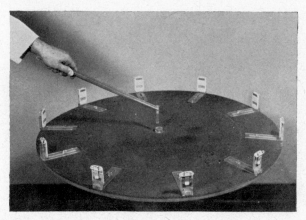

Fig. 459.—Table for calibration of monitoring films. A radium source (usually 100 mg.) is placed at the centre and the film 'badges' are arranged around the periphery and exposed for periods of time from about ½ to about 8 hr. They thus receive Exposures ranging from 0·35 R to 5·6 R.

It will be noted in this procedure that all the films received the same development procedure, and all came from the same batch, thus, to a considerable extent, eliminating the effects of processing and batch variation on the final answer.

One other necessary precaution calls for attention. The blackening of any exposed film is partly due to the radiation falling on it, but partly due to 'fog', i.e., blackening produced by the developer and independent of the Exposure. This 'fog' effect must be subtracted from the total blackening on any film if the radiation effect is to be measured. To ascertain its value a number of unexposed films are always developed along with the rest, and the blackening on these deducted from that on the exposed films. In *Fig.* 460 the values along the ordinate are, in fact, the levels of blackening *above the fog level*.

Exposure and Quality.—It will be seen that in each 'badge' there is a part of the film (which is, of course, in its light-tight wrapper) which is not covered by any filter. This 'open' part of the system has an important role. Taking the simpler badge (*Fig.* 458 A) as an example, the *ratio* of the blackening (above fog) in the 'open' part of the film to that of the region under the tin filter gives an indication of the quality of radiation to which the 'badge' has been exposed. If, for instance, the two portions are almost equally blackened, 'hard' gamma rays or high-energy X-rays would be the likely cause. On the other hand, if the blackening in the open part were four times as great as that under the tin, then 200–250-kV. X-rays are likely to have been involved, because for this sort of generating voltage the reading of curve A (*Fig.* 457) is four times that of curve B. In practice, interpretation may not be quite so simple when workers, in the course of their duties, may have been exposed to radiations of a variety of energies. However, formulae are available for use in conjunction with the modern 'badges' (*Fig.* 458 B) which enable even these complicated cases to be analysed, and thus the apparent disadvantage of the

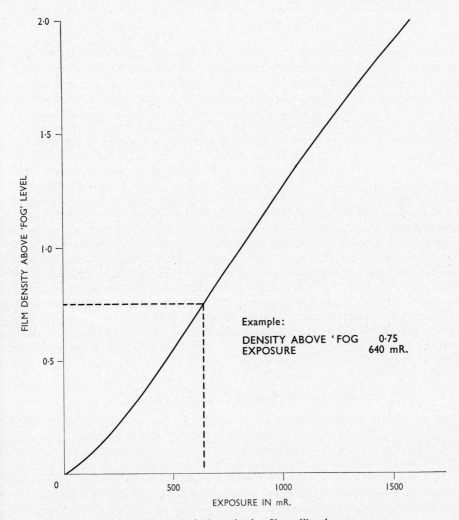

Example:

DENSITY ABOVE 'FOG   0·75
EXPOSURE   640 mR.

Fig. 460.—A typical monitoring film calibration curve.

considerable variation of sensitivity can be turned into a source of extra information and a real advantage.

Diagnostic Workers.—The tin-filter technique enables the film to be used as a satisfactory dosemeter for workers working with practically all radiations used in radiotherapy (200 kV. and upwards). What, however, of those working with radiations generated at lower voltages, and especially the range 50–120 kV. which covers

22*

most diagnostic radiology? It will be clear from *Fig*. 457 that here the response of the film under the tin filter is changing rapidly as the radiation energy falls, and is not suitable for dosage measurements. On the other hand, and happily, the variation in sensitivity of the ordinary film is not great in this region. If the value of the sensitivity of the 'open' film is taken as 20 for the whole of the diagnostic range the error introduced, as *Fig*. 457 shows, is only about ± 10 per cent. Film dosemetry may therefore also be used for monitoring diagnostic radiography workers, as well as for those working with higher-energy radiations.

Wearing the 'Badge'.—The period for which each film should be worn is not universally agreed, but the most usual period is 2 weeks, though this is sometimes increased to 4 where it is reasonably certain that the radiation hazard is very small. Should accidental high exposure be suspected the film should immediately be processed. 'Badges' such as those shown are normally worn at chest or waist level on the outside of the normal working clothes, to give an indication of the whole-body Exposure to which the worker is subjected. (If a lead rubber, or other protective, apron is worn the badge should be *underneath* the apron, since it is the Exposure to the worker's body and not to the apron that interests us.) Modified versions of the 'badges' are also available to be worn on the wrist, to indicate general hand Exposure, and on the forehead to provide an estimate of the Exposure to the eyes. A difficult problem is the measurement of the radiation received by the fingers of, for example, doctors performing radium implants, or workers manipulating radioactive isotopes. Any 'badge' must not impede the dexterity, otherwise wearing it will slow down the work and subject the worker's fingers to greater doses than if it was not being worn. Small pieces of film in light-tight wrapping have been strapped to fingers for Exposure measurement, but it would appear that for this important purpose small amounts of lithium fluoride in light-proof plastic sachets may be a more useful method. This application of radiation-induced thermo-luminescence is rapidly being developed. Lithium fluoride shows but small change in sensitivity with radiation energy change, an especial advantage over the film in this situation where filters to exploit the film's energy-dependent characteristics cannot be employed because of the smallness of the piece of film being used.

INGESTED RADIOACTIVE MATERIALS

The film badge condenser chamber or similar devices are effective methods of assessing the amount of radiation received from external radiation sources. However, they give little indication of the dose received from ingested gamma-ray emitters and much less about injected pure beta-ray emitters. This 'internal' dose can be assessed only by determining the amount of radioactive material ingested and for this reason those dealing with unsealed radioactive sources should undergo periodic checks. The tests used depend on the type of radioactive materials being used. For example, if radioactive iodine is involved routine estimates of the amount of iodine in the thyroid gland, using the technique described in CHAPTER XXVIII, will yield the required information. If the nuclide is likely to be widely distributed throughout the body and is a gamma-ray emitter the whole-body counter, also described in CHAPTER XXVIII, can be used to measure how much is present.

Pure beta-ray emitters present a much more difficult problem since their penetrating power precludes their being detected by external counters. Some form of 'biological' monitoring has to be used. One example of this concerns the detection and measurement of carbon 14, which emits low-energy beta rays (maximum 160 keV.). A fraction of any carbon 14 in the body will be exhaled as carbon dioxide and therefore the collection and testing of the exhaled breath will enable the amount of carbon 14 in the body to be estimated. To do this the difficulty of the low energy of the beta particles has to be circumvented, and one way of doing this is to introduce the gas to be measured into a Geiger-Müller counter, thus avoiding the impenetrable barrier that the tube wall would present to these radiations.

Tritium (hydrogen 3), which emits even lower-energy (maximum 5·5 kV.) beta rays, is used in a number of tests, and is widely used in the luminizing industry, whose workers have to be tested regularly to ensure that they are not ingesting undesirable amounts of the isotope. Any tritium in the body eventually becomes incorporated in water and is excreted in the urine, the tritium content of which is a good indication of the tritium content of the body. For this test another technique is usually used— that of liquid scintillation counting. To a sample of urine is added a liquid that scintillates when irradiated. This is in intimate relation to the tritium and thus the problem of the extremely small range of the beta particles is overcome. A tube containing the mixture is placed between two well-shielded photomultiplier tubes which detect the light emitted and thus the amount of tritium to be estimated.

RADIATION PROTECTION FOR THE PATIENT

Because the departmental staff are continuously being exposed, in some measure, to radiation, it is not unreasonable that their radiation safety should have received our main attention up to this point. However, just because the patient is only in a radiation department on a limited number of occasions and is deliberately being subjected to radiation during these visits, it must not be assumed that his or her radiation protection is unimportant. In fact radiation protection of the patient presents rather more problems than does the radiation protection of the worker. First, except when actually receiving the treatment or the diagnostic procedure, the patient must be protected in the same way as any other member of the general public. For example, waiting rooms and changing cubicles must be as fully protected as they would be if they were used as, say, offices—after all visitors, friends, and the patients themselves often have to stay in them for quite long periods! Secondly, there is the deliberate irradiation, which may be considered under two distinct headings—that to the region which is to be treated or investigated, and that to the rest of the body. All radiation to parts of the body outside the field of interest is undesirable and must be minimized. Within the zone of interest it must be no more than is necessary to achieve the task in hand but equally it must not be less. The dose must not be reduced so far in the interests of protection that the treatment fails or the diagnostic procedure fails to produce all the information that a rather higher dose could give.

Because their details are different it is convenient to consider separately the patient protection problems in X- and gamma-ray beam therapy, in X-ray diagnosis, and in the use of radioactive isotopes. One factor, however, they have in common: the greatest contribution to the radiation safety of the patient lies in the careful selection of the best technique for the work to be done, and in its meticulous execution.

X- and Gamma-ray Beam Therapy.—Whatever treatment technique is used the patient will be subject to radiation 'leakage' through the tube or source housing, which will irradiate part of, or the whole, body and therefore its intensity must be kept as low as possible. The I.C.R.P. recommends that the Exposure rate at 1 metre from the tube housing should not exceed 2 mR per hour and this is usually achieved with modern radiation-beam equipment. However, it must not be forgotten that, as time passes, parts wear, screws slacken, and small gaps may appear in the protective shielding near diaphragms, treatment cone carriers, or filter slides, giving leakage beams of small area but sometimes considerable intensity. Regular tests, possibly using film fastened round the suspect parts, should therefore be made.

The aim of radiotherapy is to deliver the 'correct' dose (i.e., that established by clinical experience as being most appropriate for the treatment being undertaken) to the 'right' part of the body (i.e., that which it is desired to treat) with as little radiation as possible elsewhere. Field selection and accurate 'beam direction' along lines such as have already been described are, therefore, essential, especially as field sizes must be kept to the minimum required to produce uniform irradiation of the treatment zone. Excessive, or insufficient, dosage being equally harmful, accurate dosemetry is also essential. Whenever possible, treatments should be controlled by a monitor Exposure meter, though it must never be forgotten that such devices, like all others made by man, may go wrong. Regular check calibrations must be carried out, and it is very desirable that further safeguards are taken to indicate if a faulty monitor terminates an exposure prematurely, as well as to prevent its allowing a dangerous over-exposure. Over-exposure can be minimized by adding a timer to the controls and by setting it to terminate any treatment after a time of, say, 20 per cent more than the estimated time. Actual exposure times can also be recorded by a pen recorder linked to the monitor so that delivered doses can be estimated if the control apparatus were faulty. Such protective devices are especially necessary where the output Exposure rate is very large, as, for example, with electron beams.

The effects of possible human errors must also be guarded against. The pen recorder enables simple errors of dose and time setting as well as apparatus errors to be revealed. In fractionated treatments correction for over- or under-dosage can easily be made in subsequent treatments—unless the error happens in the last of a series! Special care, of course, has to be taken where only one treatment is given. Electrical interlock devices are usually provided to prevent the wrong plain or wedge filter being used or the wedge filter inserted the wrong way round into the beam. Again, however, it must be stressed that such devices may fail and in the last resort there is no adequate substitute for having all control settings and accessories checked by an independent worker, and above all for the most careful attention to detail by the person responsible for carrying out the treatment.

Another important contribution to the prevention of unwanted irradiation is made by the compilation of accurate prescription and record forms. The radio-therapist's instructions must be set out clearly and unequivocally and precise details of all procedures carried out (including field sizes, tube-running conditions, and so on) carefully recorded. And as far as possible—in the absence of a national radiation record card—steps must be taken, including the briefing and questioning of the patient, to guard against the (admittedly unlikely) possibility of the treatment being unwittingly repeated at another place.

Finally, there are tissues of particular importance the irradiation of which should be avoided if this is at all possible. Examples of these are the gonads, the kidneys, the eyes, and the spinal cord. If they lie in the treatment zone their irradiation may be inevitable, though it is often possible to shield them from direct irradiation by using shielding blocks (as described on p. 490), without impairing the treatment. In this connexion two aspects of eye 'shielding' are of interest. For treatments of the eyelid with low-energy (60–100 kV.) X-rays it is normal to use some kind of eye-shield in between the lid and the eye. These shields are usually made of lead, and though they protect the eye they can increase the dose to the inner surface of the lid because of the electrons emitted as a result of the photo-electric effect. (For reasons already explained on p. 249 in connexion with the metal backing in a cassette, the lead reduces the amount of back-scatter.) Fortunately these electrons have relatively small penetrating power and can easily be removed by a thin layer of plastic over the lead. A simple way of applying this is to spray the lead with one of the proprietary plastics used for protecting motor-car ignition systems against damp. At the other end of the scale, when megavoltage radiations are being used and where it is necessary to irradiate through the eye, the dose to the lens can be usefully reduced by instructing the patient to keep his or her eyes open during treatment. Closing the lids over the eyes increases the superficial dose by the 'build-up' phenomenon.

None of these measures prevents irradiation due to mainly side scattered radiation, which cannot be avoided. However, it can be considerably reduced by using megavoltage radiations.

Diagnostic Radiology.—Although the doses involved are very much smaller than those used in radiotherapy this is no reason for not using any chosen technique with the greatest care and efficiency. The first question to be asked is always: 'Should a radiograph be taken?' and the answer can only be in the affirmative if the benefit to the patient from the information that might be obtained, or alternatively if the hazard to the patient if the information is not sought, outweighs the hazard (admittedly small) from the radiation effects. The small amount of radiation effect from a chest radiograph is far outweighed by the benefit that could accrue from the early diagnosis of chest disease. On the other hand, the use of radiography to aid the fitting of children's shoes seldom bestows any advantage and is, therefore, to be avoided.

The aim of diagnostic radiography is to produce an 'acceptable' radiograph (i.e., one which yields, to the radiologist concerned, as much of the desired information as is available) of the part of the body which is under review, and no more. These goals are being achieved by the selection of the most appropriate technique for the investigation being undertaken. For example, the dose to the patient is kept low by using fast films and fast screens; by using large focus–film distances (the ratio of the dose on the skin to the dose at the film decreases with increasing F.F.D.); by using as high a kilovoltage as is consistent with obtaining the required film quality; by the beam being adequately filtered (2 mm. of aluminium, say); and by accepting the minimum blackening consistent with obtaining the desired information. Using fields large enough to cover the field of interest and no more reduces the total dose effect and, because it cuts down the amount of scattered radiation, also improves radiographic quality (*see*, for example, p. 248). It should be accepted as a hall-mark of good radiography that all four edges of the film should be unexposed, thus showing that no more than the necessary tissues were irradiated.

A word of warning is, however, necessary! In striving to attain the goal of minimum radiation damage it is important that this should not lead to an unsatisfactory radiograph, i.e., one which either fails to cover the region of interest properly or, through incorrect exposure, fails to provide a film from which the information sought can be obtained. Much better to give a 25 per cent greater exposure than absolutely necessary and obtain the required information than to underexpose by 25 per cent, achieve nothing and have to make a repeat exposure (1·25 is better than 0·75+1·0!). A repeat radiograph for any of these reasons must be regarded as a reflection on the professional competence of the radiographer concerned. Nevertheless if, for any reason, the first radiograph is inadequate it must be repeated. To irradiate unnecessarily is undesirable; to attempt a diagnosis on an inadequate film is unwise but to fail to repeat when necessary is unethical.

The same basic principles apply to fluoroscopic examinations, i.e., use the minimum beam size and the most efficient detecting system. Because this type of examination aims at studying the dynamics of a system it may be carried on over several minutes, which means that low tube currents have to be used if high doses are to be avoided. If direct fluoroscopy is used the radiologist must take care to be sufficiently dark-adapted to be able to work with the low-screen brightness available. Old screens may well be replaced, with advantage, by more modern faster ones and it must not be forgotten that the lead glass backing may have to be replaced from time to time as it becomes discoloured and therefore less transparent. Whenever possible image intensification and television techniques should be exploited in so far as they reduce patient dosage or enable more information to be obtained and not simply for the convenience and increased comfort of the radiologist.

Fluoroscopic examinations should be carried out as expeditiously as possible with the beam switched on for the shortest times commensurate with obtaining the desired information. It is not uncommon nowadays to have integrating timers incorporated in fluoroscopic units. These can be very valuable to indicate to the radiologist, and perhaps emphasize to him, the time he takes over an examination. Also available are monitor ionization chambers which integrate the dose in rads × field area in square centimetres and also often indicate audibly the rate at which this product is accumulating. For example the 'peeps' will be emitted faster when a large field is being used than with a small field, and this may serve as a reminder to the radiologist that he should close down his diaphragms as much as possible. Whether this background noise is worth while or not depends largely on the personal psychology of the radiologist—in some cases it could be a distraction producing an altogether undesirable pressure of urgency. Finally, some equipment is fitted with devices which terminate the exposure when a pre-set exposure time or dose has been given. Although these are admirable in intention they may be unfortunate in operation if, for example, they operate just at that crucial moment when some important information is emerging. Once again the prime importance of obtaining the required information must be stressed, and ultimately the greatest factor in the protection of the patient is the unhurried skill of the radiologist. In this work, as in so many other ways, more haste may indeed mean less speed.

As with therapy tubes there will be some leakage of radiation through the tube housing, so that not only must this housing conform to internationally accepted standards but checks must be carried out regularly to ensure that no leaks have developed in use.

Reduction of dose to all tissues is important but the dose to the gonads deserves special attention to minimize the genetic changes which radiation can produce. When the gonads are in the field to be radiographed it may be impossible to avoid their irradiation without obscuring the region of interest. In such a case the dis-advantage of possible genetic effects has to be weighed against the importance of the information to be obtained. Sometimes shielding can be used without reducing the usefulness of the radiograph and in such cases it must be used. Gonad shielding also protects against tube leakage radiation and therefore, whenever practicable, it should be used, especially when children are being irradiated.

Scattered radiation, of course, is not eliminated by shields and, when field edges are close to the gonads, can contribute quite considerable doses to them. Radio-graphy during pregnancy, and especially during the first 12 weeks, should only be undertaken if it is regarded as essential, whilst wherever possible radiography of the pelvic region of women of child-bearing age should be restricted to the first 10 days of the menstrual cycle, to give the maximum chance of avoiding the irradiation of an, as yet, unsuspected foetus.

The subject of patient protection is an extensive one and only the main principles can be touched on here. Further and more detailed information is now available in I.C.R.P. Publication 16 entitled *Protection of the Patient in X-ray Diagnosis*. Published by Pergamon Press, it is strongly recommended.

Radioactive Isotopes.—As with the use of radiation beams the greatest contribution to the patient's safety lies in the careful selection and execution of the treatment or investigation technique. The radioactive isotope must be suitable for the region or organ being treated or studied; the detecting equipment used must be as sensitive as possible; care must be taken to ensure that there are no regions of the body (except those being investigated) where unacceptable concentrations of isotope may occur, thus leading to high local dosage; the radiation must be appropriate (ideally beta rays for radiotherapy and medium-energy gamma rays only for diagnostic tests) and the effective half-life conveniently short. Special care must be taken in radioactive isotope tests on children, since concentrations different from those in adults may easily occur (e.g. in the epiphyses), and on a pregnant, or potentially pregnant, woman.

As in the other techniques discussed, all efforts must be directed towards keeping the radiation doses as small as possible but enough radioactive isotope must be used to enable the desired end to be achieved. Having decided, for example, that a brain scan was needed it would be a serious error of judgement and an unjustified assault upon the patient if the amount of isotope used was insufficient for the obtaining of a successful picture.

General.—Sometimes the question is asked how many radiographs can be taken or radioactive isotope investigations carried out on a patient, and in some places tables of values for various sites are given. The numbers in these tables are based on some maximum dose which it is felt can be accepted. Whilst these tables are possibly useful as a guide, the answer to the question must surely be: 'As many as are needed for the benefit of the patient'—and that includes none! One unnecessary radiograph is too many; a radiograph likely to provide information important to the health or life of the patient must be taken regardless of what has previously happened.

Electrical and Mechanical Safety.—Although radiation hazards from radiological equipment have occupied all our attention so far, as is appropriate in view of their insidious nature and potential seriousness, electrical and mechanical safety must in no way be neglected. A breakdown in either may not only be more spectacular in its immediate effects but just as dangerous. Constant attention to the proper state of the equipment is necessary; the adequacy of electrical earthing and the freedom from wear and defect of cables must be checked regularly, as must the effectiveness of brakes, counterweights, and other mechanical features outlined in CHAPTER XXXIX.

Ultrasonics.—The value of ultrasonic radiations as an alternative to X-rays in some aspects of clinical diagnosis has been outlined in CHAPTER XXVII in which mention was also made of their biological effects and of the possible hazards arising from their use. At the lower levels used in diagnostic procedures it is fairly certain that these hazards are likely to be much smaller than the (small) hazards inherent in the use of X-rays for similar purposes. However, at this stage, long-term consequences, such as those that may by produced by X-rays or of a so-far unsuspected nature, cannot be ruled out entirely. It is, therefore, incumbent upon all who use ultrasonic radiations, or any other radiation for that matter, to do so only when positive value to the patient is likely to accrue, and to be ever alert for possible deleterious effects.

CONCLUSION

Ionizing radiation, if misused, could be a scourge to those on whom, and by whom, it is used, and indeed to all mankind, present and future. Properly applied it is one of the great boons, preventing, or alleviating, much suffering, bringing health where there was sickness, hope where there was despair. The equipment for this work is available; its safe use calls for trained, responsible workers with a knowledge of the properties of this type of radiation and an appreciation of its dangers. If this book has helped in providing some of that knowledge and appreciation it will not have been written in vain.

APPENDIX I

S.I. UNITS

IN 1960 the General Conference of Weights and Measurements launched the International System of Units which has become known by the initials S.I. from the French title 'Système International d'Unités'. The aim of the system was to establish a minimum number of fundamental or *base* units, which do not depend on one another and from which units of other physical quantities can logically be derived. There are seven *base* units as follows:

Quantity	S.I. Unit	Symbol
Length	metre	m
Mass	kilogramme	kg
Time	second	s
Electric current	ampere	A
Temperature	kelvin	K
Amount of substance	mol	mol
Luminous intensity	candela	cd

From these *base* units derived units can be obtained for other quantities by combining *base* units as, for example:

Quantity	S.I. Units	Base Units involved
Area	square metre	m^2
Volume	cubic metre	m^3
Velocity	metre per second	m/s or $m\,s^{-1}$
Density	kilogramme per cubic metre	kg/m^3 or $kg\,m^{-3}$

Some *derived* units are given special names (often in commemoration of some famous scientist) and symbols. These, in turn, can be used to express other *derived* units in a simpler way than in terms of *base* units. Some examples of *derived* units with special names are:

Quantity	S.I. Unit	Symbol	Relation to Base or other Units
Frequency (cycles per second)	hertz★	Hz	s^{-1}
Force	newton	N	$m\,kg\,s^{-2}$
Energy of work	joule	J	$N\,m$
Power	watt	W	J/s or $J\,s^{-1}$
Electrical potential	volt	V	W/A or $W\,A^{-1}$
Radioactivity	becquerel★	Bq	s^{-1}
Absorbed dose	gray	Gy	J/kg or $J\,kg^{-1}$

Another aim of the system is to standardize the prefixes used for multiples or sub-multiples of any unit. Some of those proposed are:

Prefix	Abbreviation	Multiplying Factor
giga	G	10^9
mega	M	10^6
kilo	k	10^3
milli	m	10^{-3}
micro	μ	10^{-6}
nano	n	10^{-9}
pico	p	10^{-12}

Thus, three million volts is written 3 MV; five-millionths of an ampere (i.e., 5 micro-amperes) is 5 μA, and 5 thousandths of a gray (i.e., 5 milli-grays) would be 5 mGy.

★ The units used for frequency and for (radio-)activity are both seconds^{-1}. The two special units of hertz and becquerel are not, however, interchangeable. Use of the special derived unit, the becquerel, is restricted to activity whilst the hertz is restricted to periodic oscillations.

APPENDIX II

THE EXPONENTIAL LAW OF RADIOACTIVE DECAY, OR OF PHOTON BEAM ATTENUATION

To illustrate the way in which the familiar exponential law arises, the case of radioactive decay will be considered. It is assumed that, at any time and at all times, every atom of a particular radioactive substance has the same chance (a probability) of undergoing radioactive decay in, say, the next second. This chance is expressed as the *transformation constant*, λ per second. Thus, if N atoms of some radioactive material are present at a particular time, t, then the number (dN) which will decay in the next, very short, interval of time dt is given by:

$$dN = -N\lambda \, dt. \qquad (1)$$

Stated in words, this means that the number which decay equals the product of the number present, the chance of decay per second, and the time interval. The negative sign indicates that dN, the change in N, is a reduction.

To find what happens over a period of time which is not short, equation (1) must be integrated, i.e., the effects of a large number of small intervals must be added together:

$$\int dN = -\int N\lambda \, dt,$$

or

$$\int dN/N = -\int \lambda \, dt,$$

or

$$\log_e N = -\lambda t + \text{a constant } C.$$

(It will be recalled that $\int dx/x = \log_e x + C$.)

If the value of N at some time is known, then C can be evaluated. For example, if there were N_0 atoms present initially (i.e., when $t = 0$) it follows that:

$$\log_e N_0 = 0 + C,$$

therefore

$$\log_e N = -\lambda t + \log_e N_0,$$

or

$$\log_e N - \log_e N_0 = -\lambda t,$$

or

$$N/N_0 = e^{-\lambda t}.$$

A similar formula showing how many X-ray photons pass through a given thickness, d, of some material can be deduced in the same way if it is assumed that the chance per centimetre of material of a photon being removed from the beam is constant. Hence

$$I/I_0 = e^{-\mu d}.$$

The evaluation of these formulae would seem to call for tables of values of the exponential function e^{-x} and these are not always available. On the other hand, it is usually possible to obtain tables of common logarithms ('logs to the base 10') and these can be used quite easily to give the desired result. In a typical practical case the value of N/N_0 at some time, or of I/I_0, after the beam has passed through some material, is known and it is necessary to find λ or μ.

Since $I/I_0 = e^{-\mu d}$ it follows that $I_0/I = e^{\mu d}$.

Therefore taking the common logarithm of each side of the equation:

$$\log_{10}(I_0/I) = \log_{10}(e^{\mu d}) = \mu d \log_{10} e$$
$$= 0.4343\mu d$$

or

$$\mu d = (\log_{10} I_0/I)/0.4343 = 2.3 \log_{10} I_0/I.$$

Examples.—
(a) Using the values taken from Example 1 of CHAPTER XLIII (p. 635), it is required to find μd if $I_0 = 0.1$ R per hour and $I = 10^{-3}$ R per hour.

$$I_0/I = 0.1/10^{-3} = 100$$
$$\therefore \quad \mu d = \log_{10}(100) \times 2.3 = 2.0 \times 2.3 = 4.60.$$

(b) Using values from Example 3 of CHAPTER XLIII (p. 636),

$$I_0 = 48 \text{ R per hour.} \quad I = 10^{-3} \text{ R per hour.}$$
$$\therefore \quad I_0/I = 48/10^{-3} = 4.8 \times 10^4,$$
$$\therefore \quad \mu d = \log_{10}(4.8 \times 10^4) \times 2.3$$
$$= 4.6812 \times 2.3 = 10.78.$$

MODULATION TRANSFER FUNCTION AND ASSOCIATED CONCEPTS

FOR various reasons (e.g., the finite size of the focal spot; the relative movement of patient, film and X-ray source during radiography; the structure of intensifying screens; optical and electronic defects in image intensifier and T.V. systems) the final radiographic or radioscopic image is not a faithful reproduction of the object which caused it. We say that the image is 'blurred' and that the system lacks 'resolution'. It is useful to be able to give a quantitative description of the unsharpness associated with the various causes, both individually and collectively. The rather mathematical, and certainly difficult, concept of Modulation Transfer Function is used to help to achieve this aim. What follows here is a descriptive and, admittedly, superficial account of this function and of some other associated concepts. For simplicity, and by way of example, the unsharpness caused by the use of intensifying screens will be discussed. The same method of analysis can be equally well applied to each other stage in the formation of the image.

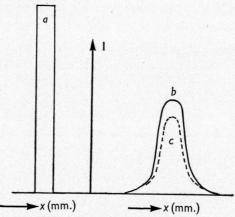

Fig. 461.—Density patterns of X-ray beam (*a*), and resulting pattern (*b*), with 'point spread function' (*c*).

Point Spread Function.—If a fine narrow pencil of X-rays is directed on to a film-screen combination the resulting pattern of density on the developed film will be spread out over a larger area than that of the X-ray beam cross-section.

The incident X-ray pattern and the resulting density pattern on the film are shown in *Fig.* 461 (curves *a* and *b* respectively), whilst the X-ray intensity pattern which would be required to produce the same pattern (curve *b*) on the film *in the absence of the screen* is shown in *Fig.* 461 (curve *c*). This is known as the 'point spread function' associated with the blurring of this particular film-screen combination. Curve *c* can be deduced from curve *b* provided the characteristic curve of the film-screen combination is known.

The usefulness of the point spread function can be appreciated by considering the pattern produced on the film when a slightly more complex pattern of X-rays is incident on the film-screen pair (*Fig*. 462). The X-ray pattern KLMN shown in *Fig*. 462 A can be considered as being made up of a large number of pencil beams (*p*) of different, appropriate amplitudes, as shown, for each of which there is a point spread function. The X-ray pattern, which corresponds to the density pattern on the film, is obtained by the addition of all the individual point spread functions. As shown in *Fig*. 462 B this corresponds to the previously discussed pattern resulting from screen blurring (*see* CHAPTER XVII, p. 201). This process of deriving the final pattern by use of the point spread function is known as 'convolution'.

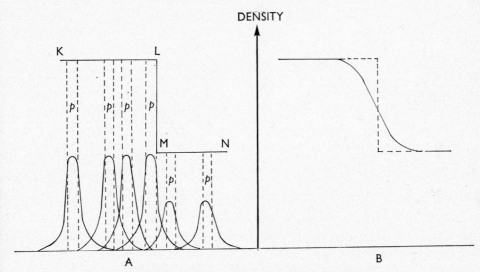

Fig. 462.—A, The beam pattern, KLMN, showing some of its constituent 'pencils' (*p*) and their line spread functions, and B, the 'convoluted' pattern.

In practice the reverse process, known as 'deconvolution', is more interesting and more useful. If the point spread function is known then, at least in theory, it can be used to deduce, from the practical unsharp pattern, the real object of interest, that is to say the pattern that actually existed, and of which the pattern on the film is an image distorted by screen, and other types of blurring. So far this exercise has not been carried out for screen blurring but it is regularly used, in radioactive isotope scanning techniques, to compensate for (i.e., remove the effect of) the blurring resulting from the inevitable imperfections of the collimator.

The ideas of convolution and deconvolution can be applied in many branches of science for the improvement of available information. For example (as illustrated in *Fig*. 463) 'Box A' represents a device which performs a certain function (e.g., converting an X-ray pattern into a visible density pattern as is done by the film-screen combination) but, because it is not absolutely perfect, 'spoils' the picture (the output) in a *known* way. By *known* is meant that, for example, the point spread function is known. In principle it is possible to design a further device (B) which 'unspoils' the output, that is to say that it 'deconvolutes' it using the known point spread function. The device for this purpose may be a piece of equipment or it may be a mathematical process carried out by a computer.

At the present time not much practical use is made of these possibilities in clinical radiology although some T.V. fluoroscopic equipment has such devices to help to minimize any deterioration of the image due to optical or electronic parts of the system.

Line Spread Function.—The point spread function is, of course, three-dimensional, referring as it does to a pencil beam or a point source. In the above descriptions diagrams are, for simplicity only, drawn to show what happens in two dimensions. The corresponding function for the truly two-dimensional situation produced by, for example, a narrow slit source giving a linear beam of radiation is the 'line spread function' (L.S.F.).

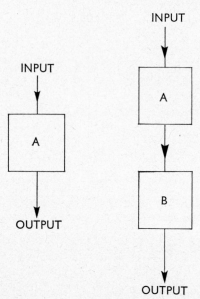

Fig. 463.—'Box' B deconvolutes the output from pattern-producing 'Box' A.

If the pattern of *Fig.* 462 A is now taken to be that produced by a semi-opaque straight-edged object placed in a uniform X-ray beam then the dotted curves are the line spread functions and the curve of *Fig.* 462 B shows the pattern of X-rays corresponding to the blurred shadow of the edge on the film. As with the point spread function, the line spread function can be used to convolute and to deconvolute patterns.

MODULATION TRANSFER FUNCTION

The modulation transfer function offers an alternative and rather more useful approach in that it gives a quantitative estimate of the 'image spoiling property' of each component part of the formation of the radiographic or radioscopic image. It is particularly useful for combining the defects of each stage in order to obtain an overall 'figure of merit'. Unfortunately the modulation transfer function involves some rather advanced mathematical ideas and techniques, though fortunately the chore of the associated calculations can now be given over to a computer. In this account of the function only the basic ideas will be described and in a simplified form.

Fourier Analysis.—It has been known for many years that any shape of pattern can be synthesized by the adding together of a (infinitely) large number of sinusoidal waves of appropriate relative frequency, amplitude, and phase. The analysis of a pattern into its component sinusoidal waves is known as 'Fourier analysis', and there exist well-known mathematical techniques for carrying out this analysis for any pattern.

As an example, consider the Fourier analysis of an infinitely long train of rectangular-shaped waves, like that depicted in *Fig.* 464. Such a pattern can be represented by the following series:—

$$\text{Amplitude} = \sin fx + \tfrac{1}{3}\sin 3fx + \tfrac{1}{5}\sin 5fx + \ldots 1/n \sin nfx,$$

where f is the spatial frequency (in this case the number of waves per millimetre) of the rectangular wave train and n is any *odd* integer.

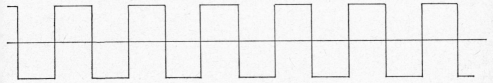

Fig. 464.—Train of 'square' waves.

Fig. 465 shows how the successive addition of the terms of this series (that is using more and more of its terms) leads to an increasingly accurate representation of the rectangular pattern.

The Line Spread Function and Sharp Pencil Beam.—In like manner a single symmetrical pattern like the line spread function for the screen-film pair (*Fig.* 461 *c*), or like the X-ray pencil beam pattern (*Fig.* 461 *a*) can be analysed into, and, therefore, synthesized from, a set of sinusoidal curves. The important difference between the analysis of the single pattern and that of the continuous train of waves, such as that shown in *Fig.* 464, is that, for the single pattern, all frequencies* (f) from zero to infinity will be present (i.e., there is a continuous spectrum) whereas for the train of waves only specific, harmonic frequencies are needed (i.e., a 'line' spectrum). Fourier analysis of a line spread function pattern such as in *Fig.* 461 *c* shows that the relative amplitudes A_f of the various frequencies f which are necessary are as shown by the full curve in *Fig.* 466. The corresponding frequencies for the X-ray pencil beam of *Fig.* 461 *a* are indicated by the dotted line in *Fig.* 466, from which it will be seen that, in order to achieve the sharp pattern, all frequencies must be present and of the same amplitude. Therefore only if the recording medium (in our example the film-screen pair) is able to record all frequencies equally well, is it possible to achieve a perfect image of the pattern in the incident beam. It turns out that the presence of the higher frequencies is necessary in order to achieve sharp patterns. If the incident pattern is not, in itself, sharp, the ability of the recording medium to reproduce faithfully the higher frequencies is not so important, though perfect reproduction of any pattern demands equal response to all frequencies.

The ratio of the amplitudes of these two curves (*Fig.* 466 *a* and *b*) at any frequency, f, is a function of the frequency and this is called the 'modulation transfer function'. A graph of the modulation transfer function for, in this case, the film-screen pair is shown in *Fig.* 467 A. It will be recognized that since, in the example given, one curve is a

---

* It must be emphasized that, as indicated earlier, the frequency referred to in this Appendix is the spatial frequency of the sinusoidal pattern and is measured in cycles per millimetre. It must not be confused with the frequency (in cycles per second) associated with the quantum energy of the X-rays.

horizontal line, the shape of the modulation transfer function curve is identical with that of the amplitude response (full line of *Fig.* 466).

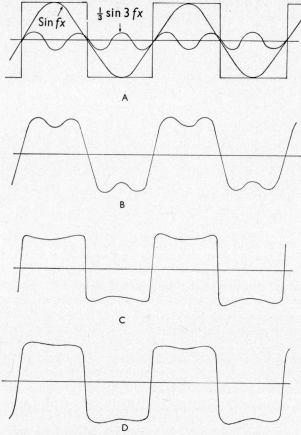

Fig. 465.—The Fourier analysis of a train of 'square' waves.
A, The square-wave train with the curves for $\sin fx$ and $\frac{1}{3}\sin 3fx$.
B, Sum of $\sin fx + \frac{1}{3}\sin 3fx$.
C, Sum of $\sin fx + \frac{1}{3}\sin 3fx + \ldots + \frac{1}{19}\sin 19fx$.
D, Sum of $\sin fx + \frac{1}{3}\sin 3fx + \ldots + \frac{1}{39}\sin 39fx$.

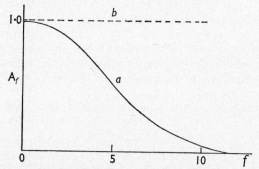

Fig. 466.—Amplitude frequency diagram for (*a*) the line spread function from *Fig.* 461 *c* and (*b*) the X-ray pencil beam of *Fig.* 461 *a*.

In practice it is usual to plot the modulation transfer function using logarithmic scales, as in the example shown in *Fig.* 467 B. Curve *a* shows the same information as in *Fig.* 467 A which is for a high definition screen. Curve *b* is the corresponding curve for a fast screen and has a much lower value of the modulation transfer function at the higher frequencies, thus demonstrating its greater unsharpness (screen blurring). The frequency at which the modulation transfer function has fallen to about 0·7 is often taken as an index of resolution; high frequency values indicating high resolution.

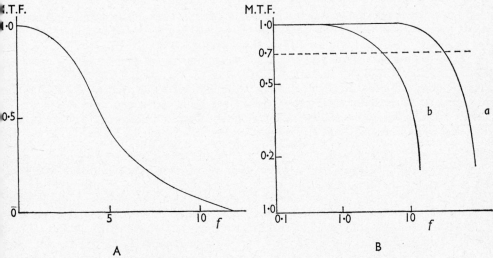

Fig. 467.—Modulation transfer functions: A, Linear plot; B, Logarithmic plot.

Unsharp Pencil Beam of X-rays.—The modulation transfer function of the film-screen pair derived above is equally applicable to an unsharp X-ray pattern. Instead of the sharp pencil of X-rays shown in *Fig.* 461*a* consider a beam which, because, of focal spot size and finite collimator to film distance, suffers from geometric unsharpness; for example such a beam as is represented by curve *a, Fig.* 468. The amplitude spectrum of this pattern as derived by Fourier analysis is shown in the full curve *b* of *Fig.* 468.

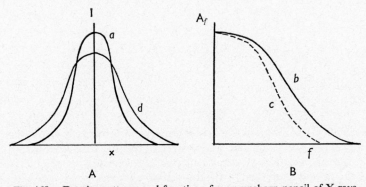

Fig. 468.—Density patterns and functions for an unsharp pencil of X-rays

If this unsharp beam is now incident upon the film-screen pair the resulting image will be even more unsharp because of the effects that have been discussed. The full curve of *Fig.* 468 can be modified to allow for this by multiplying the ordinate at each frequency by the appropriate ratio read off the modulation transfer function graph given in *Fig.* 467. This modification leads to the dotted curve *c* of *Fig.* 468, and this is the amplitude spectrum of the final image on the film. This can be transposed back (by Fourier 'synthesis') to give the pattern which will be produced on the film. This is shown as curve *d* of *Fig.* 468. As expected this is less sharp, because of screen blurring, than the already unsharp beam presented to the film; in this connexion it will be noted that there are less of the higher frequency components in the amplitude spectrum of the final pattern (*see* the dotted curve *c* of *Fig.* 468) than there were in that of the incident pattern.

Combination of Unsharpnesses.—The description given above is, to a certain extent, rather trivial but its importance lies in the fact that it illustrates that the modulation transfer function of each stage is quite independent of all other stages and of the pattern presented to the stage being considered. This means that in a multi-stage process the overall modulation transfer function (MTF) is simply the product of the individual functions of each separate stage.

$$(\text{MTF})_{\text{total}} = (\text{MTF})_1 \times (\text{MTF})_2 \times (\text{MTF})_3 \times \ldots.$$

An example of this is given in *Fig.* 469, which shows the modulation transfer functions for the film-screen pair (curve *a*), for the geometric unsharpness in the beam (curve *b*), and for the movement of the object (curve *c*) as well as for the overall effect (curve *d*, which is obtained by multiplying together the corresponding ordinates for each curve). A point made in an earlier chapter (CHAPTER XXI, p. 267) that the overall unsharpness is worse than any one of the individual unsharpnesses but not much worse than the worst is nicely illustrated in *Fig.* 469 which shows quite clearly

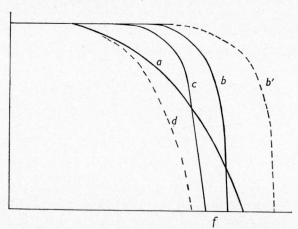

Fig. 469.—The combination of individual modulation transfer functions to produce the overall function (curve *d*).

that no benefit is to be obtained by attempting to improve just one of the unsharpnesses, for example the geometric unsharpness. Even if this were done to such an extent that the modulation transfer function associated with this unsharpness is changed to the value represented by the dotted curve *b'*, the overall modulation transfer function would remain substantially coincident with curve *d*.

Improvement of Pattern.—The modulation transfer function points a way to the possibility of correcting for defects originating in one stage of the image-forming process by the modification of, or the addition of, other stages. For example it may be decided that, in order to achieve a sufficiently faithful presentation of the ideal pattern, a particular system needs an overall modulation transfer function of the form shown in curve *a* of *Fig.* 470. Unfortunately the actual form of the function falls

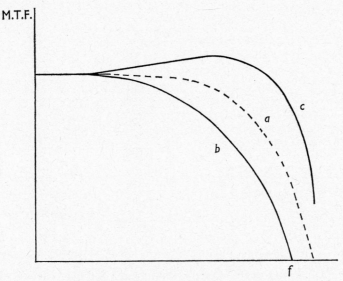

Fig. 470.—Improvement in overall effect by introduction of an extra stage with a special modulation transfer function (curve *c*).

off more rapidly at the higher frequencies (curve *b*). In principle, at least, it is possible to consider the addition to the system of an extra stage which is specially designed to have a modulation transfer function of the form shown in curve *c* of *Fig.* 470. This form is such that the average overall function (obtained by taking the product of the values from the curves *b* and *c*) corresponds sufficiently closely with the desired curve *a*. Although this is a very common technique in electronics it is only just beginning to be used in radiology, and there only in the optical–electronic parts of the system. As yet no device able, for example, to compensate for screen blurring is available.

As always a price has to be paid for such improvements in resolution—and not only in the form of more cash to the manufacturer! There is an increase in so-called 'noise' which shows itself as a loss in contrast.

Determination of Modulation Transfer Function.—The modulation transfer function is not easy to determine and this is usually done indirectly. Use is made of the fact that the amplitude spectrum of a narrow beam of X-rays produced by a fine slit is a horizontal straight line, i.e., equal amplitudes for all frequencies. Such a beam is therefore directed on to the film-screen pair being investigated and, after processing, the line spread function is determined from the film, as described below. The line spread function is then converted by Fourier analysis into the corresponding amplitude spectrum. As described above, this curve is identical with the modulation transfer function curve for the film-screen pair, since the amplitude spectrum of the incident beam is of uniform amplitude at all frequencies:

$$\text{M.T.F.}_{(f)} = \frac{\text{Amplitude of output spectrum at } f}{\text{Amplitude of input spectrum at } f}$$

$$= \text{Amplitude of output spectrum at } f$$

since the amplitude of the input spectrum is constant and can, in relative terms, be considered as equal to 1.

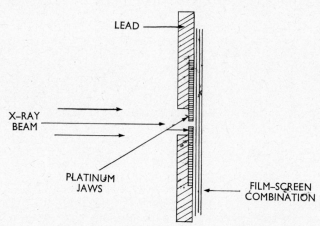

Fig. 471.—Apparatus for determination of modulation transfer function.

The practical arrangement consists of a long (20 mm.), narrow (10 μm.) slit, formed by two parallel, opaque jaws of platinum, on to which is directed a beam of X-rays from a distant source (*Fig.* 471). The film-screen pair is placed in intimate contact with the jaws, using a 'vacuum' cassette to ensure close contact. In this way geometric unsharpness is eliminated and the only cause of blurring is that due to the film-screen pair, which is what is being investigated.

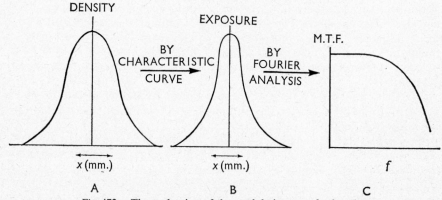

Fig. 472.—The evaluation of the modulation transfer function.

After processing, the density pattern across the film is measured by means of a microdensitometer, with an aperture width smaller than the slit width. This density pattern, shown in *Fig.* 472 A, is converted into the equivalent X-ray exposure curve (*see Fig.* 472 B) with the aid of the experimentally determined characteristic curve for the film-screen pair. This equivalent X-ray exposure curve is the exposure pattern which, in the *absence* of film-screen blurring, would have produced the density pattern (*Fig.* 472 A) actually obtained. This exposure pattern is then converted by Fourier analysis* (using the inevitable computer) and the amplitude spectrum, and hence modulation transfer function (*Fig.* 472 C) is obtained.

Direct Determination of Modulation Transfer Function.—Let it be assumed that it is possible to produce a sinusoidal pattern (as, for example, in *Fig.* 473 A) of exposure in a beam of radiation. (This is practically impossible for X-rays but it can be done for visible light.)

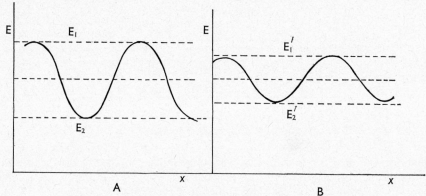

Fig. 473.—Direct determination of modulation transfer function.

This pattern can now be directed on to an imaging device (for example, a film-screen pair) and a similar sinusoidal pattern, of exactly the same frequency, will be produced (*Fig.* 473 B). The amplitude of the wave form will, however, be reduced. More precisely the 'modulation' is reduced. Using the symbols from *Fig.* 473 'modulation' (M) may be defined:—

$$M = \frac{E_1 - E_2}{\frac{1}{2}(E_1 + E_2)},$$

so that in this case

the input modulation is $M = (E_1 - E_2)/\frac{1}{2}(E_1 + E_2)$

and

the output modulation is $M' = (E_1' - E_2')/\frac{1}{2}(E_1' + E_2')$.

The ratio M'/M is, in fact, the modulation transfer function at the frequency of the sinusoidal wave employed. Repetition of the experiment over a range of frequencies enables the modulation transfer function curve to be drawn.

---

* For those interested the calculation is:—

$$A_f = \int_{-\infty}^{+\infty} (Ex) \cos 2\pi f \, dx \bigg/ \int_{-\infty}^{+\infty} E(x) \, dx,$$

where $E(x)$ is the exposure at a distance x (*Fig.* 472 B) and A_f is the amplitude of the frequency f (*Fig.* 472 C) and hence the modulation transfer function at f. Although this expression is tiresome to evaluate manually, very straightforward computer programmes exist for executing the calculation very quickly.

23

Although this method of determining the modulation transfer function can be adopted for optical systems and a corresponding method used for electronic systems, as indicated above, the method is not suitable for use with X-rays because of the impossibility of creating the required sinusoidal pattern. Very similar methods can, however, be used to determine the quantity known as the 'contrast frequency response'.

Contrast Frequency Response.—A diaphragm of equally spaced slits and opaque bars, incorporating both widely spaced and, progressively, more closely spaced slits (as depicted in *Fig.* 474), is used for the determination of contrast frequency response.

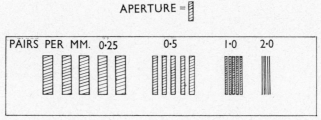

Fig. 474.—Slit pattern for determination of contrast frequency response.

The diaphragm is placed in a beam of X-rays and its image on the film (or the television tube screen) is examined—using a microdensitometer, for example. The image pattern will be found to have the form shown in *Fig.* 475.

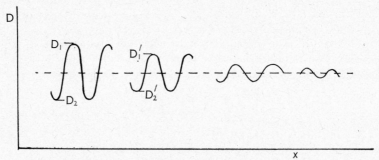

Fig. 475.—Image density patterns produced by slit pattern of *Fig.* 474.

The quantity

$$C = (D_1 - D_2)/\tfrac{1}{2}(D_1 + D_2)$$

can be regarded as a measure of the contrast, and is determined for each of the pattern frequencies. When plotted, this yields the 'contrast frequency response', as shown in *Fig.* 476.

Although this is not exactly identical to the modulation transfer function it has a very similar form and general use. Unfortunately the values determined depend not only on the properties of the system but also on the exact construction and nature of the diaphragm. Different diaphragms lead to different results, but if the same diaphragm is always used the comparative results obtained and the deductions made from them are valid and useful. The modulation transfer function does not suffer from this deficiency since it is inherent in the use of the fine slit that, provided it is small, the results are independent of it, and only depend on the system being tested. In spite of its deficiency, however, the contrast frequency response has the overriding advantage that it is, in practice, a very simple method—which cannot be said for the modulation transfer function.

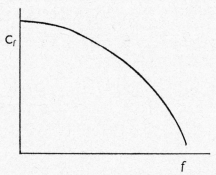

Fig. 476.—Contrast frequency response for patterns of *Fig.* 475.

Conclusion.—It must be emphasized that what has been written above about the modulation transfer function and allied concepts is intended only to give an overall impression of the purpose of the concepts. There are many gaps and simplifications in the descriptions, which may be filled in from the several textbooks and hundreds of papers already published on the subject.

INDEX